Cardiovascular Imaging

Elena Aikawa
Editor

Cardiovascular Imaging

Arterial and Aortic Valve Inflammation and Calcification

Springer

Editor
Elena Aikawa, MD, PhD, FAHA
Cardiovascular Medicine
Brigham and Women's Hospital
Harvard Medical School
Boston, MA
USA

ISBN 978-3-319-09267-6 ISBN 978-3-319-09268-3 (eBook)
DOI 10.1007/978-3-319-09268-3
Springer Cham Heidelberg New York Dordrecht London

Library of Congress Control Number: 2014954989

Printed on acid-free paper

Springer is part of Springer Science+Business Media (www.springer.com)

Foreword

Since Roentgen's day imaging has contributed to the diagnosis and understanding of cardiovascular diseases. In the first half of the twentieth century, radiographic plain films and fluoroscopy provided essential tools to the clinical cardiovascular specialist. In the latter half of the twentieth century the advent of image intensification, contrast angiography, and the introduction of cross-sectional imaging modalities such as computed tomography and magnetic resonance augmented the armamentarium of radiographic imaging tools modalities applied to cardiovascular disease. Simultaneously, the development of echocardiography beginning with M-mode, and evolving to two-dimensional and ultimately three-dimensional echocardiography, not only permitted the in vivo evaluation of ventricular function and cardiac structure but also enabled the in-depth assessment of cardiac valves. These tools opened the door to a golden era of non-invasive cardiovascular imaging that permitted the study of pathophysiology of cardiac and valvular diseases in intact humans and indeed experimental animals and, in the case of ultrasound, without using ionizing radiation. The concurrent evolution of nuclear imaging offered the opportunity to reach beyond defining structures to probe metabolism and perform quantitative and regional flow studies, further expanding the repertoire of imaging tools available to the cardiovascular specialist and investigator.

In the twenty-first century, molecular or functional imaging has provided a new frontier for advancing the field of cardiovascular imaging [1, 2]. This approach joins the traditional quest for defining structure and physiologic function with advances in understanding the cells and molecules involved in the pathogenesis of cardiovascular diseases. Molecular imaging weds basic science discoveries to imaging in a manner that promises to transform cardiovascular medicine and science.

This volume edited by Elena Aikawa provides us with an updated and comprehensive overview of this promising landscape. Much of the initial foray into the application of molecular imaging to cardiovascular diseases targeted atherosclerosis, which is the subject of Part I of this book [3]. After a masterful review of the basic pathobiological mechanisms at play in atherosclerosis (Chap. 1), a series of authoritative chapters reviews modalities ranging from contrast enhanced ultrasound (Chap. 2), magnetic resonance imaging (MRI) (Chap. 3), and optical approaches such as near-infrared fluorescence and optical coherence tomography (Chaps. 4, 5, 6, 7, and 8). Various chapters emphasize different pathophysiologic targets such as inflammation (Chap. 5), endothelial activation (Chap. 2), macrophage activity (Chap. 3), protease activity

(Chap. 4), oxidation and lipid content (Chap. 6), thrombosis (Chap. 8), and calcification (Chap. 5.) The laboratory applications of intravital microscopy that have proven of immense value to cardiovascular researchers also receive expert discussion in this part (Chap. 7).

The second part of this book delves more deeply into the imaging of calcification as applied particularly to cardiac valves, an area that has evolved far beyond the fluorographic estimation of calcification in cardiac structures by traditional roentgenography. Long-regarded as a passive degenerative process, we now appreciate the active nature of calcification, its relation to inflammation (a special interest of Dr. Aikawa herself [4, 5]), and its importance not only in atherosclerosis, but also in the growing epidemic of sclerocalcific aortic valvular disease. After an authoritative and up-to-date review of the pathobiology of aortic valve calcification (Chap. 9), a report on work from the Edinburgh group on fluoride imaging sheds new light on the investigation of calcification as an active process in humans (Chap. 10). Other chapters by established experts focus on the well-validated use of ultrasound in the imaging of aortic valve disease in humans (Chap. 11), and on experimental approaches to the imaging of microcalcification (Chap. 12.) Indeed, foci of microcalcification not only provide a nidus for the growth of calcium mineral deposits in cardiovascular structures but may also have important biomechanical consequences that relate to the stability of atherosclerotic plaques [6, 7].

The third part strives to illustrate the clinical applications of molecular and functional imaging to the cardiovascular system. This includes expert reviews on MRI of atherosclerosis (Chap. 13), positron emission tomography (PET) in coronary artery disease (Chap. 14), and the use of PET combined with computed tomography for the clinical imaging of inflammation and anti-inflammatory interventions as well as calcification (Chaps. 15 and 16.)

The timely and comprehensive compilation assembled in this volume gives an overview of the established and emerging tools provided by molecular and functional imaging. As with all emerging fields, however, a number of issues regarding their use remain unsettled. One area of application related to these techniques engenders no controversy: their use in animal and human investigation. The ability to probe pathophysiologic functions in vivo using minimally invasive approaches has transformed cardiovascular research. Well-controlled animal studies using molecular imaging now permit in vivo probing of mechanisms unraveled by studies conducted in cell culture or in excised specimens of human tissues. The nascent application of molecular imaging to patients has provided a pathway to affirming the human relevance of laboratory studies or inferences obtained from soluble biomarker studies in humans.

A major unmet investigative need revolves around resolving contemporary barriers to the clinical evaluation and development of new cardiovascular therapies [8]. In face of the efficacy of the current standard of care, for many cardiovascular diseases, event rates have fallen, raising the bar for clinical trials required to demonstrate the value of new therapies and obtain registration of new pharmacologic agents. Molecular and functional imaging provide a potential path to overcome some of the hurdles facing current cardiovascular drug development.

Before embarking on a lengthy and resource-intensive clinical endpoint trial, illumination of two critical issues would help to attenuate the risk inherent in clinical drug development. First, such programs would profit enormously from the ability to obtain signals that a novel agent actually alters the intended particular biological pathway in intact humans. Molecular imaging promises an avenue to achieving this goal. Second, many clinical trials fail because they test doses of a new agent that seem ill-chosen in hindsight. Molecular and functional imaging can furnish a way in which doses can be evaluated in a relatively small number of intact humans using imaging biomarkers to help ascertain the most appropriate dose to use in a clinical endpoint trial. Such in vivo methodologies in humans would complement the usual inferences based on pharmacokinetic modeling and observations on non-human species that may vary substantially in their responses to various doses of agents.

Beyond these clear unmet needs in investigation, the human application of molecular and functional imaging requires careful consideration regarding clinical and cost-effectiveness. For imaging modalities to prove clinically useful as additions to the current panel of validated biomarkers of prospective risk, they require rigorous evaluation. While coronary calcium scanning indubitably predicts prospective risk of cardiovascular events, adding to traditional risk and emerging biomarkers, its clinical utility remains incompletely validated. No study has yet tested whether the targeting of therapy based on coronary calcium score leads to greater cardiovascular event reduction than therapy directed by already validated markers such as the Framingham covariates or high-sensitivity C-reactive protein. The contention that imaging studies such as coronary artery calcium scores can motivate patients to adopt a healthy lifestyle or adhere to therapies has not received consistent validation when studied rigorously [9].

Much of the interest in molecular and functional imaging of the cardiovascular system over the last decade or so has focused on the quest to identify the so-called "vulnerable" plaque. This goal assumes implicitly that identification of a plaque that has characteristics associated in post-mortem studies with plaque rupture and fatal thrombosis could direct a local therapy that would forestall such complications of atherosclerosis. Multiple lines of evidence cast doubt on this simplistic notion [7]. First, plaques with thin fibrous caps, large lipid cores, and active inflammation tend to occur in clusters rather than singly within the coronary circulation. Moreover, patients who harbor such plaques in their coronary arteries likely have activated atherosclerotic plaques in other arterial beds, such as in the carotid circulation. Many plaques that have the characteristics of "vulnerability" may not rupture. Autopsy studies provide us with a numerator but not a denominator with regard to the fatal thrombotic potential of plaques with the characteristic attributed to "vulnerability". Indeed, in the PROSPECT study, during a more than 3-year observation period, fewer than 5 % of plaques, judged by intravascular ultrasound virtual histology study to have characteristics of vulnerability, actually caused clinical events [10]. Thus, the vast majority of so-called "vulnerable" plaques will not cause a clinical complication over a period of several years. These various observations suggest that systemic therapy, often directed by non-imaging biomarkers, may prove more clinically effective at targeting therapy and reducing events than the application of imaging modalities.

Likewise, as illustrated in this volume, while calcium provides an attractive imaging target, its mutability remains questionable. Although the ability to prevent or retard calcification of cardiovascular structures such as the aortic valve, the atherosclerotic plaques, or the mitral annulus might be desirable, we currently lack clinical tools to this end. Perhaps the application in investigation of the modalities described in this volume will enable research that renders the modulation of calcification a realistic therapeutic target. Molecular and functional imaging of the cardiovascular system, like any emerging tool, must overcome a number of challenges. First, while well-developed preclinically, molecular imaging must traverse the "valley of death" to clinical application for it to achieve its promise of transforming the practice of cardiovascular medicine [8, 11].

Clinical use of molecular imaging probes requires toxicologic evaluation and preparation of material according to "good manufacturing practices" (GMP) [11]. These expensive undertakings lie beyond the resources of most academic research groups. While many have made experimental animals "glow in the dark" by the use of molecular imaging modalities, the realization of the promise in patients remains rudimentary. As illustrated in the excellent chapters in Part III of this volume, some of the most mature modalities for clinical application include PET and MRI. The work with fluorodeoxyglucose and sodium fluoride uptake provide examples of the application of the principles of molecular imaging to human patients. Yet, we must remain mindful of the need to validate the interpretation of the origin of signals attributed to inflammation in the case of FDG or calcification, as in the case of sodium fluoride imaging [12]. We must also require rigorous clinical validation of the relationship between these imaging biomarkers and clinical events and patient outcomes.

The compendium of chapters in this collection provide with a proper support and guidepost to the future of realizing the promise both in investigation and in the clinic of molecular and functional imaging of the cardiovascular system.

Peter Libby
Division of Cardiovascular Medicine
Brigham and Women's Hospital
Harvard Medical School
Boston, MA 02115, USA

References

1. Jaffer FA, Libby P, Weissleder R. Molecular imaging of cardiovascular disease. Circulation. 2007;116:1052–61.
2. Libby P, Jaffer FA, Weissleder R. Molecular imaging in cardiovascular disease. In: Bonow RO, Mann DL, Zipes DP, Libby P, editors. Braunwald's heart disease: a textbook of cardiovascular medicine. Philadelphia: Elsevier Saunders; 2011:448–58.

3. Jaffer FA, Libby P. Molecular imaging of atherosclerosis. In: Weissleder R, Ross BD, Rehemtulla A, Gambhir SS, editors. Molecular imaging: principles and practice. Shelton: PMPH USA; 2010:960–79.
4. Aikawa E, Nahrendorf M, Figueiredo JL, Swirski FK, Shtatland T, Kohler RH, Jaffer FA, Aikawa M, Weissleder R. Osteogenesis associates with inflammation in early-stage atherosclerosis evaluated by molecular imaging in vivo. Circulation. 2007;116:2841–50.
5. Aikawa E, Nahrendorf M, Sosnovik D, Lok VM, Jaffer FA, Aikawa M, Weissleder R. Multimodality molecular imaging identifies proteolytic and osteogenic activities in early aortic valve disease. Circulation. 2007;115:377–86.
6. Maldonado N, Kelly-Arnold A, Vengrenyuk Y, Laudier D, Fallon JT, Virmani R, Cardoso L, Weinbaum S. A mechanistic analysis of the role of microcalcifications in atherosclerotic plaque stability: potential implications for plaque rupture. Am J Physiol Heart Circ Physiol. 2012;303:H619–28.
7. Libby P. Mechanisms of the acute coronary syndromes and their implications for therapy. N Engl J Med. 2013;368:2004–13
8. Libby P, Di Carli MF, Weissleder R. The vascular biology of atherosclerosis and imaging targets. J Nucl Med. 2010;51:1S–5S
9. Ridker PM. Coronary artery calcium scanning in primary prevention: a conversation with cardiology fellows. Arch Intern Med. 2011;171:2051–2.
10. Stone GW, Maehara A, Lansky AJ, de Bruyne B, Cristea E, Mintz GS, Mehran R, McPherson J, Farhat N, Marso SP, Parise H, Templin B, White R, Zhang Z, Serruys PW. A prospective natural-history study of coronary atherosclerosis. N Engl J Med. 2011;364:226–35.
11. Swanson D, Graham M, Heinonen TM, Libby P, Mills GQ. Current good manufacturing practices for pet drug products in the United States. J Nucl Med. 2009;50:26N–8
12. Folco EJ, Sheikine Y, Rocha VZ, Christen T, Shvartz E, Sukhova GK, Di Carli MF, Libby P. Hypoxia but not inflammation augments glucose uptake in human macrophages. Implications for imaging atherosclerosis with fdg-pet. J Am Coll Cardiol. 2011;58:603–14.

Preface

Due to population aging in Western countries, cardiovascular calcification is a growing burden and contributes significantly to cardiovascular risk. Recent evidence suggests that microcalcifications in thin fibrous caps increase the mechanical vulnerability of atherosclerotic plaques and promote acute myocardial infarction. Aortic valve macrocalcifications cause aortic stenosis and heart failure. Despite this vast clinical impact, calcification remains a neglected pathology, and the cellular mechanisms of cardiovascular calcification are poorly understood. Therefore, no effective medical therapies are available for calcification. Clinical and preclinical studies, including our own, suggest that inflammation contributes to calcification through the expression of high levels of osteogenic molecules and reactive oxygen species by activated macrophages and other inflammatory cells. Critical barriers to progress in the field include a lack of high-resolution imaging techniques that can detect preclinical calcification. Our studies demonstrated that molecular imaging can identify early stages of calcification undetectable by conventional histological and imaging methods, thus providing a potentially powerful tool for exploring microcalcifications and their association with inflammation in the clinic. The National Heart, Lung and Blood Institute of the National Institutes of Health has emphasized the importance of understanding the underlying mechanisms of calcification, particularly the identification of novel pathways, and the need to develop imaging modalities for the detection of subclinical calcification.

Cardiovascular Imaging: Arterial and Aortic Valve Inflammation and Calcification covers the contemporary understanding of the basic pathobiology and the mechanisms of atherosclerosis and calcific aortic valve disease, and provides insights into the modern imaging modalities that visualize various stages of these diseases. Preclinical studies, including our own, provided the in vivo evidence of temporal and spatial association of cardiovascular inflammation and calcification in experimental animals. Clinical studies have confirmed the feasibility of such technologies in patients. I hope that this book, written by the top experts in the fields of vascular biology and cardiovascular imaging, will enable readers to comprehend our current knowledge and focus on the possibility of preventing calcification disease progression in the near future.

I would like to acknowledge my mentors: Dr. Frederick J. Schoen, for introducing me to the exciting pathology of cardiac valve disease; Dr. Ralph Weissleder for empowering me to link cardiovascular pathology and imaging; and Dr. Peter Libby for his continuous support and inspiration. I would also like to thank my research fellows and students, whose perspicacious questions challenged me to find new answers, develop innovative hypotheses, and look into novel pathways for cardiovascular calcification. And I can never thank my family enough—especially my husband, Dr. Masanori Aikawa—for believing in me and encouraging me throughout my career.

Boston, MA, USA Elena Aikawa, MD, PhD, FAHA

Contents

Part I

Preclinical Imaging of Mechanisms of Atherosclerosis and Its Complications

Pathobiology and Mechanisms of Atherosclerosis

1

Thibaut Quillard and Kevin J. Croce

Contents

T. Quillard, PhD
INSERM, UMR957, LPRO, Nantes F-44035, France
e-mail: thibaut.quillard@univ-nantes.fr

K.J. Croce, MD, PhD (✉)
Cardiovascular Division, Interventional Cardiology, Brigham and Women's Hospital, Harvard Medical School, 77 Ave Louis Pasteur, NRB 742, Boston, MA 02115, USA
e-mail: KCROCE@PARTNERS.ORG

E. Aikawa (ed.), *Cardiovascular Imaging: Arterial and Aortic Valve Inflammation and Calcification*, DOI 10.1007/978-3-319-09268-3_1

Abbreviations

ALP	Alkaline phosphatase
CT	Computed tomography
CTA	CT angiography
CVD	Cardiovascular disease
EC	Endothelial cell
ECM	Extracellular matrix
FCH	Fluorocholine
FDG	Fluorine-labeled 2-deoxy-D-glucose
Gp IIb/IIIa	Glycoprotein IIb/IIIa
HMGCOA	3-hydroxy-3-methylglutaryl-coenzyme A
HSP	Heat shock proteins
ICAM-1	Intercellular adhesion molecule 1
IPH	Intraplaque hemorrhage
IVUS	Intravascular ultrasound
LDL	Low-density lipoprotein
LOX-1	Lectin-like oxidized LDL receptor
LSS	Low shear stress
MCP-1	Monocyte chemotactic protein 1
MDA	Malondialdehyde-lysine
MGP	Matrix Gla-protein
MI	Myocardial infarction
MMP	Matrix metalloproteinases
MPO	Myeloperoxidase
MRA	Magnetic resonance angiography
MRI	Magnetic resonance imaging
NaF	Sodium fluoride
NIR	Near infrared
NO	Nitric oxide
OCT	Optical coherence tomography
OFDI	Optical frequency domain imaging
PET	Positron emission tomography
PPARγ	Peroxisome proliferator-activated receptor γ
PS	Phosphatidylserine
RBC	Red blood cells
RGD	Arg-Gly-Asp

ROS	Reactive oxygen species
SMC	Smooth muscle cell
SPECT	Single-photon emission computed tomography
SPIO	Superparamagnetic iron oxide probes
SR	Scavenger receptors
SR-A	Scavenger receptor-A
TF	Tissue factor
TGF-β	Transforming growth factor-β
TLR	Toll-like receptor
TNF-α	Tumor necrosis factor-α
t-PA	Plasminogen activator
u-PA	Urokinase plasminogen activator
USPIO	Ultrasmall superparamagnetic iron oxide
VCAM-1	Vascular cell adhesion molecule 1
VH-IVUS	Virtual histology IVUS

Atherosclerosis is a disease of medium and large arteries in which atherosclerotic plaque narrowing of the arterial lumen causes obstruction of blood flow and tissue ischemia. Vascular inflammation is central to the pathobiology of atherosclerosis, and inflammatory processes play critical roles in early plaque formation, plaque progression, and atherothrombotic plaque complications. Advances in anatomic and molecular imaging techniques have enhanced the ability to quantify atherosclerotic plaque burden and to study the cellular and molecular processes that promote atherogenesis. This chapter provides an overview of the mechanisms of atherosclerosis and focuses on structural and physiological entities that can be evaluated by anatomic or molecular imaging techniques.

1.1 Introduction

Cardiovascular disease (CVD) is the leading cause of death worldwide. Atherosclerosis and its complications are the most common cause of CVD-related death. Atherosclerosis develops when pathogenic dysregulation of vascular and immune cell function results in altered blood vessel structure and stenotic narrowing of the lumen of large- and medium-sized arteries. Over the past two decades, a tremendous amount of basic and clinical research has emerged which supports the premise that inflammation is at the heart of atherosclerosis pathobiology. In addition, we now understand that atherosclerosis is an insidious process that can remain clinically silent for years until a complication such as plaque rupture results in arterial thrombosis and tissue ischemia.

Vascular imaging research and methods have greatly advanced our understanding of the cellular and molecular mechanisms that cause atherosclerosis, and moving forward, advanced imaging techniques have the potential to elucidate novel atherogenic mechanisms while improving diagnostic and prognostic capabilities. This chapter reviews the critical inflammatory mechanisms that underlie the pathobiology of atherosclerotic vascular disease and highlights the anatomic, cellular, and molecular targets which are the focus of vascular imaging techniques.

1.2 Plaque Formation

In healthy arteries, endothelial cells (EC), which cover the inner surface of blood vessels, regulate blood flow, control vessel wall permeability, and inhibit blood clotting and activation of circulating leukocytes and platelets [1]. In the normal or "healthy" state, endothelial cells maintain vascular homeostasis by producing protective compounds that inhibit coagulation, prevent leukocyte and platelet adhesion, and modulate the contractile and proliferative state of underlying smooth muscle cells. Nitric oxide (NO) is one of the key EC-derived molecules that control vascular health and inflammation. The pathobiology of arterial disease begins with an inciting injury that activates inflammatory mechanisms and leads to a reduction in bioavailable NO. Under normal circumstances, the cellular and molecular processes that control vascular injury responses direct repair and vascular healing. In pathological conditions, dysregulation of inflammatory responses results in persistent vascular inflammation and adverse arterial remodeling.

Atherogenic stimuli such as tobacco, hyperlipidemia, and elevated glucose levels from diabetes cause endothelial damage that is characterized by decreased NO, altered EC permeability, and increased expression of adhesion molecules that control leukocyte homing. In diabetic patients who are at risk for CV disease, hyperglycemia increases reactive oxygen species (ROS) in vascular cells and leads to the induction of proinflammatory signaling pathways and production of proinflammatory cytokines [2].

A century ago, Anitchkov and Khalatov demonstrated in rabbits that lipid consumption was strongly associated with the formation of atherosclerotic lesions. Consistently, numerous epidemiological studies have strongly linked plasma cholesterol levels with the occurrence of atherosclerotic thrombotic complications in humans. Accumulation of cholesterol-containing lipoproteins in the arterial wall is the hallmark of plaque development. This progressive process is associated with endothelial dysfunction. Sera from hypercholesterolemic human volunteers or purified low-density lipoproteins (LDL) reduce NO production by endothelial cells, promoting an atherogenic microenvironment [3]. HMGcoA (3-hydroxy-3-methylglutaryl-coenzyme A) reductase inhibitors or statins, which block cholesterol biosynthesis, have shown a major beneficial clinical impact in the prevention of atherothrombotic events, reflecting the critical importance of hyperlipidemia in the pathobiology of atheroma [4].

Tobacco smoke constituents also damage the vascular endothelium by increasing ROS. Studies have demonstrated that sera from active smokers decrease NO availability from ECs by altering the expression and activity of the endothelial NO synthase enzyme [5, 6]. Similarly, multiple studies have demonstrated that cigarette

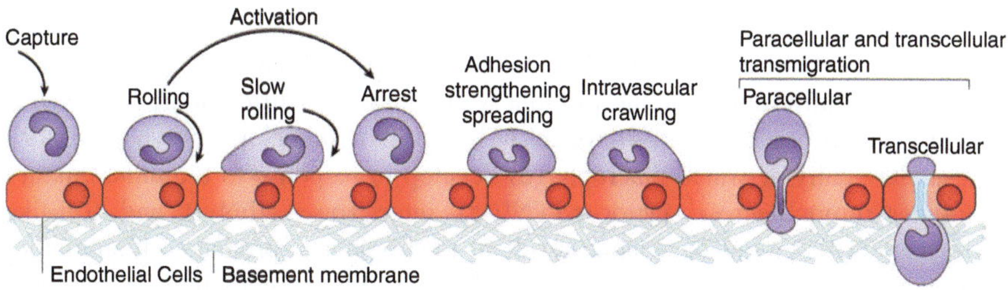

Fig. 1.1 Leukocyte adhesion cascade. Leukocytes are attracted by chemokines and recruited by activated endothelial cells. Leukocyte rolling is mediated by selectins, activation is mediated by chemokines, and arrest is mediated by integrins. Additional adhesion molecules like ESAM (endothelial cell-selective adhesion molecule), JAM (junctional adhesion molecule), cadherins, and PI3K signaling allow leukocytes firm adhesion and ultimately the transmigration of leukocytes through the endothelial layer (Adapted from Ley et al. [12])

smoke extract or isolated components, such as nicotine, decreased NO availability and promote atherogenic EC inflammation [7, 8].

Hemodynamic forces in the vasculature also play a major role in the initiation of atherosclerotic disease. Blood vessel segments that experience low shear stress (LSS) and disturbed blood flow (e.g., at inner curvatures or bifurcations) have a predilection to develop atheromatous plaques [9]. Areas of altered shear stress have reduced NO production and increased expression of atherogenic cytokines and proinflammatory leukocyte adhesion molecules [10]. In addition, low shear areas have increased EC permeability that heightens accumulation of atherogenic LDL in the subendothelial matrix [11].

By inducing endothelial inflammation and increased vessel permeability, atherogenic stimuli enable progressive accumulation of lipids such as oxidized LDL in the arterial wall. Intimal lipid deposition induces vascular and immune cell inflammatory responses. LSS and LDL specifically stimulate EC and platelet expression of leukocyte chemokines (e.g., monocyte chemotactic protein 1 [MCP-1]) and the leukocyte adhesion molecules vascular cell adhesion molecule 1 [VCAM-1], intercellular adhesion molecule 1 [ICAM-1], E-selectin, and P-selectin. These leukocyte adhesion molecules direct a well-characterized series of multistep adhesion events where leukocytes roll, arrest, and transmigrate through inflamed vascular endothelium (Fig. 1.1) [12].

In the early phases of atherosclerosis, monocytes enter the arterial intima and differentiate into macrophages. Recent work has demonstrated that hyperlipidemia increases a subpopulation of particularly proinflammatory monocytes in blood that preferentially home to nascent plaques. These proinflammatory monocytes, which are identified in mice by high expression of the surface marker Ly6C and low expression of CD43 (Ly6C^{high} CD43^{low}), produce high levels of atherogenic signaling molecules [13–17]. It is currently unclear whether similar subpopulations of atherogenic monocytes exits in humans; however, recent data suggest that mon1 monocyte subsets found in spleen and atherosclerotic lesions (CD14++ CD16- CCR2+ CX3CR1^{lo}; CD62L+ CD115+) are functionally similar to proatherogenic murine Ly6C^{high}

CD43^{low} cells. More investigation will be required to refine our understanding of the role of monocyte heterogeneity in human atherosclerotic disease.

Following infiltration into the vascular wall, monocytes differentiate into macrophages, which predominantly have an M1 proinflammatory phenotype [18, 19]. These classically activated macrophages develop in response to the inflammatory cytokines tumor necrosis factor-α (TNF-α), interferon-γ (IFN-γ), and Toll-like receptor (TLR) agonists. Plaque-resident macrophages produce inflammatory mediators, which direct recruitment of additional immune cells into the evolving atherosclerotic plaque. Macrophage differentiation is marked by an increased expression of scavenger receptors (SRs), such as scavenger receptor-A (SR-A (CD204)), CD36, macrophage receptor (MARCO), and lectin-like oxidized LDL receptor (LOX-1), which mediate macrophage internalization of LDL particles and apoptotic bodies. Macrophages also engulf cholesterol particles by micropinocytosis of native LDL and phagocytosis of aggregated LDL [20, 21]. In the setting of hyperlipidemia, intimal cholesterol deposition overwhelms the ability of monocytes/macrophages to clear these noxious molecules, and lipid-overloaded macrophages turn into "foam cells," which contain abundant cholesteryl ester droplets within the cytosol. Foam cell formation is the hallmark feature of fatty streaks which are the earliest stage of an atherosclerotic plaque. Foam cells have a highly inflamed phenotype, constitutively active NFkB inflammation pathways, and produce atherogenic cytokines and matrix metalloproteinases (MMP) [22].

1.3 Plaque Progression

As atheroma formation progresses, lipid-engorged foam cells undergo apoptosis, and the buildup of apoptotic bodies and necrotic debris results in the formation of a "necrotic" plaque core (Fig. 1.2). Inflammatory mediators stimulate plaque expression of the prothrombotic clotting protein tissue factor (TF) on cells within the plaque [23, 24].

The proinflammatory milieu within the nascent plaque stimulates migration and proliferation of smooth muscle cells (SMC) in the burgeoning atheroma. Cytokines such as transforming growth factor-β (TGF-β), which are released by vascular and immune cells, promote SMC proliferation and drive a phenotypic switch from a quiescent SMC contractile form to a proliferative and hypersynthetic phenotype. The accumulation of these SMCs in the plaque is associated with the production of several extracellular matrix (ECM) proteins (i.e., collagen, elastin), which increase plaque mass. Importantly, the plaque ECM components also create a scaffold that provides tensile strength to the atheromatous lesion [25]. In addition to ECM deposition, impaired macrophage clearance of apoptotic debris (impaired efferocytosis) also promotes plaque expansion.

Curiously, plaques often enlarge outward (outward or positive remodeling), preserving the lumen until later phases of the disease when the direction of plaque expansion shifts inward to obstruct blood flow by impinging on the vessel lumen. In this manner, the clinical manifestations of atherosclerosis often only become

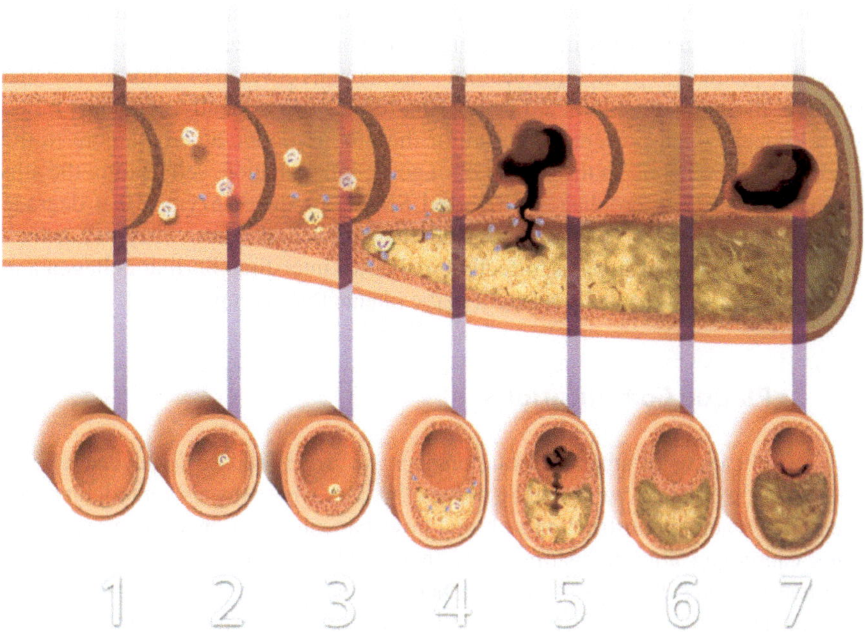

Fig. 1.2 Development and complications of atherosclerotic plaques. Illustration of longitudinal and transversal sections of an artery from the initiation of the lesion (*1*) to the thrombotic complications of atherosclerosis (*5–7*). In the early phase of plaque formation (*2*), dysfunctional endothelium induces an increased vascular permeability allowing the progressive accumulation of lipids in the artery wall. Dysfunctional endothelial cells recruit inflammatory leukocytes by releasing chemokines and expressing adhesion molecules. (*3*) Accumulating macrophages in the lesion engulf modified lipoproteins and form lipid-laden foam cells. Leukocytes and vascular cells release inflammatory cytokines that sustain and amplify the recruitment of inflammatory cells within the intima and promote smooth muscle cell migration and proliferation. (*4*) Progressive accumulation of lipids and necrotic cells forms an acellular "necrotic core" in the lesion, overlapped by a fibrous cap, composed by extracellular matrix and smooth muscle cells. Inflammation further increases the production of prothrombotic molecules and proteinases that can cleave extracellular matrix proteins of the fibrous cap and weaken its resistance from rupture. (*5*) When the fibrous cap ultimately breaks, coagulation factors in blood gain access to prothrombotic molecules in the necrotic lipid-rich core, forming a thrombus. If fibrinolytic mechanisms fail to overcome clot formation, an occlusive thrombus may form and provoke an acute coronary syndrome. (*6*) Plaques can evolve towards a more fibrous lesion, rich in extracellular matrix and smooth muscle cells, and often calcified nodules. These more "stable" lesions can however become significantly stenotic. (*7*) Superficial erosion can occur in advanced lesions. Erosion is characterized by a local desquamation of endothelial cells, exposing procoagulant signals, and associates with the formation of a mural thrombus without any visible signs of plaque rupture (Adapted from Libby [10])

apparent in the later phase of the disease when luminal obstruction and arterial insufficiency result in tissue ischemia (Fig. 1.2).

As the expanding plaque outstrips its oxygen supply, the artery wall adventitial vasa vasorum sprout new blood vessels that penetrate the media and intima to augment plaque oxygen delivery. Neoangiogenic processes may attenuate cell death and necrotic core accumulation by providing nutrients and oxygen to cells deep within the plaque. Neoangiogenic blood vessel also provides a pathway for the entry of additional immune cells into the center of inflamed plaques [26].

As the plaque progresses, the necrotic core remains covered by a fibrous cap that supports the luminal endothelial cells. This fibrous cap critically maintains blood vessel integrity and prevents exposure of the prothrombotic atheroma core to the circulating blood pool. In the setting of ongoing inflammation, cells within the atheroma (primarily macrophages, ECs, and SMCs) produce enzymes that degrade arterial ECM proteins to enable geometrical remodeling. These enzymes, which include MMPs and cathepsins, directly breakdown interstitial fibrillar collagen and elastin which provide tensile strength to the plaque fibrous cap [27, 28].

1.4 Plaque Complications

The complications of atherosclerotic plaques are largely related to adverse effects on delivery oxygen and nutrients to tissues. In cases where inward remodeling progressively results in obstruction of blood flow, patients experience ischemic symptoms caused by arterial insufficiency. In the insidious setting of stable plaque progression, the symptoms of tissue ischemia often develop gradually and may be prompted by activities which increase utilization and oxygen demand of the affected organ. Symptomatic atherosclerotic complications also occur acutely, when a previously asymptomatic atherosclerotic plaque causes sudden arterial thrombosis and tissue ischemia. Indeed, it is estimated that thrombosis of subclinical atherosclerotic plaques accounts for the majority of fatal myocardial infarctions annually [29]. Subclinical and clinical plaque-associated thrombosis and healing is also a common mechanism for plaque expansion that promotes inward remodeling and narrowing of the arterial lumen [30]. The three main types of acute plaque complications discussed below are plaque rupture, intraplaque hemorrhage, and plaque erosion.

1.4.1 Plaque Rupture

Plaque rupture is the most common form of atherosclerotic plaque complications, and it accounts for ~70 % of fatal myocardial infarcts (MI) [31]. Plaque rupture occurs when shear forces of flowing blood or microcalcification impurities cause physical rupture of the fibrous cap that underlies the endothelium and separates the prothrombotic atheroma core from luminal blood. Exposure of the TF-rich plaque core to flowing blood results in clotting cascade activation, platelet deposition, and thrombus formation that can acutely obstruct arterial blood flow.

Importantly, rupture prone or "vulnerable atherosclerotic plaques" have characteristic features that include thin fibrous caps (<65–55 um), a large lipid-rich core (>40 % of plaque's volume), and active inflammation as evidenced by extensive accumulation of macrophages [32]. Inflamed plaques produce numerous proteases that cleave the ECM proteins in the fibrous cap and weaken the cap structure, and it is well established that inflammation-induced ECM proteolysis promotes plaque rupture. The major classes of proteinases expressed in atherosclerotic plaques are MMPs (MMP1, 2, 8, 9, 13, 14), and cathepsins (S, K, L) [33–39]

As plaques expand, inflammation promotes macrophage and SMC-mediated calcium deposition within the plaque and plaque calcification heightens plaque vulnerability by increasing stiffness and biomechanical inhomogeneity [40]. Plaque calcification occurs in response to cytokines that alter local expression of the proteins that promote calcium deposition (e.g., alkaline phosphatase (ALP), osteopontin, Runx2/Cbfa1, osteocalcein, members of the Notch family) and inhibit calcium resorption (e.g., Matrix Gla-protein (MGP), fetuin, osteoprotegerin). In clinical studies, vascular calcification markedly increases the risk of acute cardiovascular events and sudden cardiovascular death [41, 42].

1.4.2 Plaque Erosion

Plaque erosion, which accounts for ~20–25 % of fatal MIs, predominantly affects young women and patients with dyslipidemia [43]. Plaque erosion occurs when there is local desquamation of luminal endothelial cells in the absence of physical signs of fibrous cap rupture. In the setting of plaque erosion, exposure of the subendothelial ECM stimulates clotting cascade activation and arterial thrombosis. Unlike plaque rupture, cap thinning, and macrophage do not appear to be associated with plaque erosion. In fact, plaques undergoing erosion tend to have a high content of SMCs and proteoglycans [44]. Although the drastic differences in composition between rupture and erosion prone plaques suggest that the two processes have different pathologic mechanisms, the molecular mechanisms of plaque erosion are largely unknown. Notably, patients with plaque erosion have high levels of circulating myeloperoxidase (MPO), and in vitro analysis has demonstrated that MPO and its associated ROS (hypochlorous acid) can trigger EC apoptosis which promotes EC sloughing and erosion [45].

1.4.3 Intraplaque Hemorrhage (IPH)

IPH is an important contributor to plaque destabilization and in some cases can promote acute plaque rupture. The neovessels which develop in complex atheroma are fragile and prone to rupture. Following neoangiogenic rupture, the influx of immune cells, red blood cells (RBC), and blood proteins dramatically influence plaque biology.

ROS, oxidized LDLs, and lipids extracted from human atheromatous plaques promote RBC lysis and hemoglobin release [46, 47]. Within the plaque, free hemoglobin amplifies the oxidative stress responses which drive EC damage, apoptosis, and accumulation of necrotic debris [48, 49]. Blood-derived proteases also act on plaque ECM components and promote fibrous cap thinning and rupture. In line with this concept, studies have demonstrated that markers of IPH associate with rupture prone vulnerable plaque morphology [50]. Plaque neutrophil infiltration also increases following IPH, and the neutrophil-derived proteases including tissue plasminogen activator (t-PA), urokinase plasminogen activator (u-PA), plasmin, gelatinase, and serine proteases also degrade fibrous cap components and increase chance of rupture [51]. In addition to directly degrading ECM component of the fibrous cap, neutrophil-derived serine proteases break down atheroprotective SMC-secreted heat shock proteins (HSP) [52, 53].

1.5 Atherosclerosis Imaging

Advanced imaging strategies have a central role in the detection, treatment, and prevention of atherosclerotic vascular disease and its ischemic complications. The insidious nature of atherosclerosis is such that plaque development continues for years until lumen obstruction or thrombotic complications result in clinically apparent symptoms. The majority of acute CV events occur in patients who were previously asymptomatic, and thus, there has been a concerted effort to develop novel diagnostic imaging strategies that can identify patients before atherosclerotic complications occur. Once identified, the goal would be to treat these patients with risk-reduction therapies. In the following section, we will describe the general categories of CV imaging techniques with a focus on the vascular pathology which can be interrogated with each method. This general introduction will frame subsequent in-depth chapters which are focused on specific imaging modalities.

1.6 Anatomic Atherosclerotic Plaque Imaging

Several types of anatomical imaging methods are available to study cardiovascular anatomy and vascular structures. These modalities can be stratified by whether they involve noninvasive or invasive imaging methods (Table 1.1). With regard to vascular imaging of atherosclerosis, anatomic imaging provides excellent assessment of blood vessel structure and lumen stenosis; however, most anatomic techniques provide little information about plaque physiology or composition (as reviewed in depth [54]).

1.6.1 X-Ray Computed Tomography

X-ray computed tomography (CT) is a noninvasive method that uses high-resolution X-ray imaging systems to generate images of cardiac and vascular structures. CT angiography (CTA) involves the intravenous administration of iodinated contrast agents to visualize luminal features of blood vessels (Fig. 1.3). Although CTA is a rapid and noninvasive method for assessment of flow-limiting peripheral and coronary artery stenosis, the spatial resolution of CTA is less than invasive coronary angiography (see below). Thus, invasive coronary angiography has superior

Table 1.1 Invasive and noninvasive imaging modalities

	Technology	Resolution	Depth	Imaging moieties
Noninvasive				
CT/CTA	X-ray	50 μm	No limit	Iodinated molecules
MRI/MRA	Magnetic	10–100 μm	No limit	Gd chelates, SPIO, USPIO
PET/SPECT	Nuclear	~2 mm	No limit	^{18}F, ^{64}Cu, ^{11}C Tracers/^{99m}Tc, $^{123/124/125/131}$I, ^{111}In tracers
Invasive				
Angiography	X-ray	~0.5–1 mm	No limit	Iodinated molecules
OCT/OFDI	Optical	~10 μm	1–3 mm	None
Angioscopy	Optical	10–50 μm	Surface imaging	None
IVUS/ IVUS-VH	Ultrasound	~150 μm	4–10 mm	None

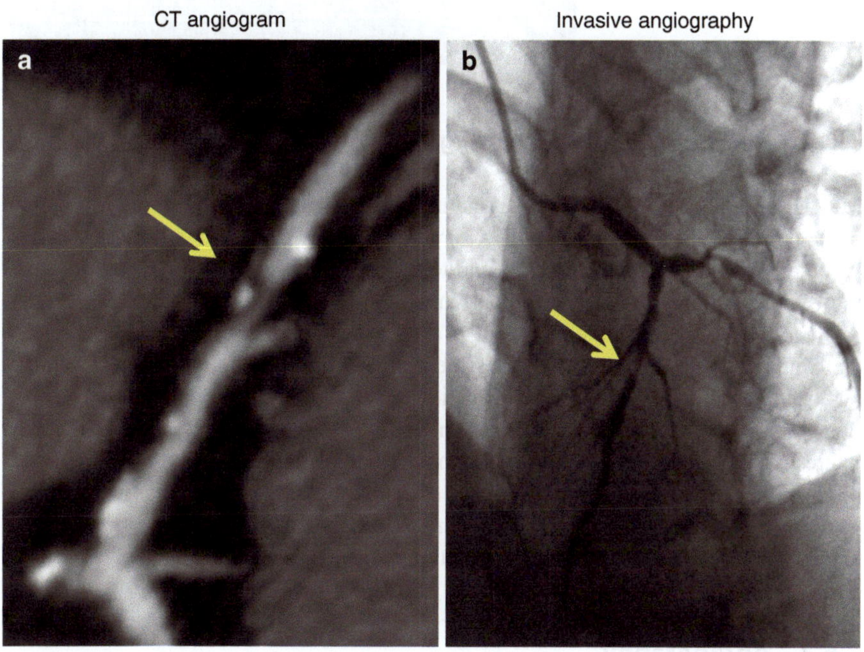

Fig. 1.3 Computed tomography coronary angiogram (**a**) and invasive coronary angiogram (**b**) in the same patient. *Yellow arrows* denote an obstructive atherosclerotic plaque in the mid-segment of the left anterior descending artery (*LAD*)

sensitivity for identifying obstructive stenosis in medium- and small-caliber blood vessels. CTA also performs poorly in calcified or previously stented arteries where imaging artifacts limit interpretation of lumen patency. When compared to invasive angiography, the sensitivity and specificity of CTA for detecting flow-limiting stenosis of 50 % or greater are typically 96 and 86 %, respectively [55].

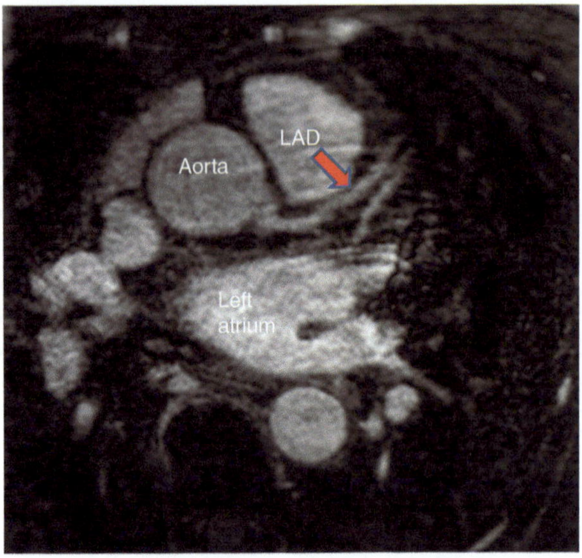

Fig. 1.4 Magnetic resonance angiogram (*MRA*) showing origin of the left main coronary artery from the aorta, giving rise to the left anterior descending artery (*LAD*), Red arrow

1.6.2 Magnetic Resonance Imaging

Magnetic resonance imaging (MRI) is another noninvasive cardiovascular imaging method that utilizes a magnetic field and radiofrequency detection to visualize cardiovascular structures with high spatial and temporal resolution. MRI frequently utilizes intravenous gadolinium-contrast enhancement to perform magnetic resonance angiography (MRA) (Fig. 1.4). Although MRA does an excellent job imaging large arteries and veins, its clinical use for the assessment of flow-limiting coronary artery stenosis has been hampered by significant limitations in visualizing distal segment and small branch disease. With the advent of advanced 3 tesla MRI systems, there is renewed interested in developing MRA for diagnostic imaging of obstructive coronary artery disease [56–58]. In research applications, combination of cardiovascular MRI with an invasive intracoronary MRI detector coil enables characterization of lipid-rich, fibrotic, and calcified plaques with favorable sensitivity and specificity [59].

1.6.3 Angiography

Angiography is an invasive cardiovascular imaging technique that involves direct injection of an iodinated radiopaque contrast agent into the blood vessel to enable imaging with an X-ray-based video fluoroscopy technique (Fig. 1.5). Historically, angiography has been the gold standard for diagnosing obstructive vascular disease because it has excellent sensitivity and specificity and is frequently coupled with invasive methods to treat obstructive vascular disease with angioplasty and stenting. Although angiography is excellent at outlining the luminal border of the vasculature, this method provides no information about blood vessel structure or size beneath the endothelial surface.

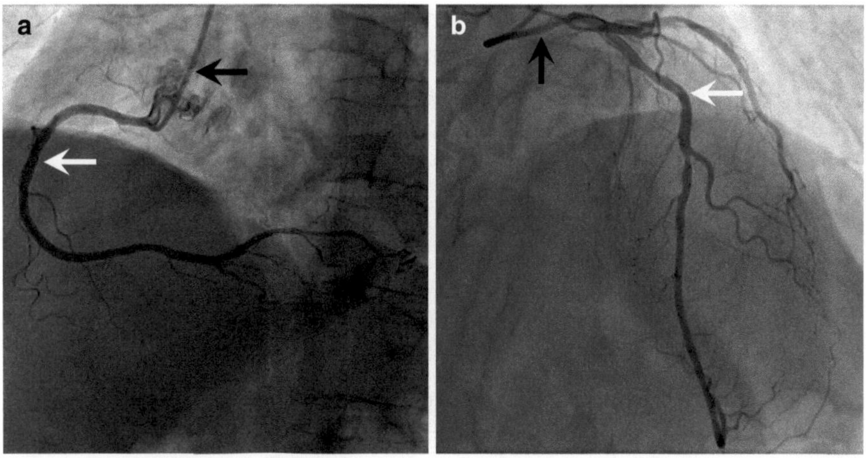

Fig. 1.5 Coronary angiogram. (**a**) Angiogram of a right human coronary artery. (**b**) Angiogram of a left human coronary artery prominently showing the left anterior descending artery (*black arrow* denotes the injection catheter; *white arrow* denotes the artery)

1.6.4 Angioscopy

Angioscopy is an invasive imaging modality that utilizes a high-intensity light source and optical imaging fibers to produce a full-color, 3-dimensional picture of the artery surface. Angioscopy requires that the imaging catheter be placed into the lumen of the artery, and because angioscopy utilizes standard light-based imaging, image acquisition cannot be done in the opaque blood medium. Thus, the angioscopy method requires occlusion of the artery with a balloon that enables arterial perfusion with a clear medium such as saline during the imaging sequence. Angioscopy generates images of the coronary artery lumen; however, it is only able to focus on a small part of the artery at a single time (Fig. 1.6). The limited imaging area and cumbersome process of balloon occlusion and saline perfusion have limited the widespread use of angioscopy in clinical practice or for research applications.

1.6.5 Intravascular Ultrasound

Intravascular ultrasound (IVUS) is an invasive vascular imaging method that utilizes an intracoronary ultrasound catheter that is placed into the lumen of the artery. The IVUS catheter contains a small ultrasound probe which employs reflected sound waves to generate an image of the blood vessel structure (Fig. 1.7). Standard clinical IVUS catheters have a spatial resolution of 150–200 μm and can image 4–10 mm deep into the blood vessel wall. IVUS can operate without balloon occlusion because the presence of blood does not impede sound wave imaging. IVUS imaging enables analysis of lumen and vessel dimensions and the distribution of

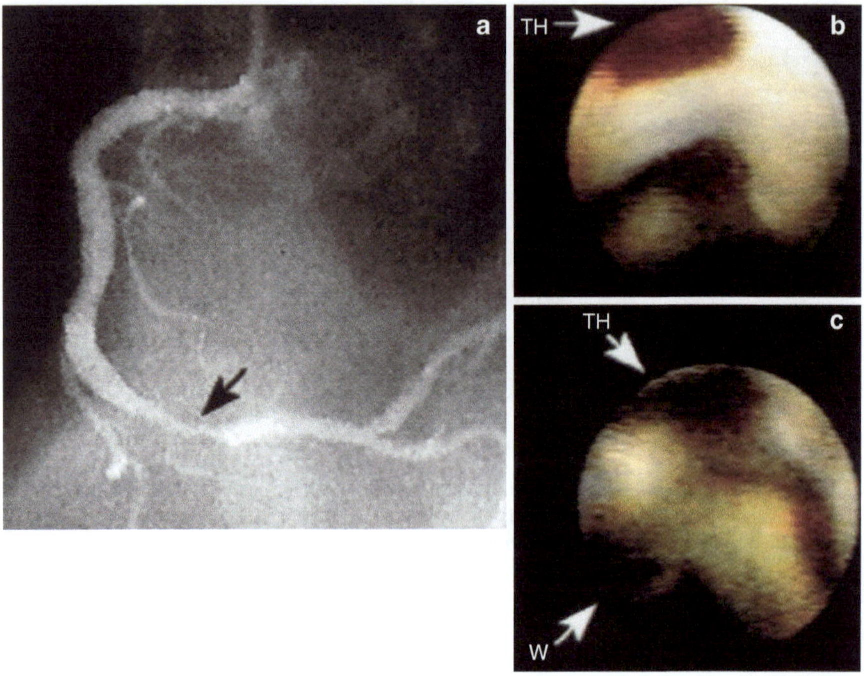

Fig. 1.6 Coronary artery angioscopy. (**a**) Angiogram of the right coronary lesion (*Black arrow*) in a patient with unstable angina. (**b**) Before percutaneous angioplasty, angioscopy shows mural thrombus (*TH*), (*White arrow*). (**c**) After percutaneous angioplasty, angioscopy shows the guidewire (*W*) in the lumen and persistent mural thrombus (*TH*) within an intimal dissection (*White arrows*) (Adapted from White et al. [187])

atherosclerotic plaques. Because of the high spatial resolution, IVUS provides information about intravascular anatomy that far exceeds the level of detail obtained from conventional contrast angiography.

A recent adaptation of IVUS imaging has been termed virtual histology IVUS (VH-IVUS). VH-IVUS utilizes radiofrequency of reflected ultrasound signals and frequency domain analysis to generate a color-coded tissue map of plaque composition which is superimposed on the standard gray scale IVUS cross-sectional images. VH-IVUS improves characterization of the lipid content and necrotic core of atheroma, and in small studies, VH-IVUS-correlated plaque lipid content increased risk of adverse embolization events during therapeutic coronary artery intervention [60].

1.6.6 Optical Coherence Tomography

Optical coherence tomography (OCT) is an invasive intravascular imaging modality that utilizes near-infrared light to generate cross-sectional blood vessel images. OCT catheters, placed into the blood vessel lumen to enable imaging, generate images of coronary arteries with 10–15 μm of spatial resolution that is an order of magnitude

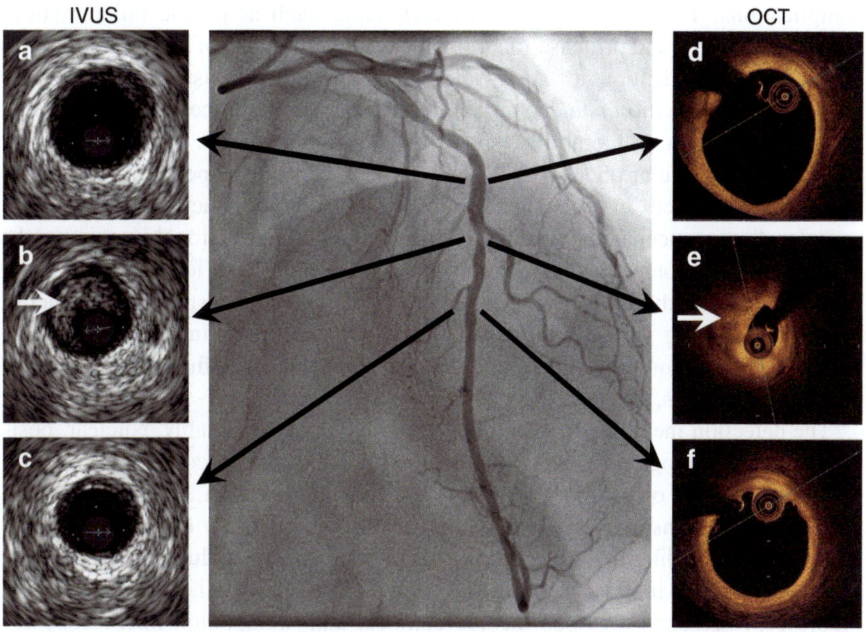

Fig. 1.7 Intravascular ultrasound and optical coherence tomography of the left anterior descending coronary artery. IVUS (*left*) and OCT (*right*). *Black arrows* denote corresponding cross section of the artery coregistered to the angiogram. Panels (*B*) and (*E*) show a stenotic atherosclerotic plaque (*white arrow*). Panel A-C, LAD IVUS images. Panel D-F LAD OCT images.

more precise than the 150–200 μm resolution of IVUS (Fig. 1.7). Although the spatial resolution of OCT is markedly superior to IVUS, near-infrared light does not penetrate tissue as effectively as sound, and thus, OCT can only image from 1 to 3 mm into the vessel wall. In addition, because near-infrared light is scattered by red blood cells, OCT is similar to angioscopy because it requires transient blood clearance during image acquisition. Importantly, recent technological advances in OCT console and catheter design (i.e., optical frequency domain imaging (OFDI)) have enabled rapid imaging element pullback that allows image acquisition to occur during the brief blood-free interval when standard angiography contrast is injected into the artery. This improvement in catheter speed eliminated the need for the arterial balloon occlusion, and OCT imaging is now a convenient, high-resolution imaging modality that is widely used in many centers. In addition, several recent studies have demonstrated that OCT is a highly effective method for identifying and quantifying thin cap fibroatheroma which are predisposed to plaque rupture [61–63].

1.7 Functional Atherosclerotic Plaque Imaging

Although anatomic imaging methods provide some insights into plaque lipid composition, fibrous cap thickness, and plaque volume, anatomic imaging methods lack the ability to define critical components of plaque physiology that predict plaque complications. These physiological characteristics such as plaque inflammation, metabolic activity, and protease function are key determinants of atheroprogression and clinical complications of atherosclerotic disease. In the past decade, we have made great strides in our understanding of the molecular processes that promote plaque progression, vulnerability, and atherothrombotic events. Plaque characterization with molecular phenotyping can now be done using a spectrum of imaging modalities. Advances in molecular imaging methods greatly facilitate research on vascular disease mechanisms, and several molecular and functional imaging techniques have the potential to be used in the clinical setting to identify vulnerable plaques, to follow disease activity, and to monitor therapeutic responses. In general, functional imaging methods employ specific molecular imaging probes that are linked to one or more detectable imaging constituents such as fluorophores, radionuclide compounds, magnetic particles, or microbubbles.

The detection methods for functional imaging vary considerably. Nuclear, positron emission tomography (PET), and single-photon emission computed tomography (SPECT) rely on radioactive tracers for imaging detection, and these method often have high sensitivity and quantitative ability but relatively low spatial resolution. Optical modalities for functional imaging typically utilize fluorescent detectors and probes that are in the near-infrared (NIR) spectrum to visualize vascular tissues. Fluorescent detection methods include confocal and multiphoton microscopy for invasive intravital imaging and fluorescent tomography for noninvasive imaging. The limited penetration of light through tissues currently prevents the noninvasive use of optical and fluorescent methods to image the human vasculature. The invasive, catheter-based, InfraRedx Lipiscan™ combines IVUS and intravascular fluorescence to define vessel architecture and plaque lipid content [64]. The following sections will highlight physiologic processes and specific targets that are the focus of current functional and molecular imaging techniques (Table 1.2, Fig. 1.8).

1.7.1 Cell Activation Imaging

Endothelial and inflammatory cell activation is an attractive target for functional imaging of atherosclerosis because vascular inflammation (1) is increased in early atherogenesis, (2) correlates with atheroprogression, and (3) is a marker of plaque vulnerability. VCAM-1 is an adhesion molecule expressed by activated ECs and macrophages at sites of vascular inflammation and within inflamed atherosclerotic lesions. Various imaging strategies have targeted VCAM-1 expression with very late antigen-4 (VLA-4) peptides, anti-VCAM-1 antibodies, or an MHCI peptide that interacts with VCAM-1. These VCAM-1 targeting moieties have been coupled to radionuclides (^{123}I, ^{99m}Tc, ^{18}F), near-infrared fluorescent dyes, superparamagnetic iron oxide (SPIO) particles, or microbubbles. After injection, these probes accumulate in inflamed tissues and on activated cells, with little or no toxicity [65–71]. Preclinical analysis in mouse models established that there is selective increase in VCAM-1 probe concentration in atherosclerotic lesions in vivo and that probe uptake correlates with lipid content and VCAM-1 expression [72–76].

Table 1.2 Molecular targets of atherosclerotic plaques and associated imaging moieties and modalities

Biological process	Molecular target	Imaging moieties	Imaging platforms
Adhesion	VCAM-1	^{123}I, ^{99m}Tc, ^{18}F, SPIO, NIRF, microbubbles	PET/SPECT, MRI, optical imaging, CEU
	ICAM-1	Gd, microbubbles	MRI, CEU
	E-selectin	SPIO	MRI
	P-selectin	SPIO, Gd, microbubbles	MRI, CEU
Phagocytic activity	–	SPIO	MRI
	–	^{64}Cu, ^{18}F-SPIO	PET/SPECT
Metabolic activity	FDG	^{18}F	PET
	FCH	^{18}F	PET
Lipid uptake	HDL/LDL	^{123}I, ^{125}I, ^{131}I, ^{111}In, ^{99m}Tc, Gd	PET/SPECT, MRI
	CD68	^{124}I	PET/SPECT
	LOX-1	^{111}In, ^{99m}Tc, Gd	SPECT, MRI
	SRs	Microbubbles	CEU
Oxidative stress	Oxidized epitopes	^{125}I, Gd, SPIO	PET/SPECT, MRI
	MPO	Gd	MRI
Cell death	Phosphatidylserine	^{123}I, ^{124}I, ^{99m}Tc, Gd, SPIO	PET/SPECT, MRI
Proteinase activity	MMPs	^{123}I, ^{99m}Tc, ^{18}F, Gd, SPIO, NIRF	PET/SPECT, MRI, optical imaging
	Cathepsins	NIRF	Optical imaging
	Collagen	Gd, NIRF	MRI, optical imaging
Neoangiogenesis	αvβ3 integrin	^{18}F, Gd, NIRF, microbubbles	PET, MRI, optical imaging, CEU
	–	MR-contrast agent (K^{trans}), microbubbles	MRI, CEU
Osteogenesis	Ca^{++} hydroxyapatite	^{18}F, NIRF	PET, optical imaging
Thrombosis	Glycoprotein IIb/IIIa	^{99m}Tc, SPIO, NIRF, microbubbles	PET, MRI, optical imaging, CEU
	Fibrin	^{64}Cu, Gd	PET, MRI
	Factor XIII	Gd, SPIO, NIRF	MRI, optical imaging

Similar strategies target other cell adhesion molecules that play a critical role in the pathobiology of atherosclerosis. Specific probes for ICAM-1, E-selectin, and P-selectin effectively identify activated endothelial cells in atherosclerotic lesions [77–81]. Theranostic imaging strategies have coupled molecular imaging with therapeutic compound delivery; ICAM-1 antibody-targeted echogenic immunoliposomes that contain NO donors deliver vasculoprotective NO to areas of inflamed EC [82]. Combination of targeting moieties for adhesion molecules increases the sensitivity

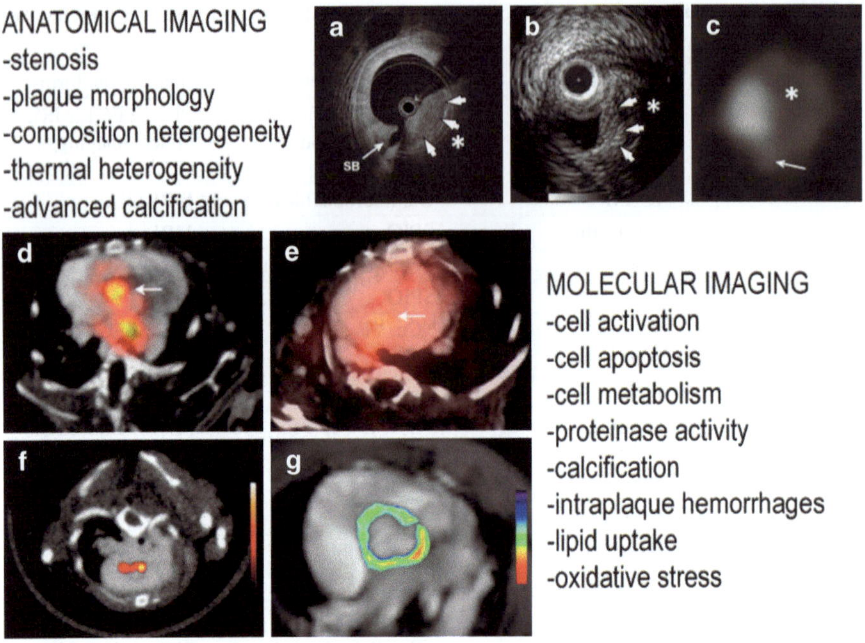

Fig. 1.8 Anatomical and molecular imaging for atherosclerosis. *Top panels*: OCT optical frequency domain imaging (*OFDI*) (**a**) shows a thick fibrous cap (*white arrows*) and a large necrotic core with typical low-intensity appearance (*). IVUS (**b**) demonstrates a narrowed coronary lumen with a focal heterogeneous plaque overlapped by a fibrous layer (*white arrows*). The signal drops out due to the plaque thickness (*). Computed tomography angiography (**c**) detects a large noncalcified plaque segment. *Bottom panels*: (**d**) VCAM-1 expression in atherosclerosis using ^{18}F –4 V PET/CT. (**e**) Lower uptake is seen in ApoE$^{-/-}$ mice treated with statins. (**f**) PET/CT with macrophage targeting nanoparticles. (**g**) MRI with pseudocolored T2-weighted signal intensity, which decreased because of accumulation of iron oxide nanoparticles (Adapted from Refs. [14, 15, 188, 189])

and specificity of inflammation imaging and can provide information about the colocalization of physiologic processes and anatomic structures in vivo [67, 83–85].

1.7.2 Phagocytosis Imaging

Macrophages are the predominant immune cells in atherosclerotic plaques and their presence correlates with plaque inflammation and risk of rupture [86]. To detect macrophage accumulation in lesions, researchers developed iron-based MRI probes (i.e., superparamagnetic iron oxide probes (SPIO, >50 nm) and ultrasmall superparamagnetic iron oxide (USPIO, <50 nm) probes) that are engulfed and concentrated in plaque-resident macrophages. These iron MRI compounds were first in class among a growing number of novel enhanced MRI nanoagents. The prototypical phagocytosis MRI agent has an iron oxide crystal core and a synthetic monomeric or polymeric polysaccharide coating [87, 88]. Phagocytic cells avidly take up these nanoparticles which causes them to accumulate preferentially in inflamed plaques that have large number of activated macrophages [89–91]. Macrophage phagocytic probes have been used to assess the effect of atherosclerosis therapies. In the ATHEROMA study (Atorvastatin Therapy: Effects on Reduction of Macrophage Activity), atorvastatin reduced plaque USPIO uptake in humans which is reflective of decreases in macrophage-mediated plaque inflammation [92]. The plaque specificity of agents that target macrophage phagocytic activity can be increased by conjugating macrophage-avid nanoparticles with lipoproteins that undergo receptor-mediated endocytosis or by conjugating particles with phosphatidylserine (PS)-coated vesicles that mimic apoptotic bodies (discussed in detail below) [93, 94].

In experimental models of atherosclerosis, dual coupling of radiolabeled elements (^{64}Cu, ^{18}F) and/or fluorescent dyes to nanoparticles allows combined multimodal optical and PET/SPECT imaging of plaque [95, 96]. Combination imaging strategy offers the benefits of high spatial anatomic resolution of fluorescence and excellent sensitivity and quantification of PET/SPECT. CT imaging also has the potential to detect plaque-resident macrophages. In experimental rabbit studies, high-resolution CT readily detects iodinated nanoparticles within inflamed macrophage-rich plaques [97].

1.7.3 Imaging of Lipid Uptake/Foam Cell Formation

Macrophage lipid uptake is critical to the pathobiology of early plaque development when foam cell formation is occurring, and heightened lipid uptake also occurs in lipid-rich plaques that are vulnerable to plaque rupture [98]. Lipid-based imaging agents can potentially identify areas of early plaque formation and progression. These probes include high-density lipoprotein (HDL) and LDL compounds conjugated to radioisotopes for nuclear imaging (^{123}I, ^{125}I, ^{131}I, ^{111}In, ^{99m}Tc) or magnetic compounds for MRI visualization [99, 100]. As discussed above, monocytes and macrophages engulf lipids using specific scavenger receptors, and thus, an alternative approach for imaging lipid uptake involves selective targeting of lipoprotein receptors such as LOX-1 or CD68. A preclinical study using ^{99m}Tc-labeled anti-LOX-1 antibody quantified rabbit atherosclerotic plaques by PET. In this study, signal enhancement colocalized strongly with postmortem LOX-1 plaque expression, albeit the signal intensity did not correlate with histological plaque grading [101]. LOX-1 targeted USPIO compounds are promising MRI agents that colocalize with plaque macrophage accumulation [102]. LOX-1 targeting moieties also function well in MR, PET, and fluorescent imaging investigations [103]. NIRF-conjugated anti-oxLDL antibodies enable imaging of plaque progression and statin-induced plaque regression by fluorescent reflectance imaging in mice [104].

1.7.4 Imaging Metabolic Activity

Plaque progression strongly correlates with vascular cell proliferative activity and with heightened metabolic activity of cells within the atheroma. Several studies demonstrate that atherosclerotic plaques have greater metabolic activity compared to healthy vascular tissue, and this increased metabolic state can be exploited to study plaque physiology [105]. Metabolically active cells readily uptake glucose and its analog, fluorine-labeled 2-deoxy-D-glucose (FDG). ^{18}F-FDG is widely used to image the myocardium by PET, and it is currently under development as a vascular imaging agent. Early work demonstrated that FDG uptake in plaques colocalizes with macrophages more than with SMCs [106, 107]. Furthermore, in vivo preclinical studies provide evidence that ^{18}F-FDG PET signal is increased in atherosclerotic rabbit aortas compared to controls [107]. Recently, experimental work using human tissues confirmed that FDG selectively accumulates in inflamed atheromatous plaques [108–116], and clinical studies have showed that FDG PET can be used to follow beneficial vascular effects of lipid or lifestyle therapies aimed at reducing atherosclerotic risk [117–125].

In order to enhance the signal to noise ratio of cardiovascular metabolism imaging, scientists are developing new metabolic biotracers that will preferentially enter plaque and/or macrophages over the metabolically active myocardium. Indeed, compared to the myocardium, macrophages have a higher avidity for the PET agent ^{18}F- fluorocholine (FCH), which incorporates into the cell membrane. In preclinical studies, macrophages in mouse atherosclerotic lesions take up FCH more readily than FDG [126]. Further investigations are needed to determine if FCH performs better than FDG for human plaque imaging.

Intravascular thermography (IV thermography) is an invasive method that examines plaque metabolic activity. Thermography is similar to angioscopy, IVUS, and OCT in that it requires placement of a catheter into the artery. The thermography catheter utilizes a miniaturized thermal sensor to measure temperature heterogeneity along the length of the blood vessel. Heightened plaque inflammation and metabolic activity are associated with increase cellular thermogenesis, and thus, inflamed or proliferative plaques can be identified because they have an increased temperature and greater thermal signals. Although elevated IV thermography temperature signals have been shown to correlate with plaque inflammation [127], this technology is still under development and is not currently approved for widespread clinical use.

1.7.5 Apoptosis Imaging

Cellular apoptosis contributes prominently to accumulation of the debris that comprise the necrotic core of advanced atheroma. In addition, plaque inflammation is associated with increased apoptosis because several inflammatory cytokines activate apoptotic pathways in vascular cells [128]. In non-apoptotic cells, there is asymmetric phospholipid distribution of the cellular membrane in which negatively charged PS is sequestered on the cytosolic (inner) layer of bilipid membrane. Upon activation of apoptotic pathways, PS becomes present on the outer surface of the cell, and thus, PS is a marker of cellular apoptosis and PS-targeted imaging agents can enable visualization of cell death.

One of the most widely used PS probes is the protein annexin V, which binds avidly to PS-containing cell membranes. Iron and radiolabeled annexin V (^{123}I, ^{124}I,

^{99m}Tc and ^{18}F) identify plaques, plaque macrophages, and vascular apoptosis by MRI and SPECT [129–133]. Notably, ^{99m}Tc-annexin V concentrates preferentially in lesions that contain macrophages and necrotic debris compared to lesions that have a non-inflamed fibrous core [132]. In a clinical study of orthotopic heart transplant patients who were suffering from rejection, there was increased uptake of ^{99m}Tc-annexin radiotracer in areas of myocardial infarction [134]. Based on early success in preclinical studies, new investigations are underway to examine whether annexin V probes can quantify the vasculoprotective anti-apoptotic effects of angiotensin inhibitory medications [135].^{124}I-hypericin is a new necrosis-avid PET agent that accumulates in areas of cell death. Preliminary studies using ^{124}I-hypericin demonstrate enhancement of carotid plaques in atherosclerotic mice [136, 137].

1.7.6 Oxidative Stress Imaging

Oxidative stress markedly increases in atherogenic conditions, and ROS promote inflammatory cell activation, lipid oxidation, and apoptosis events that drive plaque development and progression [138]. One method of oxidative stress imaging has focused on developing antibodies that detect by-products of lipid oxidation. Studies that employed radionuclide or MRI-conjugated antibodies against oxidized malondialdehyde-lysine (MDA) or oxidized phospholipid epitopes (e.g., MDA2, E06, and IK17) showed the feasibility of assessing qualitatively and quantitatively oxidative stress in atherosclerotic lesions [139, 140]. Another strategy for oxidative stress imaging involves targeting the ROS-producing enzymes that are made by cells within atherosclerotic plaques. MPO is an enzyme that generates hypochlorous acid (HOCl/OCl-) which is a marker of oxidative stress. To detect MPO activity, investigators designed a small-molecule, gadolinium-based MRI sensor for MPO activity. This MPO probe detected increased MPO activity in the infarcted myocardium of mice 2 days after coronary artery ligation. Moreover, serial imaging sessions with this MPO agent accurately reflected the therapeutic beneficial effect of statins after ischemia-reperfusion injury [141]. Similarly designed fluorescent MPO nanosensors have also been used to detect ROS in preclinical studies [142].

1.7.7 Angiogenesis Imaging

The utility of neoangiogenesis imaging extends well beyond the realm of cardiovascular disease, and much of the pioneering work in this field has been applied to the study of tumor angiogenesis in oncology. Many angiogenic imaging agents target expression of proteins that are critically involved in new blood vessel growth. The cell surface receptor $\alpha_v\beta_3$ is an integrin adhesion molecule that regulates cell migration, proliferation, and survival [143]. $\alpha_v\beta_3$ expression increases during angiogenesis, and Arg-Gly-Asp (RGD) peptides that bind to this integrin are effective angiogenesis probes. Ferromagnetic RGD MRI probes enable detection of angiogenesis in the abdominal aorta of atherosclerotic rabbits and rats [144, 145]. These imaging agents also effectively quantify reduction in angiogenesis following treatment with antiangiogenic drugs [146, 147]. Several investigations have also utilized PET-, optical-, and CEU-based $\alpha_v\beta_3$ integrin probes to assess plaque burden in animal models of atherosclerosis [148–150]. With regard to atherosclerosis imaging, it is currently unclear whether $\alpha_v\beta_3$ imaging techniques are detecting neoangiogenic process or the accumulation of macrophages in lesions, because macrophages and angiogenic cells both express $\alpha_v\beta_3$ receptors [148].

One method of angiogenesis imaging exploits the fact that atherosclerosis-associated angiogenesis results in the production of fragile blood vessels that have markedly increased vascular permeability. Because neoangiogenic vessels have increased permeability, intravascular contrast agents can detect the presence of new vessels based on the leakage of intravascular contents into the perivascular space. Dynamic contrast-enhanced MRI is an angiogenesis imaging method that detects the extravascular presence of an MRI contrast agent. This functional imaging method relies on altered blood vessel physiology rather than a singular molecular target to obtain information about angiogenic responses.

1.7.8 Proteinase Imaging

Proteinases are important catalytic enzymes that play a central role in all aspects of atherosclerotic plaque biology. These enzymes, which include matrix metalloproteinases (MMP) and cathepsins, directly break down interstitial fibrillar collagen and elastin and contribute to fibrous cap thinning and plaque rupture. Imaging "smart" probes for proteinases take advantage of their proteolytic activity because the probe signal intensity increases dramatically upon cleavage by the proteinase.

Investigators have successfully imaged vascular MMP activity in preclinical models using a NIRF MMP-cleaved smart probe [151, 152]. Pharmacotherapy experiments demonstrated that NIRF MMP smart probes can quantify the therapeutic effect of MMP-13 and peroxisome proliferator-activated receptor PPARγ inhibitors on plaque MMP activity and macrophage accumulation [153, 154]. NIRF smart probe technology has been adapted to image the activity of several plaque proteinases including MMP-2 and MMP-9 [155], and cathepsin B, C, and S [38, 156–158]. The majority of these NIRF smart probes have only been tested in animal models, and there are technical hurdles related to the fact that most smart probes have poor plaque penetration and rapidly diffuse out of the plaque once they are activated. To address the issue of probe diffusion and the overall low sensitivity of NIRF smart probes agents, investigators have developed invasive intraluminal optical imaging catheters that can detect NIRF probes with higher sensitivity and spatial resolution than noninvasive detectors [159]. New activatable, cell-penetrating NIRF peptide probes may also improve NIRF proteinase imaging because these agents are retained and concentrate within cells following proteinase cleavage [160, 161].

Researchers have labeled a variety of proteinase inhibitors with SPECT imaging isotopes (^{123}I, ^{99m}Tc, and ^{18}F) to facilitate multimodal plaque imaging. Experiments using ^{99m}Tc- or ^{111}In-labeled MMP inhibitors (MMPI) identify macrophages and activated MMP-2 and MMP-9 in atheromata and aneurysms [162, 163]. Gd-conjugated

MMP peptides are also effective imaging agents for experimental MRI-based proteinase imaging of mouse atherosclerotic lesions [164], and several studies demonstrate the feasibility of imaging gelatinase with MRI probes [165, 166]. One important point regarding the physiology of inhibitor and peptide-based probes is that they may only reflect proteinase expression, rather than activity; proteinase expression and activity can be discordant because activity is tightly controlled by posttranslational regulation and by the expression of endogenous proteinase inhibitors [167].

1.7.9 Imaging Thrombosis

As described above, atherothrombosis is a frequent mechanism of plaque complication, and sub-occlusive plaque thrombosis and intraplaque hemorrhage are major contributors to plaque progression. Molecular imaging of thrombotic process has the potential to identify high-risk plaques and facilitate diagnosis of atherothrombotic events.

Platelets play a central role in thrombotic processes, and they are viable targets for cellular and molecular plaque imaging. The platelet surface adhesion receptor P-selectin (CD62P) is an attractive target for platelet-based thrombosis imaging because this molecule is only expressed by activated platelets. SPECT- and MRI-based P-selectin binding peptides and antibodies enable imaging of plaques in animal models of atherosclerosis, and signals derived from those agents correlate with plaque progression [81, 168]. The platelet membrane glycoprotein IIb/IIIa (also called integrin $\alpha_{IIb}\beta_{IIIa}$, or Gp IIb/IIIa) is another potential platelet imaging target. Upon platelet activation, GPIIb/IIIa undergoes a conformational change that exposes ligand binding epitopes. These activation epitopes interact with specific peptides, and studies using molecular MRI with GPIIb/IIIa peptide imaging have demonstrated the presence of activated platelets on the surface of symptomatic human atherosclerotic plaques [169–171]. Although P-selectin and GPIIb/IIIa targeting approaches to thrombosis imaging are promising, these methods will require further diagnostic and prognostic validation before they can be adopted for clinical use.

Fibrin as another thrombosis imaging target and the fibrin-binding peptide, EP-2104R, identifies thrombosis in noninvasive imaging studies. When coupled to Gd for MRI or ^{64}Cu for PET, EP-2104R detects arterial and venous clots in rodents and humans [172–175]. Fibrin-based probes also successfully identify late stage atherosclerotic plaques [176]. Investigations which utilized probes that target factor XIII show promising results in preclinical studies that examined thrombus formation by PET, NIRF, and MRI [177–181].

1.7.10 Imaging Calcification

Vascular calcification is associated with adverse cardiovascular outcomes, and emerging evidence suggests that calcification promotes plaque rupture by increasing biomechanical inhomogeneity [40]. Standard imaging modalities such as CT, MRI, IVUS, and OCT can readily detect vascular macrocalcification without using molecular imaging probes. In addition, several novel molecular imaging probes have the potential to detect early vascular calcification events which are below the sensitivity of standard anatomic imaging techniques.

^{18}F-sodium fluoride (^{18}F-NaF) is readily incorporated at sites of osteogenic calcification, and this agent performed well with PET/SPECT vascular calcification imaging studies [182]. A 51-patient pilot investigation demonstrated increased ^{18}F-NaF signal in advanced plaques in coronaries and the degree of the tracer enhancement correlated with the severity of arterial stenosis [109]. Despite this early success, it is entirely unclear if ^{8}F-NaF uptake is a marker of plaque vulnerability.

Experimental studies in animal models of atherosclerosis have successfully employed novel fluorescent bisphosphonate-conjugated imaging agents to examine early vascular calcification with optical imaging methods [183, 184]. These fluorescent probes, which are incorporated at sites of calcium deposition, readily detect vascular calcification of atherosclerotic plaques and calcification of heart valves [184–186].

Conclusion

Vascular inflammation is a central mechanism in the pathobiology of atherosclerosis, and although there has been much progress in the past two decades, there are still large gaps in our understanding of the molecular mechanisms of atherosclerotic vascular disease. In addition, there is an urgent need to identify novel methods to identify and treat patients with atherosclerotic vascular disease before they develop devastating ischemic complications. Advanced imaging techniques have the potential to greatly facilitate discovery of new disease mechanisms which can be the target of novel atherosclerosis treatments, and theranostic imaging agents have the potential to simultaneously monitor progression and treat disease. In the near future, molecular imaging methods may also help clinicians identify "at risk patents" so that they can receive preventative personalized therapies before they develop symptoms.

References

1. Pober JS, Sessa WC. Evolving functions of endothelial cells in inflammation. Nat Rev Immunol. 2007;7:803–15.
2. Guerci B, Bohme P, Kearney-Schwartz A, Zannad F, Drouin P. Endothelial dysfunction and type 2 diabetes. Part 2: altered endothelial function and the effects of treatments in type 2 diabetes mellitus. Diabetes Metab. 2001;27:436–47.
3. Feron O, Dessy C, Moniotte S, Desager JP, Balligand JL. Hypercholesterolemia decreases nitric oxide production by promoting the interaction of caveolin and endothelial nitric oxide synthase. J Clin Invest. 1999;103:897–905.
4. Labreuche J, Deplanque D, Touboul PJ, Bruckert E, Amarenco P. Association between change in plasma triglyceride levels and risk of stroke and carotid atherosclerosis: systematic review and meta-regression analysis. Atherosclerosis. 2010;212:9–15.
5. Barua RS, Ambrose JA, Eales-Reynolds LJ, DeVoe MC, Zervas JG, Saha DC. Dysfunctional endothelial nitric oxide biosynthesis in healthy smokers with impaired endothelium-dependent vasodilatation. Circulation. 2001;104:1905–10.

6. Barua RS, Ambrose JA, Srivastava S, DeVoe MC, Eales-Reynolds LJ. Reactive oxygen species are involved in smoking-induced dysfunction of nitric oxide biosynthesis and upregulation of endothelial nitric oxide synthase: an in vitro demonstration in human coronary artery endothelial cells. Circulation. 2003;107:2342–7.
7. Ota Y, Kugiyama K, Sugiyama S, Ohgushi M, Matsumura T, Doi H, Ogata N, Oka H, Yasue H. Impairment of endothelium-dependent relaxation of rabbit aortas by cigarette smoke extract – role of free radicals and attenuation by captopril. Atherosclerosis. 1997;131:195–202.
8. Zhang S, Day I, Ye S. Nicotine induced changes in gene expression by human coronary artery endothelial cells. Atherosclerosis. 2001;154:277–83.
9. Chiu JJ, Chien S. Effects of disturbed flow on vascular endothelium: pathophysiological basis and clinical perspectives. Physiol Rev. 2011;91:327–87.
10. Hsieh HJ, Liu CA, Huang B, Tseng AH, Wang DL. Shear-induced endothelial mechanotransduction: the interplay between reactive oxygen species (ROS) and nitric oxide (NO) and the pathophysiological implications. J Biomed Sci. 2014;21:3.
11. Miyazaki T, Taketomi Y, Takimoto M, Lei XF, Arita S, Kim-Kaneyama JR, Arata S, Ohata H, Ota H, Murakami M, Miyazaki A. m-calpain induction in vascular endothelial cells on human and mouse atheromas and its roles in VE-cadherin disorganization and atherosclerosis. Circulation. 2011;124:2522–32.
12. Ley K, Laudanna C, Cybulsky MI, Nourshargh S. Getting to the site of inflammation: the leukocyte adhesion cascade updated. Nat Rev Immunol. 2007;7:678–89.
13. Robbins CS, Chudnovskiy A, Rauch PJ, Figueiredo JL, Iwamoto Y, Gorbatov R, Etzrodt M, Weber GF, Ueno T, van Rooijen N, Mulligan-Kehoe MJ, Libby P, Nahrendorf M, Pittet MJ, Weissleder R, Swirski FK. Extramedullary hematopoiesis generates Ly-6C(high) monocytes that infiltrate atherosclerotic lesions. Circulation. 2012;125:364–74.
14. Swirski FK, Pittet MJ, Kircher MF, Aikawa E, Jaffer FA, Libby P, Weissleder R. Monocyte accumulation in mouse atherogenesis is progressive and proportional to extent of disease. Proc Natl Acad Sci U S A. 2006;103:10340–5.
15. Swirski FK, Libby P, Aikawa E, Alcaide P, Luscinskas FW, Weissleder R, Pittet MJ. Ly-6Chi monocytes dominate hypercholesterolemia-associated monocytosis and give rise to macrophages in atheromata. J Clin Invest. 2007;117:195–205.
16. Swirski FK, Nahrendorf M, Etzrodt M, Wildgruber M, Cortez-Retamozo V, Panizzi P, Figueiredo JL, Kohler RH, Chudnovskiy A, Waterman P, Aikawa E, Mempel TR, Libby P, Weissleder R, Pittet MJ. Identification of splenic reservoir monocytes and their deployment to inflammatory sites. Science. 2009;325:612–6.
17. Tacke F, Alvarez D, Kaplan TJ, Jakubzick C, Spanbroek R, Llodra J, Garin A, Liu J, Mack M, van Rooijen N, Lira SA, Habenicht AJ, Randolph GJ. Monocyte subsets differentially employ CCR2, CCR5, and CX3CR1 to accumulate within atherosclerotic plaques. J Clin Invest. 2007;117:185–94.
18. Johnson JL, Newby AC. Macrophage heterogeneity in atherosclerotic plaques. Curr Opin Lipidol. 2009;20:370–8.
19. Stoger JL, Gijbels MJ, van der Velden S, Manca M, van der Loos CM, Biessen EA, Daemen MJ, Lutgens E, de Winther MP. Distribution of macrophage polarization markers in human atherosclerosis. Atherosclerosis. 2012;225:461–8.
20. Kruth HS. The fate of lipoprotein cholesterol entering the arterial wall. Curr Opin Lipidol. 1997;8:246–52.
21. Kruth HS. Sequestration of aggregated low-density lipoproteins by macrophages. Curr Opin Lipidol. 2002;13:483–8.
22. Newby AC, George SJ, Ismail Y, Johnson JL, Sala-Newby GB, Thomas AC. Vulnerable atherosclerotic plaque metalloproteinases and foam cell phenotypes. Thromb Haemost. 2009;101:1006–11.
23. Mach F, Schonbeck U, Bonnefoy JY, Pober JS, Libby P. Activation of monocyte/macrophage functions related to acute atheroma complication by ligation of cd40: induction of collagenase, stromelysin, and tissue factor. Circulation. 1997;96:396–9.
24. Moore KJ, Tabas I. Macrophages in the pathogenesis of atherosclerosis. Cell. 2011;145:341–55.

25. Toutouzas K, Synetos A, Nikolaou C, Tsiamis E, Tousoulis D, Stefanadis C. Matrix metalloproteinases and vulnerable atheromatous plaque. Curr Top Med Chem. 2012;12:1166–80.
26. Rademakers T, Douma K, Hackeng TM, Post MJ, Sluimer JC, Daemen MJ, Biessen EA, Heeneman S, van Zandvoort MA. Plaque-associated vasa vasorum in aged apolipoprotein e-deficient mice exhibit proatherogenic functional features in vivo. Arterioscler Thromb Vasc Biol. 2013;33:249–56.
27. Galis ZS, Khatri JJ. Matrix metalloproteinases in vascular remodeling and atherogenesis: the good, the bad, and the ugly. Circ Res. 2002;90:251–62.
28. Lutgens SP, Cleutjens KB, Daemen MJ, Heeneman S. Cathepsin cysteine proteases in cardiovascular disease. FASEB J. 2007;21:3029–41.
29. Ambrose JA, Tannenbaum MA, Alexopoulos D, Hjemdahl-Monsen CE, Leavy J, Weiss M, Borrico S, Gorlin R, Fuster V. Angiographic progression of coronary artery disease and the development of myocardial infarction. J Am Coll Cardiol. 1988;12:56–62.
30. Mann J, Davies MJ. Mechanisms of progression in native coronary artery disease: role of healed plaque disruption. Heart. 1999;82:265–8.
31. Richardson PD, Davies MJ, Born GV. Influence of plaque configuration and stress distribution on fissuring of coronary atherosclerotic plaques. Lancet. 1989;2:941–4.
32. Virmani R, Kolodgie FD, Burke AP, Farb A, Schwartz SM. Lessons from sudden coronary death: a comprehensive morphological classification scheme for atherosclerotic lesions. Arterioscler Thromb Vasc Biol. 2000;20:1262–75.
33. Galis ZS, Sukhova GK, Lark MW, Libby P. Increased expression of matrix metalloproteinases and matrix degrading activity in vulnerable regions of human atherosclerotic plaques. J Clin Invest. 1994;94:2493–503.
34. Nikkari ST, O'Brien KD, Ferguson M, Hatsukami T, Welgus HG, Alpers CE, Clowes AW. Interstitial collagenase (MMP-1) expression in human carotid atherosclerosis. Circulation. 1995;92:1393–8.
35. Herman MP, Sukhova GK, Libby P, Gerdes N, Tang N, Horton DB, Kilbride M, Breitbart RE, Chun M, Schonbeck U. Expression of neutrophil collagenase (matrix metalloproteinase-8) in human atheroma: a novel collagenolytic pathway suggested by transcriptional profiling. Circulation. 2001;104:1899–904.
36. Sukhova GK, Schonbeck U, Rabkin E, Schoen FJ, Poole AR, Billinghurst RC, Libby P. Evidence for increased collagenolysis by interstitial collagenases-1 and -3 in vulnerable human atheromatous plaques. Circulation. 1999;99:2503–9.
37. Shah PK, Falk E, Badimon JJ, Fernandez-Ortiz A, Mailhac A, Villareal-Levy G, Fallon JT, Regnstrom J, Fuster V. Human monocyte-derived macrophages induce collagen breakdown in fibrous caps of atherosclerotic plaques. Potential role of matrix-degrading metalloproteinases and implications for plaque rupture. Circulation. 1995;92:1565–9.
38. Aikawa E, Aikawa M, Libby P, Figueiredo JL, Rusanescu G, Iwamoto Y, Fukuda D, Kohler RH, Shi GP, Jaffer FA, Weissleder R. Arterial and aortic valve calcification abolished by elastolytic cathepsin s deficiency in chronic renal disease. Circulation. 2009;119:1785–94.
39. Lutgens E, van Suylen RJ, Faber BC, Gijbels MJ, Eurlings PM, Bijnens AP, Cleutjens KB, Heeneman S, Daemen MJ. Atherosclerotic plaque rupture: local or systemic process? Arterioscler Thromb Vasc Biol. 2003;23:2123–30.
40. Alexopoulos N, Raggi P. Calcification in atherosclerosis. Nat Rev Cardiol. 2009;6:681–8.
41. O'Donnell CJ, Kavousi M, Smith AV, Kardia SL, Feitosa MF, Hwang SJ, Sun YV, Province MA, Aspelund T, Dehghan A, Hoffmann U, Bielak LF, Zhang Q, Eiriksdottir G, van Duijn CM, Fox CS, de Andrade M, Kraja AT, Sigurdsson S, Elias-Smale SE, Murabito JM, Launer LJ, van der Lugt A, Kathiresan S, Krestin GP, Herrington DM, Howard TD, Liu Y, Post W, Mitchell BD, O'Connell JR, Shen H, Shuldiner AR, Altshuler D, Elosua R, Salomaa V, Schwartz SM, Siscovick DS, Voight BF, Bis JC, Glazer NL, Psaty BM, Boerwinkle E, Heiss G, Blankenberg S, Zeller T, Wild PS, Schnabel RB, Schillert A, Ziegler A, Munzel TF, White CC, Rotter JI, Nalls M, Oudkerk M, Johnson AD, Newman AB, Uitterlinden AG, Massaro JM, Cunningham J, Harris TB, Hofman A, Peyser PA, Borecki IB, Cupples LA, Gudnason V, Witteman JC. Genome-wide association study for coronary artery calcification with follow-up in myocardial infarction. Circulation. 2011;124:2855–64.

42. Folsom AR, Kronmal RA, Detrano RC, O'Leary DH, Bild DE, Bluemke DA, Budoff MJ, Liu K, Shea S, Szklo M, Tracy RP, Watson KE, Burke GL. Coronary artery calcification compared with carotid intima-media thickness in the prediction of cardiovascular disease incidence: the multi-ethnic study of atherosclerosis (mesa). Arch Intern Med. 2008;168:1333–9.
43. Arbab-Zadeh A, Nakano M, Virmani R, Fuster V. Acute coronary events. Circulation. 2012;125:1147–56.
44. Falk E, Nakano M, Bentzon JF, Finn AV, Virmani R. Update on acute coronary syndromes: the pathologists' view. Eur Heart J. 2013;34:719–28.
45. Sugiyama S, Kugiyama K, Aikawa M, Nakamura S, Ogawa H, Libby P. Hypochlorous acid, a macrophage product, induces endothelial apoptosis and tissue factor expression: involvement of myeloperoxidase-mediated oxidant in plaque erosion and thrombogenesis. Arterioscler Thromb Vasc Biol. 2004;24:1309–14.
46. van den Berg JJ, Op den Kamp JA, Lubin BH, Roelofsen B, Kuypers FA. Kinetics and site specificity of hydroperoxide-induced oxidative damage in red blood cells. Free Radic Biol Med. 1992;12:487–98.
47. Nagy E, Eaton JW, Jeney V, Soares MP, Varga Z, Galajda Z, Szentmiklosi J, Mehes G, Csonka T, Smith A, Vercellotti GM, Balla G, Balla J. Red cells, hemoglobin, heme, iron, and atherogenesis. Arterioscler Thromb Vasc Biol. 2010;30:1347–53.
48. Abraham NG, Lavrovsky Y, Schwartzman ML, Stoltz RA, Levere RD, Gerritsen ME, Shibahara S, Kappas A. Transfection of the human heme oxygenase gene into rabbit coronary microvessel endothelial cells: protective effect against heme and hemoglobin toxicity. Proc Natl Acad Sci U S A. 1995;92:6798–802.
49. Balla G, Jacob HS, Eaton JW, Belcher JD, Vercellotti GM. Hemin: a possible physiological mediator of low density lipoprotein oxidation and endothelial injury. Arterioscler Thromb. 1991;11:1700–11.
50. Tavora F, Cresswell N, Li L, Ripple M, Burke A. Immunolocalisation of fibrin in coronary atherosclerosis: implications for necrotic core development. Pathology. 2010;42:15–22.
51. Ionita MG, van den Borne P, Catanzariti LM, Moll FL, de Vries JP, Pasterkamp G, Vink A, de Kleijn DP. High neutrophil numbers in human carotid atherosclerotic plaques are associated with characteristics of rupture-prone lesions. Arterioscler Thromb Vasc Biol. 2010;30:1842–8.
52. Martin-Ventura JL, Leclercq A, Blanco-Colio LM, Egido J, Rossignol P, Meilhac O, Michel JB. Low plasma levels of HSP70 in patients with carotid atherosclerosis are associated with increased levels of proteolytic markers of neutrophil activation. Atherosclerosis. 2007;194:334–41.
53. Martin-Ventura JL, Nicolas V, Houard X, Blanco-Colio LM, Leclercq A, Egido J, Vranckx R, Michel JB, Meilhac O. Biological significance of decreased HSP27 in human atherosclerosis. Arterioscler Thromb Vasc Biol. 2006;26:1337–43.
54. Leuschner F, Nahrendorf M. Molecular imaging of coronary atherosclerosis and myocardial infarction: considerations for the bench and perspectives for the clinic. Circ Res. 2011;108:593–606.
55. Gorenoi V, Schonermark MP, Hagen A. Ct coronary angiography vs. Invasive coronary angiography in chd. GMS Health Technol Assess. 2012;8:Doc02.
56. Kelle S, Hays AG, Hirsch GA, Gerstenblith G, Miller JM, Steinberg AM, Schar M, Texter JH, Wellnhofer E, Weiss RG, Stuber M. Coronary artery distensibility assessed by 3.0 tesla coronary magnetic resonance imaging in subjects with and without coronary artery disease. Am J Cardiol. 2011;108:491–7.
57. Zhao X, Underhill HR, Zhao Q, Cai J, Li F, Oikawa M, Dong L, Ota H, Hatsukami TS, Chu B, Yuan C. Discriminating carotid atherosclerotic lesion severity by luminal stenosis and plaque burden: a comparison utilizing high-resolution magnetic resonance imaging at 3.0 tesla. Stroke. 2011;42:347–53.
58. Maroules CD, McColl R, Khera A, Peshock RM. Assessment and reproducibility of aortic atherosclerosis magnetic resonance imaging: impact of 3-tesla field strength and parallel imaging. Invest Radiol. 2008;43:656–62.
59. Larose E, Yeghiazarians Y, Libby P, Yucel EK, Aikawa M, Kacher DF, Aikawa E, Kinlay S, Schoen FJ, Selwyn AP, Ganz P. Characterization of human atherosclerotic plaques by intravascular magnetic resonance imaging. Circulation. 2005;112:2324–31.

60. Claessen BE, Maehara A, Fahy M, Xu K, Stone GW, Mintz GS. Plaque composition by intravascular ultrasound and distal embolization after percutaneous coronary intervention. JACC Cardiovasc Imaging. 2012;5:S111–8.
61. Kubo T, Ino Y, Tanimoto T, Kitabata H, Tanaka A, Akasaka T. Optical coherence tomography imaging in acute coronary syndromes. Cardiol Res Pract. 2011;2011:312978.
62. Bouki KP, Katsafados MG, Chatzopoulos DN, Psychari SN, Toutouzas KP, Charalampopoulos AF, Sakkali EN, Koudouri AA, Liakos GK, Apostolou TS. Inflammatory markers and plaque morphology: an optical coherence tomography study. Int J Cardiol. 2012;154:287–92.
63. Cilingiroglu M, Oh JH, Sugunan B, Kemp NJ, Kim J, Lee S, Zaatari HN, Escobedo D, Thomsen S, Milner TE, Feldman MD. Detection of vulnerable plaque in a murine model of atherosclerosis with optical coherence tomography. Catheter Cardiovasc Interv. 2006;67:915–23.
64. Gardner CM, Tan H, Hull EL, Lisauskas JB, Sum ST, Meese TM, Jiang C, Madden SP, Caplan JD, Burke AP, Virmani R, Goldstein J, Muller JE. Detection of lipid core coronary plaques in autopsy specimens with a novel catheter-based near-infrared spectroscopy system. JACC Cardiovasc Imaging. 2008;1:638–48.
65. McAteer MA, Schneider JE, Ali ZA, Warrick N, Bursill CA, von zur Muhlen C, Greaves DR, Neubauer S, Channon KM, Choudhury RP. Magnetic resonance imaging of endothelial adhesion molecules in mouse atherosclerosis using dual-targeted microparticles of iron oxide. Arterioscler Thromb Vasc Biol. 2008;28:77–83.
66. Broisat A, Riou LM, Ardisson V, Boturyn D, Dumy P, Fagret D, Ghezzi C. Molecular imaging of vascular cell adhesion molecule-1 expression in experimental atherosclerotic plaques with radiolabelled B2702-p. Eur J Nucl Med Mol Imaging. 2007;34:830–40.
67. Ferrante EA, Pickard JE, Rychak J, Klibanov A, Ley K. Dual targeting improves microbubble contrast agent adhesion to VCAM-1 and P-selectin under flow. J Control Release. 2009; 140:100–7.
68. Kaufmann BA, Sanders JM, Davis C, Xie A, Aldred P, Sarembock IJ, Lindner JR. Molecular imaging of inflammation in atherosclerosis with targeted ultrasound detection of vascular cell adhesion molecule-1. Circulation. 2007;116:276–84.
69. Kelly KA, Nahrendorf M, Yu AM, Reynolds F, Weissleder R. In vivo phage display selection yields atherosclerotic plaque targeted peptides for imaging. Mol Imaging Biol. 2006;8: 201–7.
70. Southworth R, Kaneda M, Chen J, Zhang L, Zhang H, Yang X, Razavi R, Lanza G, Wickline SA. Renal vascular inflammation induced by western diet in ApoE-null mice quantified by (19)F NMR of VCAM-1 targeted nanobeacons. Nanomedicine. 2009;5:359–67.
71. Liu Y, Davidson BP, Yue Q, Belcik T, Xie A, Inaba Y, McCarty OJ, Tormoen GW, Zhao Y, Ruggeri ZM, Kaufmann BA, Lindner JR. Molecular imaging of inflammation and platelet adhesion in advanced atherosclerosis effects of antioxidant therapy with NADPH oxidase inhibition. Circ Cardiovasc Imaging. 2013;6:74–82.
72. Nahrendorf M, Jaffer FA, Kelly KA, Sosnovik DE, Aikawa E, Libby P, Weissleder R. Noninvasive vascular cell adhesion molecule-1 imaging identifies inflammatory activation of cells in atherosclerosis. Circulation. 2006;114:1504–11.
73. Nahrendorf M, Keliher E, Panizzi P, Zhang H, Hembrador S, Figueiredo JL, Aikawa E, Kelly K, Libby P, Weissleder R. 18F-4V for PET-CT imaging of VCAM-1 expression in atherosclerosis. JACC Cardiovasc Imaging. 2009;2:1213–22.
74. Kaufmann BA, Carr CL, Belcik JT, Xie A, Yue Q, Chadderdon S, Caplan ES, Khangura J, Bullens S, Bunting S, Lindner JR. Molecular imaging of the initial inflammatory response in atherosclerosis: implications for early detection of disease. Arterioscler Thromb Vasc Biol. 2010;30:54–9.
75. McAteer MA, Akhtar AM, von Zur Muhlen C, Choudhury RP. An approach to molecular imaging of atherosclerosis, thrombosis, and vascular inflammation using microparticles of iron oxide. Atherosclerosis. 2010;209:18–27.

76. Khanicheh E, Qi Y, Xie A, Mitterhuber M, Xu L, Mochizuki M, Daali Y, Jaquet V, Krause KH, Ruggeri ZM, Kuster GM, Lindner JR, Kaufmann BA. Molecular imaging reveals rapid reduction of endothelial activation in early atherosclerosis with apocynin independent of antioxidative properties. Arterioscler Thromb Vasc Biol. 2013;33:2187–92.
77. Villanueva FS, Jankowski RJ, Klibanov S, Pina ML, Alber SM, Watkins SC, Brandenburger GH, Wagner WR. Microbubbles targeted to intercellular adhesion molecule-1 bind to activated coronary artery endothelial cells. Circulation. 1998;98:1–5.
78. Demos SM, Alkan-Onyuksel H, Kane BJ, Ramani K, Nagaraj A, Greene R, Klegerman M, McPherson DD. In vivo targeting of acoustically reflective liposomes for intravascular and transvascular ultrasonic enhancement. J Am Coll Cardiol. 1999;33:867–75.
79. Kang HW, Torres D, Wald L, Weissleder R, Bogdanov Jr AA. Targeted imaging of human endothelial-specific marker in a model of adoptive cell transfer. Lab Invest. 2006; 86:599–609.
80. Nakamura I, Hasegawa K, Wada Y, Hirase T, Node K, Watanabe Y. Detection of early stage atherosclerotic plaques using pet and ct fusion imaging targeting p-selectin in low density lipoprotein receptor-deficient mice. Biochem Biophys Res Commun. 2013;433: 47–51.
81. Rouzet F, Bachelet-Violette L, Alsac JM, Suzuki M, Meulemans A, Louedec L, Petiet A, Jandrot-Perrus M, Chaubet F, Michel JB, Le Guludec D, Letourneur D. Radiolabeled fucoidan as a p-selectin targeting agent for in vivo imaging of platelet-rich thrombus and endothelial activation. J Nucl Med. 2011;52:1433–40.
82. Kim H, Kee PH, Rim Y, Moody MR, Klegerman ME, Vela D, Huang SL, McPherson DD, Laing ST. Nitric oxide improves molecular imaging of inflammatory atheroma using targeted echogenic immunoliposomes. Atherosclerosis. 2013;231:252–60.
83. Jefferson A, Wijesurendra RS, McAteer MA, Digby JE, Douglas G, Bannister T, Perez-Balderas F, Bagi Z, Lindsay AC, Choudhury RP. Molecular imaging with optical coherence tomography using ligand-conjugated microparticles that detect activated endothelial cells: rational design through target quantification. Atherosclerosis. 2011;219:579–87.
84. McAteer MA, Mankia K, Ruparelia N, Jefferson A, Nugent HB, Stork LA, Channon KM, Schneider JE, Choudhury RP. A leukocyte-mimetic magnetic resonance imaging contrast agent homes rapidly to activated endothelium and tracks with atherosclerotic lesion macrophage content. Arterioscler Thromb Vasc Biol. 2012;32:1427–35.
85. Maiseyeu A, Badgeley MA, Kampfrath T, Mihai G, Deiuliis JA, Liu C, Sun Q, Parthasarathy S, Simon DI, Croce K, Rajagopalan S. In vivo targeting of inflammation-associated myeloid-related protein 8/14 via gadolinium immunonanoparticles. Arterioscler Thromb Vasc Biol. 2012;32:962–70.
86. Boyle JJ. Macrophage activation in atherosclerosis: pathogenesis and pharmacology of plaque rupture. Curr Vasc Pharmacol. 2005;3:63–8.
87. Tsuchiya K, Nitta N, Sonoda A, Nitta-Seko A, Ohta S, Takahashi M, Murata K, Mukaisho K, Shiomi M, Tabata Y, Nohara S. Evaluation of atherosclerotic lesions using dextran- and mannan-dextran-coated USPIO: Mri analysis and pathological findings. Int J Nanomedicine. 2012;7:2271–80.
88. Tsuchiya K, Nitta N, Sonoda A, Otani H, Takahashi M, Murata K, Shiomi M, Tabata Y, Nohara S. Atherosclerotic imaging using 4 types of superparamagnetic iron oxides: new possibilities for mannan-coated particles. Eur J Radiol. 2013;82:1919–25.
89. Korosoglou G, Weiss RG, Kedziorek DA, Walczak P, Gilson WD, Schar M, Sosnovik DE, Kraitchman DL, Boston RC, Bulte JW, Weissleder R, Stuber M. Noninvasive detection of macrophage-rich atherosclerotic plaque in hyperlipidemic rabbits using "positive contrast" magnetic resonance imaging. J Am Coll Cardiol. 2008;52:483–91.
90. Morishige K, Kacher DF, Libby P, Josephson L, Ganz P, Weissleder R, Aikawa M. High-resolution magnetic resonance imaging enhanced with superparamagnetic nanoparticles measures macrophage burden in atherosclerosis. Circulation. 2010;122:1707–15.

91. Ruehm SG, Corot C, Vogt P, Kolb S, Debatin JF. Magnetic resonance imaging of atherosclerotic plaque with ultrasmall superparamagnetic particles of iron oxide in hyperlipidemic rabbits. Circulation. 2001;103:415–22.
92. Tang TY, Howarth SP, Miller SR, Graves MJ, Patterson AJ, UK-I JM, Li ZY, Walsh SR, Brown AP, Kirkpatrick PJ, Warburton EA, Hayes PD, Varty K, Boyle JR, Gaunt ME, Zalewski A, Gillard JH. The atheroma (atorvastatin therapy: effects on reduction of macrophage activity) study. Evaluation using ultrasmall superparamagnetic iron oxide-enhanced magnetic resonance imaging in carotid disease. J Am Coll Cardiol. 2009;53:2039–50.
93. Jung C, Kaul MG, Bruns OT, Ducic T, Freund B, Heine M, Reimer R, Meents A, Salmen SC, Weller H, Nielsen P, Adam G, Heeren J, Ittrich H. Intraperitoneal injection improves the uptake of nanoparticle labeled HDL to atherosclerotic plaques compared to intravenous injection: a multimodal imaging study in ApoE−/− mice. Circ Cardiovasc Imaging. 2014;7(2):303–11.
94. Ogawa M, Umeda IO, Kosugi M, Kawai A, Hamaya Y, Takashima M, Yin H, Kudoh T, Seno M, Magata Y. Development of 111In-labeled liposomes for vulnerable atherosclerotic plaque imaging. J Nucl Med. 2014;55:115–20.
95. Nahrendorf M, Zhang H, Hembrador S, Panizzi P, Sosnovik DE, Aikawa E, Libby P, Swirski FK, Weissleder R. Nanoparticle pet-ct imaging of macrophages in inflammatory atherosclerosis. Circulation. 2008;117:379–87.
96. Tassa C, Shaw SY, Weissleder R. Dextran-coated iron oxide nanoparticles: a versatile platform for targeted molecular imaging, molecular diagnostics, and therapy. Acc Chem Res. 2011;44:842–52.
97. Hyafil F, Cornily JC, Feig JE, Gordon R, Vucic E, Amirbekian V, Fisher EA, Fuster V, Feldman LJ, Fayad ZA. Noninvasive detection of macrophages using a nanoparticulate contrast agent for computed tomography. Nat Med. 2007;13:636–41.
98. van der Wal AC, Becker AE. Atherosclerotic plaque rupture–pathologic basis of plaque stability and instability. Cardiovasc Res. 1999;41:334–44.
99. Lees AM, Lees RS, Schoen FJ, Isaacsohn JL, Fischman AJ, McKusick KA, Strauss HW. Imaging human atherosclerosis with 99MTC-labeled low density lipoproteins. Arteriosclerosis. 1988;8:461–70.
100. Frias JC, Lipinski MJ, Lipinski SE, Albelda MT. Modified lipoproteins as contrast agents for imaging of atherosclerosis. Contrast Media Mol Imaging. 2007;2:16–23.
101. Ishino S, Mukai T, Kuge Y, Kume N, Ogawa M, Takai N, Kamihashi J, Shiomi M, Minami M, Kita T, Saji H. Targeting of lectinlike oxidized low-density lipoprotein receptor 1 (LOX-1) with 99m TC-labeled anti-LOX-1 antibody: potential agent for imaging of vulnerable plaque. J Nucl Med. 2008;49:1677–85.
102. Wen S, Liu DF, Cui Y, Harris SS, Chen YC, Li KC, Ju SH, Teng GJ. In vivo MRI detection of carotid atherosclerotic lesions and kidney inflammation in ApoE-deficient mice by using LOX-1 targeted iron nanoparticles. Nanomedicine. 2014;10:639–49.
103. Li D, Patel AR, Klibanov AL, Kramer CM, Ruiz M, Kang BY, Mehta JL, Beller GA, Glover DK, Meyer CH. Molecular imaging of atherosclerotic plaques targeted to oxidized LDL receptor LOX-1 by SPECT/CT and magnetic resonance. Circ Cardiovasc Imaging. 2010;3:464–72.
104. Lu T, Wen S, Cui Y, Ju SH, Li KC, Teng GJ. Near-infrared fluorescence imaging of murine atherosclerosis using an oxidized low density lipoprotein-targeted fluorochrome. Int J Cardiovasc Imaging. 2014;30:221–31.
105. Hanssen NM, Wouters K, Huijberts MS, Gijbels MJ, Sluimer JC, Scheijen JL, Heeneman S, Biessen EA, Daemen MJ, Brownlee M, de Kleijn DP, Stehouwer CD, Pasterkamp G, Schalkwijk CG. Higher levels of advanced glycation endproducts in human carotid atherosclerotic plaques are associated with a rupture-prone phenotype. Eur Heart J. 2014;35:1137–46.
106. Tavakoli S, Zamora D, Ullevig S, Asmis R. Bioenergetic profiles diverge during macrophage polarization: implications for the interpretation of 18F-FDG PET imaging of atherosclerosis. J Nucl Med. 2013;54:1661–7.
107. Tawakol A, Migrino RQ, Hoffmann U, Abbara S, Houser S, Gewirtz H, Muller JE, Brady TJ, Fischman AJ. Noninvasive in vivo measurement of vascular inflammation with F-18 fluorodeoxyglucose positron emission tomography. J Nucl Cardiol. 2005;12:294–301.

108. Pedersen SF, Graebe M, Fisker Hag AM, Hojgaard L, Sillesen H, Kjaer A. Gene expression and 18FDG uptake in atherosclerotic carotid plaques. Nucl Med Commun. 2010;31: 423–9.
109. Dweck MR, Jones C, Joshi NV, Fletcher AM, Richardson H, White A, Marsden M, Pessotto R, Clark JC, Wallace WA, Salter DM, McKillop G, van Beek EJ, Boon NA, Rudd JH, Newby DE. Assessment of valvular calcification and inflammation by positron emission tomography in patients with aortic stenosis. Circulation. 2012;125:76–86.
110. Hag AM, Pedersen SF, Christoffersen C, Binderup T, Jensen MM, Jorgensen JT, Skovgaard D, Ripa RS, Kjaer A. (18)F-FDG PET imaging of murine atherosclerosis: association with gene expression of key molecular markers. PLoS One. 2012;7:e50908.
111. Myers KS, Rudd JH, Hailman EP, Bolognese JA, Burke J, Pinto CA, Klimas M, Hargreaves R, Dansky HM, Fayad ZA. Correlation between arterial FDG uptake and biomarkers in peripheral artery disease. JACC Cardiovasc Imaging. 2012;5:38–45.
112. Ogawa M, Nakamura S, Saito Y, Kosugi M, Magata Y. What can be seen by 18F-FDG PET in atherosclerosis imaging? The effect of foam cell formation on 18F-FDG uptake to macrophages in vitro. J Nucl Med. 2012;53:55–8.
113. Calcagno C, Ramachandran S, Izquierdo-Garcia D, Mani V, Millon A, Rosenbaum D, Tawakol A, Woodward M, Bucerius J, Moshier E, Godbold J, Kallend D, Farkouh ME, Fuster V, Rudd JH, Fayad ZA. The complementary roles of dynamic contrast-enhanced MRI and 18F-fluorodeoxyglucose PET/CT for imaging of carotid atherosclerosis. Eur J Nucl Med Mol Imaging. 2013;40:1884–93.
114. Duivenvoorden R, Mani V, Woodward M, Kallend D, Suchankova G, Fuster V, Rudd JH, Tawakol A, Farkouh ME, Fayad ZA. Relationship of serum inflammatory biomarkers with plaque inflammation assessed by FDG PET/CT: the dal-plaque study. JACC Cardiovasc Imaging. 2013;6:1087–94.
115. Millon A, Dickson SD, Klink A, Izquierdo-Garcia D, Bini J, Lancelot E, Ballet S, Robert P, Mateo de Castro J, Corot C, Fayad ZA. Monitoring plaque inflammation in atherosclerotic rabbits with an iron oxide (P904) and (18)F-FDG using a combined PET/MR scanner. Atherosclerosis. 2013;228:339–45.
116. Zhao QM, Zhao X, Feng TT, Zhang MD, Zhuang XC, Zhao XC, Li LQ, Li DP, Liu Y. Detection of vulnerable atherosclerotic plaque and prediction of thrombosis events in a rabbit model using 18F-FDG -PET/CT. PLoS One. 2013;8:e61140.
117. Fayad ZA, Mani V, Woodward M, Kallend D, Abt M, Burgess T, Fuster V, Ballantyne CM, Stein EA, Tardif JC, Rudd JH, Farkouh ME, Tawakol A. Safety and efficacy of dalcetrapib on atherosclerotic disease using novel non-invasive multimodality imaging (dal-PLAQUE): a randomised clinical trial. Lancet. 2011;378:1547–59.
118. Tahara N, Kai H, Ishibashi M, Nakaura H, Kaida H, Baba K, Hayabuchi N, Imaizumi T. Simvastatin attenuates plaque inflammation: evaluation by fluorodeoxyglucose positron emission tomography. J Am Coll Cardiol. 2006;48:1825–31.
119. Lee SJ, On YK, Lee EJ, Choi JY, Kim BT, Lee KH. Reversal of vascular 18F-FDG uptake with plasma high-density lipoprotein elevation by atherogenic risk reduction. J Nucl Med. 2008;49:1277–82.
120. Hacker M. Monitoring anti-inflammatory therapies in patients with atherosclerosis: FDG PET emerges as the method of choice. Eur J Nucl Med Mol Imaging. 2012;39:396–8.
121. Lobatto ME, Calcagno C, Metselaar JM, Storm G, Stroes ES, Fayad ZA, Mulder WJ. Imaging the efficacy of anti-inflammatory liposomes in a rabbit model of atherosclerosis by non-invasive imaging. Methods Enzymol. 2012;508:211–28.
122. Vucic E, Calcagno C, Dickson SD, Rudd JH, Hayashi K, Bucerius J, Moshier E, Mounessa JS, Roytman M, Moon MJ, Lin J, Ramachandran S, Tanimoto T, Brown K, Kotsuma M, Tsimikas S, Fisher EA, Nicolay K, Fuster V, Fayad ZA. Regression of inflammation in atherosclerosis by the LXR agonist R211945: a noninvasive assessment and comparison with atorvastatin. JACC Cardiovasc Imaging. 2012;5:819–28.
123. Nitta Y, Tahara N, Tahara A, Honda A, Kodama N, Mizoguchi M, Kaida H, Ishibashi M, Hayabuchi N, Ikeda H, Yamagishi S, Imaizumi T. Pioglitazone decreases coronary artery

inflammation in impaired glucose tolerance and diabetes mellitus: evaluation by FDG-PET/CT imaging. JACC Cardiovasc Imaging. 2013;6:1172–82.
124. Tawakol A, Fayad ZA, Mogg R, Alon A, Klimas MT, Dansky H, Subramanian SS, Abdelbaky A, Rudd JH, Farkouh ME, Nunes IO, Beals CR, Shankar SS. Intensification of statin therapy results in a rapid reduction in atherosclerotic inflammation: results of a multicenter fluorodeoxyglucose-positron emission tomography/computed tomography feasibility study. J Am Coll Cardiol. 2013;62:909–17.
125. Tawakol A, Singh P, Rudd JH, Soffer J, Cai G, Vucic E, Brannan SP, Tarka EA, Shaddinger BC, Sarov-Blat L, Matthews P, Subramanian S, Farkouh M, Fayad ZA. Effect of treatment for 12 weeks with rilapladib, a lipoprotein-associated phospholipase A2 inhibitor, on arterial inflammation as assessed with 18F-fluorodeoxyglucose-pet imaging. J Am Coll Cardiol. 2014;63:86–8.
126. Matter CM, Wyss MT, Meier P, Spath N, von Lukowicz T, Lohmann C, Weber B, Ramirez de Molina A, Lacal JC, Ametamey SM, von Schulthess GK, Luscher TF, Kaufmann PA, Buck A. 18F-choline images murine atherosclerotic plaques ex vivo. Arterioscler Thromb Vasc Biol. 2006;26:584–9.
127. Takumi T, Lee S, Hamasaki S, Toyonaga K, Kanda D, Kusumoto K, Toda H, Takenaka T, Miyata M, Anan R, Otsuji Y, Tei C. Limitation of angiography to identify the culprit plaque in acute myocardial infarction with coronary total occlusion utility of coronary plaque temperature measurement to identify the culprit plaque. J Am Coll Cardiol. 2007;50:2197–203.
128. Geng YJ, Wu Q, Muszynski M, Hansson GK, Libby P. Apoptosis of vascular smooth muscle cells induced by in vitro stimulation with interferon-gamma, tumor necrosis factor-alpha, and interleukin-1 beta. Arterioscler Thromb Vasc Biol. 1996;16:19–27.
129. Sosnovik DE, Garanger E, Aikawa E, Nahrendorf M, Figuiredo JL, Dai G, Reynolds F, Rosenzweig A, Weissleder R, Josephson L. Molecular MRI of cardiomyocyte apoptosis with simultaneous delayed-enhancement MRI distinguishes apoptotic and necrotic myocytes in vivo: potential for midmyocardial salvage in acute ischemia. Circ Cardiovasc Imaging. 2009;2:460–7.
130. van Tilborg GA, Mulder WJ, Deckers N, Storm G, Reutelingsperger CP, Strijkers GJ, Nicolay K. Annexin a5-functionalized bimodal lipid-based contrast agents for the detection of apoptosis. Bioconjug Chem. 2006;17:741–9.
131. Johnson LL, Schofield L, Donahay T, Narula N, Narula J. 99mtc-annexin v imaging for in vivo detection of atherosclerotic lesions in porcine coronary arteries. J Nucl Med. 2005;46:1186–93.
132. Ishino S, Kuge Y, Takai N, Tamaki N, Strauss HW, Blankenberg FG, Shiomi M, Saji H. 99mtc-annexin a5 for noninvasive characterization of atherosclerotic lesions: Imaging and histological studies in myocardial infarction-prone watanabe heritable hyperlipidemic rabbits. Eur J Nucl Med Mol Imaging. 2007;34:889–99.
133. Laufer EM, Winkens HM, Corsten MF, Reutelingsperger CP, Narula J, Hofstra L. Pet and spect imaging of apoptosis in vulnerable atherosclerotic plaques with radiolabeled annexin a5. Q J Nucl Med Mol Imaging. 2009;53:26–34.
134. Hofstra L, Liem IH, Dumont EA, Boersma HH, van Heerde WL, Doevendans PA, De Muinck E, Wellens HJ, Kemerink GJ, Reutelingsperger CP, Heidendal GA. Visualisation of cell death in vivo in patients with acute myocardial infarction. Lancet. 2000;356:209–12.
135. Zhao Y, Zhao S, Kuge Y, Strauss HW, Blankenberg FG, Tamaki N. Attenuation of apoptosis by telmisartan in atherosclerotic plaques of apolipoprotein e–/– mice: evaluation using technetium 99m-annexin a5. Mol Imaging. 2013;12:300–9.
136. De Saint-Hubert M, Bauwens M, Deckers N, Drummen M, Douma K, Granton P, Hendrikx G, Kusters D, Bucerius J, Reutelingsperger CP, Mottaghy FM. In vivo molecular imaging of apoptosis and necrosis in atherosclerotic plaques using microSPECT-CT and microPET-CT imaging. Mol Imaging Biol. 2014;16:246–54.
137. Jiang B, Wang J, Ni Y, Chen F. Necrosis avidity: a newly discovered feature of hypericin and its preclinical applications in necrosis imaging. Theranostics. 2013;3:667–76.
138. Chen K, Keaney Jr JF. Evolving concepts of oxidative stress and reactive oxygen species in cardiovascular disease. Curr Atheroscler Rep. 2012;14:476–83.

139. Briley-Saebo KC, Cho YS, Tsimikas S. Imaging of oxidation-specific epitopes in atherosclerosis and macrophage-rich vulnerable plaques. Curr Cardiovasc Imaging Rep. 2011;4:4–16.
140. Torzewski M, Shaw PX, Han KR, Shortal B, Lackner KJ, Witztum JL, Palinski W, Tsimikas S. Reduced in vivo aortic uptake of radiolabeled oxidation-specific antibodies reflects changes in plaque composition consistent with plaque stabilization. Arterioscler Thromb Vasc Biol. 2004;24:2307–12.
141. Nahrendorf M, Sosnovik D, Chen JW, Panizzi P, Figueiredo JL, Aikawa E, Libby P, Swirski FK, Weissleder R. Activatable magnetic resonance imaging agent reports myeloperoxidase activity in healing infarcts and noninvasively detects the antiinflammatory effects of atorvastatin on ischemia-reperfusion injury. Circulation. 2008;117:1153–60.
142. Panizzi P, Nahrendorf M, Wildgruber M, Waterman P, Figueiredo JL, Aikawa E, McCarthy J, Weissleder R, Hilderbrand SA. Oxazine conjugated nanoparticle detects in vivo hypochlorous acid and peroxynitrite generation. J Am Chem Soc. 2009;131:15739–44.
143. Lal H, Verma SK, Foster DM, Golden HB, Reneau JC, Watson LE, Singh H, Dostal DE. Integrins and proximal signaling mechanisms in cardiovascular disease. Front Biosci. 2009;14:2307–34.
144. Winter PM, Morawski AM, Caruthers SD, Fuhrhop RW, Zhang H, Williams TA, Allen JS, Lacy EK, Robertson JD, Lanza GM, Wickline SA. Molecular imaging of angiogenesis in early-stage atherosclerosis with alpha(v)beta3-integrin-targeted nanoparticles. Circulation. 2003;108:2270–4.
145. Burtea C, Laurent S, Murariu O, Rattat D, Toubeau G, Verbruggen A, Vansthertem D, Vander Elst L, Muller RN. Molecular imaging of alpha v beta3 integrin expression in atherosclerotic plaques with a mimetic of rgd peptide grafted to gd-dtpa. Cardiovasc Res. 2008;78:148–57.
146. Winter PM, Caruthers SD, Zhang H, Williams TA, Wickline SA, Lanza GM. Antiangiogenic synergism of integrin-targeted fumagillin nanoparticles and atorvastatin in atherosclerosis. JACC Cardiovasc Imaging. 2008;1:624–34.
147. Winter PM, Neubauer AM, Caruthers SD, Harris TD, Robertson JD, Williams TA, Schmieder AH, Hu G, Allen JS, Lacy EK, Zhang H, Wickline SA, Lanza GM. Endothelial alpha(v)beta3 integrin-targeted fumagillin nanoparticles inhibit angiogenesis in atherosclerosis. Arterioscler Thromb Vasc Biol. 2006;26:2103–9.
148. Laitinen I, Saraste A, Weidl E, Poethko T, Weber AW, Nekolla SG, Leppanen P, Yla-Herttuala S, Holzlwimmer G, Walch A, Esposito I, Wester HJ, Knuuti J, Schwaiger M. Evaluation of alphavbeta3 integrin-targeted positron emission tomography tracer 18F-galacto-RGD for imaging of vascular inflammation in atherosclerotic mice. Circ Cardiovasc Imaging. 2009;2:331–8.
149. Partovi S, Loebe M, Aschwanden M, Baldi T, Jager KA, Feinstein SB, Staub D. Contrast-enhanced ultrasound for assessing carotid atherosclerotic plaque lesions. AJR Am J Roentgenol. 2012;198:W13–9.
150. Heroux J, Gharib AM, Danthi NS, Cecchini S, Ohayon J, Pettigrew RI. High-affinity alphavbeta3 integrin targeted optical probe as a new imaging biomarker for early atherosclerosis: initial studies in watanabe rabbits. Mol Imaging Biol. 2010;12:2–8.
151. de Vries BM W, Hillebrands JL, van Dam GM, Tio RA, de Jong JS, Slart RH, Zeebregts CJ. Images in cardiovascular medicine. Multispectral near-infrared fluorescence molecular imaging of matrix metalloproteinases in a human carotid plaque using a matrix-degrading metalloproteinase-sensitive activatable fluorescent probe. Circulation. 2009;119:e534–6.
152. Razansky D, Harlaar NJ, Hillebrands JL, Taruttis A, Herzog E, Zeebregts CJ, van Dam GM, Ntziachristos V. Multispectral optoacoustic tomography of matrix metalloproteinase activity in vulnerable human carotid plaques. Mol Imaging Biol. 2012;14:277–85.
153. Quillard T, Tesmenitsky Y, Croce K, Travers R, Shvartz E, Koskinas KC, Sukhova GK, Aikawa E, Aikawa M, Libby P. Selective inhibition of matrix metalloproteinase-13 increases collagen content of established mouse atherosclerosis. Arterioscler Thromb Vasc Biol. 2011;31:2464–72.
154. Chang K, Francis SA, Aikawa E, Figueiredo JL, Kohler RH, McCarthy JR, Weissleder R, Plutzky J, Jaffer FA. Pioglitazone suppresses inflammation in vivo in murine carotid atherosclerosis: novel detection by dual-target fluorescence molecular imaging. Arterioscler Thromb Vasc Biol. 2010;30:1933–9.

155. Deguchi JO, Aikawa M, Tung CH, Aikawa E, Kim DE, Ntziachristos V, Weissleder R, Libby P. Inflammation in atherosclerosis: visualizing matrix metalloproteinase action in macrophages in vivo. Circulation. 2006;114:55–62.
156. Lin SA, Patel M, Suresch D, Connolly B, Bao B, Groves K, Rajopadhye M, Peterson JD, Klimas M, Sur C, Bednar B. Quantitative longitudinal imaging of vascular inflammation and treatment by ezetimibe in apoe mice by fmt using new optical imaging biomarkers of cathepsin activity and alpha(v)beta(3) integrin. Int J Mol Imaging. 2012;2012:189254.
157. Jaffer FA, Kim DE, Quinti L, Tung CH, Aikawa E, Pande AN, Kohler RH, Shi GP, Libby P, Weissleder R. Optical visualization of cathepsin k activity in atherosclerosis with a novel, protease-activatable fluorescence sensor. Circulation. 2007;115:2292–8.
158. Kim DE, Kim JY, Schellingerhout D, Shon SM, Jeong SW, Kim EJ, Kim WK. Molecular imaging of cathepsin b proteolytic enzyme activity reflects the inflammatory component of atherosclerotic pathology and can quantitatively demonstrate the antiatherosclerotic therapeutic effects of atorvastatin and glucosamine. Mol Imaging. 2009;8:291–301.
159. Jaffer FA, Vinegoni C, John MC, Aikawa E, Gold HK, Finn AV, Ntziachristos V, Libby P, Weissleder R. Real-time catheter molecular sensing of inflammation in proteolytically active atherosclerosis. Circulation. 2008;118:1802–9.
160. Myochin T, Hanaoka K, Komatsu T, Terai T, Nagano T. Design strategy for a near-infrared fluorescence probe for matrix metalloproteinase utilizing highly cell permeable boron dipyrromethene. J Am Chem Soc. 2012;134:13730–7.
161. Olson ES, Whitney MA, Friedman B, Aguilera TA, Crisp JL, Baik FM, Jiang T, Baird SM, Tsimikas S, Tsien RY, Nguyen QT. In vivo fluorescence imaging of atherosclerotic plaques with activatable cell-penetrating peptides targeting thrombin activity. Integr Biol (Camb). 2012;4:595–605.
162. Haider N, Hartung D, Fujimoto S, Petrov A, Kolodgie FD, Virmani R, Ohshima S, Liu H, Zhou J, Fujimoto A, Tahara A, Hofstra L, Narula N, Reutelingsperger C, Narula J. Dual molecular imaging for targeting metalloproteinase activity and apoptosis in atherosclerosis: molecular imaging facilitates understanding of pathogenesis. J Nucl Cardiol. 2009;16:753–62.
163. Razavian M, Tavakoli S, Zhang J, Nie L, Dobrucki LW, Sinusas AJ, Azure M, Robinson S, Sadeghi MM. Atherosclerosis plaque heterogeneity and response to therapy detected by in vivo molecular imaging of matrix metalloproteinase activation. J Nucl Med. 2011;52:1795–802.
164. Amirbekian V, Aguinaldo JG, Amirbekian S, Hyafil F, Vucic E, Sirol M, Weinreb DB, Le Greneur S, Lancelot E, Corot C, Fisher EA, Galis ZS, Fayad ZA. Atherosclerosis and matrix metalloproteinases: experimental molecular mr imaging in vivo. Radiology. 2009;251:429–38.
165. Olson ES, Jiang T, Aguilera TA, Nguyen QT, Ellies LG, Scadeng M, Tsien RY. Activatable cell penetrating peptides linked to nanoparticles as dual probes for in vivo fluorescence and mr imaging of proteases. Proc Natl Acad Sci U S A. 2010;107:4311–6.
166. Liu CH, You Z, Liu CM, Kim YR, Whalen MJ, Rosen BR, Liu PK. Diffusion-weighted magnetic resonance imaging reversal by gene knockdown of matrix metalloproteinase-9 activities in live animal brains. J Neurosci. 2009;29:3508–17.
167. Visse R, Nagase H. Matrix metalloproteinases and tissue inhibitors of metalloproteinases: structure, function, and biochemistry. Circ Res. 2003;92:827–39.
168. Jacobin-Valat MJ, Deramchia K, Mornet S, Hagemeyer CE, Bonetto S, Robert R, Biran M, Massot P, Miraux S, Sanchez S, Bouzier-Sore AK, Franconi JM, Duguet E, Clofent-Sanchez G. Mri of inducible p-selectin expression in human activated platelets involved in the early stages of atherosclerosis. NMR Biomed. 2011;24:413–24.
169. Duerschmied D, Meiner M, Peter K, Neudorfer I, Roming F, Zirlik A, Bode C, von Elverfeldt D, von Zur MC. Molecular magnetic resonance imaging allows the detection of activated platelets in a new mouse model of coronary artery thrombosis. Invest Radiol. 2011;46:618–23.

170. von zur Muhlen C, Peter K, Ali ZA, Schneider JE, McAteer MA, Neubauer S, Channon KM, Bode C, Choudhury RP. Visualization of activated platelets by targeted magnetic resonance imaging utilizing conformation-specific antibodies against glycoprotein iib/iiia. J Vasc Res. 2009;46:6–14.
171. von Elverfeldt D, Meissner M, Peter K, Paul D, Meixner F, Neudorfer I, Merkle A, Harloff A, Zirlik A, Schollhorn J, Markl M, Hennig J, Bode C, von zur Muhlen C. An approach towards molecular imaging of activated platelets allows imaging of symptomatic human carotid plaques in a new model of a tissue flow chamber. Contrast Media Mol Imaging. 2012;7:204–13.
172. Uppal R, Catana C, Ay I, Benner T, Sorensen AG, Caravan P. Bimodal thrombus imaging: simultaneous pet/mr imaging with a fibrin-targeted dual pet/mr probe–feasibility study in rat model. Radiology. 2011;258:812–20.
173. Vymazal J, Spuentrup E, Cardenas-Molina G, Wiethoff AJ, Hartmann MG, Caravan P, Parsons Jr EC. Thrombus imaging with fibrin-specific gadolinium-based mr contrast agent ep-2104r: results of a phase ii clinical study of feasibility. Invest Radiol. 2009; 44:697–704.
174. Wu X, Balu N, Li W, Chen Y, Shi X, Kummitha CM, Yu X, Yuan C, Lu ZR. Molecular MRI of atherosclerotic plaque progression in an apoe(–/–) mouse model with a cltl peptide targeted macrocyclic gd(iii) chelate. Am J Nucl Med Mol Imaging. 2013;3:446–55.
175. Starmans LW, van Duijnhoven SM, Rossin R, Berben M, Aime S, Daemen MJ, Nicolay K, Grull H. Evaluation of 111In-labeled EPep and FibPep as tracers for fibrin SPECT imaging. Mol Pharm. 2013;10(11):4309–21.
176. Makowski MR, Forbes SC, Blume U, Warley A, Jansen CH, Schuster A, Wiethoff AJ, Botnar RM. In vivo assessment of intraplaque and endothelial fibrin in apoe(–/–) mice by molecular MRI. Atherosclerosis. 2012;222:43–9.
177. McCarthy JR, Patel P, Botnaru I, Haghayeghi P, Weissleder R, Jaffer FA. Multimodal nanoagents for the detection of intravascular thrombi. Bioconjug Chem. 2009;20:1251–5.
178. Jaffer FA, Tung CH, Wykrzykowska JJ, Ho NH, Houng AK, Reed GL, Weissleder R. Molecular imaging of factor xiiia activity in thrombosis using a novel, near-infrared fluorescent contrast agent that covalently links to thrombi. Circulation. 2004;110:170–6.
179. Tei L, Mazooz G, Shellef Y, Avni R, Vandoorne K, Barge A, Kalchenko V, Dewhirst MW, Chaabane L, Miragoli L, Longo D, Neeman M, Aime S. Novel MRI and fluorescent probes responsive to the factor XIII transglutaminase activity. Contrast Media Mol Imaging. 2010; 5:213–22.
180. Miserus RJ, Herias MV, Prinzen L, Lobbes MB, Van Suylen RJ, Dirksen A, Hackeng TM, Heemskerk JW, van Engelshoven JM, Daemen MJ, van Zandvoort MA, Heeneman S, Kooi ME. Molecular MRI of early thrombus formation using a bimodal alpha2-antiplasmin-based contrast agent. JACC Cardiovasc Imaging. 2009;2:987–96.
181. Majmudar MD, Keliher EJ, Heidt T, Leuschner F, Truelove J, Sena BF, Gorbatov R, Iwamoto Y, Dutta P, Wojtkiewicz G, Courties G, Sebas M, Borodovsky A, Fitzgerald K, Nolte MW, Dickneite G, Chen JW, Anderson DG, Swirski FK, Weissleder R, Nahrendorf M. Monocyte-directed rnai targeting ccr2 improves infarct healing in atherosclerosis-prone mice. Circulation. 2013;127:2038–46.
182. Beheshti M, Saboury B, Mehta NN, Torigian DA, Werner T, Mohler E, Wilensky R, Newberg AB, Basu S, Langsteger W, Alavi A. Detection and global quantification of cardiovascular molecular calcification by fluoro18-fluoride positron emission tomography/computed tomography–a novel concept. Hell J Nucl Med. 2011;14:114–20.
183. Zaheer A, Murshed M, De Grand AM, Morgan TG, Karsenty G, Frangioni JV. Optical imaging of hydroxyapatite in the calcified vasculature of transgenic animals. Arterioscler Thromb Vasc Biol. 2006;26:1132–6.
184. Lee JS, Morrisett JD, Tung CH. Detection of hydroxyapatite in calcified cardiovascular tissues. Atherosclerosis. 2012;224:340–7.

185. Aikawa E, Nahrendorf M, Figueiredo JL, Swirski FK, Shtatland T, Kohler RH, Jaffer FA, Aikawa M, Weissleder R. Osteogenesis associates with inflammation in early-stage atherosclerosis evaluated by molecular imaging in vivo. Circulation. 2007;116:2841–50.
186. Aikawa E, Nahrendorf M, Sosnovik D, Lok VM, Jaffer FA, Aikawa M, Weissleder R. Multimodality molecular imaging identifies proteolytic and osteogenic activities in early aortic valve disease. Circulation. 2007;115:377–86.
187. White CJ, Ramee SR, Collins TJ, Murgo JP. Coronary angioscopy. Tex Heart Inst J. 1995;22(1):20–5.
188. Donnelly P, et al. Multimodality imaging atlas of coronary atherosclerosis. JACC Cardiovasc Imaging. 2010;3:876–80.
189. Majmudar MD, et al. Cardiovascular molecular imaging: the road ahead. J Nucl Med. 2012;53(5):673–6.

Ultrasound Molecular Imaging of Endothelial Cell Activation and Damage in Atherosclerosis

2

Tamara Atkinson and Jonathan R. Lindner

Contents

Abstract

Atherosclerosis is a gradual process that evolves over decades with variable plaque morphologies that can lead to atherothrombotic complications such as stroke and acute coronary syndromes. The ability to image the structural, cellular, or biochemical signatures of high-risk plaque phenotype has been a major goal for essentially all forms of clinical and preclinical imaging. These efforts

T. Atkinson, MD
The Knight Cardiovascular Institute, Oregon Health and Science University, Portland, OR, USA

J.R. Lindner, MD (✉)
The Knight Cardiovascular Institute, Oregon Health and Science University, Portland, OR, USA

Cardiovascular Division, UHN 62, Oregon Health and Science University,
3181 SW Sam Jackson Park Road, Portland, OR 97239, USA
e-mail: lindnerj@ohsu.edu

E. Aikawa (ed.), *Cardiovascular Imaging: Arterial and Aortic Valve Inflammation and Calcification*, DOI 10.1007/978-3-319-09268-3_2

have been based on the need to better understand pathobiology, the need to have a biologic readout for the testing of efficacy for new treatment strategies, and for the clinical purposes of potentially selecting patients for more aggressive forms of anti-atherosclerotic treatments that are in development stage. Ultrasound-based evaluation of plaque severity and plaque composition is already an integral part of the practice of cardiovascular medicine in the form of extracorporeal and intravascular imaging. New ultrasound-based techniques are being developed that may provide incremental information to structure alone. Some of these techniques are based on the ability to detect vascular inflammation by either regional abnormalities in the mechanical properties of the vessel wall or presence of plaque neovessels using contrast ultrasound imaging. Molecular imaging with acoustically active agents targeted to endothelial cell adhesion molecules, platelets, and microthrombosis has also been used to evaluate high-risk phenotype. Although clinical translation is a distant goal, the impact of ultrasound-based molecular imaging is already being felt through its application to better define pathophysiology and evaluate new therapies in atherosclerotic disease.

2.1 B-Mode Ultrasound Imaging of Atherosclerosis

2.1.1 Focused Review of Ultrasound Physics

In its simplest manifestation, sound is the propagation of pressure fluctuations that produce alternating compression and rarefaction of the medium through which it travels. Ultrasound imaging is performed by applying an electric field through piezoelectric materials which undergo mechanical vibrations at a specific frequency and secondary directional sound waves [1]. The alternating peaks and nadirs of an ultrasound wave can be defined by its propagation velocity, frequency or array of frequencies (or its inverse function wavelength), pressure amplitude, and length (pulse duration) [1–3]. The two factors, frequency and power, are the primary determinants of how ultrasound interacts with tissue with regard to acoustic reflection, scatter, attenuation, damping, and bioeffects such as heating and cavitation.

The diagnostic range of ultrasound frequencies for humans is generally between 1 and 20 MHz, whereas therapeutic ultrasound is often performed at lower acoustic frequencies [1]. High-resolution 2-D diagnostic ultrasound relies on the use of short pulses of ultrasound that can be steered and focused by altering the timing of piezoelectric element activation along a line or 2-D matrix of elements. As the focused ultrasound waves propagate through tissue, they can be influenced by tissue in many ways including wave reflection, ultrasound scatter, refraction, attenuation or damping, and frequency shift. Acoustic reflection and backscatter are the basis for images created whereby returning ultrasound energy is sensed by the piezoelectric elements and, if not filtered based on frequency and amplitude, are displayed as pixel enhancement [1].

Basic principles of acoustic physics are important in understanding the principles of contrast-enhanced and non-contrast ultrasound imaging in the assessment of endothelial activation and atherosclerosis. For example, the discrimination of different tissue types is made possible by the differences in the acoustic impedance of the tissue, angles of reflection, and scatter properties [3]. Frequency and pulse duration are important considerations for determining differences in acoustic response of different tissues as well as the axial spatial resolution for distinguishing these differences. High frequencies are optimal for axial and lateral resolution for 2-D and strain imaging and for tissue characterization. However, there is also the need for tissue penetration which is inversely related to frequency. These principles have defined the ability to evaluate intimal thickening and the presence of different plaque compositions in the vascular wall for both intravascular and surface imaging probes. Likewise, the signal generated by ultrasound contrast agents relative to tissue that have been used to evaluate atherosclerosis and spatial resolution of contrast enhancement is influenced by frequency, pulse-repetition frequency, and acoustic pressures.

Conventionally, temporal resolution for 2-D ultrasound refers to the ability to characterize tissue motion. Temporal resolution is determined by the pulse-repetition frequency, which in turn is influenced by the depth of the ultrasound field, pulse duration, and transmit frequency and by the number of ultrasound lines which for conventional imaging systems is controlled by ultrasound sector width and line density [2]. For this reason, M-mode ultrasound which is composed of single-line imaging from one or two elements is still used on occasion to structurally evaluate rapid or brief events. However M-mode imaging provides only 1-D information on tissue motion, and it cannot be used for speckle-tracking strain imaging where speckle patterns from radiofrequency data are analyzed to determine frame-to-frame differences in the rate or extent of tissue deformation. Alternatively, temporal resolution can also refer to either how often a physical or molecular event can be assessed with ultrasound. For example, temporal resolution with contrast ultrasound imaging relies on how much time is required for contrast agent injection, site-targeted attachment, and sufficient clearance of free tracer from the blood pool to distinguish attached from nonattached agent.

2.1.2 Ultrasound of Imaging of Plaque Burden

Atherosclerotic lesion formation is a gradual process that often evolves over the period of decades. In its simplest form, ultrasound can and has been used for years to evaluate the extent and rate of progression of atherosclerotic disease. Plaque dimensions and degree of luminal narrowing by carotid, peripheral, and coronary artery ultrasound imaging have been used to determine severity of stenosis and to determine whether luminal encroachment is sufficient to explain symptoms attributable to hypoperfusion at rest or during stress (angina, claudication, TIAs, left ventricular dysfunction). However, the ability to accurately assess total atherosclerotic burden also has significant clinical value [4]. Because of adverse outward remodeling of the vessel wall, atherosclerotic burden may be underestimated by simply evaluating luminal stenosis [5]. Clinical trials have clearly indicated the importance of plaque volume on prognosis for adverse cardiovascular or cerebrovascular events, and there are recent findings that indicate that plaque biology and burden are interactive features that predict adverse coronary events in patients with known coronary artery disease (CAD) [6]. The types of imaging approaches that have been used to quantify plaque burden differ according to scale and distance from the body surface. For example, carotid plaque volume can be estimated by live or post-processed 2-D or 3-D ultrasound imaging techniques using surface ultrasound at medium frequencies (5–14 MHz) [7, 8]. In contrast, coronary artery plaque volume has been quantified primarily by high-frequency intravascular ultrasound because of the smaller arterial dimension, arterial tortuosity, intervening lung, motion, and distance between the chest wall and anterior cardiac surface which limit transthoracic imaging. On ex vivo or postmortem histology, quantification of plaque or neointimal burden is best determined by measuring the area or volume that is within the confines of the internal elastic lamina. Accordingly, ultrasound-based assessment of plaque volume is based on the ability to use acoustic signatures produced by changes in composition or anisotropic transitions to define the intima-media border, and post-processing programs have been developed to automatically recognize and quantify plaque volume during calibrated transducer positioning along the axial direction of the vessel (Fig. 2.1) [9].

2.1.3 Imaging Plaque Composition

There has been extensive study of what constitutes disadvantageous plaque biology with regard to likelihood for rapid progression or susceptibility to atherothrombotic complications such as stroke and acute coronary syndromes. Some of the high-risk morphologic or cellular characteristics of a plaque include eccentricity, inflammatory cell burden and cell type, necrotic core, high lipid or foam cell content, thin fibrous cap which is defined differently for carotid and coronary vessels, microcalcifications, evidence of recent intraplaque hemorrhage, cellular apoptosis, proliferation of the vasa vasorum or plaque neovessels, and plaque ulceration or erosion [10–12].

The most basic attempts to identify high-risk plaque phenotype have been based on detecting either echolucency of plaques which have been correlated with increased lipid and necrotic core content and plaque calcification which has been associated with enhanced inflammatory activity. In cross-sectional studies, these ultrasound features have been shown to be more prevalent in unstable than stable plaques, and more recently they have been shown to provide a modest estimate of risk in prospectively followed patients [4, 10, 13]. The presence of echolucent plaques in one location (e.g., carotid artery) has also been shown to be an indicator of greater disease burden in other vascular beds [14]. With regard to calcification, the presence of a high degree of coronary calcification for age has been demonstrated to be one of the most useful markers for reclassifying risk for patients after taking into account non-imaging risk factors [15]. Although with these findings and the demonstration on histology of the relation between calcium with inflammation, it is generally accepted that lack of calcium does not necessarily denote low risk,

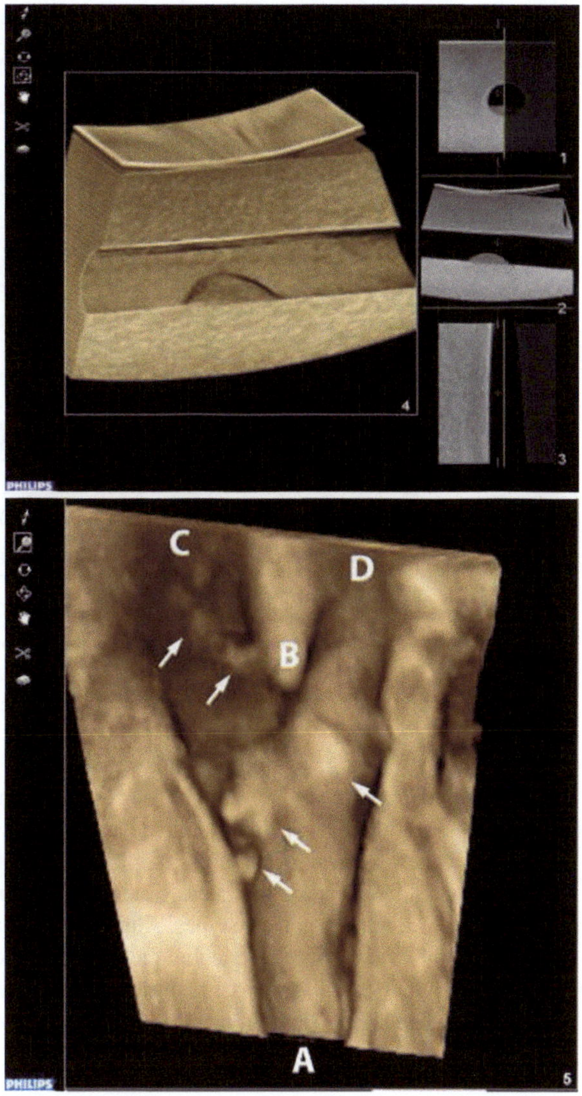

Fig. 2.1 Images obtained by mechanical 3-D acquisition. The *top panel* represents 3-D imaging of a plaque phantom with corresponding *x*-, *y*-, and *z*-plane sample acquisitions at the plaque level. The *bottom panel* illustrates a 3-D reconstruction with half-volume cutaway of a carotid artery bifurcation from a patient with lumen-encroaching plaque (From Graebe et al. [9], with permission). In the top figure, panel 4 represents the 3-D reconstruction with x-, y-, and z-planes represented in panels 1-3 to the right. In the bottom figure, arrows depict regions of plaque in different regions of the carotid including the common carotid (*A*), the bifurcation (*B*), and the internal (*D*) and external (*C*) carotid

since lipid-rich lesions with thin fibrous cap may not have much detectable calcium particularly in young individuals.

The ability to produce robust images at high transmit frequencies and the increased computational power in imaging systems have resulted in techniques that have been able to discriminate tissue types beyond simply "echolucent" and "calcified" by advance radiofrequency spectral analysis (frequency spectrum, amplitude, extinction) of backscattered signals (Fig. 2.2) [11]. Such radiofrequency analysis can characterize tissues as fibrous, fibrofatty, necrotic, and calcified with high spatial resolution and can provide a modest measure to identify plaques that may have a

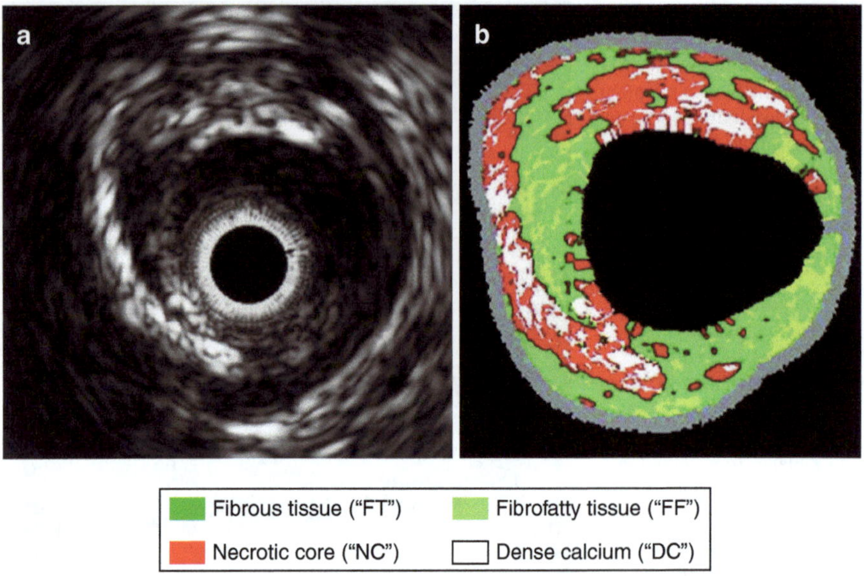

Fig. 2.2 B-mode ultrasound imaging of a coronary artery with eccentric plaque. (**a**) Gray-scale 2-D intravascular ultrasound image and (**b**) corresponding color-coded virtual histology image produced from radiofrequency spectral analysis demonstrating different plaque components according to the key at *bottom* (From Konig and Klaus [11], with permission)

high likelihood for progression or for atherothrombotic complications [11, 16, 17]. The ultrasound signatures that have been used to discriminate tissue type have been based on both modeling and radiofrequency signatures of tissue type from ex vivo vascular specimens. Some of the high-risk features of radiofrequency tissue characterization include fibrous cap thickness, volume or circumferential extent of necrotic tissue, and heterogeneity in tissue types. Although there are no prospective studies to suggest that the findings of these techniques can be used to select any therapy, they have been shown to provide a measure of risk for acute adverse atherosclerotic events particularly when paired with information on plaque size or disease burden [17].

2.1.4 Mechanical Properties

Mechanical properties are what determine the 3-D deformation of a vessel under various degrees and directions under stress. In turn, the mechanical properties are determined by the physical dimensions and composition of the vessel wall. Methods for globally assessing arterial mechanical properties in a rapid fashion have been developed, some involve ultrasound measurements such as pulse wave velocity (time delay in the onset of a systolic pulse from a proximal to more distal site in large conduit vessels) and elastic modulus which reflects stress-strain relationships by any number of mathematical approaches to correlate pulse pressure to the change vascular

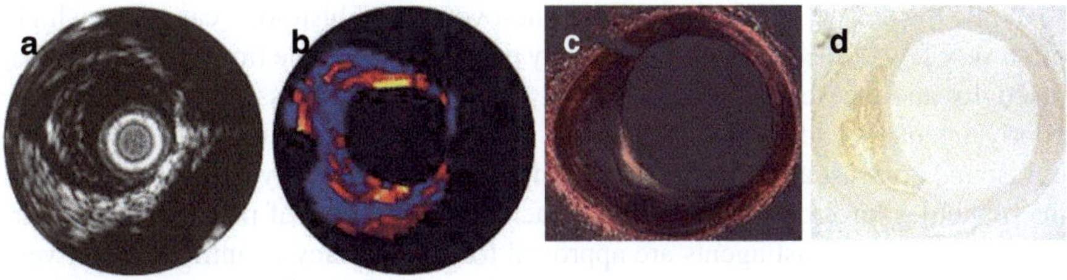

Fig. 2.3 Correlation of B-mode and elastography ultrasound with histology in a coronary artery with eccentric plaque. Ultrasound images include (**a**) intravascular ultrasound 2-D imaging and (**b**) corresponding elastogram map with *yellow* areas demonstrating a region of high strain and *blue* areas demonstrating low strain. (**c**, **d**) Histology revealing a plaque with large volume, eccentric remodeling, and thin-cap atheroma (From Schaar et al. [24], with permission)

dimension [18, 19]. Methods for spatial quantification of arterial mechanical properties have been developed but are still investigational. One approach has been to use either Doppler data or speckle-tracking echo to measure vascular strain (the degree radial or circumferential deformation) or strain rate [20–22]. This can be done in a transmural approach or just for the immediate luminal region which is sometimes referred to as palpography (Fig. 2.3) [20, 23, 24]. These approaches have been used to detect reduced vascular compliance due to longstanding hypertension [18]. They have also been used in a global or regional fashion to detect increases in vascular distension that occur in high-risk plaque due to inflammatory response, necrosis, and abnormal matrix homeostasis or in patients with high risk for unstable aortic complications from medial aortopathy (Marfan's, bicuspid aortic valve) [20, 21, 24, 25]. In particular regions with high heterogeneity of strain have been correlated with high risk for vascular rupture [24, 26, 27]. These findings suggest that shear rates within the vessel wall may be as important as shear rate at the luminal surface. Some of the limitations of the technology include that it cannot be performed for coronary vessels noninvasively, lack of studies evaluating 3-D or longitudinal strain patterns, and the inability to accurately measure focal stress (pressure) which can be influenced flow streams that become non-laminar from eccentric stenosis or at arterial branch points.

2.1.5 Vasa Vasorum and Plaque Neovessel Imaging

Expansion of the vasa vasorum (VV) and development of plaque neovessels that penetrate into the tunica media and intima have been causatively linked with risk for unstable atherosclerotic progression and plaque rupture [28]. These neovessels may promote instability in a number of ways. They can be a portal of entry for immune cells, lipoproteins, platelets, and erythrocytes that contribute to adverse plaque composition and inflammation. Conversely, VV may also be a reflection of high-risk plaque phenotype, since the growth factors, cytokines, and proteases that mediate neovascularization are in part triggered by the inflammatory response, intraplaque hemorrhage, and/or by oxidative stress [29].

While the density of VV and plaque microvessels on histology can be very high, often very few of these vessels are actively perfused at any one time. This functional inactivity and the very slow flow velocity in vasa vasoral vessels make them very poorly amenable to detection by standard Doppler-based techniques. More recently, ultrasound contrast agents which are composed of acoustically active encapsulated microbubbles have been applied to characterize the degree of plaque neovascularization. These contrast agents are approved for use in many countries for left ventricular cavity opacification on echocardiography and for liver imaging to better discriminate intrahepatic masses [30]. The degree of neovascularization in severe carotid artery plaques has been shown to be higher in those with unstable versus stable plaques based on clinical presentation and has been shown to correlate well with the number of plaque neovessels on histology from carotid endarterectomy specimens [31, 32]. The degree of plaque neovascularization on noninvasive contrast-enhanced ultrasound has also been shown to be greater in plaques that are echolucent [32, 33]. This finding is not unexpected, since the density of vessels making up the vasa vasorum by histology has been shown to increase with macrophage density and to be higher in plaques with thin-cap fibroatheromas rather than stable plaques [12].

A finding common to all studies that have compared contrast ultrasound to histology is that the degree of plaque neovascularization is much greater than one would predict from the contrast ultrasound enhancement. This finding likely reflects the low fraction of vessels that are actively perfused at any time and/or the very low blood flow through the vasa vasorum network. As a consequence, microbubble transit through plaque neovessels is in most circumstances an infrequent event compared to what is seen in the blood pool adjacent to the plaque surface. Because the presence and extent of plaque neovessels is probably more important than network flow, maximum intensity projection processing has been used which provides a more robust method for detecting these vessels even if flow and/or microbubble concentration is low (Fig. 2.4) [34, 35].

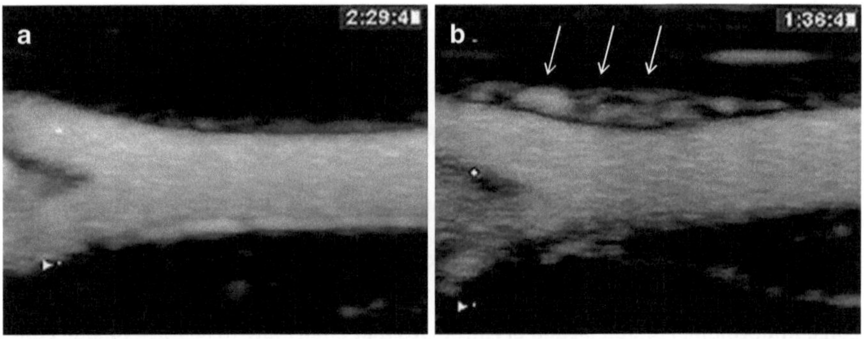

Fig. 2.4 Contrast-enhanced ultrasound imaging of rabbit femoral arteries with maximum intensity projection processing. (**a**) Normal femoral artery with minimal vaso vasorum. (**b**) Femoral artery in an atherosclerotic rabbit model of vasa vasoral proliferation (*arrows*) (From Lee et al. [34] with permission)

2.2 Ultrasound Molecular Imaging of Atherosclerosis

Molecular imaging of components of atherosclerotic plaque has become possible for all forms of noninvasive medical imaging. This advance has been based primarily on the creation of customized targeted imaging probes, although innovations in detector technology have also been important. Although a clinical application is yet to be established, molecular imaging of atherosclerosis could potentially be used to detect disease at an early and more "intervenable" stage, provide unique prognostic or pathophysiologic information that can be used to select or guide therapy, or to evaluate response to therapy. In the research realm, molecular imaging is already beginning to play an important role in the investigation of new pathophysiologic mechanisms that can be targeted for therapy or for the high throughput testing of new targeted therapies.

Key considerations when choosing a molecular imaging technique are whether it has adequate sensitivity to detect early events, whether it has adequate resolution to resolve spatial heterogeneity, and whether it is selective for the pathologic event of interest [36]. Molecular imaging of atherosclerosis with ultrasound has been used in the research realm primarily because it offers a balance between spatial resolution and sensitivity, multiple targets can be evaluated in a short imaging timespan, and the technology required to perform imaging is relatively inexpensive.

2.2.1 Basics of Ultrasound Molecular Imaging

2.2.1.1 Ultrasound Contrast Agents

Nontargeted contrast-enhanced ultrasound imaging relies on the ultrasound detection of acoustically active microbubbles or nanoparticles. Ultrasound contrast agents are currently used clinically in many countries for delineating the blood pool during echocardiography, enhancing Doppler signals, and characterizing vascular patterns and phagocytic properties in the liver [37, 38]. Ultrasound contrast agents are also used for off-label indications such as the evaluation of myocardial or tumor perfusion [39].

Ultrasound contrast agents are typically composed of gas-filled encapsulated microbubbles, liposomes, or nanoparticles. All agents that are approved for human use are composed of microbubbles that are filled with a high molecular weight gas (perfluorocarbons or sulfur hexafluoride) and have a shell composed of lipid or albumin which enhance stability. These agents are generally around 1–3 μm in diameter and do not coalesce after in vivo injection. For most vascular beds, these contrast agents are confined to the vascular compartment and they possess a rheologic profile similar to that of RBCs [40]. Accordingly, these agents transit through the microcirculation of most organs unimpeded. In general, most microbubbles are removed from the circulating blood pool by reticuloendothelial organs within 5–8 min [41, 42].

When exposed to ultrasound, microbubbles undergo volumetric oscillation with compression and expansion during the pressure peaks and nadirs of the ultrasound field [37, 43]. When stimulated at or near their ideal resonant frequency (which is

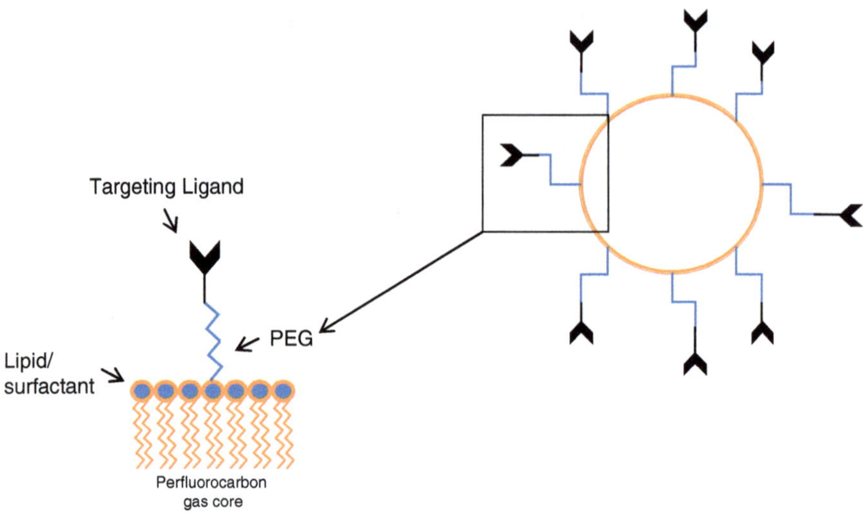

Fig. 2.5 Typical composition of targeted lipid-stabilized perfluorocarbon microbubble agent

determinated by size and shell properties), microbubbles will undergo nonlinear oscillations which produce harmonic signals (ultrasound emissions at multiples of the transmission frequency). These harmonic signals are used to enhance ultrasound imaging by increasing signal to noise ratio [44]. The tissue is less compressible and therefore produces fewer nonlinear signals and can be distinguished from the nonlinear signals generated from the microbubbles particularly when using new multipulse signal subtraction techniques that eliminate most linear signal. High acoustic pressure amplitudes result in exaggerated microbubble oscillation and subsequent microbubble destruction which is termed inertial cavitation. When this occurs, there is often formation of transient free microbubbles which also produce strong and broadband acoustic signals. Many factors affect the cavitation properties of microbubbles including shell properties, gas core compressibility, microbubble radius, temperature, and viscosity of the surrounding medium [37].

2.2.1.2 Targeted Microbubble Contrast Agents

Microbubbles can be targeted to disease-specific ligands to characterize disease phenotype. Targeting can be achieved by either chemical modification of the microbubble shell or direct attachment of ligands (e.g., antibodies, peptides, glycoproteins) to the microbubble surface which usually also involves a molecular spacer in order to reduce steric hindrance during cell-microbubble interaction (Fig. 2.5) [36, 37].

Albumin- and lipid-shelled microbubbles are capable of attachment to activated leukocytes or even activated endothelial cells via integrin or complement-mediated interactions (Fig. 2.6) [45]. The addition of negatively charged lipids, in particular phosphatidylserine, to the microbubble shell is a simple chemical modification that can amplify complement-mediated interactions for lipid-shelled agents [37, 45–47]. These nonspecific cell-microbubble interactions result in some degree

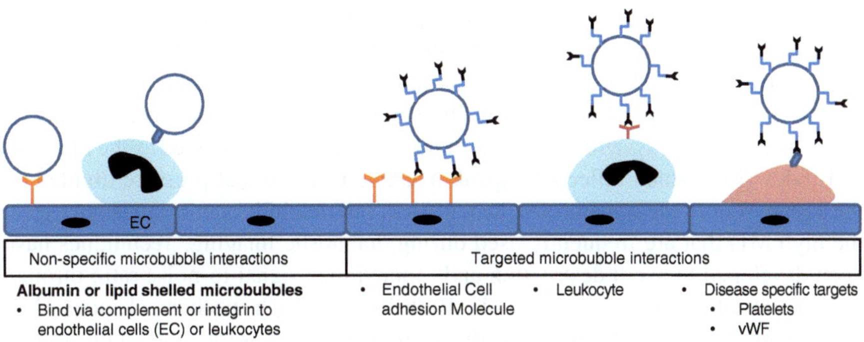

Fig. 2.6 Potential mechanisms for microbubble retention from endothelial attachment in inflamed tissues

of background signal enhancement when imaging inflammatory processes with specific ligand-directed ultrasound contrast agents.

Specific molecular targeting is achieved through surface conjugation of ligands to the surface of microbubbles or nanoscale contrast agents. In general, several thousand ligands per square micron are conjugated to the cell surface [47, 48]. Accordingly, contrast ultrasound imaging does not rely on one-to-one relation between targeted molecule and imaging tracer, but rather relies on attachment of a multivalent particle in a fashion that in many ways mimics the recruitment of circulating blood cells to the vessel surface.

Successful targeting of ultrasound contrast agents depends upon multiple considerations. For atherosclerosis imaging, these considerations include: (1) selection of a targeting ligand with high affinity and specificity for the target, (2) selection of a target molecular that is specific for the disease process of interest, (3) selection of a target molecule that is accessible by a pure intravascular tracer such as microbubbles, (4) sufficient stability of agent to generate a strong acoustic signal after attachment to target, (5) the ability to bind in vessels characterized by high shear forces, and (6) the ability to differentiate signals that come from attached versus freely circulating microbubbles [36, 49, 50]. The most important challenge when designing ultrasound molecular imaging agents is not in the preparation of the imaging probe, but rather the selection of appropriate high-performance targeting ligands that are able to bind with sufficient bond force despite the presence of endogenous competitive ligands. With regard to stability, freely circulating microbubbles are generally cleared within 5–10 min after intravenous injection. Studies have confirmed that retained microbubbles are not only able to retain their acoustic properties over this course of time but are not substantially damped through the process of attachment [51].

2.2.1.3 Targeted Contrast-Enhanced Ultrasound Molecular Imaging

Microbubble signal on ultrasound imaging is generated either by stable cavitation (stable radial oscillation which produces fundamental and harmonic frequencies) or by inertial cavitation whereby microbubbles undergo destruction from exaggerated nonlinear oscillation and transient formation of free gas nuclei which can serve as cavitation nuclei which produces not only harmonic but broadband frequencies. The type of cavitation depends on both the ultrasound frequency and acoustic amplitude. On clinical imaging systems, the ultrasound power is often displayed as the mechanical index (MI) which reflects the peak negative rarefactional pressure divided by the square root of the transmit frequency. Most microbubble agents are destroyed at the high MIs that are frequently used during diagnostic imaging. Techniques have been developed to avoid destruction and to maximize signal-to-noise ratio through elimination of tissue signals [43, 44]. Both low and high mechanical index (MI) imaging protocols have been used with different applications for contrast ultrasound imaging. In general, high MI imaging techniques can be used when signal needs to be amplified due to low contrast density.

Targeted molecular imaging using contrast-enhanced ultrasound utilizes a single bolus intravenous injection of an optimized microbubble dose according to the organ of interest, the expected adhesion density, and the magnitude of signal expected according to ultrasound frequency and power. In order to allow clearance of freely circulating bubbles, imaging is usually initiated 5–10 min after the initial bolus injection. If imaging is not delayed, then the majority of microbubble signal from most organs is attributable to the freely circulating microbubble pool. The delay in imaging allows targeted attachment and clearance of freely circulating tracer [52]. The time delay is also dictated by the tissue that is imaged. For example, a short period of time is sufficient for an organ with a low blood volume and high expected retention fraction for targeted tracer. On the other hand, targeted imaging of atherosclerosis in large blood vessels requires detection of retained agent that is directly adjacent to the blood pool so that time delay must be sufficiently long for removal of most of the freely circulating tracer.

When imaging retained tracer, signal at low or high MI can be used. If high MI is used, only the first one or two frames can be used to for analysis due to subsequent destruction of agent. Regardless of the power used to record targeted microbubble signal, the contribution from freely circulating microbubbles can be eliminated through an algorithm that has been frequently employed for in vivo imaging. The initial imaging frame signal obtained at high or low MI includes total bubble concentration of freely circulating and adhered microbubbles. All microbubbles within the imaging sector can then be destroyed by high MI imaging. After destruction the mechanical index is returned to its initial setting and the images captured post-destruction represent freely circulating bubbles. Digital subtraction of post-destruction averaged frames from the initial pre-destruction frame then creates the targeted molecular signal [52, 53]. Because in certain organs, the number of microbubbles retained depends on blood flow (which determines total number of microbubbles fluxing through tissue), methods have been developed that are able to estimate retention fraction of microbubbles [54]. This approach employs continuous low-MI imaging and deconvolution of the time-intensity curve into a gamma-variate function to reflect those microbubbles passing through after a bolus without retention and an integral of a gamma-variate to reflect the population that is retained.

Retention fraction is not necessarily germane to plaque imaging where most of the target molecules are directly adjacent to a large blood pool and, hence, flow is not a major determining factor of retention.

The methods for imaging targeted contrast ultrasound tracer discussed above have largely relied on external imaging using contrast-specific ultrasound detection schemes and low-to-medium frequency (<10 MHz). However, IVUS has also been used to assess molecular and cellular components of atherosclerosis. In these studies, echogenic liposomes or lipid-shelled perfluorocarbon nano-emulsion agents have been used based on a smaller size than microbubbles and higher likelihood to produce acoustic signal rather than attenuation at the high frequencies usually used during IVUS [55, 56]. Signal-to-noise ratios for all acoustically active agents are generally not very high for these frequencies, and, when adhered microbubble concentration is high, the degree of attenuation relative to signal enhancement is also somewhat unfavorable. Hence, newer techniques using lower frequency probes or even photoacoustic imaging are being explored.

2.2.2 Molecular Targets of Atherosclerosis Accessible to Ultrasound Contrast Agents

Target selection for molecular imaging requires clear purpose of how the information is to be used. Nowhere is this more important than in atherosclerosis where the molecular environment can vary according to stage of development. For example, evaluation for a "vulnerable plaque" or "vulnerable patient" defined as heightened susceptibility to acute atherothrombotic complication is best accomplished by imaging the specific processes that lead to plaque rupture or thrombotic occlusion. On the other hand, molecular imaging of future risk of aggressive disease decades before disease becomes symptomatic would rely on detection of events that lead to initiation and progression of plaque. For contrast ultrasound molecular imaging, the array of targets must also be honed to those that are accessible to the micro- or nanoscale contrast agents that are normally confined to the vascular compartment.

Endothelial activation is an early event in the development of atherosclerosis and plays a role in the progression of disease. One aspect of endothelial activation is the expression of adhesion molecules that participate in the recruitment of leukocytes from the blood pool [42]. Leukocyte recruitment involves a multistep process of cell capture, rolling, activation, adhesion, and transmigration [57]. All of these processes involve the cytokine-mediated expression and/or activation of endothelial cell adhesion molecules and leukocyte counter receptors. Initial capture and rolling involves primarily selectins on endothelial cells (P- and E-selectin) interacting with leukocyte glycoprotein counter receptors (e.g., P-selectin glycoprotein ligand-1 or PSGL-1) or leukocyte selectins (e.g., E-selectin). There are data that rolling can also be supported by fractalkine (CX3CL-1) on endothelial cells and its leukocyte receptor CX3CR-1, as well as endothelial vascular cell adhesion molecule-1 (VCAM-1) interaction with leukocyte VLA-4 ($\alpha_4\beta_1$ integrin) [58]. Leukocyte rolling can lead to further activation and/or expression of integrins. Integrin interactions with endothelial cell adhesion molecules such as intercellular adhesion molecule-1 (ICAM-1) and VCAM-1 are largely responsible for leukocyte adhesion followed by eventual migration into the subendothelial space. These steps are critical in the recruitment of inflammatory cells to regions of atherosclerotic plaque.

The importance of imaging adhesion molecule expression is underscored by the importance of monocytes/macrophages and T-cells that are recruited by these molecules which participate in the initiation, growth, and destabilization of plaque [59]. Inflammatory cells are present at both early and late stages of atherosclerosis, but they are also found in high concentrations in ruptured plaques demonstrating not only their role in plaque initiation but also in plaque disruption. It has also been suggested that imaging of selective monocyte subtypes may be useful in evaluating higher-risk disease [59].

Defining and identifying plaque ruptures that do not lead to overt acute coronary syndrome may represent another approach for examining unstable plaque phenotype. At the time of plaque rupture or vascular injury, thrombogenic materials such as collagen, VWF, and fibronectin are exposed which triggers a cascade of events including platelet activation, adherence, and aggregation [60]. Platelets adhere to the damaged vessel and further aggregation occurs in a large part from glycoprotein GPIIbIIIa integrin cross-linking via fibrinogen. While the role of platelets in thrombotic complications of atherosclerosis is well defined, their role in early atherosclerosis is less understood. Platelets have been identified in early stages of atherosclerosis and may be involved in the inflammatory process that initiates plaque formation [61–63]. Three mechanisms by which platelets interact with the endothelium in situations other than plaque rupture include: (1) direct platelet-endothelial interactions such as via GPIb and Mac-1, (2) platelet-vWF interactions, or (3) platelet-leukocyte interactions which are largely mediated by P-selectin. Attachment of ex vivo platelets to atherosclerotic lesions has been detected in both atherosclerotic rabbit and apolipoprotein E –/– (ApoE–/–) mouse models [63, 64]. In the latter, reduction of platelet-endothelial interactions was associated with reduced lesion formation.

2.2.3 Ultrasound Molecular Imaging of Atherosclerosis

Ultrasound molecular imaging of endothelial cell activation and atherosclerosis can be achieved via two different approaches. The first relies on nonspecific interaction between microbubble contrast agents and either endothelial cells or leukocytes in tissues where there is inflammatory activation or by direct ligand-targeting approaches.

2.2.3.1 Non-ligand Microbubble Targeting

Early studies using myocardial contrast echocardiography perfusion imaging in postischemic tissues detected the persistence of microbubble signal [65]. It was subsequently shown that albumin- and lipid-shelled microbubbles adhere to activated leukocytes on the endothelium and are retained in areas of inflammation in proportion to the degree of inflammation [41, 45, 65]. Inhibitory studies demonstrated that albumin and lipid microbubble-leukocyte interactions are mediated by leukocyte Mac-1 (β_2-integrin) and complement dependent, respectively [65]. After demonstrating the adherence of microbubbles to leukocytes, further studies were done to define microbubble-leukocyte interactions. Transmission electron and intravital microscopy studies demonstrated that microbubbles can undergo phagocytosis by activated leukocytes which results in persistent albeit damped signal generation on ultrasound imaging [41]. In order to amplify complement-mediated interactions by lipid microbubbles, phosphatidylserine has been added to the shell which results in significant signal enhancement on myocardial and renal ischemia reperfusion.

Subsequent studies used these nonspecific microbubble interactions to assess atherosclerosis. In a swine model with balloon injury-induced carotid artery endothelial dysfunction, albumin microbubbles have been found attached not only to leukocytes but to the injured endothelium [66]. These microbubble-endothelial interactions were confirmed to be complement mediated [67]. Subsequent studies in several different animal models have demonstrated the direct binding of nontargeted albumin-shelled microbubbles to damaged endothelium at early to multiple different stages of disease. Despite the simplicity of using nonspecific interactions between microbubbles and endothelial cells, signal generated from these interactions is probably not sufficiently robust for clinical use. However, this background level of adhesion serves to explain the findings in many other studies of ligand-directed molecular imaging where "control nontargeted" microbubble signal in atherosclerosis is not negligible.

2.2.3.2 Endothelial Cell Adhesion Molecules

Endothelial activation is thought to be a critical event in the initiation and progression of atherosclerotic disease and the predisposition to atherothrombotic events. The ability to examine the interface between the blood pool and endothelial surface with an intravascular ultrasound contrast agent allows interrogation for adhesion molecule expression and cell-cell interactions. Moreover, the use of a multivalent particle-based contrast agent provides some form of biologic mimicry for evaluating the actual biologic significance of adhesion molecule expression with regard to site density.

P-Selectin

P-selectin is responsible for the capture and rolling of leukocytes on endothelial cells [57]. It is released from Weibel-Palade bodies in activated endothelial cells and α granules of activated platelets [68]. It acts as an adhesion receptor for leukocytes by interacting with glycoprotein counterligands primarily on the leukocyte surface such as P-selectin glycoprotein ligand 1 (PSGL1) [68]. Studies in P-selectin deficient mice show a lack of leukocyte rolling and an extended delay in leukocyte recruitment in inflammatory tissues thus confirming the critical role of P-selectin in leukocyte-endothelial interactions [57, 68]. Histology studies have positively confirmed that P-selectin is upregulated on the endothelial luminal surface in atherosclerosis and gene-deletion studies have shown that P-selectin plays a role in lesion development and growth.

Microbubbles have been targeted to P-selectin via a variety of different surface ligands including monoclonal antibodies, sialyl lewis-X (a key carbohydrate moiety on PSGL-1), and recombinant PSGL-1. Early experiments using microbubbles bearing P-selectin antibodies employed intravital microscopy of inflamed cremaster muscles to evaluate endothelial adhesion in both wild-type mice and P-selectin knockout mice. P-selectin-targeted microbubbles adhered to activated endothelium in postcapillary venules in wild-type mice, but targeted microbubbles did not adhere in P-selectin-deficient mice demonstrating the specificity of P-selectin microbubble binding to P-selectin. Subsequent contrast ultrasound molecular imaging studies confirmed that microbubbles targeted to P-selectin were retained within the renal cortex of wild-type but not P-selectin deficient mice after renal ischemia-reperfusion injury [53]. Examination of P-selectin as a marker of vascular inflammation in atherosclerosis has been performed in murine models of age-dependent atherosclerosis [69]. In these studies, P-selectin molecular signal on contrast ultrasound imaging was strong not only at the stage of advanced inflammatory plaques but also at the stage of the earliest appearance of fatty streaks (Fig. 2.7) [69]. There was, however, an age- or stage-dependent increase in P-selectin signal relative to control agent signal. These data suggest that contrast-enhanced ultrasound molecular imaging of P-selectin can detect the inception of atherosclerosis and that the degree of signal enhancement provides some measure of disease severity.

ICAM-1 and VCAM-1

While leukocyte capture and rolling is in a large part mediated by selectins, firm adhesion is mediated primarily by the interaction between leukocyte heterodimeric integrins and endothelial cell glycoprotein adhesion molecules in the immunoglobulin family including ICAM-1 and VCAM-1. The latter have been detected on the endothelium of not only late-stage but early stage atherosclerotic lesions in animal models of atherosclerosis (e.g., rabbits, mice) and in humans [58, 70, 71]. There is evidence that VCAM-1 expression in particular can be detected even at the earliest appearance of fatty streaks. These findings as well as inhibitory studies implicate the critical role of ICAM-1 and VCAM-1 in the pathogenesis of atherosclerosis.

Early studies evaluating the feasibility of targeting ICAM-1 demonstrated that perfluorocarbon microbubbles bearing monoclonal antibodies against ICAM-1 could adhere to activated cultured human coronary artery endothelial cells [72]. In subsequent studies, acoustically active liposomes bearing ICAM-1 antibodies were shown to produce vascular contrast enhancement in a model of arterial injury in miniswine fed a high-fat diet. Acoustically reflective liposomes conjugated with antibodies to ICAM-1, when injected intra-arterially demonstrated signal enhancement in areas of early atherosclerosis using intravascular- and transvascular-targeted contrast-enhanced ultrasound [27, 73]. Echogenic immunoliposomes have been conjugated with anti-VCAM-1 and anti-ICAM-1 antibodies. Using IVUS, these immunoliposomes generated rapid significant signal enhancement at the site of endothelial injury and atherosclerotic plaque compared to unconjugated immunoliposomes allowing for identification of endothelial adhesion molecule expression at disease sites. There have been subsequent studies with the intent of improving

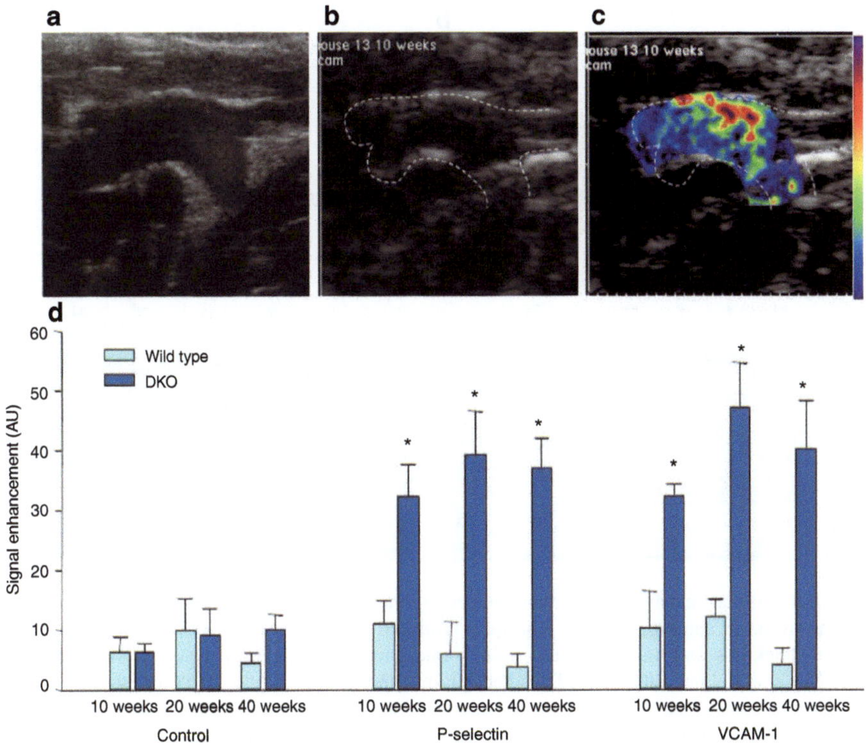

Fig. 2.7 Contrast-enhanced ultrasound imaging of endothelial cell adhesion molecule expression in progressive atherosclerosis in mice with homozygous deletion of the LDL-receptor and Apobec-1 editing peptide (DKO). The images at the top are from a 10-week-old DKO mouse illustrating (**a**) a high-frequency 2-D imaging of the thoracic aorta, (**b**) contrast-specific ultrasound imaging prior to the injection of agent (*dashed lines* illustrating aortic border), and (**c**) contrast-specific imaging 8 min after injection of a VCAM-1-targeted microbubble agent (after digital subtraction of circulating agent). (**d**) Quantitative CEU molecular imaging for control, P-selectin-targeted, and VCAM-1-targeted microbubbles in wild-type and DKO mice illustrating signal enhancement as early as 10 weeks of age. $*p<0.05$ vs wild-type (From Kaufmann et al. [69], with permission)

plaque visualization with three dimensional IVUS reconstructions [56]. While targeted immunoliposomes have had in vivo success for IVUS molecular imaging, there has been difficulty imaging microbubbles as targeted contrast agents with IVUS given the high-frequency transmission which ranges from 20 to 40 MHz and are generally above the typical resonant frequency of microbubbles [74].

Studies using aortic contrast-enhanced ultrasound (CEU) and VCAM-1 targeted microbubbles in apo-E-deficient mice were the first to demonstrate that different degrees of plaque inflammation could be evaluated with molecular imaging of an endothelial cell adhesion molecule. In these studies, there was a stepwise increase in both plaque macrophage content and VCAM-1 signal enhancement in wild-type mice fed on high-fat diet, ApoE-deficient mice on chow diet, and ApoE-deficient

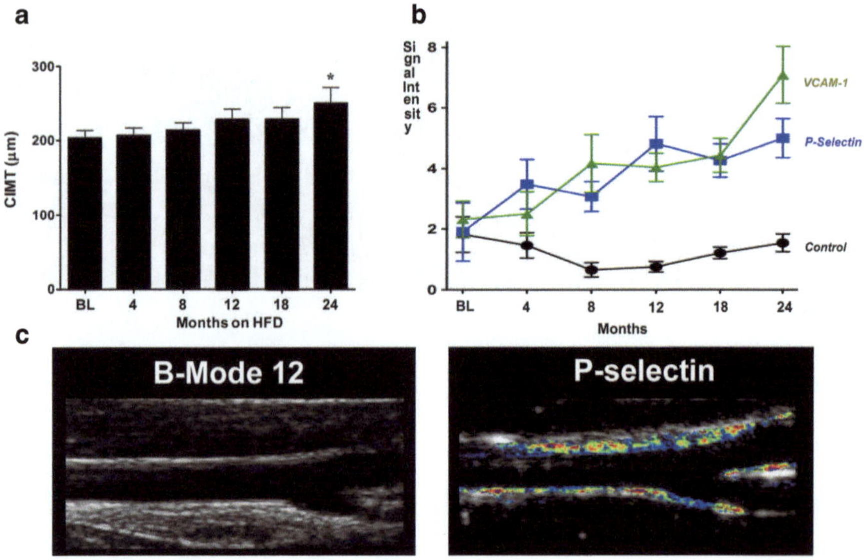

Fig. 2.8 Contrast-enhanced ultrasound molecular imaging of early endothelial activation in obese insulin-resistant adult male rhesus macaques produced by high-fat diet. (**a**) Mean carotid intima-media thickness showing very mild intimal thickening over time (*$p<0.05$ versus baseline). (**b**) Mean video intensity on CEU molecular imaging of the carotid artery using control and P-selectin-targeted and VCAM-1-targeted microbubbles. (**c**) Example of a carotid artery bifurcation using high-frequency B-mode imaging (*left*) and color-coded contrast-enhanced molecular imaging of P-selectin from a macaque after 1 year of diet (From Chadderdon et al. [75], with permission)

mice on high-fat diet. In an effort to determine whether VCAM-1 signal can detect disease at a very early stage, molecular imaging with CEU of the aortic arch was performed at various ages (10–40 weeks) in mice that develop reproducible age-dependent atherosclerosis on a chow diet due to genetic deletion of both the LDL-receptor and Apobec-1 editing peptide [69]. In these studies, the signal enhancement from VCAM-1 could be detected at the earliest stages of fatty streak formation and increased as with plaque progression [69]. It has also been shown that CEU molecular imaging of both VCAM-1 and P-selectin is able to detect the earliest stages of carotid atherosclerosis in a nonhuman primate model of the disease [75]. In these studies, signal enhancement in obese insulin-resistant rhesus macaques preceded intima-media thickening by over a year (Fig. 2.8) [75].

Molecular imaging of endothelial cell adhesion molecules has also been used to better understand the mechanisms through which new or established therapies for atherosclerosis act. In an effort to better understand how statin therapy influences endothelial activation, mice deficient for both LDL-receptor–/– and Apobec-1-editing protein were studied after treatment with 8 weeks of atorvastatin. Statin therapy resulted in less plaque burden, less VCAM-1 on western blot, and lower noninvasive CEU molecular imaging signal for VCAM-2 compared to untreated mice [76]. These data illustrate not only the capability of CEU molecular imaging to evaluate therapeutic response but also provide unique functionality, since CEU signal is attributable only to endothelial adhesion receptor expression at the blood pool interface. Novel antioxidant therapies aimed at reducing endothelial inflammation have also been evaluated using CEU molecular imaging as an in vivo readout of tissue response. Apocynin, an inhibitor of NADPH oxidase subunit transport, when given to mice deficient for both LDL-receptor−/− and Apobec-1-editing protein at late stages of disease reduced monocyte accumulation, reduced platelet adhesion on aortic histology, and improved aortic distensibility after 10 weeks of treatment compared to untreated [77]. CEU molecular imaging showed that apocynin produced a substantial decrease in aortic VCAM-1 and P-selectin signal, implying that beneficial changes in plaque phenotype and mechanical properties of the aorta were related to reduced endothelial activation. These studies indicate that molecular imaging using targeted CEU can be an important asset in the preclinical assessment of drug therapies aimed at decreasing endothelial inflammation in atherosclerosis.

Platelets and Thrombus

Early ultrasound-targeting thrombus in atherosclerotic disease focused on targeting thrombogenic processes. In some of the earliest studies, a lipid-stabilized perfluorocarbon nano-emulsion agent targeted to fibrin was shown to produce signal enhancement in canine femoral arteries where thrombus was produced by electrostimulated injury and partial ligation [78]. In a Yucatan miniswine model, echogenic liposomes targeted to both fibrin and to tissue factor have been shown to produce signal enhancement on IVUS imaging of the femoral or carotid artery after direct intra-arterial injection [55]. Tissue factor-targeted nano-emulsion particles were also shown to produce signal enhancement injured by balloon catheter overinflation. In aggregate, these studies suggested that large or small thrombi formed in response to severe vascular injury or advanced atherosclerosis can be imaged with CEU molecular imaging.

More recent studies that have focused on platelet-targeted imaging has been platelet activation, adhesion, and aggregation which are important events in most atherothrombotic complications of atherosclerosis and are initiated by exposure of subendothelial matrix to von Willebrand factor (VWF) and circulating platelets. There is also evidence that adhesive interaction between platelets and endothelial cells play role in promoting vascular inflammation and plaque formation in atherosclerosis. These interactions could potentially be mediated by platelet-endothelial interaction, binding of dysregulated VWF on the endothelium, or via platelet-leukocyte complexes. Hence, it is likely that platelet-targeted imaging may not only provide a biologic readout of highly unstable plaque phenotype in advanced disease but also likelihood for aggressive course of plaque development at much earlier stages of disease.

As mentioned previously, targeting of microbubbles to platelets has been achieved primarily through the targeting moieties that bind either GPIIb/IIIa or GPIbα. Since platelet aggregation is a critical event for the formation of occlusive thrombi and because fibrinogen cross-linking of activated platelet GPIIb/IIIa is a critical event in aggregation, microbubbles targeted to GPIIb/IIIa have been used to evaluate the presence of platelet-rich thrombosis in atherosclerosis. Abciximab, a monoclonal antibody against GPIIb/IIIa receptors, has been conjugated to immunobubbles and has been shown to produce ultrasound enhancement of human thrombi transplanted into rat carotid artery [79]. In vivo imaging of acute thrombosis in the mouse carotid artery using ferric chloride-induced injury has also been achieved using high-frequency ultrasound and microbubbles targeted to activation-specific epitopes of GPIIb/IIIa (Fig. 2.9) [80]. Results from this study were important since contrast ultrasound signal could be used for real-time assessment of the efficacy of pharmacological thrombolysis.

Molecular imaging of platelet-endothelial interactions before the formation of occlusive thrombi has been performed using microbubbles targeted to platelets via surface conjugation of the A1-domain (GPIbα-binding domain) of VWF or with microbubbles targeted to VWF via surface conjugation of recombinant GPIbα (platelet mimicry). CEU molecular imaging of these two molecular markers in mice deficient for both LDL-receptor−/− and Apobec-1-editing protein has been used to better understand the extent and mechanisms for platelet-endothelial interactions in atherosclerosis [77, 81]. Imaging of platelets with GPIbα-targeted microbubbles has also been used to show that potent antioxidant therapy can reduce platelet-endothelial interactions, presumably through less oxidative modification of VWF regulatory pathways [77].

2.3 Summary

Ultrasound-based evaluation of plaque severity and plaque composition is already an integral part of the practice of cardiovascular medicine. In particular, the catheter-based intravascular ultrasound assessment of disease is used to better define atherosclerotic lesion severity and success of percutaneous intervention. Assessment of carotid intima-media thickness to detect risk for future atherosclerotic events is beginning to lose favor because of alternative methods that can better reclassify patient risk (MESA). However, other forms of ultrasound imaging are now being applied in clinical studies to better understand plaque composition (vasa vasorum imaging) and vascular mechanical properties (palpography, pulse wave velocity). Perhaps the greatest achievement will be when ultrasound-based molecular imaging can provide unique information on plaque or vascular phenotype that can either be used to diagnose and treat aggressive disease at a more "manageable" stage or be used to select therapy based on a given molecular profile. Only the first steps have been taken toward this goal by the completion of preclinical studies illustrating feasibility of ultrasound molecular imaging to detect either proinflammatory or prothrombotic phenotype. Although clinical translation is a distant goal, the impact of ultrasound molecular imaging is already being felt through its application to better define pathophysiology and evaluate new therapies in atherosclerotic disease.

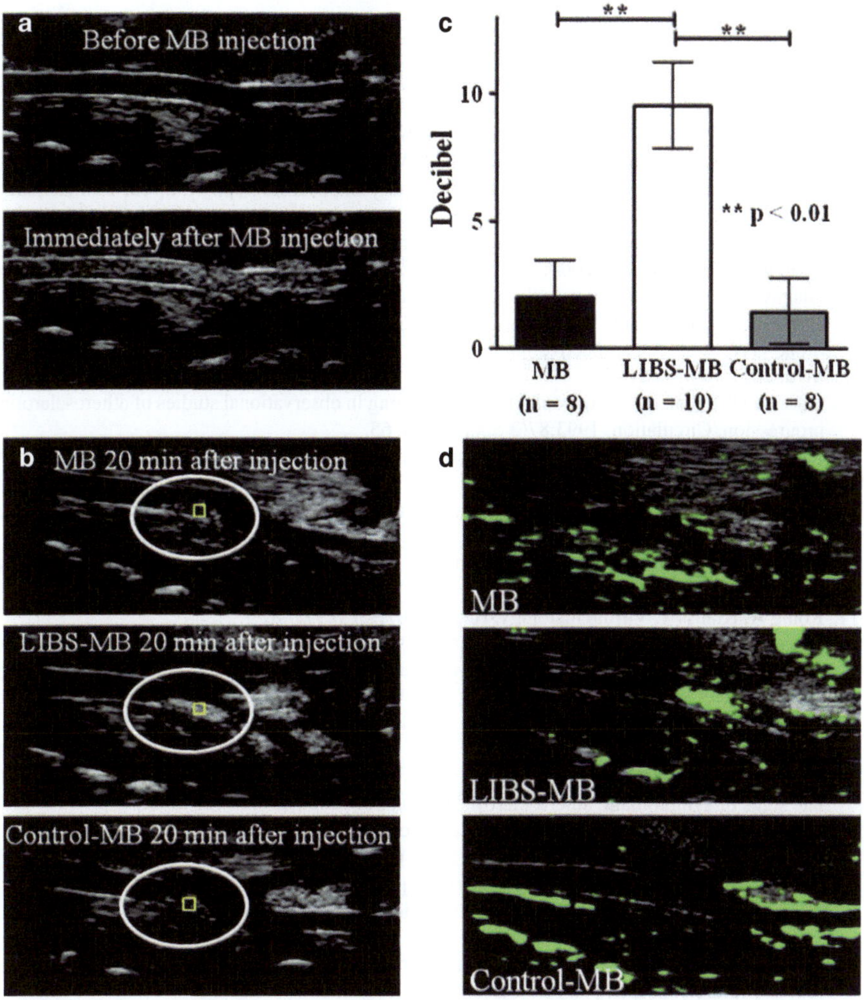

Fig. 2.9 *In vivo* imaging of acute thrombosis in the mouse carotid artery using ferric chloride-induced injury. (**a**) High-frequency ultrasound imaging of the carotid artery before and after microbubble injection showing blood pool enhancement. (**b**) Ultrasound image of thrombi 20 min after injection of nontargeted microbubbles, platelet-targeted microbubbles bearing antibodies against activation-specific epitopes of GPIIb/IIIa (LIBS-MB), and control microbubbles with nonspecific antibody. *Circles* represent the region of the distal common carotid artery. (**c**) Mean (±SD) signal intensity on CEU imaging of the carotid thrombi 20 min after microbubble injection. (**d**) Ultrasound images after digital subtraction demonstrating brighter LIBS-MB compared to control microbubble signal at the site of thrombus (From Wang et al. [80], with permission)

References

1. Lawrence JP. Physics and instrumentation of ultrasound. Crit Care Med. 2007;35(8 Suppl):S314–22.
2. Armstrong WF, Ryan T, Feigenbaum H. Feigenbaum's echocardiography. 7th ed. Philadelphia: Wolters Kluwer Health/Lippincott Williams & Wilkins; 2010. xv, 785 p.
3. Otto CM. Textbook of clinical echocardiography, Endocardiography. 5th ed. Philadelphia: Elsevier/Saunders; 2013.
4. Goldstein JA, et al. Multiple complex coronary plaques in patients with acute myocardial infarction. N Engl J Med. 2000;343(13):915–22.
5. Glagov S, et al. Compensatory enlargement of human atherosclerotic coronary arteries. N Engl J Med. 1987;316(22):1371–5.
6. Stone GW, et al. A prospective natural-history study of coronary atherosclerosis. N Engl J Med. 2011;364(3):226–35.
7. Salonen JT, Salonen R. Ultrasound B-mode imaging in observational studies of atherosclerotic progression. Circulation. 1993;87(3 Suppl):II56–65.
8. Landry A, Spence JD, Fenster A. Measurement of carotid plaque volume by 3-dimensional ultrasound. Stroke. 2004;35(4):864–9.
9. Graebe M, et al. Reproducibility of two 3-D ultrasound carotid plaque quantification methods. Ultrasound Med Biol. 2014;40:1641–9.
10. DeMaria AN, et al. Imaging vulnerable plaque by ultrasound. J Am Coll Cardiol. 2006;47(8 Suppl):C32–9.
11. Konig A, Klauss V. Virtual histology. Heart. 2007;93(8):977–82.
12. Virmani R, et al. Atherosclerotic plaque progression and vulnerability to rupture: angiogenesis as a source of intraplaque hemorrhage. Arterioscler Thromb Vasc Biol. 2005;25(10):2054–61.
13. Asakura M, et al. Extensive development of vulnerable plaques as a pan-coronary process in patients with myocardial infarction: an angioscopic study. J Am Coll Cardiol. 2001;37(5):1284–8.
14. Fleiner M, et al. Arterial neovascularization and inflammation in vulnerable patients: early and late signs of symptomatic atherosclerosis. Circulation. 2004;110(18):2843–50.
15. Polonsky TS, et al. Coronary artery calcium score and risk classification for coronary heart disease prediction. JAMA. 2010;303(16):1610–6.
16. Nasu K, et al. Accuracy of in vivo coronary plaque morphology assessment: a validation study of in vivo virtual histology compared with in vitro histopathology. J Am Coll Cardiol. 2006;47(12):2405–12.
17. Puri R, Worthley MI, Nicholls SJ. Intravascular imaging of vulnerable coronary plaque: current and future concepts. Nat Rev Cardiol. 2011;8(3):131–9.
18. Laurent S, et al. Aortic stiffness is an independent predictor of all-cause and cardiovascular mortality in hypertensive patients. Hypertension. 2001;37(5):1236–41.
19. Laurent S, et al. Expert consensus document on arterial stiffness: methodological issues and clinical applications. Eur Heart J. 2006;27(21):2588–605.
20. Schaar JA, et al. Intravascular palpography for high-risk vulnerable plaque assessment. Herz. 2003;28(6):488–95.
21. Schaar JA, et al. Characterizing vulnerable plaque features with intravascular elastography. Circulation. 2003;108(21):2636–41.
22. Maurice RL, et al. On the potential of the Lagrangian speckle model estimator to characterize atherosclerotic plaques in endovascular elastography: in vitro experiments using an excised human carotid artery. Ultrasound Med Biol. 2005;31(1):85–91.
23. Deleaval F, et al. The intravascular ultrasound elasticity-palpography technique revisited: a reliable tool for the in vivo detection of vulnerable coronary atherosclerotic plaques. Ultrasound Med Biol. 2013;39(8):1469–81.
24. Schaar JA, et al. Intravascular palpography for vulnerable plaque assessment. J Am Coll Cardiol. 2006;47(8 Suppl):C86–91.

25. Vitarelli A, et al. Aortic wall mechanics in the Marfan syndrome assessed by transesophageal tissue Doppler echocardiography. Am J Cardiol. 2006;97(4):571–7.
26. Rodriguez-Granillo GA, et al. In vivo intravascular ultrasound-derived thin-cap fibroatheroma detection using ultrasound radiofrequency data analysis. J Am Coll Cardiol. 2005;46(11): 2038–42.
27. Carr C, Lindner JR. Ultrasound imaging of atherosclerotic plaques. Curr Cardiovasc Imaging Rep. 2009;2:24–32.
28. McCarthy MJ, et al. Angiogenesis and the atherosclerotic carotid plaque: an association between symptomatology and plaque morphology. J Vasc Surg. 1999;30(2):261–8.
29. Moreno PR, et al. Neovascularization in human atherosclerosis. Curr Mol Med. 2006; 6(5):457–77.
30. Mulvagh SL, et al. American society of echocardiography consensus statement on the clinical applications of ultrasonic contrast agents in echocardiography. J Am Soc Echocardiogr. 2008;21(11):1179–201; quiz 1281.
31. Dunmore BJ, et al. Carotid plaque instability and ischemic symptoms are linked to immaturity of microvessels within plaques. J Vasc Surg. 2007;45(1):155–9.
32. Coli S, et al. Contrast-enhanced ultrasound imaging of intraplaque neovascularization in carotid arteries: correlation with histology and plaque echogenicity. J Am Coll Cardiol. 2008; 52(3):223–30.
33. Hoogi A, et al. Carotid plaque vulnerability: quantification of neovascularization on contrast-enhanced ultrasound with histopathologic correlation. AJR Am J Roentgenol. 2011;196(2):431–6.
34. Lee SC, et al. Temporal characterization of the functional density of the vasa vasorum by contrast-enhanced ultrasonography maximum intensity projection imaging. JACC Cardiovasc Imaging. 2010;3(12):1265–72.
35. Moguillansky D, et al. Quantification of plaque neovascularization using contrast ultrasound: a histologic validation. Eur Heart J. 2011;32(5):646–53.
36. Lindner JR. Molecular imaging with contrast ultrasound and targeted microbubbles. J Nucl Cardiol. 2004;11(2):215–21.
37. Kaufmann BA, Lindner JR. Molecular imaging with targeted contrast ultrasound. Curr Opin Biotechnol. 2007;18(1):11–6.
38. Lindner JR. Contrast ultrasound molecular imaging of inflammation in cardiovascular disease. Cardiovasc Res. 2009;84(2):182–9.
39. Lindner JR. Microbubbles in medical imaging: current applications and future directions. Nat Rev Drug Discov. 2004;3(6):527–32.
40. Villanueva FS, Wagner WR. Ultrasound molecular imaging of cardiovascular disease. Nat Clin Pract Cardiovasc Med. 2008;5 Suppl 2:S26–32.
41. Lindner JR, et al. Noninvasive imaging of inflammation by ultrasound detection of phagocytosed microbubbles. Circulation. 2000;102(5):531–8.
42. Lindner JR. Assessment of inflammation with contrast ultrasound. Prog Cardiovasc Dis. 2001; 44(2):111–20.
43. Kaufmann BA, Wei K, Lindner JR. Contrast echocardiography. Curr Probl Cardiol. 2007; 32(2):51–96.
44. Calliada F, et al. Ultrasound contrast agents: basic principles. Eur J Radiol. 1998;27 Suppl 2:S157–60.
45. Lindner JR, et al. Noninvasive ultrasound imaging of inflammation using microbubbles targeted to activated leukocytes. Circulation. 2000;102(22):2745–50.
46. Christiansen JP, et al. Noninvasive imaging of myocardial reperfusion injury using leukocyte-targeted contrast echocardiography. Circulation. 2002;105(15):1764–7.
47. Takalkar AM, et al. Binding and detachment dynamics of microbubbles targeted to P-selectin under controlled shear flow. J Control Release. 2004;96(3):473–82.
48. Lindner JR. Molecular imaging of cardiovascular disease with contrast-enhanced ultrasonography. Nat Rev Cardiol. 2009;6(7):475–81.

49. Choudhury RP, Fisher EA. Molecular imaging in atherosclerosis, thrombosis, and vascular inflammation. Arterioscler Thromb Vasc Biol. 2009;29(7):983–91.
50. Dayton PA, et al. Ultrasonic analysis of peptide- and antibody-targeted microbubble contrast agents for molecular imaging of alphavbeta3-expressing cells. Mol Imaging. 2004;3(2):125–34.
51. Lankford M, et al. Effect of microbubble ligation to cells on ultrasound signal enhancement: implications for targeted imaging. Invest Radiol. 2006;41(10):721–8.
52. Kaufmann BA, et al. Effect of acoustic power on in vivo molecular imaging with targeted microbubbles: implications for low-mechanical index real-time imaging. J Am Soc Echocardiogr. 2010;23(1):79–85.
53. Lindner JR, et al. Ultrasound assessment of inflammation and renal tissue injury with microbubbles targeted to P-selectin. Circulation. 2001;104(17):2107–12.
54. Carr CL, et al. Dysregulated selectin expression and monocyte recruitment during ischemia-related vascular remodeling in diabetes mellitus. Arterioscler Thromb Vasc Biol. 2011;31(11):2526–33.
55. Hamilton AJ, et al. Intravascular ultrasound molecular imaging of atheroma components in vivo. J Am Coll Cardiol. 2004;43(3):453–60.
56. Kim H, et al. In vivo volumetric intravascular ultrasound visualization of early/inflammatory arterial atheroma using targeted echogenic immunoliposomes. Invest Radiol. 2010;45(10): 685–91.
57. Ley K. Molecular mechanisms of leukocyte recruitment in the inflammatory process. Cardiovasc Res. 1996;32(4):733–42.
58. Li H, et al. An atherogenic diet rapidly induces VCAM-1, a cytokine-regulatable mononuclear leukocyte adhesion molecule, in rabbit aortic endothelium. Arterioscler Thromb. 1993;13(2):197–204.
59. Ghattas A, et al. Monocytes in coronary artery disease and atherosclerosis: where are we now? J Am Coll Cardiol. 2013;62(17):1541–51.
60. Kaplan ZS, Jackson SP. The role of platelets in atherothrombosis. Hematol Am Soc Hematol Educ Program. 2011;2011:51–61.
61. Faggiotto A, Ross R. Studies of hypercholesterolemia in the nonhuman primate. II. Fatty streak conversion to fibrous plaque. Arteriosclerosis. 1984;4(4):341–56.
62. Sevitt S. Platelets and foam cells in the evolution of atherosclerosis. Histological and immunohistological studies of human lesions. Atherosclerosis. 1986;61(2):107–15.
63. Theilmeier G, et al. Endothelial von Willebrand factor recruits platelets to atherosclerosis-prone sites in response to hypercholesterolemia. Blood. 2002;99(12):4486–93.
64. Massberg S, et al. A critical role of platelet adhesion in the initiation of atherosclerotic lesion formation. J Exp Med. 2002;196(7):887–96.
65. Lindner JR, et al. Microbubble persistence in the microcirculation during ischemia/reperfusion and inflammation is caused by integrin- and complement-mediated adherence to activated leukocytes. Circulation. 2000;101(6):668–75.
66. Tsutsui JM, et al. Detection of retained microbubbles in carotid arteries with real-time low mechanical index imaging in the setting of endothelial dysfunction. J Am Coll Cardiol. 2004;44(5):1036–46.
67. Anderson DR, et al. The role of complement in the adherence of microbubbles to dysfunctional arterial endothelium and atherosclerotic plaque. Cardiovasc Res. 2007;73(3):597–606.
68. Mayadas TN, et al. Leukocyte rolling and extravasation are severely compromised in P selectin-deficient mice. Cell. 1993;74(3):541–54.
69. Kaufmann BA, et al. Molecular imaging of the initial inflammatory response in atherosclerosis: implications for early detection of disease. Arterioscler Thromb Vasc Biol. 2010;30(1):54–9.
70. Huo Y, Hafezi-Moghadam A, Ley K. Role of vascular cell adhesion molecule-1 and fibronectin connecting segment-1 in monocyte rolling and adhesion on early atherosclerotic lesions. Circ Res. 2000;87(2):153–9.

71. Nakashima Y, et al. Upregulation of VCAM-1 and ICAM-1 at atherosclerosis-prone sites on the endothelium in the ApoE-deficient mouse. Arterioscler Thromb Vasc Biol. 1998;18(5):842–51.
72. Villanueva FS, et al. Microbubbles targeted to intercellular adhesion molecule-1 bind to activated coronary artery endothelial cells. Circulation. 1998;98(1):1–5.
73. Demos SM, et al. In vivo targeting of acoustically reflective liposomes for intravascular and transvascular ultrasonic enhancement. J Am Coll Cardiol. 1999;33(3):867–75.
74. Phillips LC, et al. Intravascular ultrasound detection and delivery of molecularly targeted microbubbles for gene delivery. IEEE Trans Ultrason Ferroelectr Freq Control. 2012;59(7):1596–601.
75. Chadderdon SM, et al. Proinflammatory endothelial activation detected by molecular imaging in obese nonhuman primates coincides with onset of insulin resistance and progressively increases with duration of insulin resistance. Circulation. 2014;129(4):471–8.
76. Khanicheh E, et al. Noninvasive ultrasound molecular imaging of the effect of statins on endothelial inflammatory phenotype in early atherosclerosis. PLoS ONE. 2013;8(3):e58761.
77. Liu Y, et al. Molecular imaging of inflammation and platelet adhesion in advanced atherosclerosis effects of antioxidant therapy with NADPH oxidase inhibition. Circ Cardiovasc Imaging. 2013;6(1):74–82.
78. Lanza GM, et al. A novel site-targeted ultrasonic contrast agent with broad biomedical application. Circulation. 1996;94(12):3334–40.
79. Alonso A, et al. Molecular imaging of human thrombus with novel abciximab immunobubbles and ultrasound. Stroke. 2007;38(5):1508–14.
80. Wang X, et al. Novel single-chain antibody-targeted microbubbles for molecular ultrasound imaging of thrombosis: validation of a unique noninvasive method for rapid and sensitive detection of thrombi and monitoring of success or failure of thrombolysis in mice. Circulation. 2012;125(25):3117–26.
81. McCarty OJ, et al. Molecular imaging of activated von Willebrand factor to detect high-risk atherosclerotic phenotype. JACC Cardiovasc Imaging. 2010;3(9):947–55.

Molecular Imaging of Macrophages in Atherosclerosis

3

Jun-ichiro Koga and Masanori Aikawa

Contents

Abstract

Activated macrophages play central roles in various stages of the pathogenesis of atherosclerosis. Particularly, the role macrophages play in the onset of acute thrombotic complications including myocardial infarction, a global health burden, has the large clinical impact. It is thus important to identify high-risk patients for these

J.-i. Koga, MD, PhD
The Center for Excellence in Vascular Biology, Department of Medicine,
Brigham and Women's Hospital, Harvard Medical School,
77 Avenue Louis Pasteur, Boston, MA 02115, USA

M. Aikawa, MD, PhD (✉)
The Center for Excellence in Vascular Biology, Department of Medicine,
Brigham and Women's Hospital, Harvard Medical School,
77 Avenue Louis Pasteur, Boston, MA 02115, USA

The Center for Excellence in Vascular Biology, Department of Medicine,
Brigham and Women's Hospital, Harvard Medical School, Boston, MA, USA
e-mail: maikawa@rics.bwh.harvard.edu

E. Aikawa (ed.), *Cardiovascular Imaging: Arterial and Aortic Valve Inflammation and Calcification*, DOI 10.1007/978-3-319-09268-3_3

thrombotic complications to improve the prognosis by detecting macrophage-rich, subclinical lesions. In addition, macrophage imaging of vascular lesions in humans would facilitate understanding of the disease mechanisms and also help to monitor the effects of new therapies in the near future. These clinical needs have driven recent efforts on the development of molecular imaging modalities to visualize macrophages. Various imaging agents which are taken up by macrophages (e.g., superparamagnetic iron oxide for magnetic resonance imaging) or target a macrophage-specific biological process (e.g., proteinase activity for optical imaging) have become available. In the field of nuclear medicine, FDG-PET already has been in the stage of clinical trials. This chapter reviews current states and future perspectives of macrophage-targeted molecular imaging.

3.1 Conventional Imaging Modalities for Atherosclerotic Vascular Diseases

Ischemic cardiovascular diseases, including acute myocardial infarction and cerebral infarction, are life-threatening disorders. In addition, peripheral arterial disease is a growing health problem due to diabetes epidemic. Atherosclerosis is a common pathological feature in these disorders. Angiography, one of the most conventional imaging modalities, is performed by injecting a radiocontrast agent into the blood vessel and imaging by X-ray-based techniques. This modality visualizes the lumen of blood vessels but not the size of atherosclerotic plaques nor their inflammatory burden such as activities of macrophages. Other modalities including computed tomography (CT) and magnetic resonance imaging (MRI) also provide anatomical information but do not visualize biological processes within the plaques.

3.2 Macrophages in Atherosclerotic Diseases

Inflammation, especially mediated by activated macrophages, is one of the central mechanisms of atherosclerotic cardiovascular diseases. Macrophages promote the pathogenesis of atherosclerosis from the initial lesion formation to advanced lesions which cause acute thrombotic complications [1]. Monocytes in peripheral blood infiltrate into the subendothelial space and differentiate into macrophages. Then, macrophage takes up oxidized low-density lipoprotein (oxLDL) and results in foam cell formation. These lipid-laden macrophages produce proinflammatory cytokines and exacerbate chronic inflammation in vessel wall. In advanced lesions, activated macrophages release proteases including matrix metalloproteinases (MMPs) and cathepsins [2, 3]. These proteases may degrade extracellular matrix, particularly fibrillar collagen, a molecular determinant of tissue stability. Collagen loss leads to thinning of the fibrous cap of plaques and impair their strength against mechanical stresses, causing physical disruption ("plaque rupture") and acute thrombotic events such as myocardial infarction and stroke [4]. Therefore, identification of subclinical inflamed atherosclerotic plaques by macrophage imaging may help to predict and prevent acute thrombotic events. Macrophage imaging in experimental animals and humans also provides new insight into the pathogenesis of atherosclerotic vascular diseases. In addition, noninvasive macrophage imaging would be useful to monitor the effects of new therapeutics in clinical trials.

3.3 Molecular Imaging

Molecular imaging visualizes various biological processes at molecular levels and is also called "functional imaging." This modality has rapidly developed in recent years in the field of cardiovascular medicine accompanied with fuller understating of the molecular pathogenesis of atherosclerotic vascular diseases. Technical innovations in MRI, nuclear medicine (e.g., single-photon emission computed tomography, SPECT; positron emission computed tomography, PET), near-infrared fluorescence (NIRF) imaging, and ultrasound have contributed to this expansion. Advances of nanotechnology also have enabled preparations and chemical modifications of small materials, facilitating the development of various new imaging probes that recognize specific cell types or biological processes.

Critical points in the development and application of novel molecular imaging probes may include: (1) The biology of target molecule/cell type is well understood. (2) Target molecules or phenomenon is not substantially seen in normal tissues and is induced in diseased organs. (3) Relatively high expression levels of target molecules. (4) The specificity and pharmacokinetics of an imaging agent are well examined from various aspects. (5) The possibility of enhancing signals. (6) Safety for human and environments.

3.4 Macrophage Imaging by Iron-Based Nanomaterials

Magnetic nanomaterials with iron cores, for example, magnetite (Fe_3O_4) or maghemite (γ-Fe_2O_3), are used as contrast agents in MRI. These iron cores are often modified with hydrophilic polymers including dextran, carboxymethylated dextran, polyvinyl alcohol, starches, chitosan, polymethyl methacrylate, polyethylene glycol (PEG), polylactic-co-glycolic acid (PLGA), polyvinylpyrrolidone, and polyacrylic acid [5]. These so-called superparamagnetic iron oxide (SPIO) nanoparticles are used as negative contrast agent in macrophage imaging in MRI. Especially, ultrasmall SPIO (USPIO) nanoparticles (<50 nm) coated with dextran remain in the blood stream for a long time by escaping from reticuloendothelial system-mediated clearance. The half-life of SPIO nanoparticle is approximately 24 h and this enables macrophage imaging in vivo. In addition, high soft-tissue contrast and resolution of MRI enables detailed observation of vessel walls [6]. Morishige et al. used 3.0 Tesla MRI and USPIO and reported in a rabbit model of atherosclerosis that (1) change in MRI signal intensity correlates with histologically evaluated macrophage accumulation, and (2) macrophage imaging with USPIO is available to monitor anti-inflammatory efficacy of lipid-lowering therapy by statins (Fig. 3.1) [7].

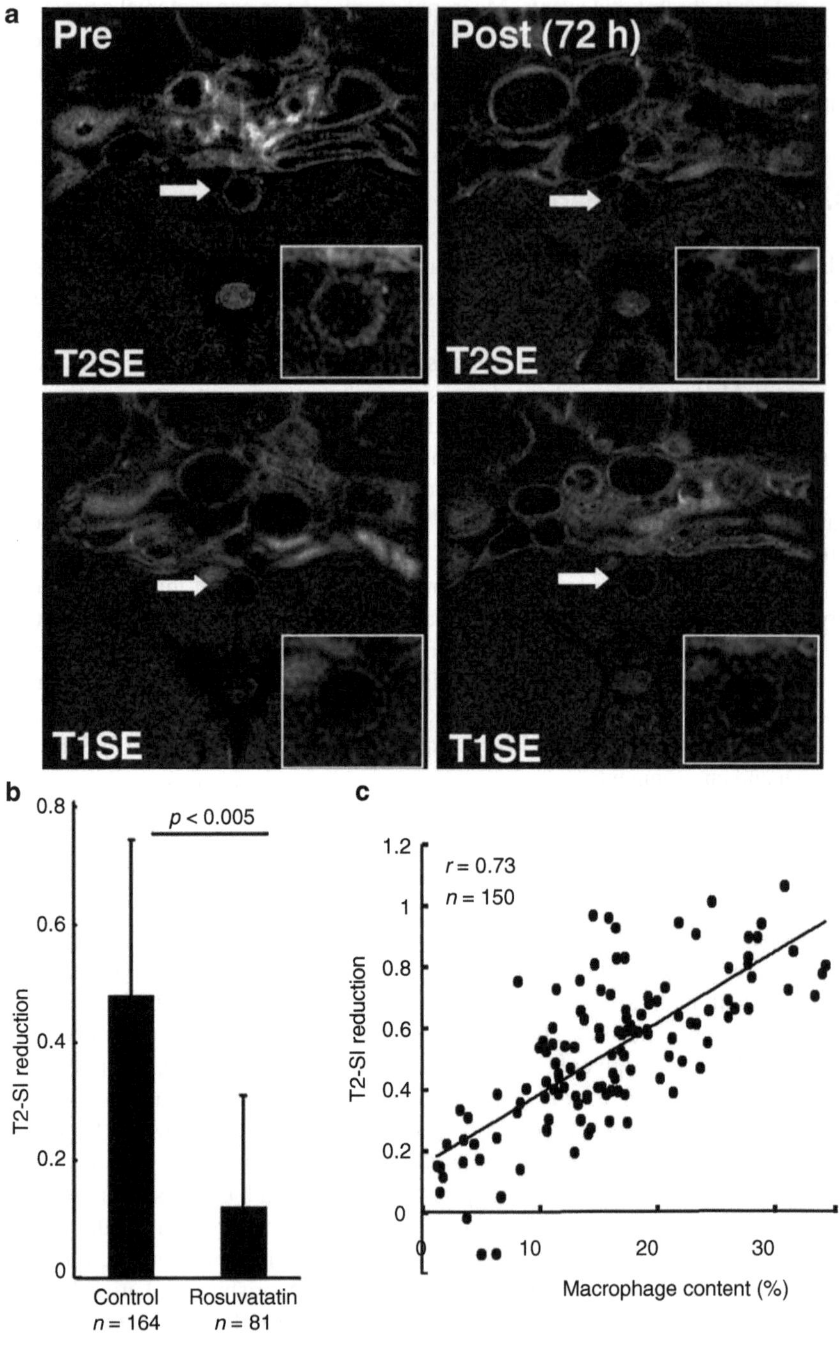

Fig. 3.1 Macrophage imaging in hyperlipidemic rabbits 6 months after balloon injury of the aorta. (**a**) MR images taken 72 h after intravenous administration of the USPIO MION-47. MION-47 administration decreased T2 signals in the aorta (*upper right*), but did not affect T1 signals (*lower right*). (**b**) Effects of lipid-lowering therapy by rosuvastatin on T2 signal reductions. MION-47-induced reduction of T2 signals was decreased by 3 months of rosuvastatin treatment. (**c**) Correlation between T2 signal reduction in MRI and histologically determined macrophage accumulation (Edited from Ref. [7])

These iron-based nanoparticles could be modified with various proteins or fluorescences. USPIO modified with peptidic scavenger receptor-AI (SR-AI) ligand showed 3.5-fold higher accumulation into atherosclerotic plaques compared to non-conjugated USPIO [8]. Lectin-like oxLDL receptor 1 (LOX-1)-targeted USPIO co-localizes with LOX-1, macrophages, and MMP-9 in atherosclerotic plaque of apolipoprotein E-deficient (ApoE−/−) mice [9]. USPIO already has been tested in humans and reported to be useful to monitor the effects of statins in carotid artery plaques [10, 11].

How these small nanoparticles are taken up by tissue macrophages or peripheral blood monocytes remains incompletely understood. Relatively large particles are taken up by phagocytosis, but the uptake of small-sized (<100 nm) particles may involve other mechanisms. For example, the uptake of cross-linked dextran iron oxide nanoparticles (CLIO) is not inhibited by phagocytosis inhibitor, cytochalasin D, but inhibited by macropinocytosis inhibitor, amiloride [5, 12]. These results suggest that these particles are taken up by macropinocytosis by monocytes/macrophages.

3.5 Macrophage Imaging by Nuclear Medicine

Nuclear medicine is one the promising modalities to visualize macrophage burden and activity in atherosclerotic plaques in patients and has dominated the field of clinical molecular imaging. PET with ^{18}F-fluorodeoxyglucose (FDG-PET) visualizes cells with active glucose metabolism, although a recent study challenged this theory by demonstrating that hypoxia promotes macrophage uptake of FDG [13]. Validation studies used histological assessment to positively correlate high FDG signals with greater macrophage accumulation [14]. Clinical studies have established that FDG-PET monitors therapeutic effects of various drugs on macrophage-rich carotid arteries, suggesting that FDG serves as a biomarker of the inflammatory burden of atherosclerotic plaques [15–18]. Interestingly, one of these studies reported that FDG-PET detected a reduction of FDG uptake as early as 4 weeks after statin treatment. The advantage that ^{18}FDG systemically circulates enables imaging of various tissues in the same patient. Bucerius et al. reported significant correlations between obesity, fat tissue inflammation, and vascular inflammation by imaging fat tissue and carotid/ascending arteries at the same time [19]. In several reports on diabetic patients, pioglitazone, an agonist of peroxisome proliferator-activated receptor-γ (PPAR-γ), reduced inflammation evaluated by FDG-PET/CT in human coronary arteries or aorta [20, 21]. Arterial FDG uptake is affected by blood glucose level before scanning and FDG circulation time [22]. Therefore, imaging protocols should be optimized for each target vessel to obtain sufficient ^{18}FDG signals.

Preclinical research has continued to actively study FDG-PET. For example, Nishimura et al. compared images of intravascular ultrasound (IVUS) and FDG-PET with histological images and reported that FDG-PET can detect foamy macrophages in atherosclerotic plaques in Watanabe heritable hyperlipidemic (WHHL) rabbits [23]. Vucic et al. reported that FDG-PET/CT evaluated anti-inflammatory effects of liver X receptor (LXR) agonist R211945 in hyperlipidemic New Zealand white rabbits [24]. Millon et al. compared sensitivity of FDG-PET and MRI with USPIO. They monitored the effects of atorvastatin on vascular inflammation and found that FDG-PET is more sensitive to detect early changes in atherosclerotic lesions [25].

Active research also has focused on the development of new FDG agents. ^{11}C-PK11195, which binds to peripheral benzodiazepine receptors (PBRs) expressed by macrophages, has been tested in a clinical trial using PET-CT as an imaging agent for plaque macrophages [26]. The study involves patients with symptomatic or asymptomatic carotid stenosis. Signals were correlated with macrophage content in carotid endarterectomy specimens and higher in symptomatic stenosis. Furthermore, new radionuclides targeting mannose receptor are reported [27]. Mannose receptors expressed on a subset of the macrophage population in high-risk plaques may be good targets for macrophage imaging. 2-deoxy-2-[^{18}F]fluoro-D-mannose (^{18}F-FDM) were taken up by cultured macrophages more efficiently than ^{18}F-FDG, suggesting that ^{18}F-FDM serves as a novel macrophage-targeting tracer [27]. Beer et al. reported PET/CT imaging which targets integrin $\alpha v\beta 3$. [^{18}F]Galacto-RGD, a novel tracer specifically binding to $\alpha v\beta 3$ integrin, increased the target/background ratio in human carotid arteries with stenosis [28]. The target/background ratio significantly correlated with histologically examined $\alpha v\beta 3$ expression. Seo et al. reported a novel tracer ^{64}Cu-Labeled LyP-1-Dendrimer. LyP-1, a cyclic 9-amino acid peptide, recognizes and binds to p32 proteins on activated macrophages. This tracer accumulated in atherosclerotic plaques in ApoE−/−mice [29]. Hatori et al. reported N-benzyl-N-methyl-2-[7,8-dihydro-7-(2-[^{18}F]fluoroethyl)-8-oxo-2-phenyl-9H-purin-9-yl]acetamide([^{18}F]FEDAC). This tracer is delivered to macrophages and neutrophils in a rat acute liver damage model [30].

3.6 Imaging of Macrophage-Derived Proteases in Atherosclerotic Plaques

Extracellular matrix such as collagen enables atherosclerotic plaques to withstand hemodynamic stresses. Matrix metalloproteinase (MMP) and cathepsins, mainly produced by plaque macrophages or smooth muscle cells, may promote plaque instability by degrading extracellular matrix. Therefore, imaging of protease activity should help to screen high-risk vessels in clinical settings. Enzyme-activatable NIRF imaging probes (excitation/emission wavelength between 600 and 900 nm) have been used to visualize proteolytic activity. Such probes have a protease-specific quenched substrate, inserted between fluorescence and carrier vehicle. Once the substrate is cleaved by target proteinases (MMP, cathepsin, etc.), the probe elaborates NIRF signals (activated state). Due to its tissue penetration, NIRF imaging has been developed to visualize inflammation in deep tissues. We used mouse models of atherosclerosis to demonstrate the feasibility of visualizing macrophage-derived MMP activity and evaluating changes due to the pharmacological inhibition (Fig. 3.2) [2, 31]. The evidence suggests that macrophage accumulation promotes cardiovascular calcification, as established by molecular imaging [32].

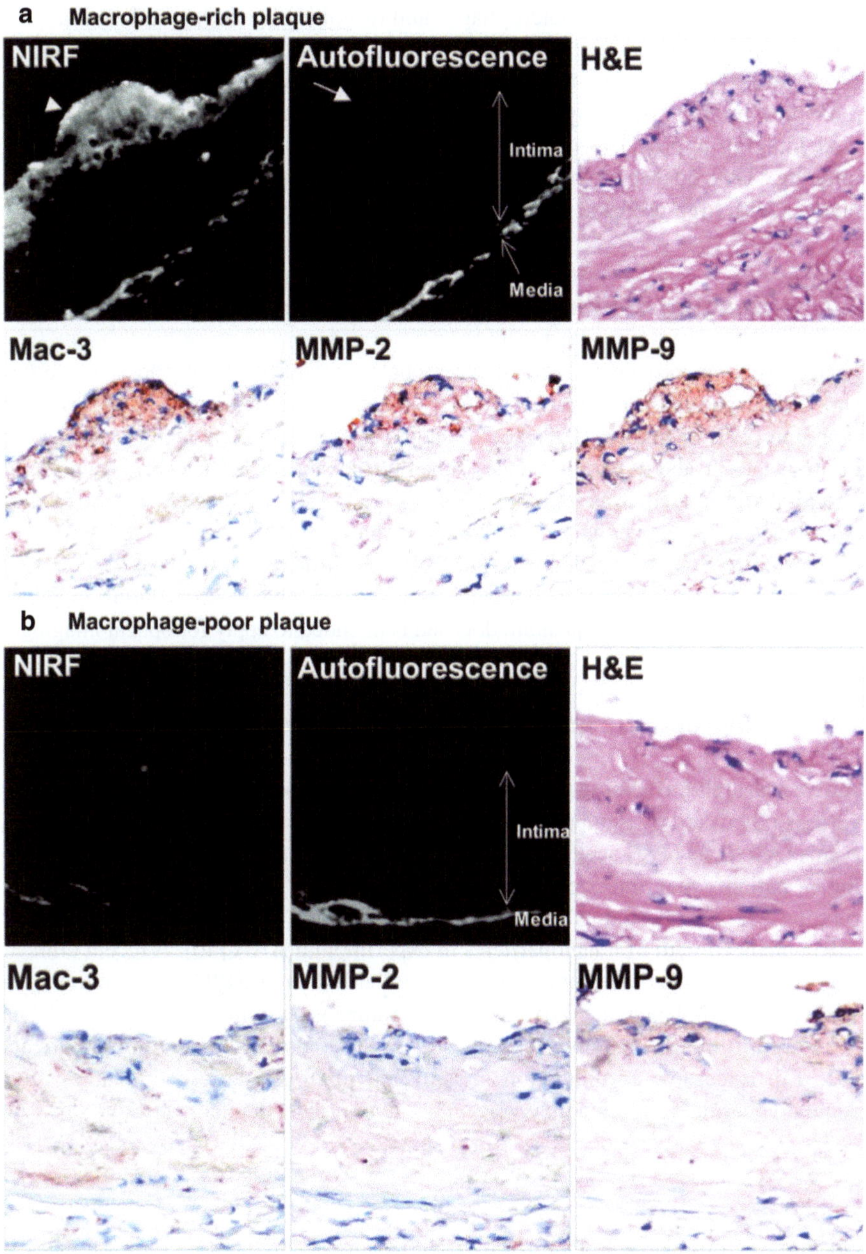

Fig. 3.2 Visualization of MMP activity by NIRF imaging in the aorta of ApoE−/− mice. Imaging agent, which is activated by gelatinase (MMP-2, MMP-9) and emits NIRF signal was injected 24 h before imaging. (**a**) In a macrophage-rich plaque, NIRF signal was detected in Mac-3-positive macrophages (*arrowhead*). Autofluorescence was observed in the media, but not in the intima (*arrow*). (**b**) NIRF imaging in a macrophage-poor plaque (Cited from Ref. [2])

NIRF imaging can co-map macrophages and osteoblastic activity and evaluate the effects of genetic manipulations or pharmacologic interventions (Fig. 3.3) [33, 34]. More recently, the Jaffer and Tearney groups have developed an intravascular molecular imaging modality [35, 36]. This technology involves a catheter-assisted dual imaging approach – optical frequency domain imaging (OFDI) and NIRF imaging. This dual-modality intra-arterial catheter can visualize atherosclerotic plaques with high protease activity in a hyperlipidemic rabbit model.

3.7 Imaging of Plaque Macrophages by HDL-Based Probes

High-density lipoprotein (HDL) mediates cholesterol efflux from cholesterol ester-enriched plaque macrophages and transfers the excessive cholesterol to the liver for excretion [37]. Therefore, HDL-based imaging agents have a possibility to visualize macrophages in atherosclerotic plaques. Macrophage-specific MRI contrast agent based on Gd-modified HDL was tested in ApoE−/− mice [38]. This agent accumulated in atherosclerotic plaque in the aorta 24 h after administration. Marrache et al. used a biodegradable HDL nanoparticle platform for the detection of macrophage apoptosis by targeting the collapse of mitochondrial membrane potential that occurs during apoptosis [39]. This particle contains quantum dots and is intended to apply for optical imaging.

3.8 Macrophage Imaging in Other Cardiovascular Diseases

Active research has attempted to establish imaging modalities for inflammation in various other cardiovascular diseases. The pathogenesis of aortic abdominal aneurysms (AAA) involves accumulation of activated macrophages. Macrophage imaging in patients may thus help identify high-risk aneurysms that may enlarge and rupture. Preclinical studies reported the feasibility of detecting macrophages by MRI enhanced with iron nanoparticles in experimental AAA [40]. A recent clinical study demonstrated that a similar approach with MRI and USPIO (ferumoxtran) can visualize macrophages in AAA and predict future growth [41]. FDG-PET/CT has been used to image macrophages in aortic or cervical artery dissection in patients [42, 43]. Excessive accumulation of activated microglia and macrophages after acute myocardial infarction may worsen tissue injuries. An interesting study by Lee

→

Fig. 3.3 Antibody blockade of the Notch ligand Delta-like 4 (*Dll4*) reduces aortic and valvular calcification in Ldlr−/− mice. (**a**) Histological assays for alkaline phosphatase activity (*top*) and calcium deposit demonstrate that Dll4 antibody administration reduced calcification in the aortas of fat-fed Ldl−/− mice. (**b**) NIRF imaging co-localized macrophages and osteogenic activity in excised aortas of Ldlr−/− mice. Dll4 blockade diminished macrophage accumulation and osteogenic activity in parallel. (**c**) Dll4 suppression reduced osteogenic activity in aortic valves of Ldl−/− mice (Cited from Ref. [34])

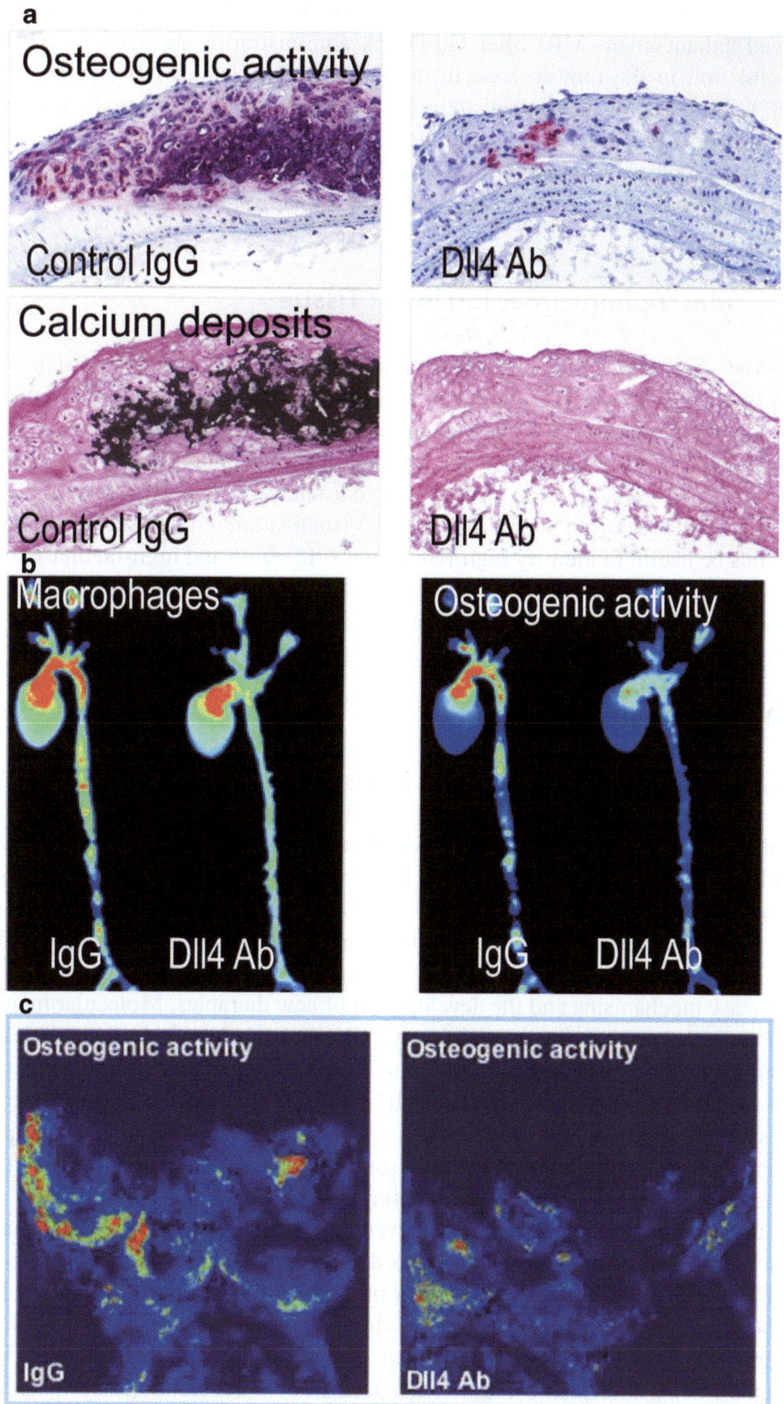
a
Osteogenic activity
Control IgG
Dll4 Ab
Calcium deposits
Control IgG
Dll4 Ab
b
Macrophages
IgG
Dll4 Ab
Osteogenic activity
IgG
Dll4 Ab
c
Osteogenic activity
IgG
Osteogenic activity
Dll4 Ab

et al. demonstrated that PET/MR imaging involving FDG-PET combined with delayed enhancement MRI after Gd-DTPA administration detected macrophage accumulation in the remote zone in infarcted hearts. Using MRI enhanced with USPIO (ferumoxytol), a clinical study showed the feasibility of visualizing macrophages after acute myocardial infarction [44]. Schroeter et al. used PET with a double tracer strategy involving ^{11}C-PK11195 and FDG to image activated microglia and macrophages in peri-infarct zones after ischemic stroke [45].

3.9 Macrophage Imaging in Fat Tissue

Recent studies suggest that fat tissue inflammation causes insulin resistance and plays important roles in the pathogenesis of metabolic syndrome [46]. Metabolic overload induces adipocyte enlargement, oxidative stress, and production of adipocytokines. These responses cause macrophage-mediated inflammation and a vicious cycle of chronic inflammation. Metabolic syndrome is recognized as one of the risk factors for atherosclerotic vascular diseases. Visualization of fat tissue inflammation may thus be useful to identify high-risk patients. In *ob/ob* and high-fat diet-induced obese mice, real-time in vivo imaging system visualized dynamic interaction between macrophage and other types of cells in fat tissues [47].

3.10 Future Perspectives

All cardiovascular diseases mentioned in this article are global health threats. We have summarized the status of preclinical and clinical development of molecular imaging of macrophages targeting such devastating diseases. In the last several decades, tremendous efforts have used histopathology, molecular and cell biology, and animal experiments to explore the mechanisms by which inflammation promotes cardiovascular disorders. Effective therapies for these diseases remain limited. Macrophage imaging, particularly in humans, would provide new insight into the disease mechanisms and the development of new therapies. Molecular imaging, particularly by noninvasive modalities, should help to identify subclinical lesions rich in activated macrophages and initiate an intense anti-inflammatory therapy as an example of personalized medicine. In addition, macrophage imaging may be used in the near future to monitor changes in vascular inflammation during clinical trials for new therapies, contributing to establishing more cost-effective and shorter clinical drug development. Whether imaging as a biomarker can add additional benefits to the current strategies using conventional risk markers, however, remains uncertain. In addition, each modality has advantages and disadvantages. Thus, the combined use of multiple modalities may play a major role in clinical imaging [48]. Furthermore, as we have witnessed in the last decade, active multidisciplinary research facilitates technological advancements of molecular imaging. More dynamic cross-sector collaboration may speed clinical translation of new technologies and preclinical findings.

References

1. Libby P, Aikawa M. Stabilization of atherosclerotic plaques: new mechanisms and clinical targets. Nat Med. 2002;8(11):1257–62. doi:10.1038/nm1102-1257.
2. Deguchi J, Aikawa M, Tung CH, Aikawa E, Kim DE, Ntziachristos V, Weissleder R, Libby P. Inflammation in atherosclerosis: visualizing matrix metalloproteinase action in macrophages in vivo. Circulation. 2006;114(1):55–62. doi:10.1161/CIRCULATIONAHA.106.619056.
3. Sukhova GK, Shi GP, Simon DI, Chapman HA, Libby P. Expression of the elastolytic cathepsins S and K in human atheroma and regulation of their production in smooth muscle cells. J Clin Invest. 1998;102(3):576–83. doi:10.1172/JCI181.
4. Libby P. The molecular mechanisms of the thrombotic complications of atherosclerosis. J Intern Med. 2008;263(5):517–27. doi:10.1111/j.1365-2796.2008.01965.x.
5. Weissleder R, Nahrendorf M, Pittet MJ. Imaging macrophages with nanoparticles. Nat Mater. 2014;13(2):125–38. doi:10.1038/nmat3780.
6. Oikawa M, Ota H, Takaya N, Miller Z, Hatsukami TS, Yuan C. Carotid magnetic resonance imaging. A window to study atherosclerosis and identify high-risk plaques. Circ J Off J Jpn Circ Soc. 2009;73(10):1765–73.
7. Morishige K, Kacher DF, Libby P, Josephson L, Ganz P, Weissleder R, Aikawa M. High-resolution magnetic resonance imaging enhanced with superparamagnetic nanoparticles measures macrophage burden in atherosclerosis. Circulation. 2010;122(17):1707–15. doi:10.1161/CIRCULATIONAHA.109.891804.
8. Segers FM, den Adel B, Bot I, van der Graaf LM, van der Veer EP, Gonzalez W, Raynal I, de Winther M, Wodzig WK, Poelmann RE, van Berkel TJ, van der Weerd L, Biessen EA. Scavenger receptor-AI-targeted iron oxide nanoparticles for in vivo MRI detection of atherosclerotic lesions. Arterioscler Thromb Vasc Biol. 2013;33(8):1812–9. doi:10.1161/ATVBAHA.112.300707.
9. Wen S, Liu DF, Cui Y, Harris SS, Chen YC, Li KC, Ju SH, Teng GJ. In vivo MRI detection of carotid atherosclerotic lesions and kidney inflammation in ApoE-deficient mice by using LOX-1 targeted iron nanoparticles. Nanomed Nanotechnol Biol Med. 2013. doi:10.1016/j.nano.2013.09.009.
10. Trivedi RA, U-King-Im JM, Graves MJ, Kirkpatrick PJ, Gillard JH. Noninvasive imaging of carotid plaque inflammation. Neurology. 2004;63(1):187–8.
11. Patterson AJ, Tang TY, Graves MJ, Muller KH, Gillard JH. In vivo carotid plaque MRI using quantitative T2* measurements with ultrasmall superparamagnetic iron oxide particles: a dose-response study to statin therapy. NMR Biomed. 2011;24(1):89–95. doi:10.1002/nbm.1560.
12. Araki N, Johnson MT, Swanson JA. A role for phosphoinositide 3-kinase in the completion of macropinocytosis and phagocytosis by macrophages. J Cell Biol. 1996;135(5):1249–60.
13. Folco EJ, Sheikine Y, Rocha VZ, Christen T, Shvartz E, Sukhova GK, Di Carli MF, Libby P. Hypoxia but not inflammation augments glucose uptake in human macrophages: Implications for imaging atherosclerosis with 18fluorine-labeled 2-deoxy-D-glucose positron emission tomography. J Am Coll Cardiol. 2011;58(6):603–14. doi:10.1016/j.jacc.2011.03.044.
14. Figueroa AL, Subramanian SS, Cury RC, Truong QA, Gardecki JA, Tearney GJ, Hoffmann U, Brady TJ, Tawakol A. Distribution of inflammation within carotid atherosclerotic plaques with high-risk morphological features: a comparison between positron emission tomography activity, plaque morphology, and histopathology. Circ Cardiovasc Imaging. 2012;5(1):69–77. doi:10.1161/CIRCIMAGING.110.959478.
15. Rudd JH, Narula J, Strauss HW, Virmani R, Machac J, Klimas M, Tahara N, Fuster V, Warburton EA, Fayad ZA, Tawakol AA. Imaging atherosclerotic plaque inflammation by fluorodeoxyglucose with positron emission tomography: ready for prime time? J Am Coll Cardiol. 2010;55(23):2527–35. doi:10.1016/j.jacc.2009.12.061.
16. Tahara N, Kai H, Nakaura H, Mizoguchi M, Ishibashi M, Kaida H, Baba K, Hayabuchi N, Imaizumi T. The prevalence of inflammation in carotid atherosclerosis: analysis with fluorodeoxyglucose-positron emission tomography. Eur Heart J. 2007;28(18):2243–8. doi:10.1093/eurheartj/ehm245.

17. Tahara N, Kai H, Yamagishi S, Mizoguchi M, Nakaura H, Ishibashi M, Kaida H, Baba K, Hayabuchi N, Imaizumi T. Vascular inflammation evaluated by [18F]-fluorodeoxyglucose positron emission tomography is associated with the metabolic syndrome. J Am Coll Cardiol. 2007;49(14):1533–9. doi:10.1016/j.jacc.2006.11.046.
18. Tawakol A, Fayad ZA, Mogg R, Alon A, Klimas MT, Dansky H, Subramanian SS, Abdelbaky A, Rudd JH, Farkouh ME, Nunes IO, Beals CR, Shankar SS. Intensification of statin therapy results in a rapid reduction in atherosclerotic inflammation: results of a multicenter fluorodeoxyglucose-positron emission tomography/computed tomography feasibility study. J Am Coll Cardiol. 2013;62(10):909–17. doi:10.1016/j.jacc.2013.04.066.
19. Bucerius J, Mani V, Wong S, Moncrieff C, Izquierdo-Garcia D, Machac J, Fuster V, Farkouh ME, Rudd JH, Fayad ZA. Arterial and fat tissue inflammation are highly correlated : a prospective F-FDG PET/CT study. Eur J Nucl Med Mol Imaging. 2014. doi:10.1007/s00259-013-2653-y.
20. Mizoguchi M, Tahara N, Tahara A, Nitta Y, Kodama N, Oba T, Mawatari K, Yasukawa H, Kaida H, Ishibashi M, Hayabuchi N, Harada H, Ikeda H, Yamagishi S, Imaizumi T. Pioglitazone attenuates atherosclerotic plaque inflammation in patients with impaired glucose tolerance or diabetes a prospective, randomized, comparator-controlled study using serial FDG PET/CT imaging study of carotid artery and ascending aorta. JACC Cardiovasc Imaging. 2011;4(10):1110–8. doi:10.1016/j.jcmg.2011.08.007.
21. Nitta Y, Tahara N, Tahara A, Honda A, Kodama N, Mizoguchi M, Kaida H, Ishibashi M, Hayabuchi N, Ikeda H, Yamagishi S, Imaizumi T. Pioglitazone decreases coronary artery inflammation in impaired glucose tolerance and diabetes mellitus: evaluation by FDG-PET/CT imaging. JACC Cardiovasc Imaging. 2013;6(11):1172–82. doi:10.1016/j.jcmg.2013.09.004.
22. Bucerius J, Mani V, Moncrieff C, Machac J, Fuster V, Farkouh ME, Tawakol A, Rudd JH, Fayad ZA. Optimizing (18)F-FDG PET/CT imaging of vessel wall inflammation: the impact of (18)F-FDG circulation time, injected dose, uptake parameters, and fasting blood glucose levels. Eur J Nucl Med Mol Imaging. 2014;41(2):369–83. doi:10.1007/s00259-013-2569-6.
23. Ishino S, Ogawa M, Mori I, Nishimura S, Ikeda S, Sugita T, Oikawa T, Horiguchi T, Magata Y. F-FDG PET and intravascular ultrasonography (IVUS) images compared with histology of atherosclerotic plaques: F-FDG accumulates in foamy macrophages. Eur J Nucl Med Mol Imaging. 2013. doi:10.1007/s00259-013-2635-0.
24. Vucic E, Calcagno C, Dickson SD, Rudd JH, Hayashi K, Bucerius J, Moshier E, Mounessa JS, Roytman M, Moon MJ, Lin J, Ramachandran S, Tanimoto T, Brown K, Kotsuma M, Tsimikas S, Fisher EA, Nicolay K, Fuster V, Fayad ZA. Regression of inflammation in atherosclerosis by the LXR agonist R211945: a noninvasive assessment and comparison with atorvastatin. JACC Cardiovasc Imaging. 2012;5(8):819–28. doi:10.1016/j.jcmg.2011.11.025.
25. Millon A, Dickson SD, Klink A, Izquierdo-Garcia D, Bini J, Lancelot E, Ballet S, Robert P, Mateo de Castro J, Corot C, Fayad ZA. Monitoring plaque inflammation in atherosclerotic rabbits with an iron oxide (P904) and (18)F-FDG using a combined PET/MR scanner. Atherosclerosis. 2013;228(2):339–45. doi:10.1016/j.atherosclerosis.2013.03.019.
26. Gaemperli O, Shalhoub J, Owen DRJ, Lamare F, Johansson S, Fouladi N, Davies AH, Rimoldi OE, Camici PG. Imaging intraplaque inflammation in carotid atherosclerosis with C-11-PK11195 positron emission tomography/computed tomography. Eur Heart J. 2012;33(15):1902–10. doi:10.1093/eurheartj/ehr367.
27. Tahara N, Mukherjee J, de Haas HJ, Petrov AD, Tawakol A, Haider N, Tahara A, Constantinescu CC, Zhou J, Boersma HH, Imaizumi T, Nakano M, Finn A, Fayad Z, Virmani R, Fuster V, Bosca L, Narula J. 2-deoxy-2-[F]fluoro-d-mannose positron emission tomography imaging in atherosclerosis. Nat Med. 2014. doi:10.1038/nm.3437.
28. Beer AJ, Pelisek J, Heider P, Saraste A, Reeps C, Metz S, Seidl S, Kessler H, Wester HJ, Eckstein HH, Schwaiger M. PET/CT imaging of integrin alphavbeta3 expression in human carotid atherosclerosis. JACC Cardiovasc Imaging. 2014. doi:10.1016/j.jcmg.2013.12.003.
29. Seo JW, Baek H, Mahakian LM, Kusunose J, Hamzah J, Ruoslahti E, Ferrara KW. Cu-labeled LyP-1-dendrimer for PET-CT imaging of atherosclerotic plaque. Bioconjug Chem. 2014. doi:10.1021/bc400347s.

30. Hatori A, Yui J, Xie L, Yamasaki T, Kumata K, Fujinaga M, Wakizaka H, Ogawa M, Nengaki N, Kawamura K, Zhang MR. Visualization of acute liver damage induced by cycloheximide in rats using PET with [(18)F]FEDAC, a radiotracer for translocator protein (18 kDa). PLoS One. 2014;9(1):e86625. doi:10.1371/journal.pone.0086625.
31. Quillard T, Tesmenitsky Y, Croce K, Travers R, Shvartz E, Koskinas KC, Sukhova GK, Aikawa E, Aikawa M, Libby P. Selective inhibition of matrix metalloproteinase-13 increases collagen content of established mouse atherosclerosis. Arterioscler Thromb Vasc Biol. 2011;31(11):2464–72. doi:10.1161/ATVBAHA.111.231563.
32. New SE, Aikawa E. Molecular imaging insights into early inflammatory stages of arterial and aortic valve calcification. Circ Res. 2011;108(11):1381–91. doi:10.1161/CIRCRESAHA.110.234146.
33. Aikawa E, Aikawa M, Libby P, Figueiredo JL, Rusanescu G, Iwamoto Y, Fukuda D, Kohler RH, Shi GP, Jaffer FA, Weissleder R. Arterial and aortic valve calcification abolished by elastolytic cathepsin S deficiency in chronic renal disease. Circulation. 2009;119(13):1785–94. doi:10.1161/CIRCULATIONAHA.108.827972.
34. Fukuda D, Aikawa E, Swirski FK, Novobrantseva TI, Kotelianski V, Gorgun CZ, Chudnovskiy A, Yamazaki H, Croce K, Weissleder R, Aster JC, Hotamisligil GS, Yagita H, Aikawa M. Notch ligand delta-like 4 blockade attenuates atherosclerosis and metabolic disorders. Proc Natl Acad Sci U S A. 2012;109(27):E1868–77. doi:10.1073/pnas.1116889109.
35. Yoo H, Kim JW, Shishkov M, Namati E, Morse T, Shubochkin R, McCarthy JR, Ntziachristos V, Bouma BE, Jaffer FA, Tearney GJ. Intra-arterial catheter for simultaneous microstructural and molecular imaging in vivo. Nat Med. 2011;17(12):1680–4. doi:10.1038/nm.2555.
36. Jaffer FA, Calfon MA, Rosenthal A, Mallas G, Razansky RN, Mauskapf A, Weissleder R, Libby P, Ntziachristos V. Two-dimensional intravascular near-infrared fluorescence molecular imaging of inflammation in atherosclerosis and stent-induced vascular injury. J Am Coll Cardiol. 2011;57(25):2516–26. doi:10.1016/j.jacc.2011.02.036.
37. Zheng C, Morishige K, Aikawa M. Functional molecular imaging linking macrophages to reverse cholesterol transport. Circ J Off J Jpn Circ Soc. 2013;77(6):1403–6.
38. Cormode DP, Frias JC, Ma Y, Chen W, Skajaa T, Briley-Saebo K, Barazza A, Williams KJ, Mulder WJ, Fayad ZA, Fisher EA. HDL as a contrast agent for medical imaging. Clin Lipidol. 2009;4(4):493–500. doi:10.2217/clp.09.38.
39. Marrache S, Dhar S. Biodegradable synthetic high-density lipoprotein nanoparticles for atherosclerosis. Proc Natl Acad Sci U S A. 2013;110(23):9445–50. doi:10.1073/pnas.1301929110.
40. Miyama N, Dua MM, Schultz GM, Kosuge H, Terashima M, Pisani LJ, Dalman RL, McConnell MV. Bioluminescence and magnetic resonance imaging of macrophage homing to experimental abdominal aortic aneurysms. Mol Imaging. 2012;11(2):126–34.
41. Richards JM, Semple SI, MacGillivray TJ, Gray C, Langrish JP, Williams M, Dweck M, Wallace W, McKillop G, Chalmers RT, Garden OJ, Newby DE. Abdominal aortic aneurysm growth predicted by uptake of ultrasmall superparamagnetic particles of iron oxide: a pilot study. Circ Cardiovasc Imaging. 2011;4(3):274–81. doi:10.1161/CIRCIMAGING.110.959866.
42. Pfefferkorn T, Saam T, Rominger A, Habs M, Gerdes LA, Schmidt C, Cyran C, Straube A, Linn J, Nikolaou K, Bartenstein P, Reiser M, Hacker M, Dichgans M. Vessel wall inflammation in spontaneous cervical artery dissection: a prospective, observational positron emission tomography, computed tomography, and magnetic resonance imaging study. Stroke J Cereb Circ. 2011;42(6):1563–8. doi:10.1161/STROKEAHA.110.599548.
43. Reeps C, Pelisek J, Bundschuh RA, Gurdan M, Zimmermann A, Ockert S, Dobritz M, Eckstein HH, Essler M. Imaging of acute and chronic aortic dissection by 18F-FDG PET/CT. J Nucl Med Off Publ Soc Nucl Med. 2010;51(5):686–91. doi:10.2967/jnumed.109.072298.
44. Alam SR, Shah AS, Richards J, Lang NN, Barnes G, Joshi N, MacGillivray T, McKillop G, Mirsadraee S, Payne J, Fox KA, Henriksen P, Newby DE, Semple SI. Ultrasmall superparamagnetic particles of iron oxide in patients with acute myocardial infarction: early clinical experience. Circ Cardiovasc Imaging. 2012;5(5):559–65. doi:10.1161/CIRCIMAGING.112.974907.

45. Schroeter M, Dennin MA, Walberer M, Backes H, Neumaier B, Fink GR, Graf R. Neuroinflammation extends brain tissue at risk to vital peri-infarct tissue: a double tracer [11C]PK11195- and [18F]FDG-PET study. J Cereb Blood Flow Metab Off J Int Soc Cereb Blood Flow Metab. 2009;29(6):1216–25. doi:10.1038/jcbfm.2009.36.
46. Donath MY, Dalmas E, Sauter NS, Boni-Schnetzler M. Inflammation in obesity and diabetes: islet dysfunction and therapeutic opportunity. Cell Metab. 2013;17(6):860–72. doi:10.1016/j.cmet.2013.05.001.
47. Nishimura S, Manabe I, Nagasaki M, Seo K, Yamashita H, Hosoya Y, Ohsugi M, Tobe K, Kadowaki T, Nagai R, Sugiura S. In vivo imaging in mice reveals local cell dynamics and inflammation in obese adipose tissue. J Clin Invest. 2008;118(2):710–21. doi:10.1172/JCI33328.
48. Jolesz FA. Intraoperative imaging in neurosurgery: where will the future take us? Acta Neurochir Suppl. 2011;109:21–5. doi:10.1007/978-3-211-99651-5_4.

Intravascular Molecular Imaging of Proteolytic Activity

4

Eric A. Osborn and Farouc A. Jaffer

Contents

E.A. Osborn
Cardiology Division, Cardiovascular Research Center, Massachusetts General Hospital, Harvard Medical School, Simches Research Building 3206, 185 Cambridge Street, Boston, MA 02114, USA

Cardiology Division, Beth Israel Deaconess Medical Center, Harvard Medical School, Boston, MA, USA

F.A. Jaffer, MD, PhD (✉)
Cardiology Division, Cardiovascular Research Center, Massachusetts General Hospital, Harvard Medical School, Simches Research Building 3206, 185 Cambridge Street, Boston, MA 02114, USA
e-mail: fjaffer@mgh.harvard.edu

E. Aikawa (ed.), *Cardiovascular Imaging: Arterial and Aortic Valve Inflammation and Calcification*, DOI 10.1007/978-3-319-09268-3_4

Abstract

Atherosclerotic plaque disruption leads to myocardial infarction and stroke, but current clinical diagnostic tests lack the ability to predict which patients will suffer these complications. New strategies to define high-risk plaque biology in vivo hold promise to differentiate stable from vulnerable atherosclerotic plaques. Plaque proteolytic activity has emerged as a key target for identifying vulnerable plaques given its association with plaque inflammation and role in mechanical destabilization of plaques. Protease activity can now be evaluated in vivo with intravascular molecular imaging, a leading technology to identify inflammation in high-risk atherosclerotic plaques in coronary-sized arteries. In particular, hybrid catheters combining micrometer-resolution optical frequency domain structural imaging and high-sensitivity near-infrared fluorescence molecular imaging are proving to be powerful tools to investigate plaque biology in living subjects with clear translational potential for human use. Ultimately, through additional validation in human clinical trials, intravascular imaging of proteolytic activity and inflammation could inform new treatment strategies for atherosclerotic vascular disease that are likely to have significant impact on cardiovascular health.

4.1 Background

Complications of atherosclerotic vascular disease, mainly evident as myocardial infarction and stroke, continue to be a leading cause of morbidity and mortality throughout the world [1]. Recent decades have witnessed major advances in the diagnosis and treatment of atherosclerosis, including the development of improved diagnostic tests and pharmacologic agents that have greatly improved clinical outcomes. Despite these significant gains, the ability to identify high-risk "vulnerable" atherosclerotic plaques in coronary arteries of patients remains elusive [2].

Traditionally, coronary atherosclerosis severity is determined with x-ray angiography by calculating the percent vessel lumen stenosis. A major pitfall of angiographic plaque risk assessment includes an inability to assess the atherosclerotic plaque beyond the lumen, which substantially limits its ability for plaque risk prediction. Before causing lumen narrowing, many plaques exhibit positive vessel remodeling in which the plaque expands outward while maintaining the lumen diameter [3]. Angiographic mild or moderately stenosed plaques may harbor high-risk features and are the suspected culprit lesions in the majority of acute coronary syndromes by autopsy studies [4].

Clinical intravascular imaging modalities such as intravascular ultrasound (IVUS) and optical coherence tomography (OCT) can visualize plaque structures beyond the lumen border outlined by angiography but are primarily able to describe plaque anatomy [5]. Therefore, stand-alone IVUS and OCT lack the ability to determine important biological aspects within the plaque that may promote vulnerability. While plaque structural composition can be discriminated further through analysis of the backscattered IVUS signal [6] or by near-infrared spectroscopy to identify lipid pools [7], the clinical use of these technologies remains under investigation.

Cardiovascular molecular imaging strategies, built on synergistic advances in chemistry, molecular biology, nanomaterials, and imaging technology, aim to move beyond anatomy and structure to characterize plaque biology in vivo [8,9]. In atherosclerosis, specialized molecular imaging agents that can detect high-risk vulnerable plaque features such as inflammation, neovascularization, apoptosis, and oxidative stress in preclinical studies have been developed on multiple imaging modalities including magnetic resonance imaging (MRI), positron emission tomography (PET), computed tomography (CT), and optical and ultrasound platforms. Increasingly, molecular imaging approaches are being translated to human cardiovascular clinical trials [10], primarily employing noninvasive 18-fluorodeoxyglucose (FDG) PET imaging to report on inflammation in large arteries (e.g., carotids, aorta). Although noninvasive approaches for coronary molecular imaging have been pursued [11,12], they are significantly limited by suboptimal spatial resolution and sensitivity. To overcome these obstacles, an intravascular molecular imaging approach that provides comprehensive plaque assessment could be invaluable.

Intravascular molecular imaging of important plaque biology, such as proteolytic activity that destabilizes plaque collagen and elastin, holds promise to enhance detection of high-risk coronary artery plaques and provide additive risk stratification that surpasses anatomic plaque burden. If high-risk plaques can be identified in advance, then preventative treatment with intensified medical therapy or mechanical interventions may be instituted earlier. The evolution of concerning plaques in response to treatment can then be followed by serial studies to determine stabilization of the high-risk phenotype. In this chapter, we discuss emerging intravascular imaging approaches to identify coronary plaque inflammatory protease activity in vivo using near-infrared fluorescence (NIRF) optical molecular reporters.

4.2 High-Risk Plaque Features

Atherosclerosis is a chronic, systemic, and progressive disease involving medium- to large-sized arteries in the cerebral, coronary, and peripheral beds [13]. Affected vessels develop lesions comprised of variable amounts of lipid, inflammatory cells, fibrous tissue, and calcium that can grow over time triggered by ongoing lipid deposition, oxidation, and local inflammation. Atherosclerotic plaques initiate at sites of low wall fluid shear stress and endothelial cell dysfunction, attracting circulating monocytes to migrate into the vessel wall and become activated tissue macrophages, the key cellular mediator of atherosclerotic plaque inflammation and progression. Chapter 1 provides additional detailed information on mechanisms of atherosclerotic plaque formation.

Once resident, atherosclerotic plaques are highly heterogeneous and encompass different risk phenotypes based on their underlying composition and biological framework [14,15]. Structurally, thin-cap fibroatheromas (TCFA) are the prototypical vulnerable plaques consisting of a dense lipid-rich core sealed by a thin,

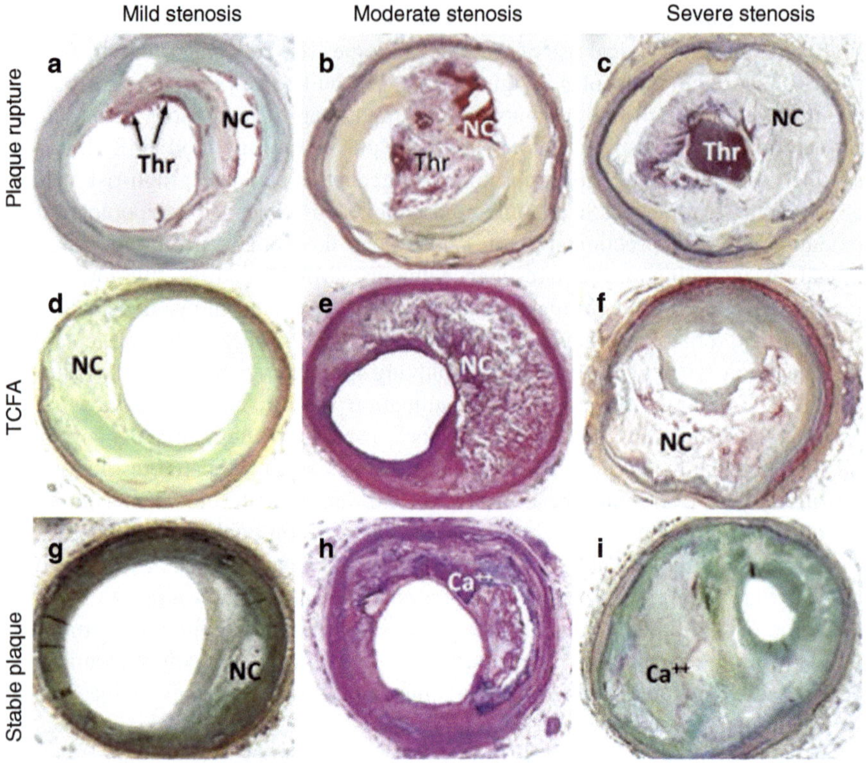

Fig. 4.1 Stable and unstable human coronary artery atherosclerotic plaque histopathology. Example cross-sectional photomicrographs from human coronary artery autopsy specimens with mild to severe luminal stenosis demonstrating plaque rupture, prototypical high-risk "vulnerable" plaques known as thin-cap fibroatheroma (*TCFA*), and stable plaques. Ruptured plaques exhibit intraluminal thrombus (*Thr*) that may be (**a**) nonocclusive, (**b**) partially occlusive, or (**c**) completely occlusive. (**d–f**) TCFA are notable for the presence of a large necrotic core (*NC*) separated from the lumen by a thin-walled fibrous cap, without intraluminal thrombus formation as observed in ruptured plaques. (**g–i**) Stable plaques, also known as fibroatheroma, reveal relatively smaller necrotic core with regional calcification (Ca^{++}) (Reprinted with permission from Narula et al. [15])

rupture-prone fibrotic cap (Fig. 4.1). Other types of high-risk lesions include plaque erosion, where the endothelium has denuded often with the formation of overlying thrombus, and superficial microscopic calcified nodules that can precipitate focal plaque disruption.

Biologically, autopsy studies following sudden cardiac death have identified enhanced inflammation, neovascularization, and apoptosis as histological markers associated with plaque disruption [4,16]. Inflammation is of particular interest given its potential as a treatment target in high-risk individuals. Macrophages function as the primary effector cells in inflamed atherosclerotic plaques, where they orchestrate the release of cytokines and proteases that cause plaque growth and destabilization and undergo apoptosis and necrosis to expand the necrotic core [17].

4.2.1 Plaque Proteolytic Activity

Proteases liberated from plaque macrophages have been heavily evaluated with respect to plaque vulnerability [18,19]. Precursor proteases mobilized to the macrophage surface become activated and mediate degradation of the collagen and elastin extracellular matrix network, thus structurally weakening the plaque in general and compromising the integrity of the overlying protective fibrotic cap [20]. This sequence of events has been implicated in the development and evolution of high-risk TCFA from more stable plaque phenotypes [21] and with mechanical instability of the rupture-prone fibrous cap shoulder regions that experience high wall stresses [22,23].

In vascular disease, activated serine and cysteine proteases, as well as matrix metalloproteinases (MMP), have been shown to be critical elements in plaque destabilization [19,24]. Histologic studies of inflamed plaques demonstrate overexpression of cathepsins, a family of cysteine proteases [25,26], and MMPs [18,27,28]. Given their association with plaque rupture and remodeling, proteases have proven to be a rich source of high-value plaque imaging targets [29–34], and hold particular promise as agents for intravascular coronary artery imaging applications [35].

4.3 Coronary Artery Molecular Imaging

Compared to larger-sized arteries, imaging the coronary arteries poses special challenges. First, most epicardial coronary arteries of interest are 2–4 mm luminal diameter necessitating imaging platforms with high spatial resolution to resolve local phenomena. To enable interrogation of individual plaques, resolution demands increase significantly, on the order of tens of micrometers. Second, cardiac and respiratory motion requires high temporal resolution systems and often gating to the electrocardiogram, in order to sample rapidly enough to avoid blurring. In comparison, large arteries such as the carotids are relatively fixed in space, making motion artifacts less problematic. Overall, meeting the stringent requirements for successful coronary artery imaging remains a major challenge.

4.3.1 Clinical Trials

Current efforts to apply molecular imaging strategies to human coronary arteries have employed noninvasive techniques with PET imaging of FDG and ^{18}F-sodium fluoride (NaF) to measure coronary plaque metabolism/inflammation and osteogenesis, respectively. FDG PET has preliminarily identified a subset of inflamed coronary plaques in pilot studies of patients with acute coronary syndromes, stable angina, and following coronary stenting (Fig. 4.2) [12,36–38]. NaF PET, historically used in bone scans, has more recently been employed in small studies to detect coronary artery osteogenesis in different patient populations and has the advantage of having minimal myocardial background uptake compared to FDG [11]. Ultrasmall

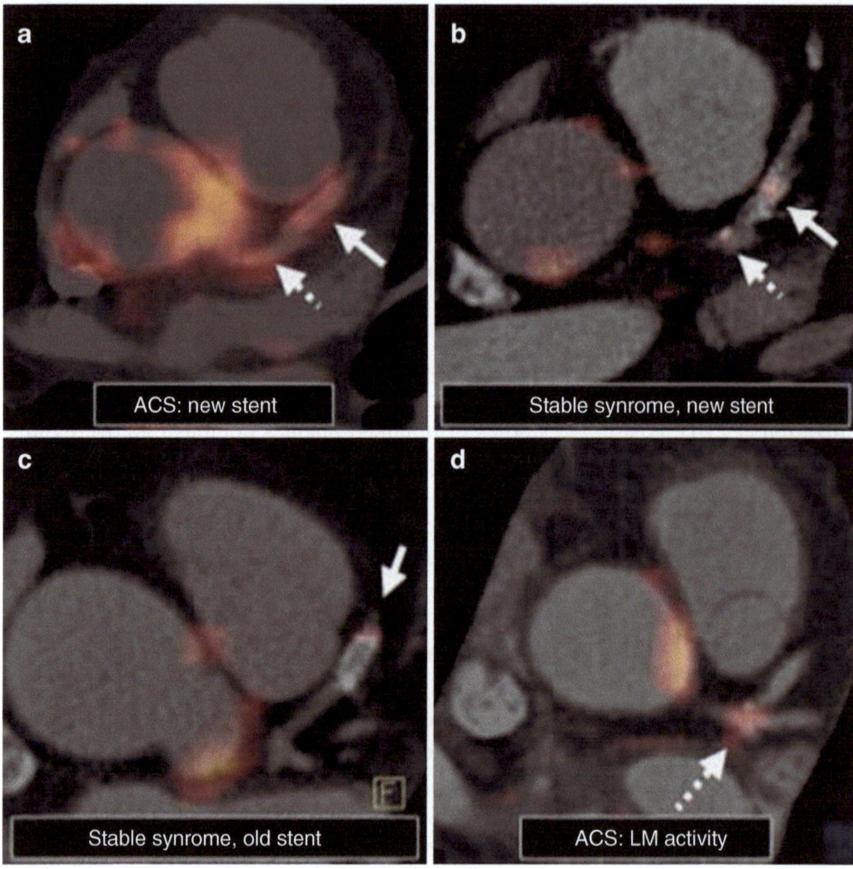

Fig. 4.2 Noninvasive coronary artery hybrid FDG-PET/CT imaging of inflammation in patients presenting with stable angina or acute coronary syndrome (*ACS*). (**a**, **d**) ACS subjects demonstrate increased FDG uptake in the left main (*LM*) coronary artery (*hatched arrows*) and at a newly placed stent (*solid arrows*). (**b**, **c**) While FDG activity is present in stable syndrome patients, it is of lower intensity than ACS. Furthermore, a more recently placed "healing" stent exhibits relatively greater FDG signal than an older "healed" stent that was implanted months earlier. *CT* computed tomography, *FDG* fluorodeoxyglucose, *PET* positron emission tomography (Reproduced with permission from Rogers et al. [12])

superparamagnetic iron oxide (USPIO) nanoparticles, another clinically tested macrophage-targeted agent detectable by MRI, have shown utility for large-artery inflammation imaging [39–41], but the relatively lower temporospatial resolution of MRI to image-small plaques in the highly dynamic coronary environment has limited its utility.

Coronary plaque imaging with FDG-PET and NaF-PET has important limitations, however, as they both possess lower spatial resolution and require ionizing radiation. Furthermore, due to intense FDG uptake in the highly metabolically active myocardium that obscures coronary wall FDG signal, only the left main and most proximal coronary artery segments can be reliably evaluated by FDG [12]. Attempts to suppress myocardial FDG uptake with high-fat dietary protocols have met moderate success [38], but still a significant number of segments remain uninterpretable.

Given the challenges of noninvasive clinical coronary molecular imaging, new approaches to evaluate coronary inflammation in vivo are being investigated. A particularly promising translational imaging technique that can detect inflammation and protease activity in coronary-sized arteries involves intravascular optical imaging using near-infrared fluorescence (NIRF) [42,43].

4.4 Intravascular NIRF Imaging

Offering high resolution and good sensitivity to fluorescence imaging agents, NIRF molecular imaging has advantageous technical specifications to enable atherosclerotic plaque imaging in coronary arteries. NIRF employs light wavelengths in the near-infrared window (700–900 nm) with relatively low blood absorbance and reduced tissue autofluorescence at a reasonable depth penetration [44,45]. These properties are highly favorable for intravascular NIRF imaging of the 2–4 mm diameter epicardial coronary arteries, which can be obtained through blood without the need to displace blood from the imaging field by vessel occlusion and flushing [46]. Furthermore, light-based NIRF imaging is safe and does not expose the patient to the hazards of ionizing radiation associated with CT and nuclear imaging (e.g., PET, SPECT). On the other hand, catheter placement for intravascular imaging carries risk to the subject (e.g., vessel spasm, perforation, dissection), and, therefore, decision tools for appropriate selection of patients that may benefit from intravascular NIRF imaging will be important for clinical translation of this technology.

NIRF has been utilized extensively in preclinical and clinical imaging studies in cardiovascular disease and oncology, illuminating important in vivo pathobiology not previously available for interrogation by structural imaging modalities. A broad and versatile range of NIRF molecular imaging agents have now been established, utilizing the latest advances in nanotechnology and bioengineering [10,47]. Specifically for atherothrombosis applications, in vivo NIRF agents have successfully exposed enhanced endothelial adhesion molecule expression, upregulated macrophage inflammation, thrombin activity, and plaque proteolysis.

4.4.1 Intravascular NIRF Imaging Platforms

Recent technological advances have witnessed a growing presence of optical intravascular imaging systems available for clinical use [5,35,48,49]. Currently, physicians have access to two FDA-approved catheters for light-based atherosclerosis imaging, optical coherence tomography (OCT), and near-infrared spectroscopy (NIRS). OCT, and its second-generation high-speed counterpart termed optical frequency domain imaging (OFDI), generates excellent axial resolution (~10 μm) structural images of the vessel wall by analyzing reflected near-infrared light [50]. OCT/OFDI can visualize all three layers of the artery wall, thrombus, stent struts, and plaques with lipid pools, calcification, and thin fibrous caps. OCT is limited by relatively arterial wall penetration depth (1–2 mm), and the need for a blood-free imaging field. NIRS is a newer spectroscopic approach that can identify lipid within the vessel wall based on near-infrared cholesterol absorbance patterns [51–53]. Since intravascular NIRF is also a light-based imaging approach utilizing flexible optical fibers that can be housed in a catheter design similar to the currently FDA-approved devices, the development of NIRF imaging catheter systems applicable for human coronary artery imaging is feasible. Recently, promising translational intravascular NIRF molecular imaging platforms have been developed and tested in vivo in large animal models of atherosclerosis and stent healing.

4.4.1.1 One-Dimensional In Vivo Intravascular NIRF Sensing

A first-generation intravascular NIRF imaging prototype was developed in 2008 to test the feasibility of detecting NIRF activity in living subjects [54]. This early system was constructed from a near-infrared optical sensing fiber that was manually pulled back through the vessel to identify local NIRF signal (Fig. 4.3). Performance characteristics demonstrated NIRF detection in a 40 μm diameter focal spot approximately 2 mm from the catheter imaging source. However, without automated translation and rotation capabilities, this one-dimensional NIRF system lacked comprehensive 360° vessel NIRF detection and therefore could only collect data from a localized sector of the vessel wall. In addition, this stand-alone NIRF imaging system did not provide anatomic information and therefore required the use of a sequential structural intravascular imaging platform (e.g., IVUS, OCT/OFDI) to attempt localizing NIRF signal to endovascular regions of interest.

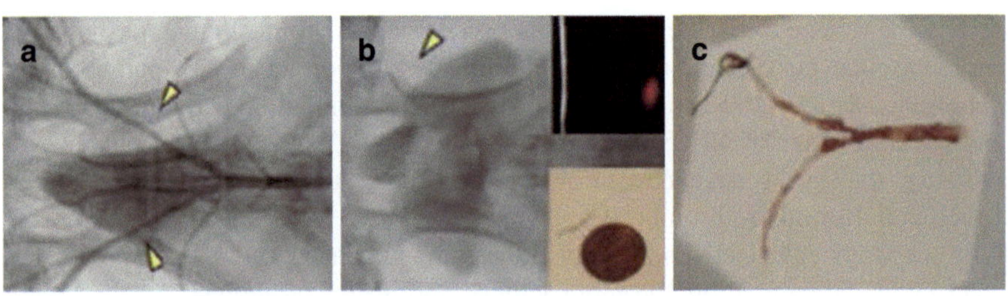

Fig. 4.3 One-dimensional intravascular NIRF catheter prototype. (**a**) Atherosclerotic-prone rabbits developed iliac artery plaques (*arrowheads*) following balloon injury. (**b**) A 90° NIRF-sensing guidewire without rotational capability (*lower inset*), fabricated to specifications of 0.48 mm/0.019 inch maximum outer diameter with a 0.036 mm/0.014 inch radiopaque tip, was easily maneuvered across the stenoses within the iliac artery (*arrowhead*). As a working distance of 2±1 mm, phantom testing revealed a 40±15 μm NIRF spot size (*upper inset*). (**c**) Resected tissue grossly confirms the presence of iliac atherosclerosis in the balloon-injured areas (Reproduced with permission from Jaffer et al. [54])

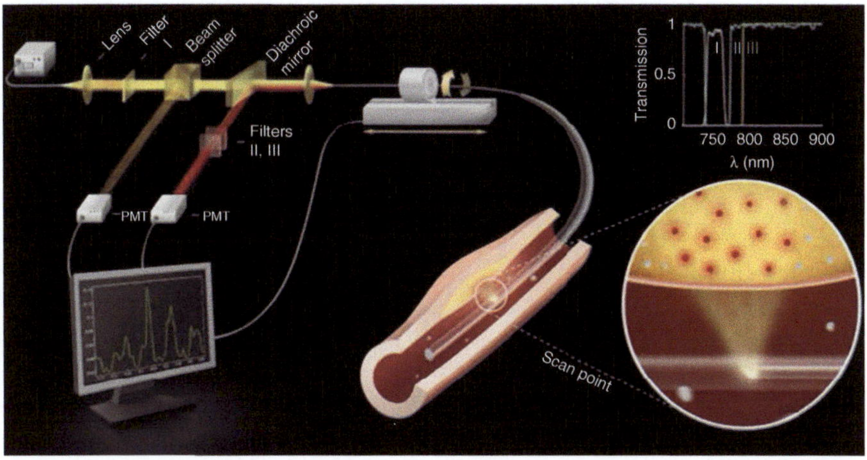

Fig. 4.4 Two-dimensional intravascular NIRF catheter schematic. Near-infrared light is delivered from a laser through specialized optical fibers within the catheter and then redirected 90° by a coated prism at the fiber tip to illuminate the artery wall (*bottom right circular inset*). Fluorescent light emissions from molecules excited by the near-infrared laser are collected via the prism, transmitted through the fiber, filtered by wavelength-selective mirrors (*top right inset* show filter spectra), and detected by a photomultiplier tube (*PMT*) for computer display and analysis. The catheter position is controlled by an automated pullback motor with rotational and translational capabilities (Reproduced with permission from Jaffer et al. [46])

4.4.1.2 Two-Dimensional In Vivo Intravascular NIRF Imaging

To overcome the lack of circumferential NIRF detection and inability for precise longitudinal anatomic localization in the one-dimensional NIRF catheter design, a second-generation NIRF imaging system was engineered [46]. This two-dimensional NIRF catheter was coupled to computer-controlled motors for automatic 360° rotation and 0.5 mm/s translation pullback (Fig. 4.4). In fluorescent phantom experiments submerged in an artificial blood-like media, the two-dimensional NIRF system had an angular resolution of 35–42° (i.e., ability to resolve >8 sectors) and longitudinal resolution of 1.0 mm at catheter-to-phantom distances of 3.0 and 2.0 mm, respectively. Although the two-dimensional intravascular NIRF imaging system marked a major step forward toward achieving detailed, comprehensive plaque characterization, it suffered from the same drawback as the one-dimensional NIRF prototype – being a stand-alone modality without accompanying structural imaging information.

4.4.1.3 In Vivo Intravascular NIRF-OFDI Molecular-Structural Imaging

In a major advance for intravascular NIRF imaging, NIRF was recently paired with OCT/OFDI in a hybrid catheter system to overcome the limitations of earlier one- and two-dimensional stand-alone NIRF catheter systems [55]. As intravascular NIRF imaging lacks anatomical information, the addition of exactly co-registered

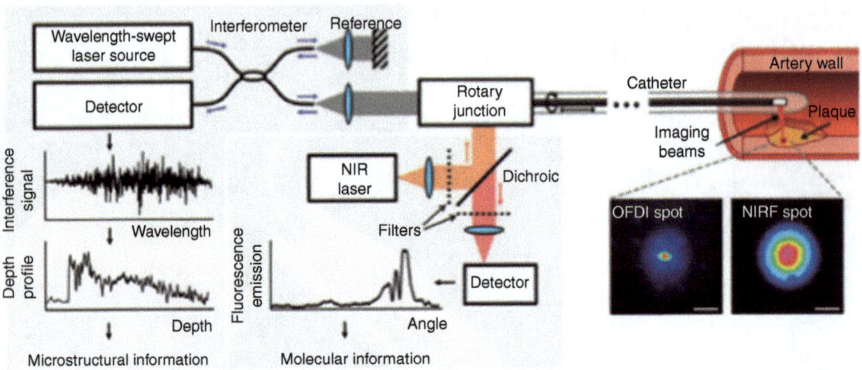

Fig. 4.5 Integrated NIRF-OFDI molecular-structural imaging catheter design. Coupled by a custom-engineered rotary junction to allow automated rotation and translation, NIRF and OFDI imaging systems are combined within a specialized dual-clad optical fiber housed in a clinical-grade intravascular imaging catheter to simultaneously deliver NIRF and OFDI laser light to image the artery wall. The dual-clad fiber contains concentric rings with different optical properties to separate the NIRF and OFDI light paths, and a custom-fabricated ball lens at the fiber tip that focuses incident light to a small spot and redirects it 90° into the tissue (scale bars, 100 μm). Returning light from the tissue collected by the ball lens is transmitted through the optical fiber and selectively filtered for detection by sensitive photomultipliers. OFDI microstructural information (depth profile) is constructed by analyzing the interference pattern between the back-reflected light with a reference arm as the laser wavelength source is rapidly cycled. Quantitative NIRF molecular information (fluorescence emission) is simultaneously acquired at every OFDI depth profile acquisition (Reproduced with permission from Yoo et al. [55])

OFDI allows precise mapping of the local NIRF signal with plaque microstructure. The design of the NIRF-OFDI system employs specialized fiber optics that can simultaneously transmit NIRF through the outer fiber cladding and OFDI through the central core. The distal end of the imaging fiber is coupled to a hand-drawn ball lens that directs light into the tissues at 90° to the optical fiber axis. At the back end, the optical fiber is coupled to the image-processing interface by a customized rotary junction that allows high-speed image acquisition simultaneously from both NIRF and OFDI channels during catheter pullback (Fig. 4.5). In benchmark testing, the NIRF-OFDI system performance was excellent at approximately 7 and 30 μm axial and transverse resolution, respectively, 25.4 frames per second image acquisition, up to 20 mm per second automated pullback speed, a 4.6 mm imaging field depth in saline, and <1 nM sensitivity for near-infrared fluorochromes. Overall, the NIRF-OFDI imaging system offers distinct advantages for enhanced diagnosis over either imaging platform alone and holds great promise for clinical use.

4.4.1.4 In Vivo Intravascular NIRF-IVUS Imaging

New catheter designs pairing intravascular NIRF with IVUS are also being developed, given the longstanding experience with IVUS in modern-day cardiac catheterization laboratories, where IVUS has been the clinical standard intravascular imaging modality [56,57]. Furthermore, NIRF-IVUS holds technical advantages over NIRF-OFDI in certain areas, despite OFDI exhibiting higher spatial resolution than IVUS. Compared to OCT/OFDI that requires rapid flushing with saline or, more commonly, iodinated contrast to displace blood from the imaging field, both IVUS and NIRF can image the vessel wall through blood without the need for flushing. Eliminating coronary artery flushing by using a NIRF-IVUS system can be time saving, decreases the small incremental risk of vessel trauma and arrhythmias associated with flushing, and lessens the overall contrast load that can result in acute kidney injury. Furthermore, IVUS has improved tissue depth penetration over OCT/OFDI and the ability to image coronary ostia that cannot be evaluated with OCT/OFDI due to difficulty effectively flushing blood from these locations. In evaluation of the left main coronary artery, these characteristics give IVUS a distinct competitive advantage over OCT/OFDI [58].

4.4.2 Intravascular NIRF Imaging Applications to Atherosclerosis

NIRF molecular imaging has the ability to uncover critical in vivo biological aspects of high-risk, "vulnerable" atherosclerotic plaques. The fundamental assumption underlying this approach to plaque imaging is that through in vivo detection of high-risk features previously linked to plaque rupture and progression by detailed histopathology that the morbidity and mortality associated with atherosclerosis complications may be lessened through early pharmacological or mechanical interventions. For example, these interventions may take the form of more aggressive medical management with traditional lipid-lowering agents or employ new anti-inflammatory and plaque-stabilizing therapeutics currently being benchmarked in preclinical and early phase clinical trials. In select cases, there may be opportunities for invasive treatment with catheter-based local drug delivery or even preventative stenting. While the opportunities for atherosclerosis management based on intravascular NIRF molecular imaging reporters are yet to be established and will require large-scale outcomes trials for validation, there is significant expectation that the biological information garnered from intravascular NIRF will inform new treatment targets and the development of goal-directed strategies.

4.4.2.1 NIRF Imaging of Cysteine Protease Activity in Inflamed Plaques

Complications related to atherosclerotic plaques prototypically involve rupture of the overlying protective fibrous cap, exposing thrombogenic elements to the circulating bloodstream [16,59]. Enhanced plaque proteolytic activity, which results in degradation of structurally important collagen and elastin fiber networks, has been mechanistically linked to plaque rupture [19]. In particular, cathepsins, a well-described cysteine protease family, have been implicated in important atherosclerosis pathology [25]. Cathepsins S and K are present at sites of plaque rupture at autopsy in humans [26], and other cathepsin family members such as cathepsin B associate with atherosclerotic plaque complications [60–63]. Therefore, cathepsins represent high-value molecular imaging targets for identifying high-risk atherosclerotic plaques.

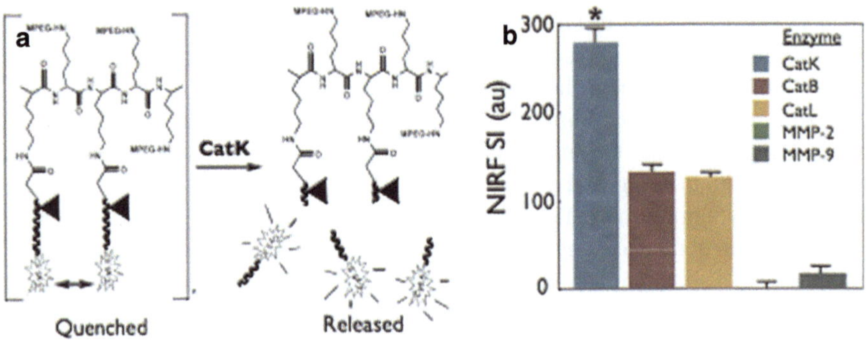

Fig. 4.6 Example of a protease-activatable NIRF molecular imaging biosensor. (**a**) Schematic of the protected graft copolymer backbone containing a peptide sequence substrate (Gly-His-Pro-Gly-Gly-Pro-Gln-Gly-Lys-Cys-NH2) specific for cathepsin K (*CatK*) linked to tightly packed nonfluorescent (quenched) NIRF reporters. In the presence of activated CatK, fluorescent probes are released by CatK substrate cleavage to liberate NIRF signaling. (**b**) In vitro testing with different cathepsin and matrix metalloproteinase (*MMP*) enzymes demonstrated preferential cleavage of the targeted agent by CatK ($*p<0.05$) (Reproduced with permission from Jaffer et al. [31])

In a significant technological achievement, smart tissue-activatable cathepsin protease NIRF molecular imaging agents have been developed [31,64,65], preclinically tested for cathepsin imaging [29,46,54,61], and commercialized (ProSense/VM110, PerkinElmer, Waltham MA). These specialized agents tightly pack 15–20 near-infrared fluorochromes onto an inert protected graft copolymer scaffold that causes the fluorochromes to be "quenched" and thus nonfluorescent at baseline [65,66]. The polymer scaffold backbone is comprised of the amino acid polylysine covalently bound to methoxypoly (ethylene glycol) chains, which in the presence of protease activity is cleaved to liberate individual fluorochromes detectable by NIRF imaging systems (Fig. 4.6). Compared to constitutively reporting agents, these smart bioreporters have major signal-to-noise advantages, since they exhibit minimal background at baseline, emit NIRF only when active tissue proteolysis is present, contain an intrinsic signal amplification strategy that liberates multiple fluorochromes from each nanosensor, and have proven to be nontoxic. To date, NIRF protease-activatable molecular imaging agents have been engineered to report on cathepsin B [65], cathepsin D [67], cathepsin K [31], and MMP 2 and 9 [68]. For further development potential, the oligopeptide, graft copolymer design of these agents form a versatile platform, enabling linkage of additional drugs or molecules.

4.4.2.2 Stand-Alone In Vivo Intravascular NIRF Sensing

Using the early prototype one-dimensional intravascular NIRF imaging system, cathepsin protease activity was assessed in the balloon-injured atherosclerotic iliac arteries of hypercholesterolemic rabbits [54]. Prosense VM110 injected 24 h prior

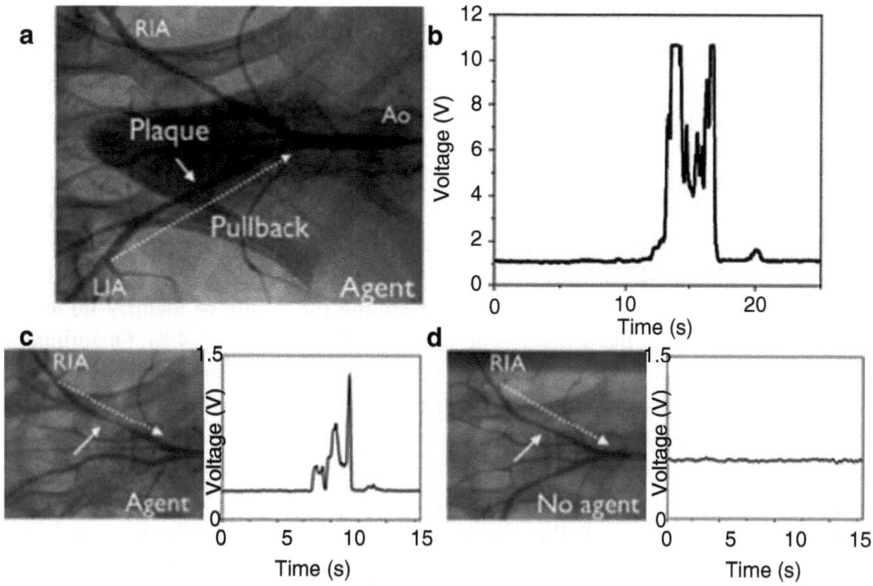

Fig. 4.7 In vivo NIRF sensing of plaque proteolytic activity with the one-dimensional intravascular NIRF catheter. (**a**) X-ray angiography of the aortoiliac vasculature in a balloon-injured atherosclerotic rabbit demonstrates the presence of left iliac artery (*LIA*) atherosclerotic plaque (white solid arrow in panels a, c, and d). Twenty-four hours after administration of a protease-activatable NIRF reporter (Prosense VM110), replicate manual NIRF catheter pullbacks from the distal LIA to the aorta (*Ao*) were performed through the blood without flushing over approximately 20 s each (*White dotted arrow* indicates catheter pullback trajectory in panels a, c, and d). (**b**) Strong NIRF protease signal was repeatedly detected at the location of the LIA plaque. (**c**) Similar findings of elevated plaque NIRF activity were observed in a different rabbit with right iliac artery (*RIA*) atherosclerosis given Prosense VM110 the day prior, but (**d**) not in those administered saline control that exhibited only background NIRF signal (Reproduced with permission from Jaffer et al. [54])

to NIRF imaging revealed increased cathepsin protease activity at sites of atheroma formation by manual catheter pullback that was confirmed by ex vivo macroscopic fluorescence reflectance imaging (FRI) and matched histopathology (Fig. 4.7). Significantly, NIRF plaque detection was accomplished through flowing blood without the need for vessel flushing of occlusion, demonstrating the advantageous in vivo light transmission properties of NIRF light wavelengths. Normal, healthy rabbits injected with Prosense VM110 and atherosclerotic rabbits injected with a saline control vehicle exhibited minimal tissue NIRF signal consistent with background autofluorescence, thus demonstrating the specificity of this agent for NIRF protease detection. Since the rabbit iliac artery is of similar caliber to a small coronary artery (2.0–2.5 mm), this study demonstrated the feasibility of NIRF catheter detection systems to imaging human coronary plaques.

Atherosclerotic plaque cathepsin proteolytic activity in the high-cholesterol rabbit model was assessed more comprehensively with the second-generation, two-dimensional NIRF imaging catheter that provides automated pullback with circumferential imaging capabilities [46]. Furthermore, this study extended in vivo NIRF imaging to the larger 3.0–4.0 mm diameter aorta, more consistent with the typical size range of proximal epicardial human coronary arteries. Eight weeks after aortic balloon injury, rabbits were administered i.v. Prosense VM110 or saline control 24 h prior to performing in vivo NIRF imaging. Anatomic plaque information was evaluated by x-ray angiography and grayscale IVUS and then carefully matched to the NIRF data set using side branches and other fiducial markers. Fusion images revealed co-localization of enhanced NIRF cathepsin protease activity with aortic atherosclerotic plaques, demonstrating the ability to identify inflamed plaques in vivo using the second-generation NIRF system (Fig. 4.8). Quantitative analysis of the plaque NIRF signal revealed excellent performance characteristics with significantly greater signal-to-noise (SNR) and target-to-background (TBR) ratios in aortic plaques from rabbits receiving Prosense VM110 compared to saline control (SNR 12.6 vs. 1.3, $p=0.02$; TBR 6.3 vs. 1.1, $p=0.02$). Ex vivo tissue analysis confirmed the in vivo NIRF findings, including the presence of histological plaque inflammation (i.e., cathepsins and macrophages) in all balloon-injured animals regardless of whether they were administered saline as a control injection with minimal in vivo NIRF signal or Prosense VM110. Notably, immunohistochemistry for plaque cathepsin proteases may be positive in regions without Prosense VM110 NIRF signal, since Prosense VM110 reports only on *biologically active* cathepsin protease activity rather than total (inactive plus active) protease content.

4.4.2.3 In Vivo Intravascular NIRF-OFDI

Building on prior experiments with earlier-generation stand-alone NIRF imaging systems, inflamed aortic atherosclerotic plaques in cholesterol-fed, balloon-injured rabbits were assessed with integrated NIRF-OFDI molecular-structural imaging using Prosense VM110 injected 24 h beforehand [55]. OFDI-defined plaques revealed enhanced NIRF cathepsin protease signal that was absent in normal vessel segments. Within a single plaque, heterogeneous NIRF proteolysis was observed at high spatial resolution and precisely mapped to the OFDI microstructure (Fig. 4.9). At histopathology, NIRF-positive aortic plaques exhibited increased macrophage infiltration and cathepsin B expression. By combining exact anatomically matched biological and structural plaque information as demonstrated in this feasibility study, intravascular NIRF-OFDI is poised to inform upon previously unappreciated and inaccessible high-risk atherosclerotic plaque features in vivo such as cysteine protease activity, with the possibility to perform serial imaging studies that evaluate drug treatment effects on plaque inflammation in living subjects. Furthermore, as OFDI signal standard deviation threshold measurements can detect resident plaque macrophages in macrophage-dense lesions [69], ongoing studies are attempting to understand whether adding NIRF imaging of proteolytic activity can identify a subset of the OFDI macrophage population that represent activated or M1-type macrophages.

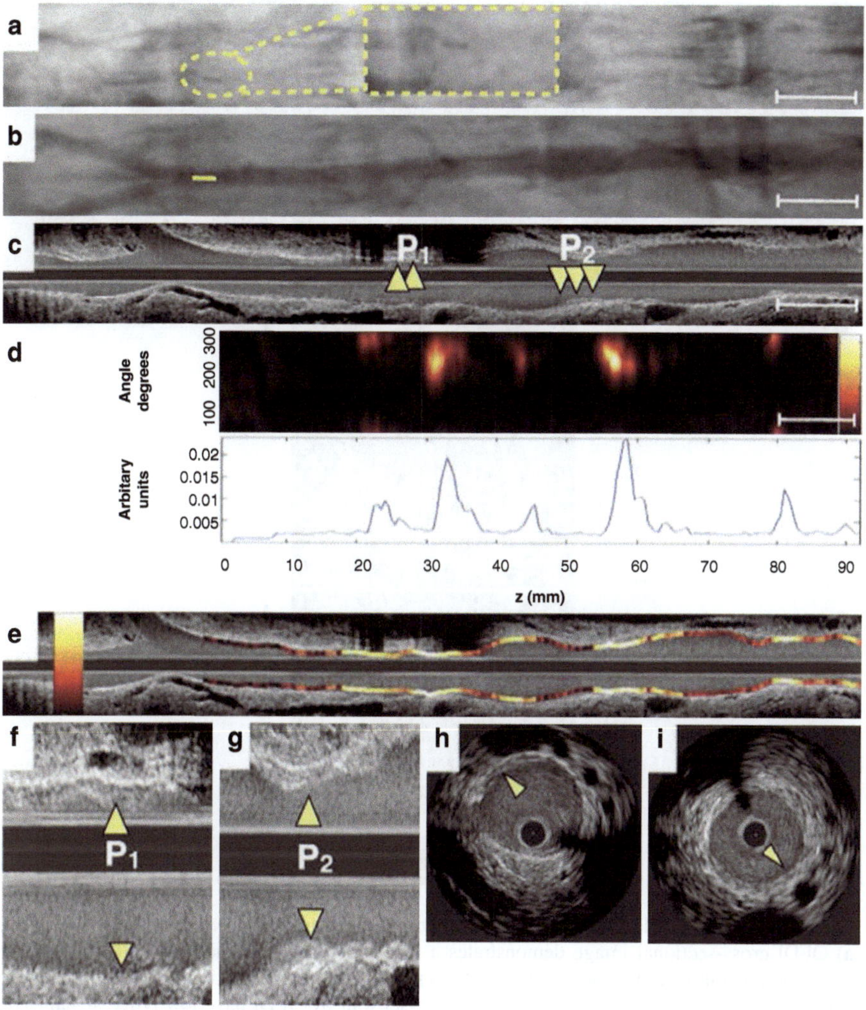

Fig. 4.8 In vivo molecular imaging of atherosclerosis protease inflammation with the two-dimensional intravascular NIRF catheter in a coronary-sized artery. (**a**) Non-contrast angiography shows placement of the two-dimensional NIRF catheter in the rabbit abdominal aorta (*dotted yellow inset* highlights radiopaque marker at the catheter tip). (**b**) Contrast angiography of the aortoiliac vasculature with mild atherosclerotic disease (*yellow line* indicates catheter tip location). (**c**) Mild plaques (P1, P2; *arrowheads*) are observed on the longitudinal IVUS, with more detail on (**f, g**) higher magnification long view and (**h, i**) axial IVUS images. (**d**) Two-dimensional NIRF map (*top panel*) aligned with angiography and IVUS demonstrates elevated plaque NIRF proteolytic activity, displayed as one-dimensional angle-averaged NIRF signal (*bottom panel*). (**e**) NIRF signal superimposed on longitudinal IVUS co-localizes elevated NIRF protease inflammation (*yellow/white* = high-intensity NIRF signal, *red/black* = low intensity NIRF signal) to regions of IVUS-defined plaque (Reproduced with permission from Jaffer et al. [46])

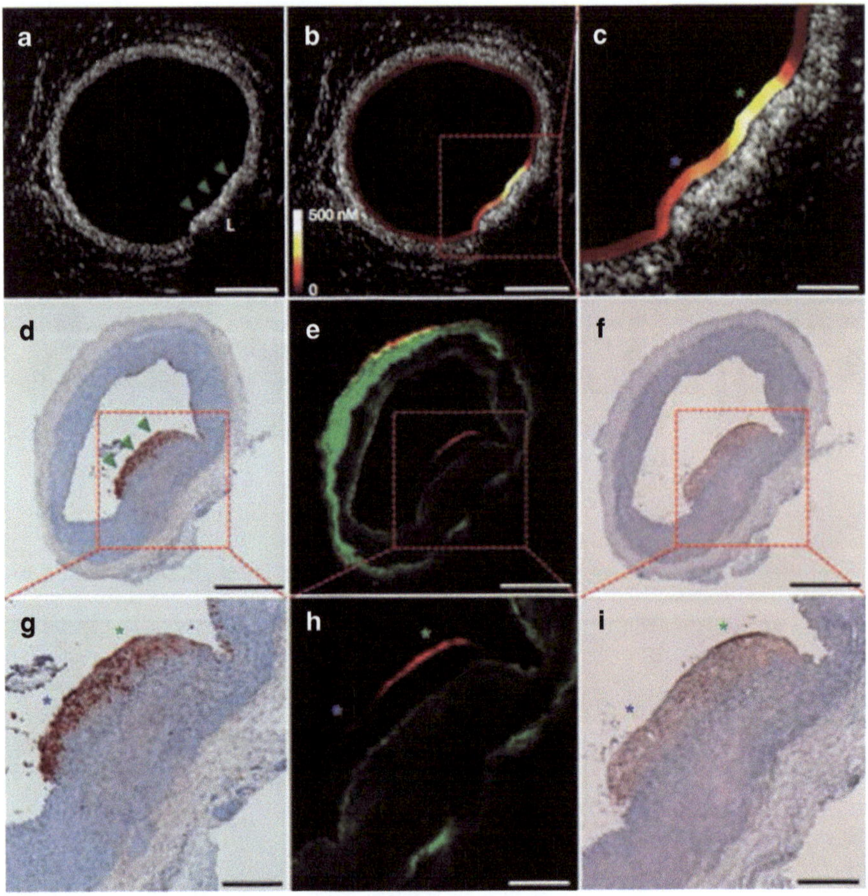

Fig. 4.9 In vivo NIRF-OFDI molecular-structural imaging of atheroma protease activity. (**a**) OFDI cross-sectional image demonstrates a focal lipid-rich (*L*) plaque (*arrowheads*) in an atherosclerotic rabbit aorta associated with (**b**, **c**) strong quantitative NIRF protease inflammation (*yellow/white*). In comparison, areas of normal vessel wall by OFDI have low NIRF signal (*red/black*). Immunochemistry staining for (**d**, **g**) RAM-11 and (**f**, **i**) cathepsin B shows dense macrophage and cysteine protease infiltration, respectively, throughout the atheroma. (**e**, **h**) Fluorescent microscopy revealed plaque NIRF signal (*red*) in a similar pattern (i.e., greater NIRF at the *green asterisk* compared to the *blue asterisk*) to the matched in vivo NIRF-OFDI axial image from (**c**) that was distinct from tissue autofluorescence (*green*). Scale bars, 200 μm (**c**, **g**–**i**) and 500 μm (**a**, **b**, **d**–**f**) (Reproduced with permission from Yoo et al. [55])

4.4.2.4 NIRF Imaging of Lipid-Rich, Inflamed Plaques with Indocyanine Green

For clinical translation of intravascular NIRF imaging technology, targeted NIRF molecular imaging agents for patient administration must be made available. At present, Prosense VM110 is not approved for human use, and therefore, alternative NIRF inflammation-sensing molecular probes have been pursued to speed clinical translation. Indocyanine green (ICG) is a candidate near-infrared fluorochrome already approved by the Food and Drug Administration (FDA) for intravascular blood flow measurements in ophthalmic retinal imaging and for assessment of cardiac output and hepatic function [70,71]. ICG is an amphiphilic fluorescent dye that binds circulating plasma proteins including atherogenic low-density lipoprotein (LDL) [72] and has been reported to localize within inflamed tissues [73].

Given these promising attributes, ICG was selected for further evaluation of its ability to identify inflamed atheroma and plaque lipid accumulation in vivo with one-dimensional stand-alone NIRF imaging [74]. Eight weeks following aortoiliac balloon injury, hyperlipidemic rabbits were injected with an FDA-approved ICG dose (1.5 mg/kg) prior to in vivo NIRF imaging. Automated pullbacks matched with IVUS for plaque topography revealed locally increased ICG signal in atheroma that was durable for up to 45 min after ICG administration (Fig. 4.10). Ex vivo FRI macroscopically corroborated the in vivo NIRF ICG signal. Detailed fluorescence microscopy and histopathology matched to NIRF and IVUS was then performed to localize the tissue source of ICG plaque signal. Within atheroma, ICG co-localized with lipid (Oil Red O neutral triglyceride staining) and macrophages (RAM-11 antibody). Extending this association further to human tissues, in vitro testing revealed ICG binding to acetylated LDL and ingestion by human macrophages and experimentally derived foam cells, and ex vivo incubation of resected carotid endarterectomy specimens with ICG demonstrated ICG uptake in plaque regions with increased lipid and macrophage content. Therefore, although additional mechanisms of ICG binding to lipid populations and macrophage subsets need to be elucidated, ICG appears to be a promising clinically available NIRF molecular imaging agent for inflamed, lipid-rich atherosclerotic plaques that may accelerate human translation of intravascular NIRF imaging studies.

4.4.3 Intravascular NIRF Imaging of Proteolytic Activity in Coronary Stents

Coronary stent procedures in the United States alone are performed in greater than one million patients annually [1] and carry measurable risks of future stent thrombosis and stent restenosis [75]. Although occurring relatively infrequently at rates from 0.3 to 4 % per year depending on the patient population studied, stent thrombosis is a major adverse event that often results in sudden cardiac death [76,77]. Even in survivors of stent thrombosis, a 30-day mortality is reported as high as 10–25 %. While generally less catastrophic, stent restenosis is a more common phenomenon (5–20 %), particularly in diabetic patients, and a significant contributor to recurrent angina, myocardial infarction, and repeat invasive procedures [78,79]. While the development of drug-eluting stents (DES) with antiproliferative coatings to antagonize smooth muscle cell ingrowth has diminished stent restenosis, DES heal slower than uncoated bare-metal stents (BMS) thus leaving metal exposed to flowing blood that may trigger local thrombosis [80–82]. Furthermore, the drug itself and/or polymer coating has been implicated in promoting stent struts that lack

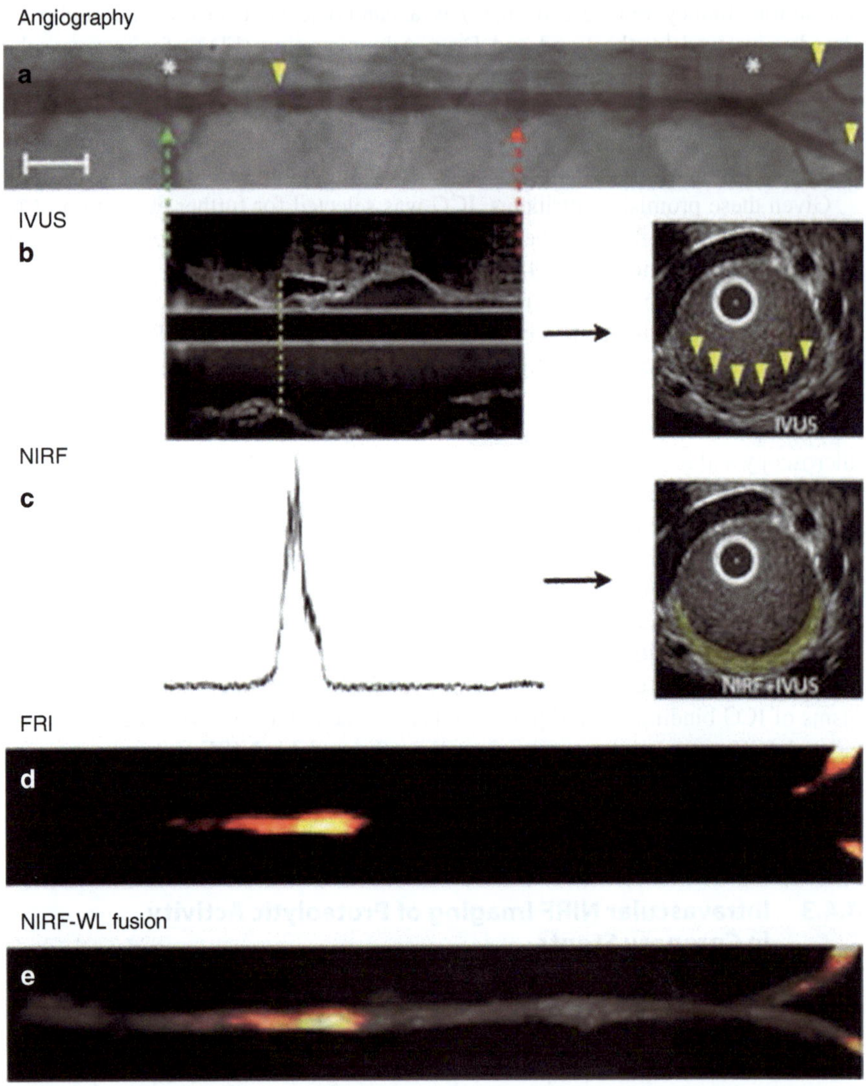

Fig. 4.10 In vivo NIRF sensing of indocyanine green (*ICG*) uptake in lipid-rich, inflamed plaques with the one-dimensional intravascular NIRF catheter. (**a**) Contrast angiography shows multiple sites of rabbit aortic and iliac artery atherosclerosis (*arrowheads*). Automated NIRF catheter pullback was performed between the *green* and *red dotted arrows*, and fiducial markers (e.g., renal and iliac artery branch points; *asterisks*) were used to anatomically register NIRF signal with IVUS for plaque structural characterization. Scale bar, 1 cm. (**b**) Longitudinal IVUS revealed small plaques (*dotted line*) that were eccentric on cross-sectional images (*arrowheads*). (**c**) Fifteen minutes after injection, in vivo ICG NIRF signal mapped to the location of IVUS atheroma (*yellow pseudocolor*). (**d**, **e**) Ex vivo fluorescence reflectance imaging (*FRI*) confirmed plaque ICG uptake (fire look-up table) within atherosclerotic segments on white light (*WL*) fusion images (Reproduced with permission from Vinegoni et al. [74])

endothelial coverage, are inflamed, and develop fibrin deposition [83]. Stent restenosis is routinely visualized with IVUS and OCT/OFDI [50,56,84], and stent strut endothelial coverage can be identified with good accuracy by OCT/OFDI given its high-resolution images [85,86]. However, despite these structural guideposts, there is great need to better understand the in vivo pathobiology that predisposes particular stents and patients to stent thrombosis or stent restenosis.

Intravascular NIRF molecular imaging approaches are ideally situated to improve understanding of the complex microenvironment present during stent healing that has been previously undetectable in vivo. Identification of overtly inflamed or fibrin-covered stents may facilitate early detection of stents at risk of stent thrombosis or aggressive restenosis and allow preventative measures to be undertaken to lessen this risk. Of particular interest is hybrid intravascular NIRF-OFDI [48,55], given the superior in vivo structural resolution of OFDI to resolve individual stent struts including the degree of stent strut coverage (i.e., endothelialization) that marks stent healing. In this way, stent-associated inflammation and fibrin deposition can be detected with NIRF-OFDI imaging strategies, revealing new biological insights into the stent healing response with potentially important clinical implications.

4.4.3.1 NIRF Imaging of Stent Inflammatory Proteolytic Activity

Efforts to understand the role of inflammation on stent healing in vivo with intravascular NIRF imaging have been undertaken in preclinical animal models. Clinical-grade BMS implanted in the rabbit aorta for 1 week were imaged with two-dimensional intravascular NIRF following intravenous Prosense VM110 injection 24 h earlier [46]. For anatomical information, IVUS and angiography were performed in serial fashion. Increased cathepsin protease NIRF activity was greatest at the stent edges, identified surrounding stent struts by in vivo NIRF and fluorescence microscopy, and also noted beyond the stent boundaries likely related to arterial injury from extension of the stent delivery balloon (Fig. 4.11). Based on this early demonstration, intravascular NIRF detection of stent inflammation is feasible in living subjects, may allow serial assessment of stent inflammation during the healing process and response to therapeutic intervention, and holds great potential for translation to human coronary stent risk assessment including informing the engineering of next-generation safer stent designs. Intravascular NIRF-OFDI molecular-structural imaging of stent NIRF protease inflammation and OFDI structural healing (i.e., endothelialization and neointimal formation, respectively) is also being actively pursued in preclinical BMS and DES stent healing studies. Given its advantageous technical properties, NIRF-OFDI is likely to propel the interrogation of coronary stent healing to the next level by enabling high-resolution longitudinal assessment of stent healing and biology with exact anatomical co-registration.

4.4.3.2 NIRF Imaging of Stent Fibrin Deposition

Stent strut fibrin accumulation has been implicated as a precursor of stent thrombosis [76,80] and therefore represents a potential high-value in vivo molecular imaging target. Given the need to interrogate individual stent struts, the high-resolution integrated intravascular NIRF-OFDI system is an ideal tool to evaluate the ability to visualize uncovered stent struts with associated fibrin deposition. In initial testing, BMS coated with exogenously NIRF-labeled fibrin was implanted in a cadaveric human coronary artery and ex vivo NIRF-OFDI performed [55]. NIRF fibrin signal overlapped with OFDI-detected thrombi on simultaneously acquired images, and

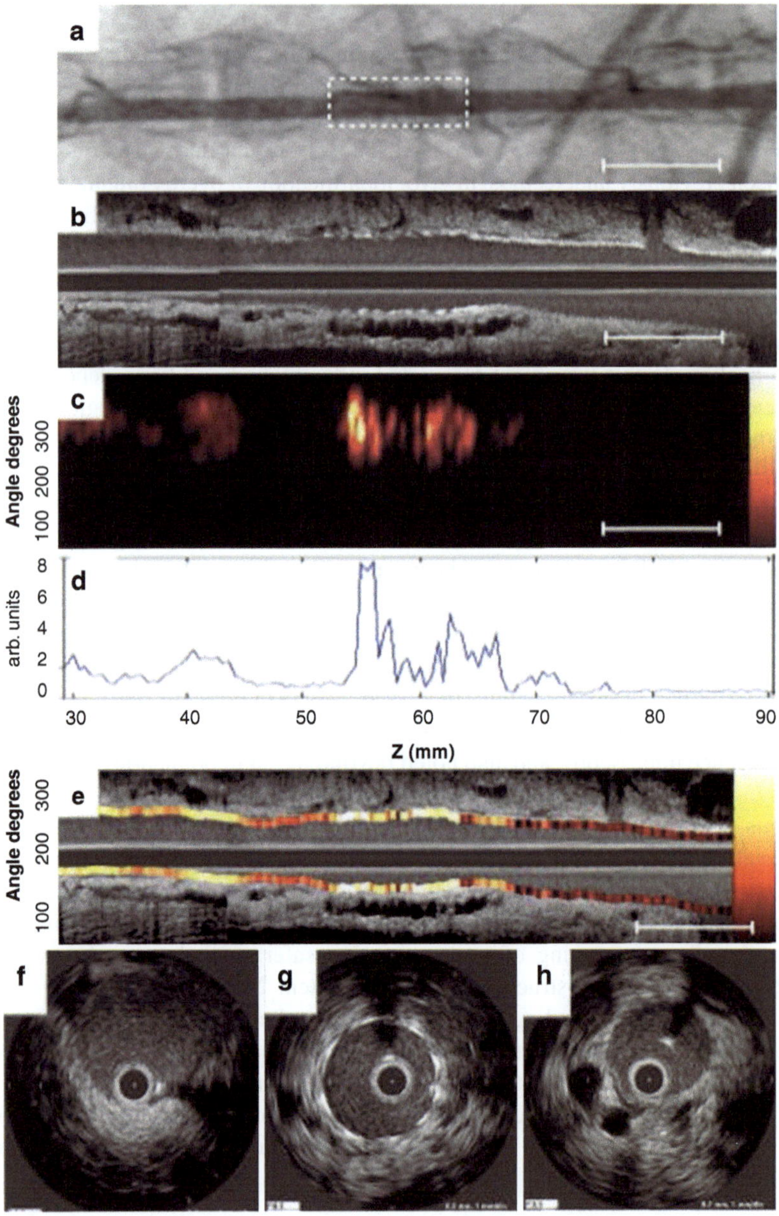

Fig. 4.11 In vivo NIRF molecular imaging of stent protease activity with the two-dimensional intravascular NIRF catheter. (**a**) X-ray angiography delineates the position of a bare-metal stent (*dotted rectangle*) implanted in a rabbit abdominal aorta 7 days earlier. (**b**, **c**) Twenty-four hours following intravenous injection of Prosense VM110, co-registered IVUS and NIRF maps obtained through blood without flushing reveal a stent strut-based pattern of NIRF protease inflammation. (**d**) One-dimensional angle-averaged NIRF signal plot of each axial NIRF acquisition. (**e**) NIRF and long view IVUS fusion image (*yellow/white* = high-intensity NIRF; *red/black* = low intensity NIRF) highlighting enhanced stent NIRF protease activity. (**f**–**h**) Respective IVUS cross-sectional images from zones of balloon angioplasty, bare-metal stent placement, and the normal artery (Reproduced with permission from Jaffer et al. [46])

NIRF fibrin signal at stent strut zones was verified by en face FRI. Next, BMS incubated with NIRF fibrin were implanted in the iliac arteries of living rabbits and in vivo NIRF-OFDI performed. As in the cadaveric coronary artery, NIRF fibrin deposition co-localized with OFDI thrombus, but NIRF fibrin imaging also detected a population of stent strut NIRF-positive microthrombi that were resolved beyond OFDI capabilities, demonstrating the improved sensitivity of targeted NIRF molecular imaging over OFDI structural imaging alone for fibrin detection (Fig. 4.12).

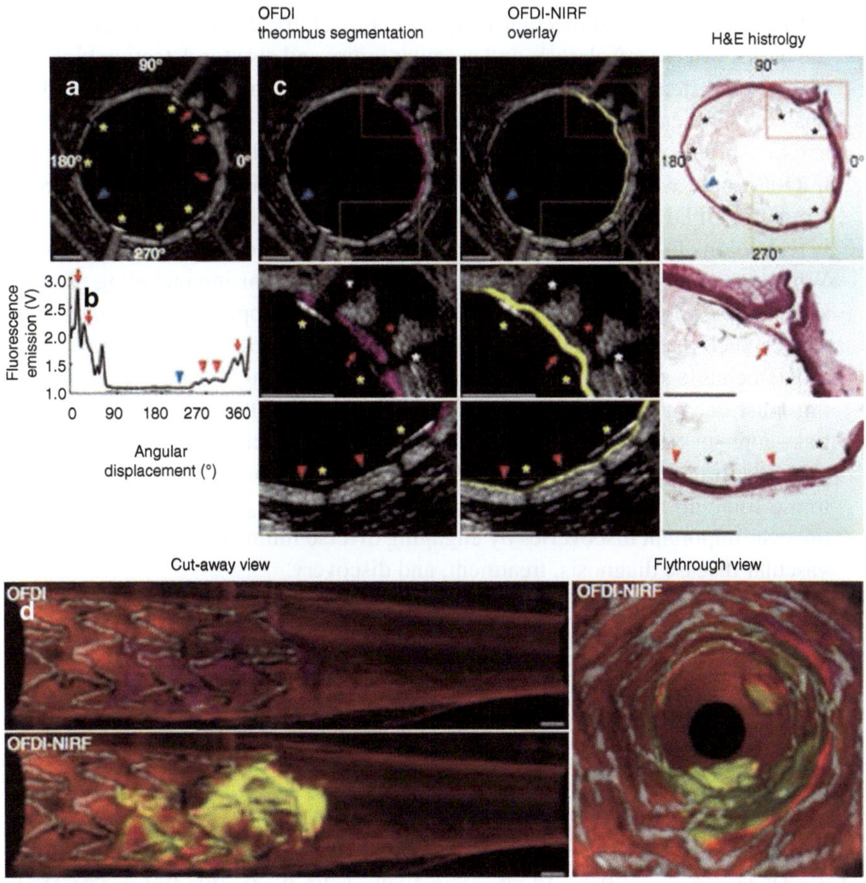

Fig. 4.12 In vivo NIRF-OFDI molecular-structural imaging of stent fibrin deposition. (**a**) A bare-metal stent coated ex vivo with a fibrin-reporting NIRF probe and implanted in the iliac artery of a rabbit was imaged in vivo with the dual-modality NIRF-OFDI catheter system. In cross-section, OFDI microstructural thrombus (*red arrows*) and stent struts (*yellow asterisks*) are apparent. (**b**) Angular NIRF plot with high-intensity NIRF fibrin signal (*red arrows*) co-localized at locations with visual OFDI thrombus. Zones without OFDI thrombus (*blue arrowheads* in **a–c**) lacked detectable NIRF fibrin signal. (**c**) OFDI thrombus segmentation (*left column*, *purple*) closely paralleled NIRF fibrin localization (*middle column*, *yellow*) anatomically matched with histological H&E staining (*right column*; *red asterisk* = side branch, *yellow* or *black asterisks* = stent struts, *white asterisks* = stent strut shadows, thrombus = *red arrows*). Insets are high-magnification views of *red-* or *yellow*-bordered rectangular regions of interest. (**d**) Three-dimensional rendered images of the NIRF-OFDI data set illustrating extensive overlap of OFDI thrombus (*purple*) and NIRF fibrin (*yellow*) deposition. Scale bars, 500 μm (Reproduced with permission from Yoo et al. [55])

As new clinical NIRF fibrin biosensors emerge, such as NIRF-labeled FTP-11 that is based on an MRI fibrin agent already tested and shown to be safe in humans [87–90], intravascular NIRF-OFDI evaluation of stent strut fibrin deposition is positioned to gain clinical traction as an intriguing novel method for stent thrombosis risk prediction.

Conclusion

Intravascular NIRF imaging of arterial proteolytic activity represents a promising new translational molecular imaging approach for the in vivo assessment of the biology of atherosclerosis and vascular injury and also for detecting high-risk plaques and stents. Early preclinical studies using prototype systems have demonstrated the feasibility of intravascular NIRF to detect plaque cysteine protease activity, lipid- and macrophage-rich plaques, stent inflammation, healing, and microthrombi with good sensitivity. The addition of high-resolution integrated structural OFDI to stand-alone NIRF imaging systems has spurred a major leap in technology to enable detailed investigation of stent and plaque biology in vivo. While a number of NIRF agents are translationally promising including protease sensors, preliminary data suggests that existing FDA-approved NIRF molecular probes such as ICG may allow even earlier human testing with intravascular NIRF technology. Going forward, however, intravascular NIRF molecular imaging must demonstrate improved risk prediction that extends beyond traditional risk scores in order to make a NIRF imaging approach clinically viable. Overall, given the broad appeal of molecular imaging to illuminate biology beyond anatomic imaging modalities, intravascular NIRF imaging has great potential to uncover important discoveries by engaging diverse future applications in cardiovascular disease diagnosis, treatment, and discovery.

Acknowledgements NIH R01 HL 108229 and American Heart Association Scientist Development Grant #0830352N (FJ); Harvard Catalyst KL2/Medical Research Investigator Training Award NIH 1UL1 TR001102-01 and Beth Israel Deaconess Medical Center Cardiovascular Division (EO).

References

1. Go AS, Mozaffarian D, Roger VL, Benjamin EJ, Berry JD, Borden WB, Bravata DM, Dai S, Ford ES, Fox CS, Franco S, Fullerton HJ, Gillespie C, Hailpern SM, Heit JA, Howard VJ, Huffman MD, Kissela BM, Kittner SJ, Lackland DT, Lichtman JH, Lisabeth LD, Magid D, Marcus GM, Marelli A, Matchar DB, McGuire DK, Mohler ER, Moy CS, Mussolino ME, Nichol G, Paynter NP, Schreiner PJ, Sorlie PD, Stein J, Turan TN, Virani SS, Wong ND, Woo D, Turner MB, Subcommittee AHASCaSS. Heart disease and stroke statistics – 2013 update: a report from the American Heart Association. Circulation. 2013;127(1):e6–245. doi:10.1161/CIR.0b013e31828124ad.
2. Fleg JL, Stone GW, Fayad ZA, Granada JF, Hatsukami TS, Kolodgie FD, Ohayon J, Pettigrew R, Sabatine MS, Tearney GJ, Waxman S, Domanski MJ, Srinivas PR, Narula J. Detection of high-risk atherosclerotic plaque: report of the NHLBI Working Group on current status and future directions. JACC Cardiovasc Imaging. 2012;5(9):941–55. doi:10.1016/j.jcmg.2012.07.007.

3. Glagov S, Weisenberg E, Zarins CK, Stankunavicius R, Kolettis GJ. Compensatory enlargement of human atherosclerotic coronary arteries. N Engl J Med. 1987;316(22):1371–5. doi:10.1056/NEJM198705283162204.
4. Virmani R, Burke AP, Farb A, Kolodgie FD. Pathology of the vulnerable plaque. J Am Coll Cardiol. 2006;47(8 Suppl):C13–8. doi:10.1016/j.jacc.2005.10.065.
5. Osborn EA, Jaffer FA. Imaging atherosclerosis and risk of plaque rupture. Curr Atheroscler Rep. 2013;15(10):359. doi:10.1007/s11883-013-0359-z.
6. García-García HM, Mintz GS, Lerman A, Vince DG, Margolis MP, van Es G-A, Morel M-AM, Nair A, Virmani R, Burke AP, Stone GW, Serruys PW. Tissue characterisation using intravascular radiofrequency data analysis: recommendations for acquisition, analysis, interpretation and reporting. EuroIntervention. 2009;5(2):177–89.
7. Waxman S, Dixon SR, L'allier P, Moses JW, Petersen JL, Cutlip D, Tardif JC, Nesto RW, Muller JE, Hendricks MJ, Sum ST, Gardner CM, Goldstein JA, Stone GW, Krucoff MW. In vivo validation of a catheter-based near-infrared spectroscopy system for detection of lipid core coronary plaques. JCMG. 2011;2(7):858–68. doi:10.1016/j.jcmg.2009.05.001.
8. Jaffer F, Libby P, Weissleder R. Molecular imaging of cardiovascular disease. Circulation. 2007;116(9):1052–61.
9. Sanz J, Fayad Z. Imaging of atherosclerotic cardiovascular disease. Nature. 2008;451(7181): 953–7.
10. Osborn EA, Jaffer FA. The advancing clinical impact of molecular imaging in CVD. JACC Cardiovasc Imaging. 2013;6(12):1327–41. doi:10.1016/j.jcmg.2013.09.014.
11. Dweck MR, Chow MWL, Joshi NV, Williams MC, Jones C, Fletcher AM, Richardson H, White A, McKillop G, van Beek EJR, Boon NA, Rudd JHF, Newby DE. Coronary arterial 18F-sodium fluoride uptake: a novel marker of plaque biology. J Am Coll Cardiol. 2012;59(17):1539–48. doi:10.1016/j.jacc.2011.12.037.
12. Rogers IS, Nasir K, Figueroa AL, Cury RC, Hoffmann U, Vermylen DA, Brady TJ, Tawakol A. Feasibility of FDG imaging of the coronary arteries: comparison between acute coronary syndrome and stable angina. JACC Cardiovasc Imaging. 2010;3(4):388–97. doi:10.1016/j.jcmg.2010.01.004.
13. Hansson GK. Inflammation, atherosclerosis, and coronary artery disease. N Engl J Med. 2005;352(16):1685–95. doi:10.1056/NEJMra043430.
14. Naghavi M, Libby P, Falk E, Casscells SW, Litovsky S, Rumberger J, Badimon JJ, Stefanadis C, Moreno P, Pasterkamp G, Fayad Z, Stone PH, Waxman S, Raggi P, Madjid M, Zarrabi A, Burke A, Yuan C, Fitzgerald PJ, Siscovick DS, de Korte CL, Aikawa M, Juhani Airaksinen KE, Assmann G, Becker CR, Chesebro JH, Farb A, Galis ZS, Jackson C, Jang I-K, Koenig W, Lodder RA, March K, Demirovic J, Navab M, Priori SG, Rekhter MD, Bahr R, Grundy SM, Mehran R, Colombo A, Boerwinkle E, Ballantyne C, Insull W, Schwartz RS, Vogel R, Serruys PW, Hansson GK, Faxon DP, Kaul S, Drexler H, Greenland P, Muller JE, Virmani R, Ridker PM, Zipes DP, Shah PK, Willerson JT. From vulnerable plaque to vulnerable patient: a call for new definitions and risk assessment strategies: part I. Circulation. 2003;108(14):1664–72. doi:10.1161/01.CIR.0000087480.94275.97.
15. Narula J, Nakano M, Virmani R, Kolodgie FD, Petersen R, Newcomb R, Malik S, Fuster V, Finn AV. Histopathologic characteristics of atherosclerotic coronary disease and implications of the findings for the invasive and noninvasive detection of vulnerable plaques. J Am Coll Cardiol. 2013;61(10):1041–51. doi:10.1016/j.jacc.2012.10.054.
16. Arbab-Zadeh A, Nakano M, Virmani R, Fuster V. Acute coronary events. Circulation. 2012;125(9):1147–56. doi:10.1161/CIRCULATIONAHA.111.047431.
17. Libby P. Inflammation in atherosclerosis. Arterioscler Thromb Vasc Biol. 2012;32(9):2045–51. doi:10.1161/ATVBAHA.108.179705.
18. Galis ZS, Khatri JJ. Matrix metalloproteinases in vascular remodeling and atherogenesis: the good, the bad, and the ugly. Circ Res. 2002;90(3):251–62.
19. Silvestre-Roig C, de Winther MP, Weber C, Daemen MJ, Lutgens E, Soehnlein O. Atherosclerotic plaque destabilization: mechanisms, models, and therapeutic strategies. Circ Res. 2014;114(1):214–26. doi:10.1161/CIRCRESAHA.114.302355.

20. Shah PK, Falk E, Badimon JJ, Fernandez-Ortiz A, Mailhac A, Villareal-Levy G, Fallon JT, Regnstrom J, Fuster V. Human monocyte-derived macrophages induce collagen breakdown in fibrous caps of atherosclerotic plaques. Potential role of matrix-degrading metalloproteinases and implications for plaque rupture. Circulation. 1995;92(6):1565–9.
21. Falk E, Nakano M, Bentzon JF, Finn AV, Virmani R. Update on acute coronary syndromes: the pathologists' view. Eur Heart J. 2013;34(10):719–28. doi:10.1093/eurheartj/ehs411.
22. Slager CJ, Wentzel JJ, Gijsen FJ, Schuurbiers JC, van der Wal AC, van der Steen AF, Serruys PW. The role of shear stress in the generation of rupture-prone vulnerable plaques. Nat Clin Pract Cardiovasc Med. 2005;2(8):401–7.
23. Wentzel JJ, Chatzizisis YS, Gijsen FJ, Giannoglou GD, Feldman CL, Stone PH. Endothelial shear stress in the evolution of coronary atherosclerotic plaque and vascular remodelling: current understanding and remaining questions. Cardiovasc Res. 2012;96(2):234–43. doi:10.1093/cvr/cvs217.
24. Dollery CM, Libby P. Atherosclerosis and proteinase activation. Cardiovasc Res. 2006;69(3):625–35. doi:10.1016/j.cardiores.2005.11.003.
25. Liu J, Sukhova GK, Sun J-S, Xu W-H, Libby P, Shi G-P. Lysosomal cysteine proteases in atherosclerosis. Arterioscler Thromb Vasc Biol. 2004;24(8):1359–66. doi:10.1161/01.ATV.0000134530.27208.41.
26. Sukhova GK, Shi GP, Simon DI, Chapman HA, Libby P. Expression of the elastolytic cathepsins S and K in human atheroma and regulation of their production in smooth muscle cells. J Clin Invest. 1998;102(3):576–83. doi:10.1172/JCI181.
27. Jones CB, Sane DC, Herrington DM. Matrix metalloproteinases: a review of their structure and role in acute coronary syndrome. Cardiovasc Res. 2003;59(4):812–23.
28. Newby AC. Metalloproteinase expression in monocytes and macrophages and its relationship to atherosclerotic plaque instability. Arterioscler Thromb Vasc Biol. 2008;28(12):2108–14. doi:10.1161/ATVBAHA.108.173898.
29. Chen J, Tung C-H, Mahmood U, Ntziachristos V, Gyurko R, Fishman MC, Huang PL, Weissleder R. In vivo imaging of proteolytic activity in atherosclerosis. Circulation. 2002;105(23):2766–71.
30. Deguchi J-o, Aikawa M, Tung C-H, Aikawa E, Kim D-E, Ntziachristos V, Weissleder R, Libby P. Inflammation in atherosclerosis: visualizing matrix metalloproteinase action in macrophages in vivo. Circulation. 2006;114(1):55–62. doi:10.1161/CIRCULATIONAHA.106.619056.
31. Jaffer F, Kim D, Quinti L, Tung C, Aikawa E, Pande A, Kohler R, Shi G, Libby P, Weissleder R. Optical visualization of cathepsin K activity in atherosclerosis with a novel, protease-activatable fluorescence sensor. Circulation. 2007;115(17):2292–8.
32. Lancelot E, Amirbekian V, Brigger I, Raynaud J-S, Ballet S, David C, Rousseaux O, Le Greneur S, Port M, Lijnen HR, Bruneval P, Michel J-B, Ouimet T, Roques B, Amirbekian S, Hyafil F, Vucic E, Aguinaldo JGS, Corot C, Fayad ZA. Evaluation of matrix metalloproteinases in atherosclerosis using a novel noninvasive imaging approach. Arterioscler Thromb Vasc Biol. 2008;28(3):425–32. doi:10.1161/ATVBAHA.107.149666.
33. Quillard T, Croce K, Jaffer FA, Weissleder R, Libby P. Molecular imaging of macrophage protease activity in cardiovascular inflammation in vivo. Thromb Haemost. 2011;105(5):828–36. doi:10.1160/TH10-09-0589.
34. Zhang J, Nie L, Razavian M, Ahmed M, Dobrucki LW, Asadi A, Edwards DS, Azure M, Sinusas AJ, Sadeghi MM. Molecular imaging of activated matrix metalloproteinases in vascular remodeling. Circulation. 2008;118(19):1953–60. doi:10.1161/CIRCULATIONAHA.108.789743.
35. Suter MJ, Nadkarni SK, Weisz G, Tanaka A, Jaffer FA, Bouma BE, Tearney GJ. Intravascular optical imaging technology for investigating the coronary artery. JACC Cardiovasc Imaging. 2011;4(9):1022–39. doi:10.1016/j.jcmg.2011.03.020.
36. Cheng VY, Slomka PJ, Le Meunier L, Tamarappoo BK, Nakazato R, Dey D, Berman DS. Coronary arterial 18F-FDG uptake by fusion of PET and coronary CT angiography at sites of percutaneous stenting for acute myocardial infarction and stable coronary artery disease. J Nucl Med. 2012;53(4):575–83. doi:10.2967/jnumed.111.097550.

37. Saam T, Rominger A, Wolpers S, Nikolaou K, Rist C, Greif M, Cumming P, Becker A, Foerster S, Reiser MF, Bartenstein P, Hacker M. Association of inflammation of the left anterior descending coronary artery with cardiovascular risk factors, plaque burden and pericardial fat volume: a PET/CT study. Eur J Nucl Med Mol Imaging. 2010;37(6):1203–12. doi:10.1007/s00259-010-1432-2.
38. Wykrzykowska J, Lehman S, Williams G, Parker JA, Palmer MR, Varkey S, Kolodny G, Laham R. Imaging of inflamed and vulnerable plaque in coronary arteries with 18F-FDG PET/CT in patients with suppression of myocardial uptake using a low-carbohydrate, high-fat preparation. J Nucl Med. 2009;50(4):563–8. doi:10.2967/jnumed.108.055616.
39. Howarth SPS, Tang TY, Trivedi R, Weerakkody R, U-King-Im J, Gaunt ME, Boyle JR, Li ZY, Miller SR, Graves MJ, Gillard JH. Utility of USPIO-enhanced MR imaging to identify inflammation and the fibrous cap: a comparison of symptomatic and asymptomatic individuals. Eur J Radiol. 2009;70(3):555–60. doi:10.1016/j.ejrad.2008.01.047.
40. Kooi ME, Cappendijk VC, Cleutjens KBJM, Kessels AGH, Kitslaar PJEHM, Borgers M, Frederik PM, Daemen MJAP, van Engelshoven JMA. Accumulation of ultrasmall superparamagnetic particles of iron oxide in human atherosclerotic plaques can be detected by in vivo magnetic resonance imaging. Circulation. 2003;107(19):2453–8. doi:10.1161/01.CIR.0000068315.98705.CC.
41. Tang TY, Howarth SPS, Miller SR, Graves MJ, Patterson AJ, U-King-Im J-M, Li ZY, Walsh SR, Brown AP, Kirkpatrick PJ, Warburton EA, Hayes PD, Varty K, Boyle JR, Gaunt ME, Zalewski A, Gillard JH. The ATHEROMA (Atorvastatin Therapy: Effects on Reduction of Macrophage Activity) Study. Evaluation using ultrasmall superparamagnetic iron oxide-enhanced magnetic resonance imaging in carotid disease. J Am Coll Cardiol. 2009;53(22):2039–50. doi:10.1016/j.jacc.2009.03.018.
42. Calfon MA, Vinegoni C, Ntziachristos V, Jaffer FA. Intravascular near-infrared fluorescence molecular imaging of atherosclerosis: toward coronary arterial visualization of biologically high-risk plaques. J Biomed Opt. 2010;15(1):011107. doi:10.1117/1.3280282.
43. Thukkani AK, Jaffer FA. Intravascular near-infrared fluorescence molecular imaging of atherosclerosis. Am J Nucl Med Mol Imaging. 2013;3(3):217–31.
44. Jaffer FA, Libby P, Weissleder R. Optical and multimodality molecular imaging: insights into atherosclerosis. Arterioscler Thromb Vasc Biol. 2009;29(7):1017–24. doi:10.1161/ATVBAHA.108.165530.
45. Weissleder R, Ntziachristos V. Shedding light onto live molecular targets. Nat Med. 2003;9(1):123–8. doi:10.1038/nm0103-123.
46. Jaffer FA, Calfon MA, Rosenthal A, Mallas G, Razansky RN, Mauskapf A, Weissleder R, Libby P, Ntziachristos V. Two-dimensional intravascular near-infrared fluorescence molecular imaging of inflammation in atherosclerosis and stent-induced vascular injury. J Am Coll Cardiol. 2011;57(25):2516–26. doi:10.1016/j.jacc.2011.02.036.
47. Osborn EA, Jaffer FA. The year in molecular imaging. JACC Cardiovasc Imaging. 2012;5(3):317–28. doi:10.1016/j.jcmg.2011.12.011.
48. Bourantas CV, Garcia-Garcia HM, Naka KK, Michalis LK, Serruys PW. Hybrid intravascular imaging: current applications and prospective potential in the study of coronary atherosclerosis. J Am Coll Cardiol. 2013;61(13):1369–78. doi:10.1016/j.jacc.2012.10.057.
49. Suh WM, Seto AH, Margey RJP, Cruz-Gonzalez I, Jang I-K. Intravascular detection of the vulnerable plaque. Circ Cardiovasc Imaging. 2011;4(2):169–78. doi:10.1161/CIRCIMAGING.110.958777.
50. Tearney GJ, Regar E, Akasaka T, Adriaenssens T, Barlis P, Bezerra HG, Bouma B, Bruining N, Cho J-M, Chowdhary S, Costa MA, de Silva R, Dijkstra J, Di Mario C, Dudeck D, Falk E, Feldman MD, Fitzgerald P, Garcia H, Gonzalo N, Granada JF, Guagliumi G, Holm NR, Honda Y, Ikeno F, Kawasaki M, Kochman J, Koltowski L, Kubo T, Kume T, Kyono H, Lam CCS, Lamouche G, Lee DP, Leon MB, Maehara A, Manfrini O, Mintz GS, Mizuno K, Morel M-A, Nadkarni S, Okura H, Otake H, Pietrasik A, Prati F, Räber L, Radu MD, Rieber J, Riga M, Rollins A, Rosenberg M, Sirbu V, Serruys PWJC, Shimada K, Shinke T, Shite J, Siegel E,

Sonada S, Suter M, Takarada S, Tanaka A, Terashima M, Troels T, Uemura S, Ughi GJ, van Beusekom HMM, van der Steen AFW, van Es G-A, van Soest G, Virmani R, Waxman S, Weissman NJ, Weisz G. Consensus standards for acquisition, measurement, and reporting of intravascular optical coherence tomography studies: a report from the international working group for intravascular optical coherence tomography standardization and validation. J Am Coll Cardiol. 2012;59(12):1058–72. doi:10.1016/j.jacc.2011.09.079.
51. Gardner CM, Tan H, Hull EL, Lisauskas JB, Sum ST, Meese TM, Jiang C, Madden SP, Caplan JD, Burke AP, Virmani R, Goldstein J, Muller JE. Detection of lipid core coronary plaques in autopsy specimens with a novel catheter-based near-infrared spectroscopy system. JACC Cardiovasc Imaging. 2008;1(5):638–48. doi:10.1016/j.jcmg.2008.06.001.
52. Garg S, Serruys PW, van der Ent M, Schultz C, Mastik F, van Soest G, van der Steen AFW, Wilder MA, Muller JE, Regar E. First use in patients of a combined near infra-red spectroscopy and intra-vascular ultrasound catheter to identify composition and structure of coronary plaque. EuroIntervention. 2010;5(6):755–6.
53. Madder RD, Smith JL, Dixon SR, Goldstein JA. Composition of target lesions by near-infrared spectroscopy in patients with acute coronary syndrome versus stable angina. Circ Cardiovasc Interv. 2012;5(1):55–61. doi:10.1161/CIRCINTERVENTIONS.111.963934.
54. Jaffer FA, Vinegoni C, John MC, Aikawa E, Gold HK, Finn AV, Ntziachristos V, Libby P, Weissleder R. Real-time catheter molecular sensing of inflammation in proteolytically active atherosclerosis. Circulation. 2008;118(18):1802–9. doi:10.1161/CIRCULATIONAHA.108.785881.
55. Yoo H, Kim JW, Shishkov M, Namati E, Morse T, Shubochkin R, Mccarthy JR, Ntziachristos V, Bouma BE, Jaffer FA, Tearney GJ. Intra-arterial catheter for simultaneous microstructural and molecular imaging in vivo. Nat Med. 2011;17(12):1680–4. doi:10.1038/nm.2555.
56. McDaniel MC, Eshtehardi P, Sawaya FJ, Douglas JS, Samady H. Contemporary clinical applications of coronary intravascular ultrasound. JACC Cardiovasc Interv. 2011;4(11):1155–67. doi:10.1016/j.jcin.2011.07.013.
57. Mintz GS, Nissen SE, Anderson WD, Bailey SR, Erbel R, Fitzgerald PJ, Pinto FJ, Rosenfield K, Siegel RJ, Tuzcu EM, Yock PG. American College of Cardiology Clinical Expert Consensus Document on Standards for Acquisition, Measurement and Reporting of Intravascular Ultrasound Studies (IVUS). A report of the American College of Cardiology Task Force on Clinical Expert Consensus Documents. J Am Coll Cardiol. 2001;37(5):1478–92.
58. Puri R, Kapadia SR, Nicholls SJ, Harvey JE, Kataoka Y, Tuzcu EM. Optimizing outcomes during left main percutaneous coronary intervention with intravascular ultrasound and fractional flow reserve: the current state of evidence. JACC Cardiovasc Interv. 2012;5(7):697–707. doi:10.1016/j.jcin.2012.02.018.
59. Libby P. Mechanisms of acute coronary syndromes and their implications for therapy. N Engl J Med. 2013;368(21):2004–13. doi:10.1056/NEJMra1216063.
60. Cheng XW, Huang Z, Kuzuya M, Okumura K, Murohara T. Cysteine protease cathepsins in atherosclerosis-based vascular disease and its complications. Hypertension. 2011;58(6):978–86. doi:10.1161/HYPERTENSIONAHA.111.180935.
61. Kim D-E, Kim J-Y, Schellingerhout D, Kim E-J, Kim HK, Lee S, Kim K, Kwon IC, Shon S-M, Jeong S-W, Im S-H, Lee DK, Lee MM, Kim G-E. Protease imaging of human atheromata captures molecular information of atherosclerosis, complementing anatomic imaging. Arterioscler Thromb Vasc Biol. 2010;30(3):449–56. doi:10.1161/ATVBAHA.109.194613.
62. Lutgens SP, Cleutjens KB, Daemen MJ, Heeneman S. Cathepsin cysteine proteases in cardiovascular disease. FASEB J. 2007;21(12):3029–41. doi:10.1096/fj.06-7924com.
63. Papaspyridonos M, Smith A, Burnand KG, Taylor P, Padayachee S, Suckling KE, James CH, Greaves DR, Patel L. Novel candidate genes in unstable areas of human atherosclerotic plaques. Arterioscler Thromb Vasc Biol. 2006;26(8):1837–44. doi:10.1161/01.ATV.0000229695.68416.76.
64. Blum G, von Degenfeld G, Merchant MJ, Blau HM, Bogyo M. Noninvasive optical imaging of cysteine protease activity using fluorescently quenched activity-based probes. Nat Chem Biol. 2007;3(10):668–77. doi:10.1038/nchembio.2007.26.

65. Weissleder R, Tung CH, Mahmood U, Bogdanov A. In vivo imaging of tumors with protease-activated near-infrared fluorescent probes. Nat Biotechnol. 1999;17(4):375–8. doi:10.1038/7933.
66. Bogdanov Jr AA, Mazzanti M, Castillo G, Bolotin E. Protected Graft Copolymer (PGC) in imaging and therapy: a platform for the delivery of covalently and non-covalently bound drugs. Theranostics. 2012;2(6):553–76. doi:10.7150/thno.4070.
67. Tung CH, Bredow S, Mahmood U, Weissleder R. Preparation of a cathepsin D sensitive near-infrared fluorescence probe for imaging. Bioconjug Chem. 1999;10(5):892–6.
68. Bremer C, Tung CH, Weissleder R. In vivo molecular target assessment of matrix metalloproteinase inhibition. Nat Med. 2001;7(6):743–8. doi:10.1038/89126.
69. Tearney GJ, Yabushita H, Houser SL, Aretz HT, Jang I-K, Schlendorf KH, Kauffman CR, Shishkov M, Halpern EF, Bouma BE. Quantification of macrophage content in atherosclerotic plaques by optical coherence tomography. Circulation. 2003;107(1):113–9.
70. Dzurinko VL, Gurwood AS, Price JR. Intravenous and indocyanine green angiography. Optometry. 2004;75(12):743–55.
71. Polom K, Murawa D, Rho YS, Nowaczyk P, Hunerbein M, Murawa P. Current trends and emerging future of indocyanine green usage in surgery and oncology: a literature review. Cancer. 2011;117(21):4812–22. doi:10.1002/cncr.26087.
72. Yoneya S, Saito T, Komatsu Y, Koyama I, Takahashi K, Duvoll-Young J. Binding properties of indocyanine green in human blood. Invest Ophthalmol Vis Sci. 1998;39(7):1286–90.
73. Fischer T, Gemeinhardt I, Wagner S, Stieglitz DV, Schnorr J, Hermann KG, Ebert B, Petzelt D, Macdonald R, Licha K, Schirner M, Krenn V, Kamradt T, Taupitz M. Assessment of unspecific near-infrared dyes in laser-induced fluorescence imaging of experimental arthritis. Acad Radiol. 2006;13(1):4–13. doi:10.1016/j.acra.2005.07.010.
74. Vinegoni C, Botnaru I, Aikawa E, Calfon MA, Iwamoto Y, Folco EJ, Ntziachristos V, Weissleder R, Libby P, Jaffer FA. Indocyanine green enables near-infrared fluorescence imaging of lipid-rich, inflamed atherosclerotic plaques. Sci Transl Med. 2011;3(84):84ra45. doi:10.1126/scitranslmed.3001577.
75. Bavry AA, Bhatt DL. Appropriate use of drug-eluting stents: balancing the reduction in restenosis with the concern of late thrombosis. Lancet. 2008;371(9630):2134–43. doi:10.1016/S0140-6736(08)60922-8.
76. Holmes DR, Kereiakes DJ, Garg S, Serruys PW, Dehmer GJ, Ellis SG, Williams DO, Kimura T, Moliterno DJ. Stent thrombosis. J Am Coll Cardiol. 2010;56(17):1357–65. doi:10.1016/j.jacc.2010.07.016.
77. Witzenbichler B, Mehran R, Guagliumi G, Dudek D, Huber K, Kornowski R, Stuckey TD, Fahy M, Parise H, Stone GW. Impact of diabetes mellitus on the safety and effectiveness of bivalirudin in patients with acute myocardial infarction undergoing primary angioplasty: analysis from the HORIZONS-AMI (Harmonizing Outcomes with RevasculariZatiON and Stents in Acute Myocardial Infarction) trial. JACC Cardiovasc Interv. 2011;4(7):760–8. doi:10.1016/j.jcin.2011.04.008.
78. Roffi M, Topol EJ. Percutaneous coronary intervention in diabetic patients with non-ST-segment elevation acute coronary syndromes. Eur Heart J. 2004;25(3):190–8. doi:10.1016/j.ehj.2003.10.027.
79. Serruys PW, de Jaegere P, Kiemeneij F, Macaya C, Rutsch W, Heyndrickx G, Emanuelsson H, Marco J, Legrand V, Materne P. A comparison of balloon-expandable-stent implantation with balloon angioplasty in patients with coronary artery disease. Benestent Study Group. N Engl J Med. 1994;331(8):489–95. doi:10.1056/NEJM199408253310801.
80. Finn AV, Joner M, Nakazawa G, Kolodgie F, Newell J, John MC, Gold HK, Virmani R. Pathological correlates of late drug-eluting stent thrombosis: strut coverage as a marker of endothelialization. Circulation. 2007;115(18):2435–41. doi:10.1161/CIRCULATIONAHA.107.693739.
81. Joner M, Finn AV, Farb A, Mont EK, Kolodgie FD, Ladich E, Kutys R, Skorija K, Gold HK, Virmani R. Pathology of drug-eluting stents in humans: delayed healing and late thrombotic risk. J Am Coll Cardiol. 2006;48(1):193–202. doi:10.1016/j.jacc.2006.03.042.

82. Nakazawa G, Finn AV, Joner M, Ladich E, Kutys R, Mont EK, Gold HK, Burke AP, Kolodgie FD, Virmani R. Delayed arterial healing and increased late stent thrombosis at culprit sites after drug-eluting stent placement for acute myocardial infarction patients: an autopsy study. Circulation. 2008;118(11):1138–45. doi:10.1161/CIRCULATIONAHA.107.762047.
83. Lüscher TF, Steffel J, Eberli FR, Joner M, Nakazawa G, Tanner FC, Virmani R. Drug-eluting stent and coronary thrombosis: biological mechanisms and clinical implications. Circulation. 2007;115(8):1051–8. doi:10.1161/CIRCULATIONAHA.106.675934.
84. Mintz GS, Nissen SE, Anderson WD, Bailey SR, Erbel R, Fitzgerald PJ, Pinto FJ, Rosenfield K, Siegel RJ, Tuzcu EM, Yock PG. J Am Coll Cardiol. 2001 Apr;37(5):1478–92.
85. Murata A, Wallace-Bradley D, Tellez A, Alviar C, Aboodi M, Sheehy A, Coleman L, Perkins L, Nakazawa G, Mintz G, Kaluza GL, Virmani R, Granada JF. Accuracy of optical coherence tomography in the evaluation of neointimal coverage after stent implantation. JACC Cardiovasc Imaging. 2010;3(1):76–84. doi:10.1016/j.jcmg.2009.09.018.
86. Nakano M, Vorpahl M, Otsuka F, Taniwaki M, Yazdani SK, Finn AV, Ladich ER, Kolodgie FD, Virmani R. Ex vivo assessment of vascular response to coronary stents by optical frequency domain imaging. JACC Cardiovasc Imaging. 2012;5(1):71–82. doi:10.1016/j.jcmg.2011.09.015.
87. Botnar RM, Buecker A, Wiethoff AJ, Parsons EC, Katoh M, Katsimaglis G, Weisskoff RM, Lauffer RB, Graham PB, Gunther RW, Manning WJ, Spuentrup E. In vivo magnetic resonance imaging of coronary thrombosis using a fibrin-binding molecular magnetic resonance contrast agent. Circulation. 2004;110(11):1463–6. doi:10.1161/01.CIR.0000134960.31304.87.
88. Hara T, Bhayana B, Thompson B, Kessinger CW, Khatri A, McCarthy JR, Weissleder R, Lin CP, Tearney GJ, Jaffer FA. Molecular imaging of fibrin deposition in deep vein thrombosis using fibrin-targeted near-infrared fluorescence. JACC Cardiovasc Imaging. 2012;5(6):607–15. doi:10.1016/j.jcmg.2012.01.017.
89. Spuentrup E, Botnar RM, Wiethoff AJ, Ibrahim T, Kelle S, Katoh M, Ozgun M, Nagel E, Vymazal J, Graham PB, Günther RW, Maintz D. MR imaging of thrombi using EP-2104R, a fibrin-specific contrast agent: initial results in patients. Eur Radiol. 2008;18(9):1995–2005. doi:10.1007/s00330-008-0965-2.
90. Vymazal J, Spuentrup E, Cardenas-Molina G, Wiethoff AJ, Hartmann MG, Caravan P, Parsons EC. Thrombus imaging with fibrin-specific gadolinium-based MR contrast agent EP-2104R: results of a phase II clinical study of feasibility. Invest Radiol. 2009;44(11):697–704. doi:10.1097/RLI.0b013e3181b092a7.

Optical Molecular Imaging of Inflammation and Calcification in Atherosclerosis

5

Joshua D. Hutcheson and Elena Aikawa

Contents

Abstract

Atherosclerotic plaque development is characterized by the presence of active inflammation, collagen remodeling, and the deposition of calcific mineral, and these processes have proven to be the main determinants of the biomechanical stability of the plaque. Collagen degradation due to proteases from inflammatory cells and/or the formation of spotty microcalcifications within the atherosclerotic

J.D. Hutcheson, PhD
Division of Cardiovascular Medicine, Center for Interdisciplinary Cardiovascular Sciences, Brigham and Women's Hospital, Harvard Medical School, 3 Blackfan St., Room 1736, Boston, MA 02115, USA

E. Aikawa, MD, PhD (✉)
Division of Cardiovascular Medicine, Center for Interdisciplinary Cardiovascular Sciences, Brigham and Women's Hospital, Harvard Medical School, 3 Blackfan St., Room 1736, Boston, MA 02115, USA

Division of Cardiovascular Medicine, Center for Excellence in Vascular Biology, Brigham and Women's Hospital, Harvard Medical School, Boston, MA 02114, USA
e-mail: eaikawa@partners.org

E. Aikawa (ed.), *Cardiovascular Imaging: Arterial and Aortic Valve Inflammation and Calcification*, DOI 10.1007/978-3-319-09268-3_5

fibrous cap can lead to plaque rupture and subsequent myocardial infarction or stroke. Therefore, the ability to monitor inflammation and calcification in situ could inform patient treatment options and prevent serious acute cardiovascular events. Commonly utilized imaging techniques lack the resolution to image these processes. In this chapter, we will discuss the promise of optical molecular imaging in imaging inflammation and calcification within atherosclerotic plaques. We will focus on data from preclinical studies performed in animal models of atherosclerosis, and we will extend our discussion into how these techniques may be fully realized in a clinical setting.

5.1 Imaging Criteria for Atherosclerotic Inflammation and Calcification

Growing epidemiological evidence conclusively demonstrates that arterial calcium burden is a significant predictor of cardiovascular morbidity and mortality. These findings have challenged previously held notions that arterial calcification serves as a biomechanical stabilizer of atherosclerotic plaques. Rupture of vulnerable atherosclerotic plaques and subsequent vessel occlusion via thrombus formation is the leading cause of myocardial infarction and stroke. Classically, atherosclerotic plaque vulnerability has been attributed to a reduction/degradation of collagen in the fibrous cap [1]; however, recent studies have identified that microcalcifications in the cap of vulnerable plaques may also contribute to its biomechanical failure [2, 3]. The presence of microcalcifications leads to significant stress accumulation resulting in plaque instability, whereas larger calcifications within the plaque may serve to stabilize the plaque. This presents a challenge for imaging vascular calcifications that contribute to plaque rupture. Due to their small size, dangerous microcalcifications are beneath the detection resolution of traditional CT-based imaging modalities that are commonly utilized to detect vascular calcification.

Calcific mineralization that forms both microcalcifications and larger calcifications within atherosclerotic plaques may be an irreversible endpoint of plaque development [4]. This mineralization is preceded by active inflammation within the plaque, and histopathological characterization of vulnerable and ruptured plaques reveals high levels of proinflammatory leukocytes within the growing neointimal region of the vessel wall [5]. These inflammatory cells release collagen-degrading proteases, compromising the biomechanical integrity of the fibrous cap [1]. Emerging evidence suggests that inflammatory macrophages may also directly contribute to the deposition of calcium phosphate mineral [6] in addition to releasing inflammatory cytokines that induce calcific phenotypic changes in vascular smooth muscle cells (SMC) [7, 8]. In contrast, stable atherosclerotic plaques contain few markers of active inflammation and are characterized by the presence of SMC with a synthetic phenotype that is responsible for the formation of a collagen-rich fibrous cap [9]. These stable plaques also often contain large calcifications that form beneath the fibrous cap.

In addition to their lipid-lowering benefits, the anti-inflammatory action of statins is believed to be responsible for their role in preventing acute cardiovascular events

[10]. By reducing inflammation within the plaque, these drugs favor the SMC-rich stable plaque phenotype. Many patients develop vulnerable plaques that lead to subsequent cardiovascular morbidity and mortality independent of traditional risk factors that would necessitate statin prescription. Updated guidelines set by the American Heart Association and American College of Cardiology are aimed at preventative treatment of these patients [11], but the clinical decision to begin statin treatment must currently be made without the benefit of positive identification of vulnerable plaque development within patients. Therefore, these guidelines will result in a portion of patients being prescribed statins unnecessarily. Additionally, a large number of patients fail to respond to statins [12]; however, currently clinicians are not able to assess changes in plaque vulnerability in patients taking statins.

Imaging modalities are needed that can monitor atherosclerotic plaque development to delineate vulnerable plaques with microcalcifications and inflammation versus collagen-rich stable plaque phenotypes. In this way, new criteria can be generated to target patients most at risk for plaque rupture, and clinicians can gauge the success of patients taking statins or other drugs that are intended to enhance plaque stability. Further, imaging techniques that are sensitive enough to detect the earliest stages of plaque development may present the opportunity to reverse and/or prevent atherosclerosis. Optical molecular imaging has exhibited promise in detecting all phases of plaque development including endothelial dysfunction and lipid accumulation, subsequent leukocyte infiltration into the plaque neointima, matrix remodeling resulting from inflammation and SMC migration, and finally the deposition of calcium phosphate mineral forming macrocalcification and microcalcification. Therefore, the advent of these techniques may lead to new paradigms in the detection and treatment of cardiovascular disease.

5.2 Optical Molecular Imaging Strategies

Both fluorescent and bioluminescent techniques are often utilized in optical molecular imaging of atherosclerotic plaques [13]. For fluorescent imaging, fluorophores are attached to the molecular probe, and light from an excitation source leads to an emission of fluorescent light where the molecules are present [14]. Bioluminescent probes employ similar targeting concepts; however, no excitation light is needed to observe sight produced by these molecules [15]. In both cases, the bioluminescent or fluorescent compounds may be directly attached to a targeting moiety, whereupon accumulation of the probes and targeting construct at the site of interest yields a signal that is detectable above the background. Alternatively, to detect enzymatic activity, the probes may be attached to a cleavable sequence in close proximity to quenchers that inhibit the output of detectable signal. Cleavage of these sequences by the enzyme of interest liberates these probes to reveal detectable signal. Three common detection modalities are utilized to receive the signal from the probes. Fluorescence reflectance imaging is the term used when the light source and detector lie on the same side of the imaged object [16]. When the detection and illumination sources are on opposite sides, it is termed transillumination fluorescence imaging

[17]. Finally, fluorescence-mediated tomography is the term used when the detector is set at a fixed position relative to a light source that is at a different location [18]. Near-infrared fluorescent (NIRF) dyes have emerged as a powerful tool for optical molecular imaging. Near-infrared light has relatively low absorption in biological tissues, allowing for a greater detectable penetration depth into tissues. Further, the advent of catheter-based modalities for intravascular detection of molecular imaging agents circumvents the limitations of tissue penetration depth that has traditionally limited optical molecular imaging in cardiovascular tissues [14].

5.3 Leukocyte Infiltration via Endothelial Cell Activation

Leukocyte infiltration into the vesicle wall and subsequent inflammation has long been known to play a role in plaque development and stability [9]. Activation of endothelial cells in regions of disturbed blood flow (e.g., arterial branch points) is believed to be an initiating event in the development of atherosclerotic plaques. Activated endothelial cells exhibit elevated expression of adhesion molecules on the apical surface (proximal to the lumen) that directs the infiltration of leukocytes into the vessel wall [19]. The leukocytes adhere to these adhesion proteins and migrate into the underlying intima. These adhesion proteins offer easily targetable sites [20] for optical molecular imaging of locations of plaque development. Due to the expression of these molecules on endothelial cells in direct contact with blood flow, molecular imaging agents designed for the detection of adhesion proteins do not have to diffuse into the vessel wall to bind to the intended target [21]. In a mouse model of atherosclerosis, injection of a magneto-optical reporter agent targeted to a specific adhesion protein, vascular cell adhesion molecule-1 (VCAM-1), was shown to identify plaque regions in vivo using MRI and ex vivo by employing NIRF imaging [19, 21]. NIRF VCAM-1 signal was validated using traditional immunohistological techniques, and endothelial expression of this protein was found to be associated with underlying leukocytes as shown by the expression of the macrophage protein Mac-3 (Fig. 5.1). Similarly, an in vitro study utilizing activated human umbilical vein endothelial cells subjected to physiologically relevant shear showed that iron oxide microparticles dually conjugated to antibodies against VCAM-1 and another adhesion molecule, E-selectin, exhibited significantly greater retention and signal-to-noise properties by optical coherence tomography compared to microparticles conjugated to antibodies against either adhesion molecule alone [22]. Similar techniques may be utilized in vivo to enhance sensitivity and specificity of plaque identification [23].

Following adhesion to the endothelial cells and migration from the lumen to the subendothelial space, monocytes give rise to macrophages that play a central role in the growth of the neointimal atherosclerotic plaque. Scavenger receptors on the plasma membrane allow these macrophages to phagocytose, or engulf, cholesterol within the early lesion forming foam cells that serve as a means of cholesterol clearance from the plaque. Molecular probes targeting macrophage scavenger receptors have shown the ability to detect inflammation by accumulating in macrophage-rich atherosclerotic plaques of mice with the amount of detectable signal proportional to

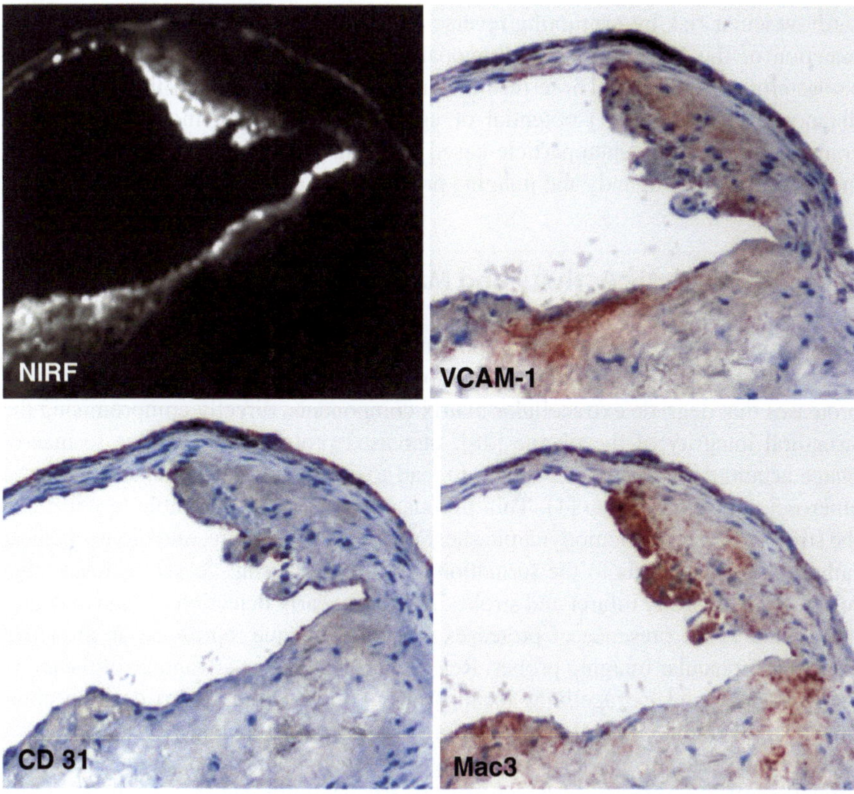

Fig. 5.1 Molecular imaging of endothelial VCAM-1 expression. A VCAM-1-targeted NIRF probe shows co-localization with VCAM-1 staining by immunohistochemistry in mouse aorta. This signal is also associated with CD31 expression, indicating the presence of endothelium, and Mac-3 expression that reveals underlying macrophages. Original magnification ×400. Bar = 50 μm (Figure is courtesy of Dr. M. Nahrendorf)

the degree of macrophage number [24]. Similarly, due to their phagocytic action, dextran-coated magnetofluorescent nanoparticles were shown to exhibit the highest uptake in plaque macrophages compared to other cell types within the plaque [25]. The specificity of these nanoparticles can be further enhanced using ligands to known macrophage markers.

Inefficiency in removing apoptotic foam cells leads to the formation of a necrotic core within the plaque that has been shown to be associated with plaque destabilization. Therefore, the identification of macrophage apoptosis within lesions would allow the detection of potentially vulnerable plaques prior to rupture. High-density lipoprotein (HDL) mimicking polymer nanoparticles with a quantum dot core and a cationic ligand that targets the mitochondria of apoptotic cells and a quantum dot core were recently developed [26]. The fluorescent quantum dots allowed optical imaging of macrophage apoptosis in vitro as the nanoparticles accumulated in the mitochondria of dying cells. Elevated plasma HDL has been shown to reduce cardiovascular risk by promoting reverse cholesterol transport. In a mouse model, injection of the HDL-mimicking nanoparticles led to a reduction in total serum cholesterol in the mice. These results demonstrate the combined therapeutic and diagnostic ("theranostic") potential of agents designed with molecular imaging components. Further, nanoparticle-based imaging strategies provide an efficient means of targeting ligands and imaging probes to the atherosclerotic plaque [27].

5.4 Proteolytic Activity and Matrix Remodeling

In addition to – and perhaps more importantly than – their role in plaque destabilization associated with necrotic core formation, macrophages within the plaque release proteases that degrade extracellular matrix components, directly compromising the structural integrity of the plaque [28]. Increased protease activity due to macrophage accumulation has been shown to lead to a reduction of collagen within the atherosclerotic fibrous cap [1]. Thin fibrous cap atheroma is not able to withstand the stresses caused by hemodynamic shear and systolic pressure, and biomechanical failure of the cap leads to the formation of thrombi causing vessel occlusion that results in myocardial infarct and stroke. Therefore, early detection of matrix degradation due to the presence of proteases within the plaque represents an attractive target for molecular imaging probes. Researchers have taken advantage of the enzymatic activity and extracellular localization of these proteases to develop compounds that exhibit NIRF signal following proteolytic activation.

Cysteine protease activity was the target of the first generation of enzymatically activated NIRF molecular probe agents [29, 30]. These probes were synthesized by incorporating NIRF molecules on cysteine peptide chains. The close proximity of the NIRF agents quenches the fluorescent signal due to fluorescence resonance energy transfer. Cleavage of the chains by cysteine proteases liberates the NIRF molecules, leading to observable fluorescent signal. Cysteine proteases include members of the cathepsin family of enzymes, namely, cathepsins B, K, and S that are the most relevant targets for atherosclerosis [30, 31]. An activatable cathepsin B-targeted NIRF agent shows lysosomal uptake and accumulation in plaque inflammatory cells [30]. Similarly, catheter-based intravascular imaging of cysteine protease activity following injection of these agents in a rabbit model of arteriosclerosis revealed strong NIRF signal in inflamed plaques that was associated with cathepsin B activity [32]. Incorporating peptide sequences targeted to enzymes of interest (rather than the nonspecific cysteine peptide chain) enables the detection of specific proteases within the plaque and can give insight into biomolecular mechanisms of plaque development. Using this strategy, cathepsin S, an elastolytic cysteine protease, was found to be increased in atherosclerotic plaques of a mouse model of chronic renal disease (CRD) with a strong association to calcification [33] (Fig. 5.2a). Osteogenic activity and mineral deposition were abolished in mice lacking cathepsin S activity, demonstrating a causative link between cathepsin S and calcification (Fig. 5.2b).

In a similar manner to the probe for cathepsin S, second-generation activatable NIRF agents were developed to measure collagen-degrading matrix metalloprotease (MMP) activity by replacing the cysteine chain with a gelatinase substrate

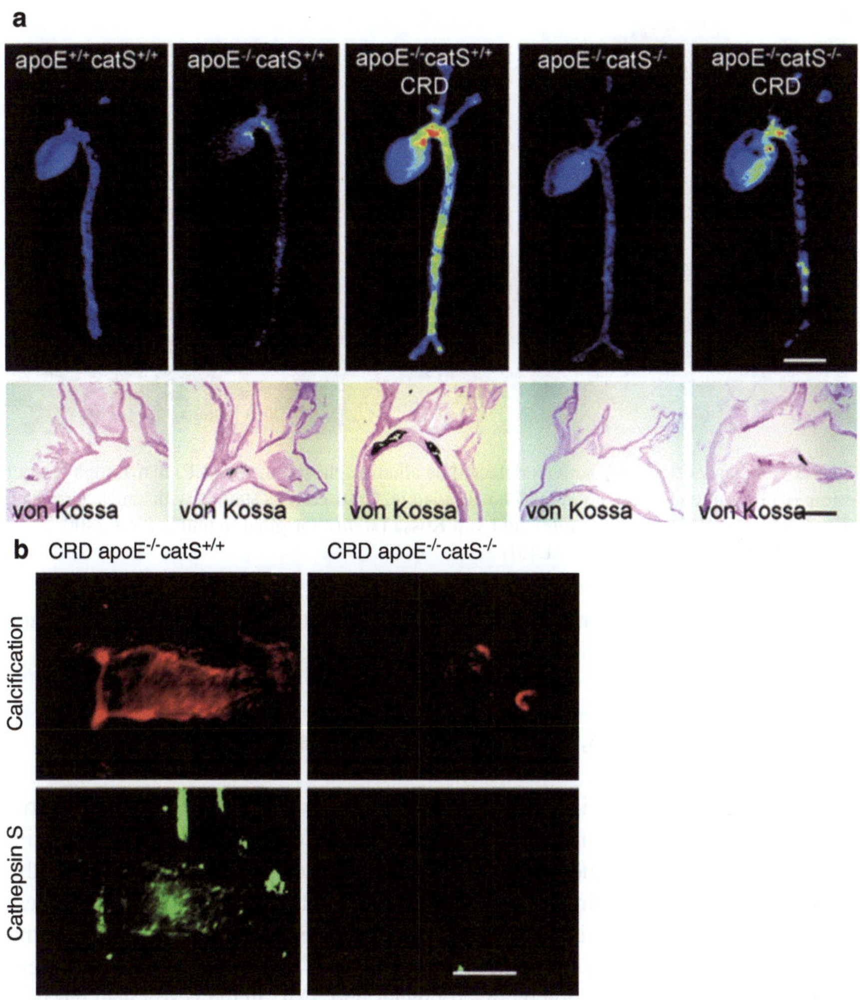

Fig. 5.2 Molecular imaging of cathepsin S and calcification. (**a**) Fluorescence reflection imaging of a NIRF probe targeted to cathepsin S revealed the highest cardiovascular activity in an $ApoE^{-/-}$ mouse model of chronic renal disease (CRD). This increased activity was also associated with aortic calcification as identified by von Kossa staining of histological sections. (**b**) Using the NIRF cathepsin S probe in combination with a NIRF probe for calcification showed a strong association between the two. Further, by knocking out cathepsin S in the mice, calcification of the aorta was mitigated (Modified from Aikawa et al. [33])

(collagenase MMPs also recognize gelatin as a substrate) [34]. An atherosclerotic mouse model on a high-cholesterol diet was given injection of the MMP-sensitive NIRF agent 24 h prior to imaging with fluorescence-mediated tomography revealing significant signal in the aortic root, arch, and thoracic aorta corresponding to sites of atheroma. These agents may provide a means for early identification of particularly vulnerable plaques. MMPs have been shown to mediate collagen degradation within the atherosclerotic fibrous cap, leading to diminished biomechanical

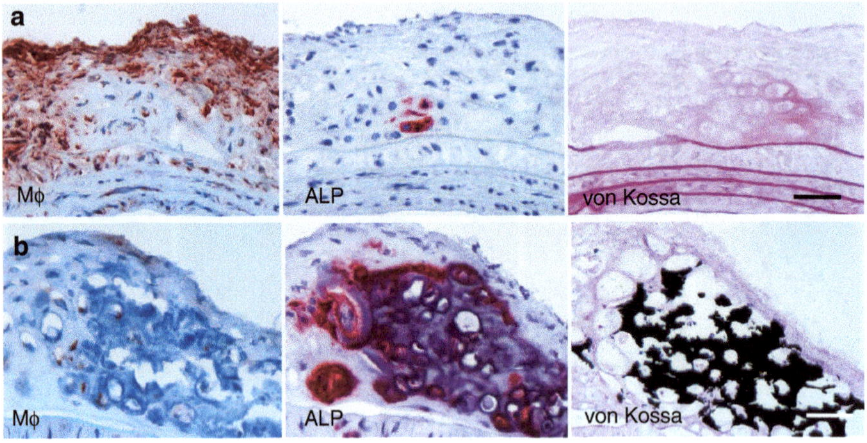

Fig. 5.3 (**a**) Early osteogenic activity detected by alkaline phosphatase (ALP) in macrophage-rich lesion. (**b**) Prominent calcification in advances plaque. Cryosections stained with anti-macrophage Mac-3 antibody (*left*), ALP (*middle*), and von Kossa (*right*). Original magnification ×400. Bar = 50 μm (Modified from Aikawa et al. [5])

integrity, plaque rupture, and thrombosis. Therefore, imaging MMP activity in early atheromas could allow clinicians to identify areas of concern prior to rupture.

5.5 Inflammation, Osteogenesis, and Calcification

In addition to their participation in plaque remodeling via the release of matrix-degrading enzymes, inflammatory cells also contribute to the formation of calcific deposits within the plaque (Fig. 5.3). In vitro studies have demonstrated that macrophage-derived cytokines (e.g., IL-1β, IL-6, IL-8, TNF-α, IGF-1, and TGF-β) can induce osteogenic differentiation of vascular SMC [7, 8]. Evidence also suggests that macrophages can actively participate in the nucleation of calcium phosphate mineral [6]. Imaging mineral deposition by macrophages and SMC in the vessel wall has been achieved using bisphosphonates conjugated to NIRF molecules [35]. Bisphosphonates have a structure similar to the calcification inhibitor pyrophosphate and are believed to bind to calcium and accumulate in mineralized crystals [35, 36]. The accumulation of NIRF-bisphosphonates in calcific regions of atherosclerotic plaques yields detectable NIRF signal that is spectrally distinct from the protease agents discussed in the previous section [37]. Imaging these processes in parallel has provided new insight into the relationship between inflammation and calcification [5, 38].

Whether by priming the matrix, stimulating SMC, or actively depositing mineral, inflammation is closely linked with calcification within the atherosclerotic plaque and ultimately to plaque stability [39]. This point was shown in an atherosclerotic mouse model, wherein fluorescence reflection imaging of explanted aortae from the mice revealed a strong association between inflammation and calcification [5] (Fig. 5.4). NIRF signals from both processes were noted in regions associated with high shear stress including the aortic arch and root, the innominate artery, and the

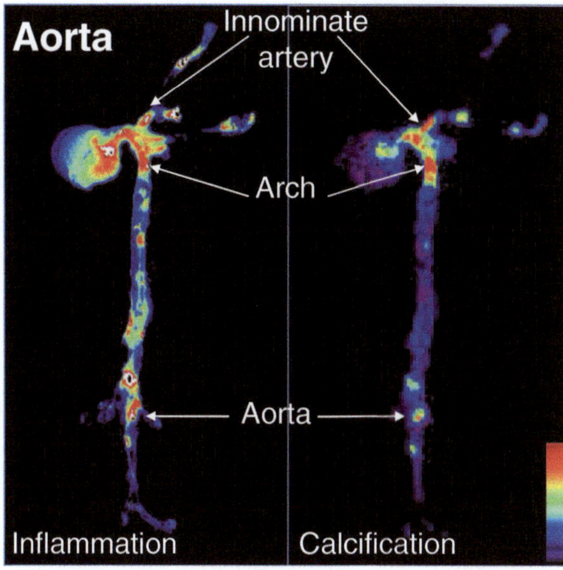

Fig. 5.4 Fluorescence reflection imaging of NIRF-conjugated iron nanoparticles that target macrophages revealed a co-localization between areas of inflammation and calcification in an excised mouse aorta (Modified from Aikawa et al. [5])

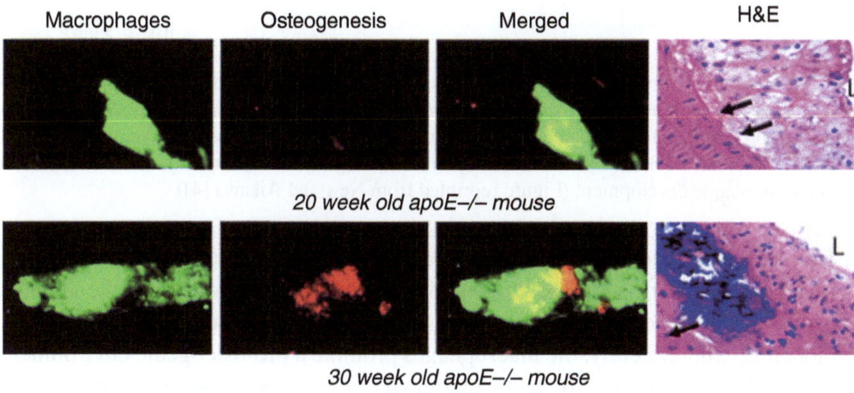

Fig. 5.5 Longitudinal study: NIRF probes with different emission wavelengths allow for simultaneous imaging of inflammation (*green fluorescence*) and calcification (*red fluorescence*). Using this technique in an $ApoE^{-/-}$ mouse model of atherosclerosis, it was shown that inflammation not only co-localizes with calcification, but also seemed to precede calcific mineral deposition. Twenty-week-old mice exhibited high arterial signal corresponding to the macrophage-targeted probe but did not exhibit signs of calcification. In 30-week-old mice, inflammatory cells and calcification were either within close proximity or co-localized (*yellow fluorescence*). Representative histomorphological images shown on the right. Hematoxylin and eosin. Magnification ×400. Bar = 50 μm. *L* depicts lumen; *arrows* depict internal elastic lamina (Modified from Aikawa et al. [5])

carotid bifurcation. The elevated mechanical stress in these regions has been shown to associate with plaque development in both mouse and humans. Longitudinal studies in Apolipoprotein E (ApoE) deficient mice further demonstrated that not only do the inflammation and calcification signals overlap but also the inflammation seemed to necessarily precede calcific mineral deposition [5] (Fig. 5.5). Therefore,

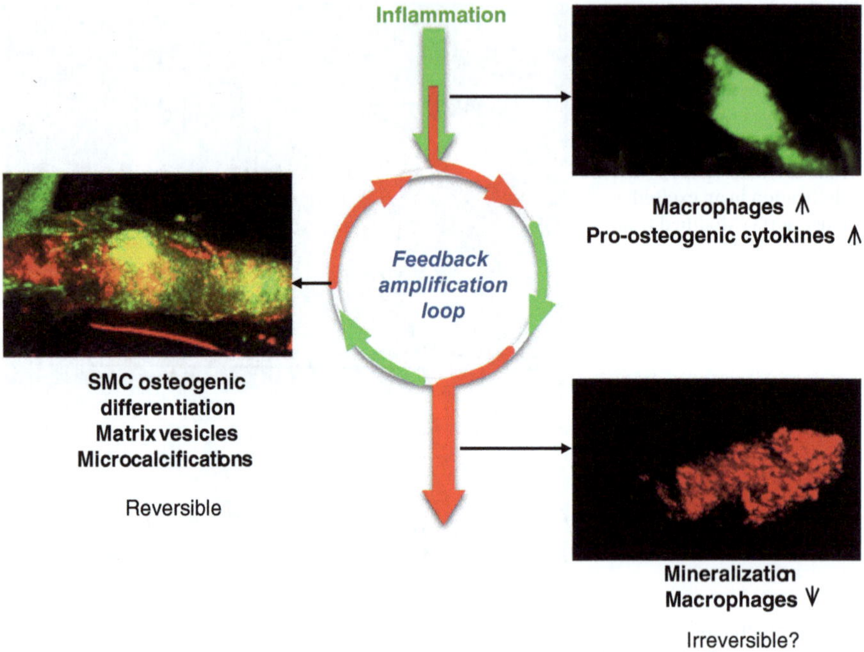

Fig. 5.6 Atherosclerotic plaque development initiates with the infiltration of proinflammatory macrophages that stimulate propagation of plaque development through matrix remodeling and the release of pro-osteogenic cytokines. The initiation and propagation phases may provide the most appropriate window for therapeutic intervention. End-stage calcification may be an irreversible endpoint of plaque development (Figure reprinted from New and Aikawa [4])

it has been proposed that inflammation-dependent calcification in the atherosclerotic plaque can be divided into three phases: initiation, propagation, and end-stage calcification [4]. The initiation phase consists of macrophage infiltration and matrix remodeling. Subsequently, the macrophages promote a pro-osteogenic environment where both SMC and macrophages participate in the propagation of plaque development through the deposition of calcium phosphate mineral. Once the mineralization begins, the final phase, end-stage calcification, progresses quickly and may be an irreversible endpoint of plaque development (Fig. 5.6).

5.6 Future Perspectives

As mentioned in the introduction to this chapter, plaque phenotype determines the biomechanical integrity of the atheroma, and both inflammation and calcification play a major role in the biomechanical state of the plaque. The persistence of inflammation in the plaque leads to both heightened protease activity resulting in thinning of collagen in the fibrous cap and the progression of calcification. Further, the presence of macrophages seems to be associated with the formation of microcalcifications within the fibrous cap. Cellular-derived matrix vesicles are believed to serve as nucleating foci for the formation of microcalcifications, and these matrix vesicles may be derived from both the macrophages themselves or from SMC stimulated to undergo osteogenic reprogramming by macrophage releasing proinflammatory cytokines. Though their role in plaque destabilization is now clear, much remains unknown about the mechanisms of microcalcification formation. As we learn more about these mechanisms, new molecular targets for imaging probes may be created to visualize the absolute earliest phases of the calcification process.

Recent advancements using positron emission tomography/CT (PET/CT) with ^{18}F-sodium fluoride (^{18}F-NaF), an established PET tracer for bone formation and remodeling, and ^{18}F-fluorodeoxyglucose (18-FDG), shown to accumulate in regions of inflammation, may provide new strategies for honing in on regions of plaque vulnerability [40]. Coronary uptake of ^{18}F-NaF was found overlaying, adjacent to, and distal from regions of CT-identified calcifications [41]. Additionally, large areas of calcification with no ^{18}F-NaF uptake were observed. This suggests that, as with bone, ^{18}F-NaF uptake in the vasculature is a marker of ongoing calcific remodeling [41]. Large, stable calcifications do not exhibit ^{18}F-NaF update, whereas active regions of mineralization accumulate ^{18}F-NaF. The ^{18}F-NaF regions faraway from the CT-identified calcific regions may represent the dangerous microcalcifications that cannot be detected by traditional imaging modalities [41]. In support of this hypothesis, a prospective clinical trial showed high ^{18}F-NaF accumulation in the culprit coronary plaques in cases of myocardial infarction and in ruptured carotid artery plaques [42]. Histological evaluation of these plaques revealed active calcification processes. These PET/CT techniques exhibit promise in identifying particularly vulnerable regions within the vasculature; however, they still do not have the resolution necessary to identify specific microcalcifications that may contribute to plaque rupture.

Owing to the lack of tissue penetration depth of optical molecular imaging, these techniques are and will continue to be invasive for the near future. New fluorescence-mediated tomography techniques are increasing the tissue depths at which optical signals may be resolved. In the future, these techniques may provide the most noninvasive means of atherosclerotic plaque detection. However, in the meantime one strategy may be to first employ PET/CT imaging to identify particularly prone atherosclerotic regions. These regions could then be further probed using catheter-based optical molecular imaging techniques [43] to further assess the morphology of the plaque in order to determine the best approach to stabilize the plaque and, with the advent of a better understanding of the molecular understanding of the disease and resultant therapeutic strategies, potentially reverse atherosclerosis.

In addition to the potential for in situ plaque detection, molecular probes can be readily employed for preclinical research and ex vivo diagnostics. NIRF probes for hydroxyapatite, the calcium phosphate-based mineral involved in calcification, allow earlier detection of calcification in human plaques than light microscopy techniques currently used by pathologists (Fig. 5.7a) [5]. This enhanced resolution may allow researchers to understand the nucleation of

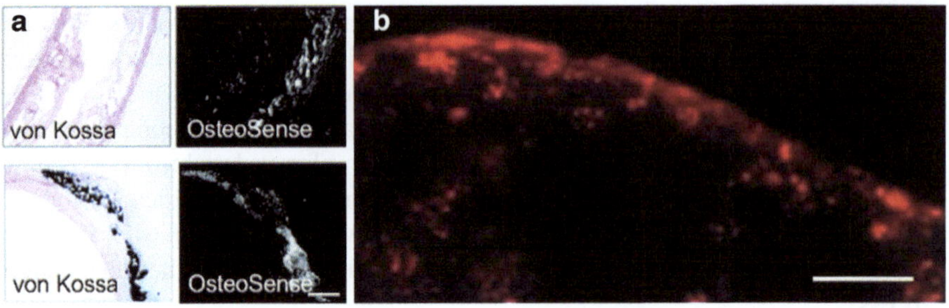

Fig. 5.7 Histological staining of calcific tissues with NIRF molecular probes. (**a**) A commercially available bisphosphonate NIRF probe, OsteoSense, exhibited greater sensitivity in detecting regions of calcification than the traditionally used von Kossa stain. Magnification ×200. Bar = 200 μm (Modified from Aikawa et al. [5]). (**b**) OsteoSense labeling of a mouse atherosclerotic plaque revealed numerous spotty microcalcifications throughout the plaque. Magnification ×400. Bar = 50 μm (Image modified from [6])

microcalcifications and allow pathologists to readily identify the presence of microcalcifications in subclinical atherosclerotic plaques from autopsy or tissues excised for other indications (Fig. 5.7b). Findings from these types of studies may provide new insight that could be used to design future iterations of optical molecular imaging strategies.

Sources of Funding Dr. Aikawa is supported by grants from the National Institutes of Health (R01HL114805; R01HL109506) and Harvard Catalyst Reactor Program.

References

1. Libby P. Collagenases and cracks in the plaque. J Clin Invest. 2013;123:3201–3.
2. Maldonado N, Kelly-Arnold A, Cardoso L, Weinbaum S. The explosive growth of small voids in vulnerable cap rupture; cavitation and interfacial debonding. J Biomech. 2013;46:396–401.
3. Kelly-Arnold A, Maldonado N, Laudier D, Aikawa E, Cardoso L, Weinbaum S. Revised microcalcification hypothesis for fibrous cap rupture in human coronary arteries. Proc Natl Acad Sci U S A. 2013;110:10741–6.
4. New SE, Aikawa E. Molecular imaging insights into early inflammatory stages of arterial and aortic valve calcification. Circ Res. 2011;108:1381–91.
5. Aikawa E, Nahrendorf M, Figueiredo JL, Swirski FK, Shtatland T, Kohler RH, Jaffer FA, Aikawa M, Weissleder R. Osteogenesis associates with inflammation in early-stage atherosclerosis evaluated by molecular imaging in vivo. Circulation. 2007;116:2841–50.
6. New SE, Goettsch C, Aikawa M, Marchini JF, Shibasaki M, Yabusaki K, Libby P, Shanahan CM, Croce K, Aikawa E. Macrophage-derived matrix vesicles: an alternative novel mechanism for microcalcification in atherosclerotic plaques. Circ Res. 2013;113:72–7.
7. Watson KE, Bostrom K, Ravindranath R, Lam T, Norton B, Demer LL. Tgf-beta 1 and 25-hydroxycholesterol stimulate osteoblast-like vascular cells to calcify. J Clin Invest. 1994;93:2106–13.
8. Tintut Y, Patel J, Parhami F, Demer LL. Tumor necrosis factor-alpha promotes in vitro calcification of vascular cells via the camp pathway. Circulation. 2000;102:2636–42.
9. Libby P. The interface of atherosclerosis and thrombosis: basic mechanisms. Vasc Med. 1998;3:225–9.
10. Libby P, Sasiela W. Plaque stabilization: can we turn theory into evidence? Am J Cardiol. 2006;98:26P–33.

11. Stone NJ, Robinson J, Lichtenstein AH, Bairey Merz CN, Lloyd-Jones DM, Blum CB, McBride P, Eckel RH, Schwartz JS, Goldberg AC, Shero ST, Gordon D, Smith Jr SC, Levy D, Watson K, Wilson PW. 2013 ACC/AHA guideline on the treatment of blood cholesterol to reduce atherosclerotic cardiovascular risk in adults: a report of the American College of Cardiology/American Heart Association Task Force on Practice Guidelines. J Am Coll Cardiol. 2013;63:2889–934.
12. Libby P. The forgotten majority: unfinished business in cardiovascular risk reduction. J Am Coll Cardiol. 2005;46:1225–8.
13. Subramanian S, Jaffer FA, Tawakol A. Optical molecular imaging in atherosclerosis. J Nucl Cardiol. 2010;17:135–44.
14. Ntziachristos V. Fluorescence molecular imaging. Annu Rev Biomed Eng. 2006;8:1–33.
15. Welsh DK, Kay SA. Bioluminescence imaging in living organisms. Curr Opin Biotechnol. 2005;16:73–8.
16. Waldeck J, Hager F, Holtke C, Lanckohr C, von Wallbrunn A, Torsello G, Heindel W, Theilmeier G, Schafers M, Bremer C. Fluorescence reflectance imaging of macrophage-rich atherosclerotic plaques using an alphavbeta3 integrin-targeted fluorochrome. J Nucl Med. 2008;49:1845–51.
17. Shirmanova M, Zagaynova E, Sirotkina M, Snopova L, Balalaeva I, Krutova I, Lekanova N, Turchin I, Orlova A, Kleshnin M. In vivo study of photosensitizer pharmacokinetics by fluorescence transillumination imaging. J Biomed Opt. 2010;15:048004.
18. Soubret A, Ntziachristos V. Fluorescence molecular tomography in the presence of background fluorescence. Phys Med Biol. 2006;51:3983–4001.
19. Nahrendorf M, Jaffer FA, Kelly KA, Sosnovik DE, Aikawa E, Libby P, Weissleder R. Noninvasive vascular cell adhesion molecule-1 imaging identifies inflammatory activation of cells in atherosclerosis. Circulation. 2006;114:1504–11.
20. Dunehoo AL, Anderson M, Majumdar S, Kobayashi N, Berkland C, Siahaan TJ. Cell adhesion molecules for targeted drug delivery. J Pharm Sci. 2006;95:1856–72.
21. Kelly KA, Allport JR, Tsourkas A, Shinde-Patil VR, Josephson L, Weissleder R. Detection of vascular adhesion molecule-1 expression using a novel multimodal nanoparticle. Circ Res. 2005;96:327–36.
22. Jefferson A, Wijesurendra RS, McAteer MA, Digby JE, Douglas G, Bannister T, Perez-Balderas F, Bagi Z, Lindsay AC, Choudhury RP. Molecular imaging with optical coherence tomography using ligand-conjugated microparticles that detect activated endothelial cells: rational design through target quantification. Atherosclerosis. 2011;219:579–87.
23. Weissleder R, Kelly K, Sun EY, Shtatland T, Josephson L. Cell-specific targeting of nanoparticles by multivalent attachment of small molecules. Nat Biotechnol. 2005;23:1418–23.
24. Tawakol A, Castano AP, Gad F, Zahra T, Bashian G, Migrino RQ, Ahmadi A, Stern J, Anatelli F, Chirico S, Shirazi A, Syed S, Fischman AJ, Muller JE, Hamblin MR. Intravascular detection of inflamed atherosclerotic plaques using a fluorescent photosensitizer targeted to the scavenger receptor. Photochem Photobiol Sci. 2008;7:33–9.
25. Jaffer FA, Nahrendorf M, Sosnovik D, Kelly KA, Aikawa E, Weissleder R. Cellular imaging of inflammation in atherosclerosis using magnetofluorescent nanomaterials. Mol Imaging. 2006;5:85–92.
26. Marrache S, Dhar S. Biodegradable synthetic high-density lipoprotein nanoparticles for atherosclerosis. Proc Natl Acad Sci U S A. 2013;110:9445–50.
27. Douma K, Prinzen L, Slaaf DW, Reutelingsperger CP, Biessen EA, Hackeng TM, Post MJ, van Zandvoort MA. Nanoparticles for optical molecular imaging of atherosclerosis. Small. 2009;5:544–57.
28. Naghavi M, Libby P, Falk E, Casscells SW, Litovsky S, Rumberger J, Badimon JJ, Stefanadis C, Moreno P, Pasterkamp G, Fayad Z, Stone PH, Waxman S, Raggi P, Madjid M, Zarrabi A, Burke A, Yuan C, Fitzgerald PJ, Siscovick DS, de Korte CL, Aikawa M, Airaksinen KE, Assmann G, Becker CR, Chesebro JH, Farb A, Galis ZS, Jackson C, Jang IK, Koenig W, Lodder RA, March K, Demirovic J, Navab M, Priori SG, Rekhter MD, Bahr R, Grundy SM, Mehran R, Colombo A, Boerwinkle E, Ballantyne C, Insull Jr W, Schwartz RS, Vogel R, Serruys PW, Hansson GK, Faxon DP, Kaul S, Drexler H, Greenland P, Muller JE, Virmani R, Ridker PM, Zipes DP, Shah PK, Willerson JT. From vulnerable plaque to vulnerable patient: a call for new definitions and risk assessment strategies: part ii. Circulation. 2003;108:1772–8.

29. Weissleder R, Tung CH, Mahmood U, Bogdanov Jr A. In vivo imaging of tumors with protease-activated near-infrared fluorescent probes. Nat Biotechnol. 1999;17:375–8.
30. Chen J, Tung CH, Mahmood U, Ntziachristos V, Gyurko R, Fishman MC, Huang PL, Weissleder R. In vivo imaging of proteolytic activity in atherosclerosis. Circulation. 2002;105:2766–71.
31. Jaffer FA, Kim DE, Quinti L, Tung CH, Aikawa E, Pande AN, Kohler RH, Shi GP, Libby P, Weissleder R. Optical visualization of cathepsin k activity in atherosclerosis with a novel, protease-activatable fluorescence sensor. Circulation. 2007;115:2292–8.
32. Yoo H, Kim JW, Shishkov M, Namati E, Morse T, Shubochkin R, McCarthy JR, Ntziachristos V, Bouma BE, Jaffer FA, Tearney GJ. Intra-arterial catheter for simultaneous microstructural and molecular imaging in vivo. Nat Med. 2011;17:1680–4.
33. Aikawa E, Aikawa M, Libby P, Figueiredo JL, Rusanescu G, Iwamoto Y, Fukuda D, Kohler RH, Shi GP, Jaffer FA, Weissleder R. Arterial and aortic valve calcification abolished by elastolytic cathepsin s deficiency in chronic renal disease. Circulation. 2009;119:1785–94.
34. Deguchi JO, Aikawa M, Tung CH, Aikawa E, Kim DE, Ntziachristos V, Weissleder R, Libby P. Inflammation in atherosclerosis: visualizing matrix metalloproteinase action in macrophages in vivo. Circulation. 2006;114:55–62.
35. Kozloff KM, Volakis LI, Marini JC, Caird MS. Near-infrared fluorescent probe traces bisphosphonate delivery and retention in vivo. J Bone Miner Res. 2010;25:1748–58.
36. Fleisch H. Development of bisphosphonates. Breast Cancer Res. 2002;4:30–4.
37. Zaheer A, Murshed M, De Grand AM, Morgan TG, Karsenty G, Frangioni JV. Optical imaging of hydroxyapatite in the calcified vasculature of transgenic animals. Arterioscler Thromb Vasc Biol. 2006;26:1132–6.
38. Aikawa E, Nahrendorf M, Sosnovik D, Lok VM, Jaffer FA, Aikawa M, Weissleder R. Multimodality molecular imaging identifies proteolytic and osteogenic activities in early aortic valve disease. Circulation. 2007;115:377–86.
39. Libby P, Tabas I, Fredman G, Fisher EA. Inflammation and its resolution as determinants of acute coronary syndromes. Circ Res. 2014;114:1867–79.
40. Chen W, Dilsizian V. Targeted pet/ct imaging of vulnerable atherosclerotic plaques: microcalcification with sodium fluoride and inflammation with fluorodeoxyglucose. Curr Cardiol Rep. 2013;15:364.
41. Dweck MR, Chow MW, Joshi NV, Williams MC, Jones C, Fletcher AM, Richardson H, White A, McKillop G, van Beek EJ, Boon NA, Rudd JH, Newby DE. Coronary arterial 18f-sodium fluoride uptake: a novel marker of plaque biology. J Am Coll Cardiol. 2012;59:1539–48.
42. Joshi NV, Vesey AT, Williams MC, Shah AS, Calvert PA, Craighead FH, Yeoh SE, Wallace W, Salter D, Fletcher AM, van Beek EJ, Flapan AD, Uren NG, Behan MW, Cruden NL, Mills NL, Fox KA, Rudd JH, Dweck MR, Newby DE. 18f-fluoride positron emission tomography for identification of ruptured and high-risk coronary atherosclerotic plaques: a prospective clinical trial. Lancet. 2014;383:705–13.
43. Jaffer FA, Vinegoni C, John MC, Aikawa E, Gold HK, Finn AV, Ntziachristos V, Libby P, Weissleder R. Real-time catheter molecular sensing of inflammation in proteolytically active atherosclerosis. Circulation. 2008;118:1802–9.

Molecular Imaging of Oxidation-Specific Epitopes to Detect High-Risk Atherosclerotic Plaques

6

Karen Briley-Saebo, Calvin Yeang, Joel R. Wilson, and Sotirios Tsimikas

Contents

Abstract

The oxidation of lipoproteins is a critical factor in the initiation, progression, and destabilization of atherosclerotic lesions. Reactive oxygen species and enzymes in the vessel wall modify lipoproteins to generate a variety of oxidation-specific epitopes (OSE). OSE are pro-inflammatory, immunogenic, and pro-atherogenic by activating macrophages leading to foam cell formation, apoptosis, and necrotic cores. OSE activate the innate and adaptive immune systems that lead to

K. Briley-Saebo, PhD
Division of Radiology, New York University, New York, NY, USA

C. Yeang • J.R. Wilson • S. Tsimikas, MD (✉)
Division of Cardiovascular Medicine, University of California San Diego, BSB-1080, La Jolla, CA 92093-0682, USA
e-mail: stsimikas@ucsd.edu

E. Aikawa (ed.), *Cardiovascular Imaging: Arterial and Aortic Valve Inflammation and Calcification*, DOI 10.1007/978-3-319-09268-3_6

pro-inflammatory responses. The immunological properties of OSE have facilitated the generation and characterization and modification of murine and human monoclonal antibodies as imaging agents. Nuclear and magnetic resonance techniques have been used to visualize OSE in preclinical models. OSE-targeted antibodies have been derivatized with radioisotopes or complexed with gadolinium, manganese, and iron oxide nanoparticles to facilitate in vivo imaging of atherosclerotic lesions. OSE-targeted antibody uptake in the vessel wall is proportional to plaque burden in early and intermediate lesions allowing quantitation of the extent of atherosclerosis. In intervention studies, imaging of OSE allows the detection of atherosclerosis regression and features of plaque stabilization. Translation of these approaches to humans may provide sensitive techniques to image, diagnose, and monitor high-risk atherosclerotic lesions, guide optimal therapeutic interventions, and evaluate efficacy of novel therapeutic agents.

6.1 Introduction

It is well established that oxidized stress plays a key role in the initiation, progression, and destabilization of atherosclerosis [1–6]. The concept of oxidative stress as it relates to cardiovascular disease encompasses the overproduction of reactive oxygen species (ROS) and upregulation of prooxidant enzymes in the vessel wall that are generated in response to physiologic and metabolic disturbances and potentiated by genetic predisposition [7], leading to the formation of atherosclerotic lesions [8]. ROS modify polyunsaturated fatty acids, amino acids, and lipoproteins, thereby producing a variety of pro-atherogenic and pro-inflammatory oxidation-specific epitopes (OSE) [3]. Oxidized phospholipids (OxPL) are a subset of OSE that induce the upregulation of pro-inflammatory genes and mediate localized inflammatory responses in the arterial wall [3, 9].

OxPL, malondialdehyde (MDA) epitopes, and oxidized cholesteryl esters are well-characterized OSE that are present on lipoproteins and in atherosclerotic lesions of preclinical models of atherosclerosis [10], in humans with vulnerable coronary and carotid plaques [11], and in patients undergoing percutaneous interventions [12–14]. OSE upregulate adhesion molecules that attract monocytes to the arterial wall, upregulate pro-inflammatory genes releasing cytokines, and mediate macrophage retention [3, 9, 15–17]. Intra-plaque macrophages in atherosclerotic mice take up OSE via a variety of scavenger receptors leading to foam cell formation, macrophage apoptosis, plaque progression and plaque rupture, and ultimately to clinical events [18].

In direct response to this pro-inflammatory cascade, immune effector proteins, such as natural antibodies and acquired autoantibodies directed to OSE, are produced by activated T and B cells [2, 19]. Strong experimental and clinical evidence demonstrates that IgM autoantibodies are atheroprotective, as manifested by accelerated atherosclerosis in mouse models of IgM knockout mice [20, 21] and by studies showing that patients with higher levels of IgM autoantibodies at baseline have

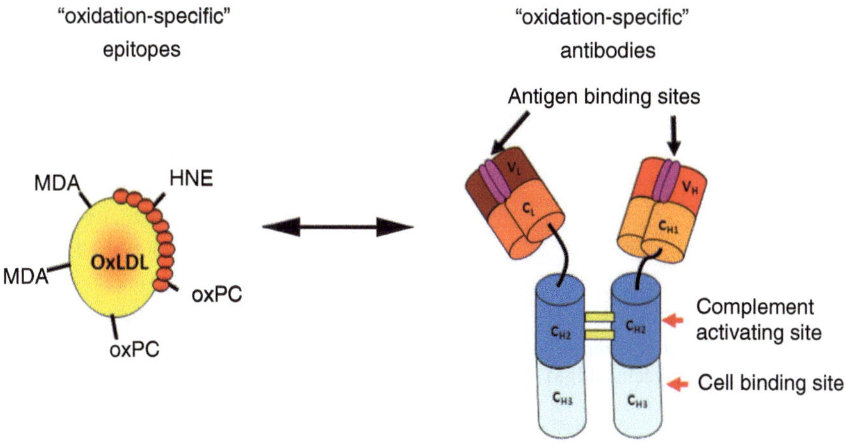

Fig. 6.1 Representations of well-characterized oxidation-specific epitopes and antibodies. Oxidation-specific antibodies recognize protein and lipid epitopes on oxidized LDL (*OxLDL*). These epitopes include malondialdehyde (*MDA*), phosphocholine-containing oxidized phospholipids (*PC-OxPL*), and 4-hydroxynonenal (*HNE*)

a reduced risk of subsequent anatomical cardiovascular disease (CVD) and CVD clinical events [22–24]. In addition, a large number of studies have also shown that OxPL are present on lipoprotein (a) [Lp(a)], which functions as a preferential lipoprotein carrier of OxPL, and that the content of OxPL on Lp(a) is a major driver of CVD risk [6, 24–27]. Lp(a) is an independent, causal risk factor for CVD and aortic valve calcification and stenosis [28–34].

We have taken advantage of the immunological properties of OSEs and their influence on generation of antibodies to OSE to generate, characterize, and evaluate murine and human monoclonal antibodies as molecular imaging agents. Below we highlight the antibodies generated and their diagnostic utility for in vivo detection of OSE (Fig. 6.1).

6.2 Antibodies and Peptides to Oxidation-Specific Epitopes

Table 6.1 summarizes the murine and human OSE autoantibodies and peptides with potential in clinical diagnostic imaging applications.

MDA2 was one of the first monoclonal antibodies (IgG2a type) isolated and generated against OSEs that are formed during the oxidative modification of LDL [35]. MDA2 was generated from hybridomas derived from mice immunized with homologous murine malondialdehyde(MDA)-modified LDL. MDA2 is a hapten-specific antibody that recognizes MDA-modified proteins, such as MDA-LDL and other modified proteins present within atherosclerotic lesions, without any binding to native LDL, high-density lipoprotein, or very low-density lipoproteins [10, 36, 37].

Table 6.1 Properties of murine and human OSE autoantibodies and peptides proposed for imaging applications

Antibody	Source	Epitopes bound	Conjugated labels
MDA2	Murine monoclonal IgG	MDA-LDL MDA-modified proteins	^{125}I, ^{99}Tc Gd micelles Mn micelles Mn dendrimers LUSPIO micelles LSPIO micelles Rhodamine micelles
E06	Natural murine monoclonal IgM	PC on oxidized phospholipids	Gd micelles Mn micelles LUSPIO micelles LSPIO micelles Rhodamine micelles
IK17 (scFv)	Human monoclonal IgG	MDA-LDL Copper OxLDL	Gd micelles Mn micelles LUSPIO micelles LSPIO micelles Rhodamine micelles
IK17 (scFab)	Human monoclonal IgG	MDA-LDL Copper OxLDL	Gd micelles Rhodamine micelles
Mimotope	**Characteristic**	**Epitopes mimicked**	**Antibodies bound**
P1	12-mer linear peptide	MAA MDA-LDL Copper OxLDL	LR04 IK17 Human IgG autoantibodies Human IgM autoantibodies
P2	7-mer cyclic peptide	MAA MDA-LDL Copper OxLDL	LR04 IK17 Human IgG autoantibodies Human IgM autoantibodies

The "natural" monoclonal antibody E06 (IgM type) antibody was discovered and characterized from splenic lymphocytes of apoE$^{-/-}$mice [38, 39]. E06 binds to the phosphocholine (PC) head group of oxidized, but not native, phospholipids [40]. E06 effectively blocks the uptake of OxLDL and apoptotic cells by mouse macrophages [41] and protects mice against atherosclerosis [42], thereby demonstrating potential therapeutic benefit [14]. Interestingly, the variable region of E06 is structurally identical to "natural" murine T15 IgA antibodies that bind unoxidized PC of pneumococcus PC and protect mice against lethal infection [43]. It is believed that this class of autoantibodies may have evolved and been preserved through natural selection in response to defense against PC-containing organisms such as pneumococci and clearance of apoptotic cells [3].

IK17 Fab, the first fully human OSE monoclonal antibody, was generated from lymphocytes of a patient with coronary artery disease [44]. Total RNA was isolated from the patient's peripheral blood mononuclear cells and was used to synthesize cDNA. Reverse transcription-polymerase chain reactions were performed, and the polymerase chain reaction products pooled according to isotype. The isotypes were then cloned into the phage display vector, pComb3H, to generate 2 phage display libraries, VH/Vκ and VH/Vλ. The resultant phagemid DNA was transformed into XL-1 blue Escherichia coli, rescued with a helper phage, and panned against MDA-LDL. The phagemid DNA was then prepared from infected bacteria and manipulated to express IK17 by removing gene III, which is fused to the C-terminus of the heavy chain gene and is essential for anchoring the Fab on the phage surface. IK17 binds to an advanced MDA-like epitope, malondialdehyde-acetaldehyde (MDA-MAA), which is expressed during extensive oxidative modification and in advanced human atherosclerotic lesions and vulnerable and ruptured plaques [11, 44–48]. IK17 has been shown to inhibit the uptake of OxLDL and apoptotic cells by macrophages similar to E06 [44]. For diagnostic imaging, both the Fab fragment and the lower-molecular-weight single-chain Fv (scFv) fragment have been used [44–47]. Overexpression of scFv IK17 with adenovirus or infusion of IK17 Fab results in reduced progression of atherosclerosis in susceptible mouse models [48]. The discovery of this human autoantibody has clinical implications not only from a diagnostic standpoint (reduced immunological concerns relative to the clinical use of murine antibodies) but also as a therapeutic agent.

Peptides are advantageous from a clinical and commercial point of view as they are less immunogenic and are more cost-effective to produce, relative to their antibody counterparts. However, in order for a peptide to maintain the efficacy of the native antibody, the functional group of the antibody needs to be fully understood and sequenced. Currently 12-mer linear (P1) and one 7-mer cyclic (P2) peptides have been identified using phage display libraries and screened using binding specificity to murine and human anti-MDA monoclonal antibodies [49]. Additionally, these peptides mimic MDA and related epitopes that are present on the surface of murine apoptotic cells. Immunization of mice with the cyclic P2 peptides resulted in the generation of MDA-LDL-specific autoantibodies. In human studies, mimotopes will provide standardized, chemically defined antigens and are a paradigm in the generation of potential antibody mimics for diagnostic imaging.

Overall, these findings suggest that the OSE-targeted antibodies and mimotopes may have significant potential in biotheranostic (biomarker, diagnostic imaging, and therapeutic) applications [14, 50]. Table 6.2 summarizes the characteristics of all OSE molecular probes.

Table 6.2 Compilations of imaging studies targeting oxidation-specific epitopes

Date	Authors	Modality	Label/dose	Platform	Antibodies	Animal models	Summary of key findings
1999	Tsimikas et al [37]	Planar/ SPECT	^{99}Tc/ 90 μCi ^{125}I ^{125}I	Direct conjugation	In vivo imaging MDA2 pKa MDA2 Halb (control Ab to human albumin) Biodistribution MDA2 alone MDA2 with MDA-LDL	In vivo imaging 7 WHHL rabbits 2 NZW rabbits (controls) pKa 7 WHHL and 2 NZW rabbits 5 WHHL and 2 NZW rabbits Biodistribution 5 WHHL rabbits = 7 WHHL rabbits	MDA2 specifically images atherosclerotic plaques in vivo First demonstration that oxidation-specific epitopes can be imaged in live animals
2001	Tsimikas et al [51–53]	Autoradiography	^{125}I	Direct conjugation	In vivo imaging MDA2 Halb (control Ab to human albumin)	In vivo imaging 16 WHHL rabbits 8 NZW rabbits (controls) Progression/regression study 81 LDLR–/– mice	In vivo uptake of radiolabeled MDA2 provides an accurate measure of atherosclerotic lesions rich in oxidized LDL and is highly sensitive to their regression and plaque stabilization. Autoantibodies to OxLDL correlate with atherosclerosis progression and regression

2008	Briley-Saebo et al [47]	MRI	Gd/0.075–mol/kg Gd/0.075–mol/kg	Micelles	In vivo imaging	In vivo imaging	MRI nanoparticles containing Gd-labeled MDA2, IK17, and E06 enhance the aorta of mice with atherosclerosis
			Gd/ 0.075–mol/kg		MDA2	8 apoE$^{-/-}$ mice	Unlabeled MDA2 competitively inhibits enhancement with Gd-MDA2
					IK17	3 apoE$^{-/-}$ mice	Targeted micelles co-localized with macrophages by confocal imaging
					E06	8 apoE$^{-/-}$ mice	
					IgG (control)	3 apoE$^{-/-}$ mice	
					pKa	pKa	
					MDA2	30 apoE$^{-/-}$ and 14 WT mice	
					IK17		
					E06		
					IgG (control)		
					Biodistribution	Biodistribution	
					MDA2	Total of 30 apoE$^{-/-}$ mice	
					IK17		
					E06		
					IgG (control)		

(continued)

Table 6.2 (continued)

Date	Authors	Modality	Label/dose	Platform	Antibodies	Animal models	Summary of key findings
2011	Briley-Saebo et al [45]	MRI	Fe/3.9 mg/kg	Lipid-coated, ultrasmall superparamagnetic iron oxide particles (LUSPIOs)	In vivo imaging	In vivo imaging	Specific signal accentuation within the aorta observed following administration of labeled MDA2, IK17, and E06 but not untargeted LUSPIOs
			Fe/3.9 mg/kg		MDA2	8 apo$E^{-/-}$ mice	Signal effect is competitively inhibited by unlabeled MDA2
			Fe/3.9 mg/kg		IK17	3 apo$E^{-/-}$ mice	LUSPIOs co-localize with intra-plaque macrophages, assessed by immunohistochemistry and confocal imaging
					E06	8 apo$E^{-/-}$ mice	LSPIOs are too large to enter plaques and cannot image lesion adequately
					Untargeted (control)	8 apo$E^{-/-}$ mice	
				Lipid-coated, superparamagnetic iron oxide particles (LSPIOs)	In vivo imaging	In vivo imaging	
					MDA2	8 apo$E^{-/-}$ mice	
					IK17	3 apo$E^{-/-}$ mice	
					E06	8 apo$E^{-/-}$ mice	
					Untargeted (control)	8 apo$E^{-/-}$ mice	
				LUSPIO and LSPIO	pKa	pKa	
					MDA2	8–10 apo$E^{-/-}$ and 8–10 WT mice in each group	
					IK17		
					Untargeted (control)		

2011	Vucic et al [54]	PET	^{18}F-FDG/1 mCi/kg	None	None	6 NZW rabbits for each imaging modality	Pioglitazone decreased PET and DCE-MRI signal in the aorta associated with decreased macrophages and OxPL immunostaining
		DCE-MRI	None				
2012	Briley-Saebo et al [46]	MRI	Mn/0.050 mol/kg	Micelle	In vivo imaging	In vivo imaging	Labeled OSE antibodies enhance the aorta in both apoE$^{-/-}$ and LDLR$^{-/-}$ mice. MDA2-Mn micelles are located within intra-plaque macrophages on confocal imaging
					MDA2	8 apoE$^{-/-}$ mice and 8 LDLR$^{-/-}$ mice	97 % of MDA2-Mn micelles cleared within 1 week postinjection, compared to 72.9 % clearance for MDA2-Gd micelles
					IK17	8 apoE$^{-/-}$ mice	
					Untargeted (control)	8 apoE$^{-/-}$ mice and 8 LDLR$^{-/-}$ mice	
			Gd/0.050 mol/kg		MDA2	8 apoE$^{-/-}$ mice	
					Untargeted (control)	8 apoE$^{-/-}$ mice	
			Mn/0.050 mol/kg		pKa	pKa	
					MDA2	3 apoE$^{-/-}$ and 3 WT mice in each group	
					IK17	Biodistribution	
					Untargeted (control)	45 apoE$^{-/-}$ mice (N=3 for each antibody/time point)	
			Mn/0.050 mol/kg		Biodistribution		
					MDA2		
					IK17		
					Untargeted (control)		

(continued)

Table 6.2 (continued)

Date	Authors	Modality	Label/dose	Platform	Antibodies	Animal models	Summary of key findings
2012	Vucic et al [55]	PET	^{18}F-FDG/1 mCi/kg	None	None	6 NZW rabbits for each imaging modality	LXR agonist, but not atorvastatin, was associated with decreased PET and DCE-MRI signal and decreased macrophage and OxPL immunoreactivity
		DCE-MRI	None				
2014	Nguyen et al [56]	MRI	Mn/0.050 mol/kg	G8 dendrimers	In vivo imaging	In vivo imaging	G8 dendrimers contain a large payload of Mn compared to micelles (768 ions on a dendrimer vs. 50 in a micelle)
					MDA2	4 apoE$^{-/-}$ mice	Mn G8 dendrimers circulate with a half-life of 2.9 h, compared to Mn micelles, which have a half-life of 16.4 h
					Untargeted (control)	3 apoE$^{-/-}$ mice	Labeled MDA2, but not untargeted G8 dendrimers, enhance the aorta apoE$^{-/-}$ mice on MRI
					pKa	pKa	
					MDA2 Untargeted (control)	3 apoE$^{-/-}$ and 3 WT mice in each group	
					Biodistribution	Biodistribution	
					MDA2 Untargeted (control)	18 apoE$^{-/-}$ mice (N=3 for each antibody/time point)	

6.3 The Role of OSE in Atherogenesis and Disease Progression

The direct correlation between OSE generation and deposition in the arterial wall and the presence of atherosclerosis and plaque progression has been demonstrated using direct extraction of modified LDL from the vessel wall [35, 57] and with immunostaining techniques in a variety of atherosclerotic animal models, including different strains of mice and rabbits, as well as monkeys and humans [11–13, 35–37, 39, 43–46, 48, 51–55, 58–60]. In general, these studies document the strong presence of oxidized lipids in early and late atherosclerotic lesions and in lesion progression. Furthermore, in dietary regression studies in $LDLR^{-/-}$ mice and cynomolgus monkeys, the deposition of OSE was greatly reduced in the arterial wall during atherosclerosis regression [53, 58]. Reduced OSE by immunostaining within the atheroma correlated strongly with features of plaque stabilization, including reduced macrophage content and increased collagen and smooth muscle cell content.

In humans with sudden cardiac death, there is evidence of differential expression of OSEs and apolipoprotein (a) [apo(a)] in different stages of plaque progression and plaque rupture [11]. In the normal coronary artery, OSEs and apo(a) could not be detected using the current immunostaining techniques. In early lesions, only nominal OSEs and apo(a) deposition was observed. Interestingly, as the lesions progressed, apoB and MDA epitopes did not significantly increase. However, OxPL and IK17 epitope expression increased linearly with advancing plaque stage. These OSEs were mainly associated with foam cell-rich areas, lipid pools, and necrotic cores that are associated with advanced, unstable, and/or ruptured plaques. Correlations have also been observed with iron deposition and IK17 epitopes in human abdominal aortic lesions in patients with the Hp2-2 genotype associated with increased oxidative stress [60]. Finally, in humans undergoing coronary, carotid, renal, and peripheral procedures, direct evidence of the presence of specific OxPL and typo, as identified by liquid chromatography and tandem mass spectrometry, was documented in distal protection devices (Fig. 6.2) [12, 13].

6.4 Molecular Imaging Probes for In Vivo OSE Detection

Table 6.3 summarizes the imaging studies using OSE-specific antibodies.

For nuclear imaging techniques such as PET and SPECT, probe design is focused on specificity, pharmacokinetics, biodistribution, and radioactive tracer half-life. Typically, an antibody or peptide is directly labeled with a radioactive tracer, and PET or SPECT imaging is performed once the antibody or peptide has cleared circulation, so that background signal from blood does not interfere with accurate imaging. When designing a probe for these modalities, it is critical that the antibody or peptide has a blood clearance that is faster than the half-life associated with the radioactive tracer. Additionally, the antibody must exhibit specificity to the target tissue. In the case of OSE imaging, the antibody or peptide can bind to and

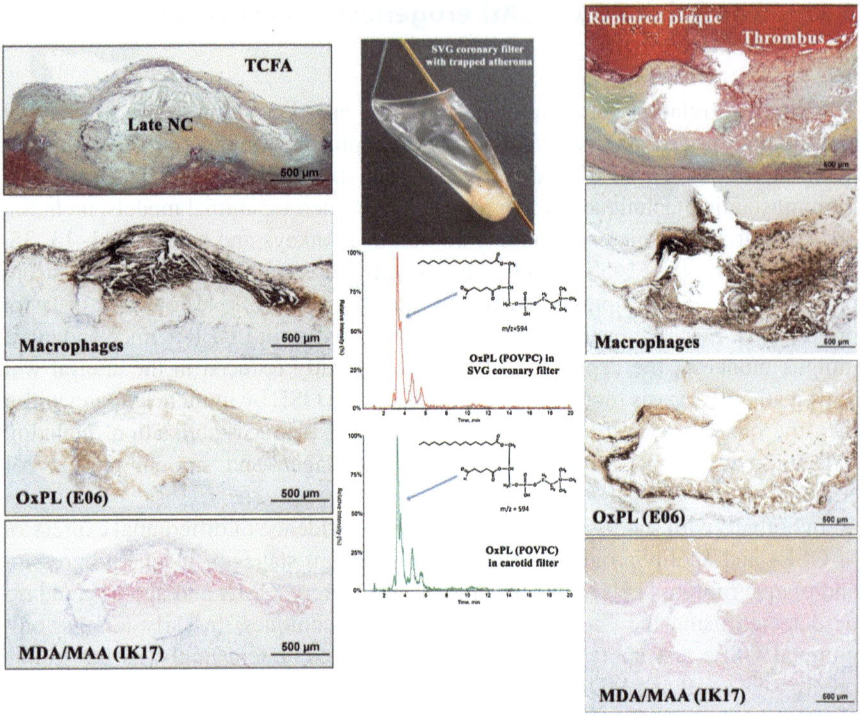

Fig. 6.2 The presence of macrophages and oxidation-specific epitopes in thin cap fibroatheroma (TCFA, *left* panels) and ruptured coronary plaques (*right* panels) detected by immunohistochemistry and coronary and carotid distal protection devices (*middle* panels) detected by LC-MS/MS (Reprinted with permission from van Dijk et al. [11])

accumulate in the extracellular space and also can be taken up by the scavenger receptors associated with intra-plaque macrophages, but with limited uptake in tissue associated with the reticular endothelial system (RES, such as spleen and liver) and mononuclear phagocytic system (MPS, such as lymph, lung, and bone).

Preclinical studies using ^{125}I-MDA2 were performed in atherosclerotic mice and rabbits, and imaging was performed 24 h after intravenous injection of the radiolabeled antibody [37, 44, 51], showing accumulation of ^{125}I-MDA2 in atherosclerotic lesions, as confirmed by autoradiography, ex vivo imaging, lipid staining, and immunohistochemistry. The uptake of ^{125}I-MDA2, evaluated as the percent of the injected dose determined by autoradiography, was highest in the aorta compared to all other tissues examined. Additionally, the uptake of ^{125}I-MDA2 in the arterial wall was directly proportional to plaque burden, as measured by en face % plaque area as well as aortic weight which is an excellent surrogate of plaque burden, as measured by autoradiography (Fig. 6.3) [51].

This initial approach also provided novel insights into the changes in OSE during plaque progression and regression induced by dietary changes in mice, rabbits, and monkeys in a series of experimental studies [51–53, 58]. It was observed that during

Table 6.3 Characteristics of various magnetic resonance nanoparticles targeting oxidation-specific epitopes

Formulation	Size (nm)	Relaxivity 60 MHz, 40 °C s^{-1} mM^{-1}	Blood half-life (h)		%ID Liver 24 h p.i. apoE–/– mice	Enhancement in the arterial wall at the optimal time point p.i. apoE–/– mice	Optimal time point for imaging and dose
			apoE–/– mice	WT mice			
Gd Micelles		*r1*				*%NENH, 9.4 T*	72 h
MDA2	22±2	9.3	14.3*	1.7	18	125	0.075-mmol Gd/kg
IK17	16±3	10.5	16.5*	1.8	18	138**	
E06	16±3	10.8	20.1*	1.7	32	231**	
IgG	16±4	10.4	1.4	1.3	18	–0.6	
Untargeted	14±2	11.6	1.5	1.5	12	15	
Mn Micelles		*r1*				*%NENH, 9.4 T*	48 h
MDA2	18±3	4.1	16.4*,+	NA	5	141**	0.05-mmol Mn/kg
IK17	12±2	3.8	12.3*,+	NA	5	135**	
E06	NA	NA	NA	NA	NA	NA	
IgG	NA	NA	NA	NA	NA	NA	
untargeted	10±2	4.1	3.4*,+	NA	4	12	
MDA2-intracellular		*45*					
Mn dendrimers		*r1*				*%NENH, 3 T*	48 h
MDA2	13±1	3.5	1.9*	0.9	11	62**	
IK17	NA	NA	NA	NA	NA	NA	0.05-mmol Mn/kg
E06	NA	NA	NA	NA	NA	NA	
IgG	NA	NA	NA	NA	NA	NA	
Untargeted	12±1	3.4	0.8	0.8	1	16	
Iron Oxides		*r2*				*$\Delta R2^{*(\%)}$, 9.4 T*	24 h

(continued)

Table 6.3 (continued)

Formulation	Size (nm)	Relaxivity 60 MHz, 40 °C s^{-1} mM^{-1}	Blood half-life (h)		%ID Liver 24 h p.i. apoE–/– mice	Enhancement in the arterial wall at the optimal time point p.i. apoE–/– mice	Optimal time point for imaging and dose
			apoE–/– mice	WT mice			
MDA2	14±3	37	9.01*	1.55	31	56**	3.9 mg Fe/kg
IK17	12±2	35	9.12	NA	31	58**	
E06	16±4	38	9.32	NA	30	62**	
IgG	NA	NA	NA	NA	NA	NA	
Untargeted	10±3	35	1.52	1.41	25	0.5	

Comparison of the physical and chemical properties of the various OSE-targeted formulations. The size represents the mean hydrated diameter as determined by light scattering. The blood half-lives were determined in apoE–/– and background wild-type mice following i.v. injection at the specified dose administered (last column of table). The percent injected dose (%ID) in the liver is also shown, 24 h after i.v. injection of the specified dose. The enhancement in the arterial wall is reflected in either the percent-normalized enhancement (%ENH) or the percent relative change in $R2^*$ at the optimal imaging time p.i. The optimal imaging time was determined based upon when maximum %ENH or delta$R2^*$ values were obtained. The field strength used to obtain the in vivo MR images is also specified. MR imaging for all studies, except the dendrimers, was performed at 9.4 T using a specialized mouse coil. For the dendrimers, imaging was performed using a clinical 3-T system

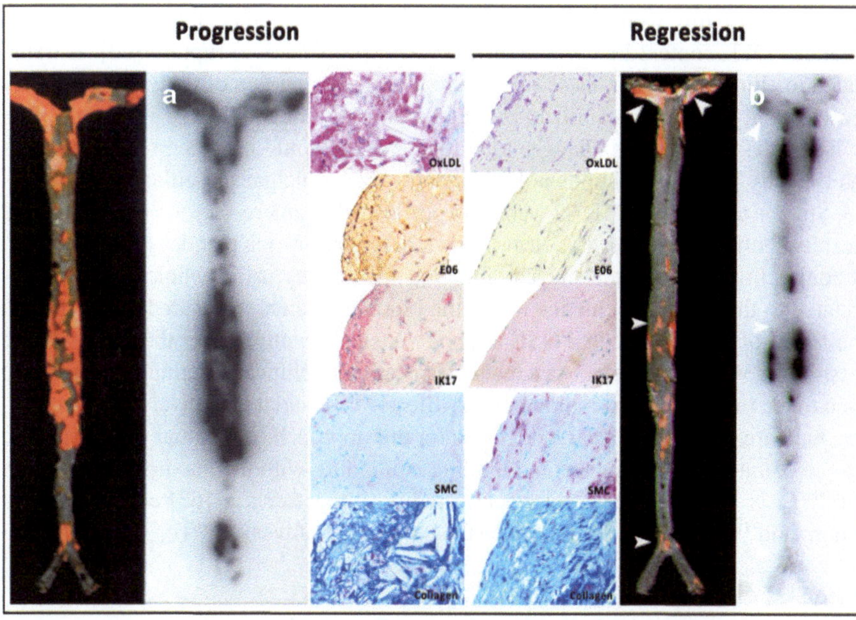

Fig. 6.3 Autoradiographic and immunohistochemistry representations of ^{125}I-MDA2 accumulation in Sudan-stained aortas of LDLR$^{-/-}$mice undergoing progression and regression diets. Representative en face mouse aortas stained with Sudan red and corresponding autoradiographs of ^{125}I-MDA2 accumulation in mouse aortas following intravenous injection, in progression (**a**) and regression. (**b**) groups. Arrowheads display discordance between lipid stained plaque and 125I-MDA2 accumulation during dietary regression. Representative aortic atherosclerotic lesions from LDLR$^{-/-}$mice from progression (*left middle* panel) and regression (*right middle* panel) groups. Immunostaining for OxLDL, SMCs, and IK17 appears *pink/purple*. Collagen is stained with Masson Trichrome and appears *bright blue*. E06 staining appears as brown product of peroxidase reaction (Reprinted with permission from Tsimikas et al. [51] and Torzewski et al. [53])

atherosclerosis progression induced by western diet (high fat, high cholesterol), OSE deposition in the vessel wall is relatively proportional to plaque burden, with evidence of strong expression of several unique OSE, along with macrophage markers and reduced smooth muscle cell and collagen content. However, when the western diets were removed and the animal placed on a normal chow diet (typically ~5 % fat and no added cholesterol), atherosclerosis progression was either reduced or regression induced. However, despite the fact that many lesions were unchanged in size, there was evidence of significant loss of OSE and macrophages, along with substantial gain in smooth muscle cells and collagen (Fig. 6.3) [53], accepted markers of plaque stabilization [61]. Furthermore, there was evidence that with loss of OxPL in the vessel wall, OxPL/apoB in plasma were increased [58], suggesting, but not proving, a reverse flux of OxPL from the vessel wall to the circulation. Finally, reduced immunostaining for OSE with concomitantly reduced ^{125}I-MDA2 uptake was noted in aged (~4 years old) Watanabe heritable hyperlipidemic rabbits with extensive (essentially 100 % of aortic surface area) atherosclerosis but with reduced OSE staining due to the presence of fibrotic and calcified lesions [53]. A clinical equivalent of this would be an obstructive, heavily calcified fibrotic lesion with reduced OSE content that would have a lower propensity to rupture [62]. If translated to clinical imaging, these observations suggest that loss of OSE may be a very early event in plaque stabilization, before any significant change in plaque size. Ultimately, linking such changes to clinical events would provide proof that this is a clinically relevant pathophysiological pathway for plaque surveillance.

Studies using ^{99m}Tc-MDA2 were also performed in atherosclerotic rabbits and the results confirm the ability to detect lipid-rich, oxidation-rich plaques [37]. However, a major limitation of the nuclear imaging techniques using whole antibodies is related to the pharmacokinetics where the blood clearance (measured as the plasma half-life) of the radiolabeled OSE antibody is significantly longer than the half-life associated with the isotope. As a result, translation to clinical imaging is not feasible due to the relatively short radiolabel half-life of ^{99m}Tc and the relatively long biological half-life of antibody clearance. Thus, for this approach, an optimal window where the maximal antibody uptake and binding coinciding with the maximal photon flux of ^{99m}Tc is not possible. Longer-acting radioisotopes such as [63] copper, ^{89}zirconium, and ^{111}indium have not been evaluated as alternatives to ^{99m}Tc.

6.5 Paramagnetic Probes for In Vivo OSE Imaging

Due to the limitations associated with the plasma half-lives of the radiolabeled OSE antibodies, alternatives to nuclear imaging techniques were sought. MRI was considered optimal due to its submillimeter resolution, intrinsic tissue contrast, and the ability to void the signal of blood by altering the MRI pulse sequences used. However, despite the potential of MRI for in vivo OSE detection, the full utility of this method may be limited by factors such as resolution (i.e., signal-to-noise ratio [SNR]), partial volume effects, and the fact that the molecular targets (scavenger receptors associated with intra-plaque macrophages) are present in very small numbers (10^{-9}–10^{-13} M/g tissue). To overcome these limitations, novel molecular imaging probes were designed to deliver a high payload of MR active metal to the molecular targets. The probes are separated into two classes: paramagnetic and superparamagnetic (SPIO) molecular imaging agents. Both classes have advantages and limitations associated with their magnetic properties and ability to detect in vivo OSE in the arterial wall of atherosclerotic animals.

However, despite which class the probe resides, all molecular imaging agents for MRI must meet the following criteria for clinical translation:

1. *Safety.* The probe must be safely metabolized or excreted without any safety issues related to the active MRI metal (such as gadolinium (Gd) or iron) or the nanoparticle/scaffolding material. The active MRI metal must be metabolized or excreted within an acceptable time frame, postinjection. This time frame is dependent upon the metal, but in all cases, intra-arterial macrophages should excrete or metabolize the metal within 3 weeks postinjection. This is critical not only from a safety point of view but also will allow for longitudinal studies to be performed.

2. *Specificity*. There should be no or limited unspecific uptake of the molecular imaging probe. This means that the untargeted nanoparticle or scaffold exhibits limited uptake within the arterial wall of atherosclerotic animals.
3. *Small particle size*. Studies have clearly shown that if nanoparticles are used to deliver the active MRI metal, the size must be less than 25 nm, preferably in the range of 5–20 nm [45]. This is due to the fact that the probes must penetrate the arterial wall in order to meet their targets, which are scavenger receptors associated with the intra-plaque macrophages. Particles that are too large are not able to penetrate the arterial wall, thereby never reaching their target. It should be mentioned that some nanoparticles are more flexible than others, so that the 25-nm cutoff is for rigid iron oxide-type materials. Micelles and other lipid-based particles may have a degree of flexibility allowing them to squeeze through the non-normal fenestrae associated with the plaque, despite their larger size. However, size is a real limitation when designing probes for OSE imaging.
4. *Pharmacokinetics*. Preclinical studies have shown that the probes must exhibit some degree of prolonged circulation (half-lives, t1/2, >4 h) to allow for adequate uptake into the arterial wall. However, excessive circulation times (t1/2 >24 h) are not desirable either, as they require scanning to be performed at late time points postinjection. The MR signal of the blood should be close to baseline during the postinjection scans of the arterial wall. There are, however, ways to reduce the wait time required postinjection by either optimizing the MR imaging sequences (to void out the signal of blood) and/or by creating probes that only modulate MR signal when they reach their molecular targets.
5. *Efficacy and payload*. MR signal will be modulated by the payload of the MRI active metal. For paramagnetic materials, typically the larger the number of metal ions associated with the nanoparticle or scaffolding, the better the signal modulation in the desired tissue. However, there are some considerations when creating paramagnetic OSE probes that will be discussed further in the paramagnetic probe section. For superparamagnetic materials, the MR signal modulation is directly linked to the size and quality of the iron oxide crystalline core. To maintain superparamagnetic properties, the core must be mono-domain. However, the larger the core, the higher saturation magnetization, and the greater the MRI signal efficacy. Iron oxide cores for OSE imaging are crystals of magnetite (spindle form) with a core of 4–5 nm. To allow for targeting and to hinder aggregation, the cores are coated with a lipid, as discussed in the superparamagnetic section.

Phospholipids are naturally occurring amphiphilic molecules that contain both a hydrophilic head group and a hydrophobic tail. Due to the energetically unfavorable contact between the lipid tails and water, amphiphiles self-associate into aggregates. The length of the hydrophobic chains and the size of the head group determine if micelle-like structure (single layer) or a bilayer (liposome) structure is formed. The rationale for using a lipid-based nanoparticle for OSE imaging is related to the ability to deliver a high payload of paramagnetic metal to the intra-plaque macrophages. For in vivo OSE imaging, we used a combination of the following lipids to allow for the self-assembly of paramagnetic micelles that

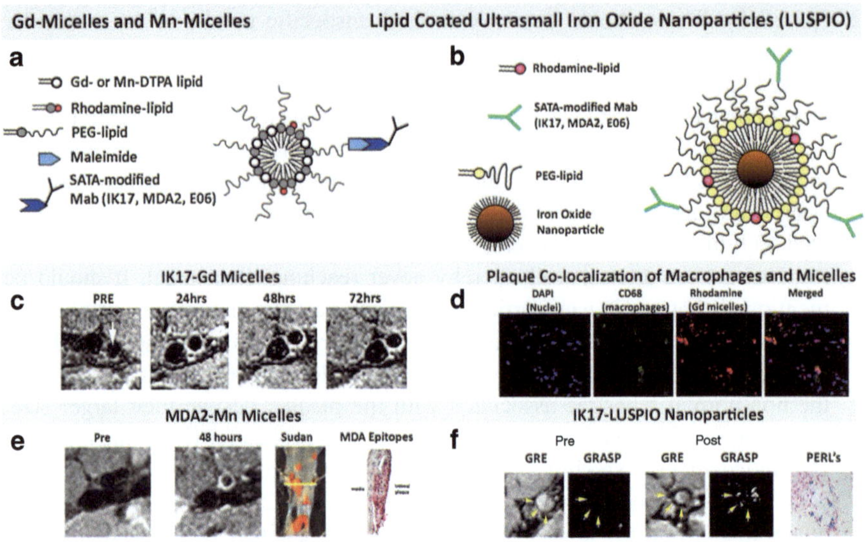

Fig. 6.4 (Panel **a**) is a schematic of Gd- and Mn-containing micelles with respective antibodies attached to the micelles using S-acetylthioglycolic acid N-hydroxysuccinimide ester (SATA). (Panel **b**) shows lipid-coated, ultrasmall, iron oxide nanoparticles (LUSPIO) attached to respective SATA-modified antibodies. (Panel **c**) shows representative noninvasive MRI of abdominal aortas of LDLR-/- mice using IK17-Gd micelles. There is no signal at the preinjection scan and maximum signal (*white contrast*) at 48–72 h. (Panel **d**) shows confocal microscopy of apoE$^{-/-}$mouse aortic atherosclerotic plaque after intravenous administration of MDA2 micelles demonstrating nuclei (*blue*), macrophages (*green*), and micelles (*red*). (Panel **e**) shows noninvasive MRI with Mn-MDA2 micelles with the accompanying panels showing the Sudan (lipid) and MDA-immunostained aortas. (Panel **f**) shows noninvasive MRI with IK17-LUSPIO micelles displaying GRE and GRASP images pre and post Ik17-USPIO injection with accompanying panel H&E-stained apoE–/– mouse aorta with Perl's stain for iron oxide and lumen associated with the abdominal aorta (*yellow arrow*). Iron oxide causes signal loss and it can be seen that the abdominal aorta plaque becomes darker following injection. The gradient echo acquisition for superparamagnetic particles with positive contrast (GRASP) sequence differentiates between iron oxide deposition (now shown as *white* signal) and artifacts that are often present when imaging the arterial wall (Reprinted with permission from Briley-Saebo et al. [45–47])

exhibited a hydrated particle size of 14 nm: PEG-DSPE (1,2-distearoyl-sn-glycero-3-phosphoethanolamine-n-methoxy(polyethylene glycol-2000), Gd or Mn DTPA-bis(stearyl-amid) (GdDTPA-BSA or MnDTPA-BSA), and PEG-maleimide-DSPE (molar ratio of 49:50:1). Targeted nanoparticles were created by covalently attaching the antibodies (MDA2, E06, or IK17) to the micelles by using SATA modification techniques (Fig. 6.4a, b) [46, 47]. Chemiluminescent ELISA showed that the activity (ability to bind OSEs) of the antibodies were not hindered by the association with the nanoparticles. Characterization of the micelles revealed that there were approximately 50 Gd or Mn ions per micelle. For the targeted formulations, approximately 1 out of 30 micelles was conjugated with an antibody. After association with the antibodies a slight increase in hydrated size was observed (15–20 nm, depending on the antibody used).

6.5.1 Gd OSE-Targeted Micelles

Gd was used as the active MR metal ion due to the fact that Gd is the most effective of all paramagnetic metal ions for the enhancement of the MR signal (increase the longitudinal relaxation rate, R1). The efficacy of paramagnetic probes is defined by the R1, and is defined as the slope of the correlation between the R1 values and metal ion concentration. These values are often obtained in vitro in aqueous solution at 40 °C. The Gd micelles exhibited in vitro R1 values that were three times greater than GdDTPA (the linear chelate not bound to the nanoparticle) at clinical imaging field strengths [64]. Additionally, the blood half-life was ≈1.5 h for both targeted and untargeted formulations in wild-type non-atherosclerotic mice following i.v. administration of a 0.075-mmol Gd/kg dose. However, in atherosclerotic mice (cholesterol fed apoE$^{-/-}$ mice) the MDA2, IK17, and E06 micelles exhibited significantly longer half-lives (14–20 h) relative to the untargeted and nonspecific IgG micelles (1.3–1.5 h). Although the mechanism of this is not clear, it is a consistent effect of all antibody-nanoparticle formulations and suggests a delayed clearance, possibly by binding to circulating OSE and remaining in plasma longer.

The diagnostic efficacy of the OSE-targeted micelles was evaluated over a 3-week time period postinjection. Due to the residual circulating micelles in atherosclerotic mice at 24 h postinjection, black-blood T1-weighted sequences were used to remove any signal from blood (repetition time, 600 ms; echo time, 8.6 ms; flip angle, 30°; number of excitations, 14; field of view, 2.6×2.6 cm) with 16 contiguous 500-μm-thick slices with a microscale in-plane resolution of 101 μm. An inflow saturation band of 3–5 mm was used with a slice gap of 3 mm for additional luminal flow suppression. Fourteen signal averages were used for a total imaging time of 36 min per scan. A saturation pulse was used to eliminate signal from fat tissue, to better delineate the boundary of the aortic wall, and to minimize chemical shift artifacts. At each time point after injection, the slices were matched to the baseline preinjection scans by using the unique vertebral anatomy and paraspinous muscular anatomy as anatomic landmarks.

To quantitatively analyze the MRI results, signal intensity measurements were obtained from regions of interest on the aortic wall and liver on slices ($n>5$) exhibiting signal modulation after contrast. The mouse aorta is typically four pixels thick, so only 10–20 pixels will make up any given region of interest. Because of the small number of pixels involved, the areas associated with the regions of interest were kept constant between the before and after images. Signal intensity measurements of the aortic lumen, muscle, and noise also were obtained for each slice. The percent-normalized enhancement (%NENH) relative to muscle was then determined for the aortic vessel wall and liver according to established methods. The %NENH values reflect the percent change in the contrast-to-noise ratios obtained before and after injection as follows:

$$\%\text{NENH} = \left(\text{CNR}_{\text{post}} / \text{CNR}_{\text{pre}}\right) - 1 \times 100,$$

where CNR is the contrast-to-noise ratio defined as $CNR=SNR_{wall}/SNR_{muscle}$ (SNR is the signal-to-noise ratio). CNR_{post} is the CNR value obtained after injection; CNR_{pre} is the CNR value obtained before administration of the micelles.

The biodistribution and confocal microscopy results show significant accumulation of the targeted micelles within atherosclerotic lesions with peak aortic wall concentration at 24 h but optimal enhancement at 72 h. In addition, co-localization of targeted micelles with macrophages in atherosclerotic plaques was observed 24 h to 3 weeks postinjection of the OSE-targeted formulations. At 72 h postinjection, the OSE-targeted micelles demonstrated higher signal enhancement (125–231 %, depending on the OSE antibody used), relative to adjacent muscle. Nonspecific IgG and untargeted micelles exhibited nominal (<15 %) signal enhancement (Fig. 6.4c). Consistent with a specific targeting mechanism, preinjection of unlabeled OSE antibody before intravenous injection of the OSE-targeted micelles resulted in ≈6-fold reduction in %NENH at 72 h postinjection. Histology and confocal microscopy (rhodamine label associated with the micelles) shows the high specificity of the OSE-targeted micelles to intra-plaque macrophages (Fig. 6.4d). Additionally, ICP-MS of $apoE^{-/-}$ mice injected with OSE-targeted micelles revealed maximum uptake in the aorta at 48 h after injection (24 h, 0.30%ID; 48 h, 0.48%ID; 72 h, 0.12%ID). No Gd was detected in the aortas of $apoE^{-/-}$ mice after the administration of either the untargeted or IgG micelles.

Although chelated Gd is 99.9 % renally excreted, bioretention and in vivo biotransformation of Gd(III) micelles was observed due to the prolonged blood half-life of the OSE-targeted micelles in atherosclerotic mice. Studies have clearly demonstrated that prolonged circulation of linear Gd chelates (such as GdDTPA) may lead to systemic toxicity in renally impaired patients. In vitro vascular stability studies were performed on the untargeted and OSE-targeted micelle formulations. The results of these studies show 3–4 % transmetallation of the Gd formulations following a 24-h incubation in 2 % bovine serum albumin spiked with 10 μmol/L of zinc and copper (clinical human range for these metal cations that is known to compete with Gd for the DTPA ligand). The biodistribution data showed significant uptake of the untargeted and OSE-targeted micelles in the liver (20–30 % ID at 24 h postinjection) and spleen (1–2 % ID). Any bioretention or biotransformation of Gd may be problematic, as studies have reported that intracellular uptake of Gd chelates might result in de-metallation and subsequent cell apoptosis. Cell viability studies were performed on ex vivo macrophages over a 48-h time frame following uptake of the OSE-targeted Gd micelle's. These studies clearly show increased apoptosis of ex vivo macrophages when compared to OSE-targeted micelles that do not contain Gd (67 % vs. 23 %). The prolonged (>3 week) MR signal enhancement within the arterial wall following administration of the OSE-targeted Gd micelles strongly suggests the transmetallation of the Gd metal ion and the formation of toxic Gd salts [47, 65]. No significant differences in the %NENH values were observed between 72 h and 3 weeks postinjection. Due to these issues potentially interfering with the safety of this agent, it was apparent that Gd is not ideal as the active MR label for in vivo OSE imaging.

6.5.2 Manganese OSE-Targeted Micelles

Manganese (Mn(II)) is an endogenous biocompatible paramagnetic metal ion. The Food and Drug Administration (FDA) has already approved the use of MnDPDP (Teslascan) as a contrast agent for MR liver indications. It should be noted that the MR efficacy of MnDPDP is linked to the Mn that is able to de-chelate from the DPDP ligand thereby allowing for uptake into normal hepatocytes [63, 66]. All Mn that remains bound to DPDP is renally excreted and does not contribute to the MR efficacy for liver indications. Experimental studies have shown that a bolus injection of MnC12 causes cardiotoxicity and even death due to competition of the "free" Mn metal ions with the calcium channels in cardiomyocytes. However, slow infusion of MnC12 does not result in cardiotoxicity as there is never a high concentration of "free" Mn metal ions. Mn metal ions will bind proteins in the plasma thereby reducing their ability to compete with calcium. The DPDP ligand in the Teslascan formation allows for the slow release of Mn metal ions, so that there is never a high concentration of free Mn metal ions (that are present in the bolus phase of MnC12). As a result, MR liver efficacy is possible without any toxic effects. Additionally, studies have shown that "free" Mn metal ions can cross the blood-brain barrier thereby inducing neurotoxicity. Again, as long as there is a slow release of Mn from a chelate, the "free" Mn metal ions will bind with components in the plasma. These endogenous Mn proteins do not cross the blood-brain barrier so that the risk of neurotoxicity by Mn is limited.

Although Mn is safe as long as the metal ion is not injected as a bolus, it is typically not used as the MR active metal. This is due to the fact that Mn(II) has a low magnetic moment (relative to Gd) that limits MR signal enhancement. However, if Mn is delivered into a cell, interaction with intracellular components and metalloproteinase results in significant (>20-fold) increases in MR efficacy. As a result, we decided to design a novel OSE-targeted Mn probe that would stay primarily chelated in the vascular phase (with limited biotransformation and de-chelation) and would release the Mn(II) once taken up by intra-plaque macrophages. It was anticipated that the intracellular release of Mn would enhance the MR signal by increasing the number of water exchange sites between the metal ion and water protons (defined as q) and by decreasing the molecular tumbling rates due to interaction with macromolecules and cell membranes. Chelation in the vascular phase has two significant effects: (1) it reduces potential cardiotoxicity and neurotoxicity associated with bolus injection of free Mn (MnC12), and (2) the background signal from blood will be nominal if chelates such as DTPA are used that completely bind the Mn metal ion so that there is no inner sphere water exchange sites available ($q=0$). The OSE antibody associated with the surface of the particle will allow for binding of the targeted Mn micelles to endogenous OSE found in circulation and/or within the arterial wall. The Mn micelle-Ab-OxLDL complex is then taken up by intra-plaque foam cells/macrophages, as shown with Gd micelles. This degradation was expected to result in the intracellular release of the Mn metal ions that are then either taken up by metalloproteinase or interact with the cell membrane.

To test this hypothesis, OSE-targeted Mn micelles were synthesized, characterized, and tested in preclinical models of atherosclerosis [46]. The micelles were prepared using the same synthesis as the Gd micelles, as described previously [47]. The results showed that the hydrated particle size of the OSE-targeted Mn micelles were slightly less (12 nm) than that of the equivalent Gd micelles. As expected, the in vitro saline and plasma R1 values were two to three times less (depending of matrix) than that of the Gd micelles due to the magnetic properties of Mn as well as the fact that MnDTPA is $q=0$ and GdDTPA is $q=1$. Once taken up by macrophages, the R1 of the OSE-targeted Mn micelles increased dramatically from 4 to 45 s^{-1} mM^{-1}. No significant intracellular R1 values were observed for the untargeted Mn micelle formulation; thereby supporting the specific uptake mechanism observed previously for OSE-targeted micelles. Only 1.5 % de-transmetallation was observed for the OSE-targeted Mn micelles 24 h after incubation in plasma spike with Cu and zinc. This suggests that the vascular biotransformation will be relatively low. Interestingly, the Gd formulation exhibited higher transmetallation (3.5 %) as discussed previously. As a result the MR signal from black blood will be nominal and with no issues related to cardiotoxicity. Neurotoxicity was evaluated using Dy OSE-targeted micelles, with no Dy found in the brain of mice at any time point postinjection, as determined by ICP-MS [46]. It should be noted that Dy was used instead of Mn, due to the high endogenous concentration of Mn in tissue. Dy is a lanthanide metal similar to Gd and can be detected with great sensitivity by ICP-MS. The results confirm that the OSE-targeted micelles cannot cross the blood-brain barrier. Since the Mn remains primarily chelated in the vascular phase (so that the concentration of vascular "free" Mn is nominal), issues related to neurotoxicity are not anticipated.

Most cells quickly metabolize or utilize soluble Mn either via integration into Mn-specific metalloproteins or interaction with other cellular components such as the cell membrane. The in vivo biodistribution data showed 97 % clearance of the MDA2-Mn micelles within 1 week postinjection [46]. The MDA2-Gd micelles, however, exhibited only 72.9 % clearance within 1 week postinjection. The variation in the retention is due to differences in the rate of metabolism of Mn and Gd micelles. For example, confocal studies show that the targeted PEG micelles were completely degraded within intra-plaque macrophages 72 h after injection (rhodamine signal is no longer present). However, as confirmed by ICP-MS as well as MR imaging, Gd is still present within the arterial wall. These data illustrate that the targeted micelles and Gd or Mn label track together at early time points postinjection (<72 h). However, as the intra-plaque macrophages internalize and degrade the particles, the lipids forming the micelles and MR label are no longer co-localized within the arterial wall. During intracellular metabolism, the cells degrade the particles, and the MR label is released from the chelate. Released from micelles, the Mn interacts with cellular components and eventually is either exocytosed or integrated into the endogenous Mn pool. However, de-metallation of Gd results in the formation of insoluble Gd salts that remains within the intracellular vesicles. So, whereas the half-life of Mn within the arterial wall was approximately 60 h (or 2.5 days), MDA2-Gd micelles exhibit prolonged retention of Gd (>3 weeks).

A comparison was made of the MR efficacy of OSE-targeted Mn and Gd micelles (Fig. 6.4e). In short, all animals underwent a preinjection MR scan within 24 h prior to the administration of the various micelle formulations. MRI was performed over a 1-week time interval after tail vein injection of either a 0.050-mmol Mn/kg dose or a 0.075-mmol Gd/kg dose of micelles. MRI of the abdominal aorta was performed using a T1-weighted black-blood spin-echo sequence, as described for the Gd micelles previously. The %NENH values were determined for each formulation at each time point. Significant and robust MR signal enhancement was observed in the arterial wall of atherosclerotic mice following administration of a 0.05-mmol Mn/kg dose of OSE-targeted Mn micelles, relative to untargeted formulations. Maximum signal enhancement was observed 48–72 h after administration of the OSE-targeted Mn micelles. Although MDA2-Mn micelles were administered at a dose that was 33 % lower than that of Gd, equivalent MR signal enhancement was observed for the OSE-targeted Mn and Gd formulations at the optimal imaging time points postinjection. For targeted Mn micelles, maximum signal enhancement was observed 48–72 h postinjection %NENH = 141 ± 20 %), with no significant signal observed after 1 week. MDA2-Gd micelles, however, exhibited maximum enhancement after 1 week postinjection (%NENH = 156 ± 21 %). The shorter time frame between injection and optimal time point postinjection of the Mn formulations is yet another reason the Mn may be preferred over Gd. The study clearly demonstrated that OSE-targeted Mn micelles allow for the detection of OxLDL-rich intraplaque macrophages without the safety concerns associated with Gd formulations.

6.5.3 OSE-Targeted, Lipid-Coated, Superparamagnetic Iron Oxide Particles (SPIOs)

Unlike the OSE-targeted paramagnetic micelles and dendrimers that promote MR signal increase (T_1 contrast agents), superparamagnetic iron oxide (SPIO) particles induce proton dephasing that results in MR signal loss (T2*or negative contrast agents). SPIO agents are composed of iron oxide crystals (primarily magnetite) and a coating material that prevents aggregation of the iron cores. As long as the core crystal size is less than a Weiss domain, the iron oxide will exhibit superparamagnetic properties with no magnetic magnetization (or remanence) observed at zero field. Typically SPIOs used for MRI have core diameters of 4–6 nm. In the absence of an external magnetic field, the individual magnetic moments that make up the superparamagnetic SPIO are randomly oriented and no net magnetization is observed. Application of a magnetic field causes the individual magnetizations to align with the magnetic field so that the net magnetization increases with increasing magnetic field until the magnetization is saturated, as defined by the saturation magnetization. The ability of iron oxide particles to induce MR signal loss is characterized by properties associated with both the iron oxide core and interactions between the iron oxide core crystals due to aggregation or agglomeration. As a result, the effective transverse relaxivity (r2* s-1 M-1) is modulated by the magnetization of the iron oxide core at the imaging field strength, the diffusion of water protons in the local magnetic field generated by the SPIO, and aggregation or agglomeration of the iron oxide particles. For OSE imaging, the intra-plaque macrophages will take up the targeted SPIO particles. Compartmentalization within the cells as well as the possibility for intracellular agglomeration causes significant MR signal loss.

The sensitivity of SPIOs, relative to similar paramagnetic formulations is roughly ten times greater due to the high magnetization associated with SPIOS at clinical imaging field strengths. The increased sensitivity makes OSE-targeted SPIOs and attractive platform relative to the paramagnetic micelle and dendrimer approaches. Additionally, iron oxide particles are considered safe in that macrophages safely metabolize iron oxide particles. These particles are degraded within the endosomes and lysosomes associated with the cells, and the iron is bond to transferrin or other proteins and is eliminated by the cell. Once eliminated the iron enters the endogenous iron pool. The FDA has approved the use of iron oxide particles for MR liver indications as well as anemia. It should be pointed out, however, in the case of the arterial wall, the degradation of the iron oxide particles in the pro-inflammatory environment of the plaque may lead to increased oxidation of lipids, in a similar way that heme iron promotes peroxidase. This has yet to be confirmed, but it is a concern worth mentioning.

OSE-targeted SPIOs were synthesized and characterized and the preclinical efficacy evaluated. To eliminate in vitro aggregation or agglomeration, the 4 nm iron oxide cores were coated with PEG lipids (Fig. 6.4f) [45]. The OSE antibodies were attached to the modified PEG using the same methods described for the paramagnetic micelles (SATA modification). The resultant OSE-targeted SPIOs exhibited a mean hydrated diameter of 14–16 nm, which is not significantly different from the size of the paramagnetic formulations. ELISA showed that conjugation did not affect their binding specificity to OxLDL. The blood half-life of the OSE-targeted SPIOS in atherosclerotic mice was approximately 9 h following the administration of a 3.9-mg Fe/kg dose. This half-life is shorter than that observed for the paramagnetic micelles, but longer than that observed by dendrimers (discussed in the next section). ICP-MS, confocal microscopy, and Perl's staining confirmed the uptake of the OSE-targeted SPIOs in the arterial wall, specifically within intra-plaque macrophages/foam cells, of atherosclerotic mice. No uptake of the untargeted SPIO was observed. Approximately 30 % of the injected dose was present in the liver 24 h postinjection.

All MRIs were performed at 9.4-T using the same system that was used for the paramagnetic micelles. Imaging was performed before and 24 h after the administration of a 3.9-mg Fe/kg dose. To obtain in vivo R2* maps, multiple gradient echo (GRE) sequences with the following pulse sequence parameters were applied: repetition time =29.1 ms, echo time = 5.1–10 ms ($n=5$), flip angle = 30°, number of signal averages = 6, in-plane resolution = 0.098 mm^2, and 100 % z-rephasing gradient. Twenty slices were acquired from the level of the renal arteries to the iliac bifurcation. The R2* maps were generated for the matched pre- and post-images on a pixel-by-pixel basis using a custom Matlab. The R2* values were obtained with regions of interest drawn on the arterial wall on slices ($n=5$) exhibiting either R2* modulation after contrast or arterial wall thickening, indicative of plaque deposition. The relative percentage change in the R2* values was determined as: % change = [R2*post-R2*pre]/R2*post) 100. Immediately after GRE acquisition, a gradient echo acquisition for superparamagnetic particles with positive contrast (GRASP) sequence was applied using 50 % of the z-rephasing gradient. The GRASP sequence is extremely useful when trying to determine whether MR signal loss is due to iron oxide deposition or other endogenous artifacts (motion, partial voluming, and perivascular effects) that might also promote signal loss. The GRASP sequence cannot be used alone, however, because this sequence does not provide adequate anatomic information. In similarity to GRE sequences, GRASP signal might be observed in lymphatic tissue that might also sequester the iron oxide particles. However, this sequence is extremely useful to differentiate between iron oxide deposition and artifacts that are often present when imaging the arterial wall. Because equivalent imaging geometry was used for both GRE and GRASP, the imaging results obtained from these sequences were directly matched and compared. The results are shown in Fig. 6.4f, and it was clearly demonstrated that OSE-targeted SPIOs allowed for in vivo detection of OSE-rich atherosclerotic plaques, as confirmed by confocal microscopy and Perl's staining. No significant MR signal loss was observed 24 h after the administration of the untargeted material.

6.5.4 Manganese OSE-Targeted Dendrimers

Although the OSE-targeted Mn micelles were safe and effective, there was a desire to increase the payload of Mn so that imaging may potentially be performed at even earlier time point postinjection (within 24 h). However, increasing the Mn payload using lipid-based constructs will result in the formation of nanoparticles that are too large (>20 nm) for intra-plaque imaging. Poly(amido amine) (PAMAM) dendrimers are synthetic macromolecules composed of repeating beta-alanine subunits. The rationale for using dendrimers is related to the ability to load large amounts of Mn while keeping the particle size small enough (<20 nm) to allow for luminal diffusion and intra-plaque macrophage uptake. Reported studies show that dendrimers can be easily modified to allow for the addition of both paramagnetic ions (such as GdDTPA) and antibodies for targeted delivery. Since in vivo MR efficacy is directly related to the delivery of Mn payloads, it was hypothesized that dendrimers would be ideal carriers since generation eight dendrimers (G8) contain 1,024 primary amine groups that may be modified and labeled with MnDTPA. This would be a significant improvement over the MnDTPA micelles where there are only ≈ 50 gadolinium or manganese ions per micelle.

Again, the use of DTPA as a chelating agent for Mn was not random. DTPA completely binds Mn so that $q=0$. Although cyclic chelating agents, such as DOTA, may increase the vascular stability (thermodynamic stability constant of MnDOTA = 19.89), it is uncertain if the high affinity to Mn would limit intracellular de-chelation. The OSE-targeted dendrimers were prepared by concentrating G8 PAMAM dendrimers to 10 mg/ml and diafiltering against 0.1 M sodium phosphate buffer (pH 9), as described in the literature [67]. A 256-fold molar excess of isothiocyanatobenzyl diethylenetriaminepentaacetic acid (ITC-Bz-DTPA) (Macrocyclics, Dallas Tx) was added, and the solution incubated at 40 °C and for 48 h (maintained at pH 9). Note that an excess of ITC-Bz-DTPA was added in order to ensure optimal labeling. The solution was then purified by diafiltration using a Centricon 30 and stochiometric amounts of $MnCl_2$ were added. A 1-mole equivalent of tetramethylrhodamine-ITC (TRITC) was added drop wise to G8-MnDTPA in DMSO. The resultant G8 MnDTPA-TRITC-dendrimer was then purified (diafiltration), lyophilized, and stored at −40 °C under N_2 to prevent oxidation of the Mn. Based upon elemental analysis, 75 % (768 MnDTPA/1,024 surface amines) of the available amines on the dendrimer surface covalently attached to MnDTPA. In addition, 10 % (102 TRITC/1,024) of the surface amines were covalently attached to the fluorescent probe. The remaining 154 surface amine groups associated with the G8 dendrimer were used to covalently link the OSE antibody to the dendrimer via interaction between thiol and maleimide (Fig. 6.5).

The OSE-targeted Mn dendrimers were characterized with respect to Mn content, hydrated particle size, in vitro MR efficacy, binding specificity, and in vitro macrophage uptake [56]. The pKa and biodistribution was determined in atherosclerotic and WT following injection of a 0.05-mmol Mn/kg dose. All MRI was performed using a clinical 3-T hybrid time-of-flight PET/MR system (Philips Gemini MRI) and a specialized mouse coil in the prone position. Mice underwent a preinjection MR scan within 24 h prior to the administration of the OSE-targeted dendrimers, and MR imaging was then performed over a 72-h time interval after tail vein injection of a 0.050-mmol Mn/kg dose. MR imaging of the abdominal aorta was performed using a T1-weighted black-blood spin-echo sequence (TR/TE = 667 ms/9.9 ms, number of averages = 10, FOV = 2.5×2.5 cm, slice thickness = 0.5 mm, 30 slices, and total scan time of 59 min) with a microscale in-plane resolution of 0.15 mm^2. At each time point postinjection, the slices were matched to the baseline preinjection scans by using the unique vertebral anatomy and paraspinous muscular anatomy as anatomic landmarks. In order to evaluate the MR data, signal intensity (SI) measurements were obtained using regions of interest (ROIs) within the aortic wall on slices exhibiting signal modulation post contrast using OsiriX software (Pixmeo Geneva, Switzerland). SI measurements of adjacent muscle and the standard deviation associated with noise were also obtained. The percent-normalized enhancement (%NENH), relative to muscle, was then determined.

The hydrated particle diameter and in vitro R1 values associated with the OSE-targeted dendrimers were similar to the values reported for the targeted Mn micelles (13.34 ± 1.2 nm, R1 saline = 3.5 s^{-1} mM^{-1}). Enzyme-linked immunosorbent assay (ELISA) showed that OSE antibody was successfully conjugated to the dendrimers without effecting OxLDL binding specificity. ICP-MS results showed limited uptake of the untargeted dendrimers in J744A.1 macrophages. In wild-type mice, the OSE-targeted dendrimers exhibited a blood half-life of 2.9 h. This is significantly lower than the half-life observed for the OSE-targeted Mn micelles in atherosclerotic mice (16.4 h). Biodistribution studies in atherosclerotic mice show strong uptake of the OSE-targeted dendrimers within the arterial wall 24–48 h postinjection.

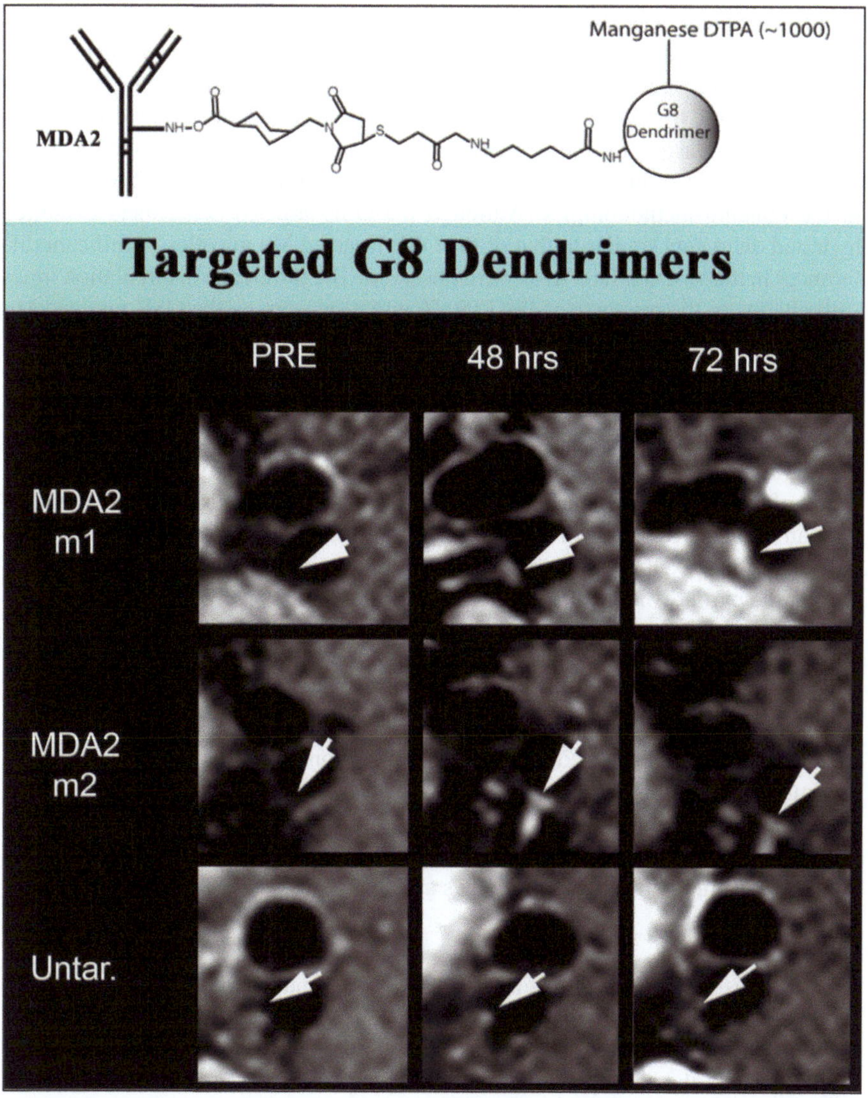

Fig. 6.5 Schematic of dendrimer which covalently attached to MnDTPA and MDA (*top*). Representative MRI images from two apoE−/− mice are shown (M1 = mouse1 and M2 = mouse2). The *arrows* point to regions within the abdominal aorta. There is increased scan signal (*white contrast*) compared to preinjection of MDA2 dendrimers (Reprinted with permission from Nguyen et al. [56])

Representative MR images obtained prior to and after the administration untargeted and OSE-targeted dendrimers (0.05-mmol Mn/kg) (Fig. 6.5). The OSE-targeted dendrimers exhibited significantly greater arterial wall enhancement at all time points postinjection, relative to the untargeted material. The maximum arterial wall enhancement was observed 48 h postinjection (62 ± 3 %), with residual signal present 72 h postinjection. The presence of Mn within atherosclerotic lesions was confirmed using spectroscopic methods (>8-μg Mn/g vs. <1-μg Mn/g, $P<0.001$). When compared to OSE-targeted Mn micelles, MR efficacy of Mn dendrimers was reduced. The reasons for the decreased efficacy of the dendrimers, relative to the micelles, may be summarized as: (1) differences in pKa values and (2) differences in the imaging methodologies. Although the OSE-targeted dendrimers exhibited hydrated diameters similar to that of the OSE-targeted Mn micelles, significant differences in the vascular half-lives were observed. The difference in circulation times is likely due to the presence of PEG (50 % wt/wt) present on the OSE-targeted Mn micelles. Studies have indicated that prolonged circulation times allow for greater accumulation of molecular probes within or on a target. As a result, the shorter circulation times exhibited by the dendrimers may limit the efficacy of this platform to some extent. Finally, MR imaging of the OSE-targeted Mn micelles was performed using a high-resolution mouse MR scanner at 9.4 T with a microscale in-plane resolution of 0.098 mm^2. In the current study, a clinical imaging system (3 T) was used with an in-plane resolution of 0.15 mm^2. The arterial wall of the mouse is very small (typically four pixels) so that the larger the volume imaged (larger voxel size), the greater the partial volume effects. It should be noted that on pre-imaging scans, the arterial wall is visible at 9.4 T (using black-blood T1-weighted sequences). At 3 T, however, the arterial wall is not visible (due to the lower resolution) when similar pulse sequences are applied. Despite the limitations related to spatial resolution and partial voluming at 3 T, significant MR enhancement was still observed following administration of the targeted dendrimers. Relaxation theory, however, predicts that the imaging efficacy of the Mn micelles will be reduced at 9.4 T, relative to 3 T. In order to allow for direct comparison, future studies will be performed to evaluate the efficacy of targeted Mn dendrimers and micelles at both 9.4 and 3 T.

Table 6.4 summarizes the advantages and disadvantages of each MRI platform.

Conclusions

The robustness of OSE imaging by OSE-targeted nanoparticles is demonstrated by the fact that all the platforms tested (^{99m}Tc, Gd micelles, Mn micelles, Mn dendrimers, SPIOs) resulted in the ability to detect OSE in vivo. From a clinical perspective, the best approach relates to safety, efficacy, and ease of use. If one considers safety first, then the Gd micelles are suboptimal due to significant and prolonged bioretention in tissues. Regarding efficacy, the preclinical results indicate that the Mn micelles may be more effective than the Mn dendrimers due to the more favorable pKa. Since the safety of the dendrimer scaffold itself is not fully determined, the Mn micelle formulation may be considered optimal compared to the dendrimers. OSE-targeted Mn micelles and SPIOs may both be considered safe and result in good visualization of the arterial wall in atherosclerotic mice. Since optimal imaging time postinjection for the SPIOs is lower than that of the micelles (24 h vs. 48 h), the SPIOs may be considered optimal from an ease point of view. However, the ability to evaluate GRE signal loss is not trivial, requiring the use of GRASP sequences [45]. Several factors result in MR signal

Table 6.4 Summary of the advantages and disadvantages of the MRI platforms

Platform	Advantages	Disadvantages
Gd micelles	Able to detect OSE in the arterial wall of atherosclerotic mice	Toxicity-related issues due to bioretention and biotransformation
	Positive MR signal enhancement (T1 agent)	Optimal imaging time point >72 h p.i.
	Easy and reproducible synthesis	
Mn micelles	Able to detect OSE in the arterial wall of atherosclerotic mice. The agent is a switch, with little or no signal in the vascular phase and strong signal enhancement (T1 agent) in the arterial wall	Nontraditional approach Optimal imaging time point at 48 h p.i.
	No issues related to toxicity as Mn is an endogenous metal ion that is safe when chelated in the bolus phase	
	Easy and reproducible synthesis	
Mn dendrimers	Able to detect OSE in the arterial wall of atherosclerotic mice	Potential safety/toxicity of dendrimers still not established
	Dendrimers offer a high payload of Mn relative to the micelles (1,024 vs. 300 Mn ions/particle)	Blood half-life may be too low for optimal arterial wall imaging (may need PEG in formulation)
	Positive MR signal enhancement (T1 agent)	Optimal imaging time point at 48 h p.i.
	No issues related to metal ion toxicity, as Mn is an endogenous metal that is safe when chelated in the bolus phase	
Iron oxides	Able to detect OSE in the arterial wall of atherosclerotic mice	Causes MR signal loss (T2* agent)
	Iron oxides have better sensitivity than paramagnetic agents due to the their increased magnetic moment (10 times more sensitive)	Iron in the arterial wall may induce oxidation
	No issues related to toxicity, as Fe is an endogenous metal ion	
	Optimal imaging time point at 24 h p.i.	

loss, such as motion, partial voluming, perivascular effect, etc. As a result, most radiologists prefer paramagnetic contrast agents that give signal enhancement over those that induce signal loss. Additionally, it is not known how long the OSE-targeted SPIOs stay in the arterial wall after administration of a single dose. Since the macrophages need to degrade and export the iron, this time may be substantial, thereby limiting the ability to perform longitudinal studies pre- and posttreatment. With all these considerations, the OSE-targeted Mn micelles may allow for the best clinical translation of this platform. Efforts to optimize these approaches and translate them to patients are ongoing.

References

1. Hansson GK, Hermansson A. The immune system in atherosclerosis. Nat Immunol. 2011;12:204–12.
2. Hartvigsen K, Chou MY, Hansen LF, Shaw PX, Tsimikas S, Binder CJ, Witztum JL. The role of innate immunity in atherogenesis. J Lipid Res. 2009;50(Suppl):S388–93.
3. Miller YI, Choi SH, Wiesner P, Fang L, Harkewicz R, Hartvigsen K, Boullier A, Gonen A, Diehl CJ, Que X, Montano E, Shaw PX, Tsimikas S, Binder CJ, Witztum JL. Oxidation-specific epitopes are danger-associated molecular patterns recognized by pattern recognition receptors of innate immunity. Circ Res. 2011;108:235–48.
4. Navab M, Ananthramaiah GM, Reddy ST, Van Lenten BJ, Ansell BJ, Fonarow GC, Vahabzadeh K, Hama S, Hough G, Kamranpour N, Berliner JA, Lusis AJ, Fogelman AM. Thematic review series: the pathogenesis of atherosclerosis: the oxidation hypothesis of atherogenesis: the role of oxidized phospholipids and HDL. J Lipid Res. 2004;45:993–1007.
5. Steinberg D, Witztum JL. Oxidized low-density lipoprotein and atherosclerosis. Arterioscler Thromb Vasc Biol. 2010;30:2311–6.
6. Tsimikas S, Miller YI. Oxidative modification of lipoproteins: mechanisms, role in inflammation and potential clinical applications in cardiovascular disease. Curr Pharma Des. 2011;17:27–37.
7. Tsimikas S, Duff GW, Berger PB, Rogus J, Huttner K, Clopton P, Brilakis E, Kornman KS, Witztum JL. Pro-inflammatory interleukin-1 genotypes potentiate the risk of coronary artery disease and cardiovascular events mediated by oxidized phospholipids and lipoprotein (a). J Am Coll Cardiol. 2014;63:1724–34.
8. Glass CK, Witztum JL. Atherosclerosis: the road ahead. Cell. 2001;104:503–16.
9. Seimon TA, Nadolski MJ, Liao X, Magallon J, Nguyen M, Feric NT, Koschinsky ML, Harkewicz R, Witztum JL, Tsimikas S, Golenbock D, Moore KJ, Tabas I. Atherogenic lipids and lipoproteins trigger cd36-tlr2-dependent apoptosis in macrophages undergoing endoplasmic reticulum stress. Cell Metab. 2010;12:467–82.
10. Rosenfeld ME, Palinski W, Yla-Herttuala S, Butler S, Witztum JL. Distribution of oxidation specific lipid-protein adducts and apolipoprotein b in atherosclerotic lesions of varying severity from whhl rabbits. Arteriosclerosis. 1990;10:336–49.
11. van Dijk RA, Kolodgie F, Ravandi A, Leibundgut G, Hu PP, Prasad A, Mahmud E, Dennis E, Curtiss LK, Witztum JL, Wasserman BA, Otsuka F, Virmani R, Tsimikas S. Differential expression of oxidation-specific epitopes and apolipoprotein(a) in progressing and ruptured human coronary and carotid atherosclerotic lesions. J Lipid Res. 2012;53:2773–90.
12. Ravandi A, Leibundgut G, Hung MY, Patel M, Hutchins PM, Murphy RC, Prasad A, Mahmud E, Miller YI, Dennis E, Witztum JL, Tsimikas S. Release and capture of bioactive oxidized phospholipids and oxidized cholesteryl esters during percutaneous coronary and peripheral arterial interventions in humans. J Am Coll Cardiol. 2014;63:1961–71.
13. Choi SH, Yin H, Ravandi A, Armando A, Dumlao D, Kim J, Almazan F, Taylor AM, McNamara CA, Tsimikas S, Dennis EA, Witztum JL, Miller YI. Polyoxygenated cholesterol ester hydroperoxide activates tlr4 and syk dependent signaling in macrophages. PLoS One. 2013;8:e83145.
14. Leibundgut G, Witztum JL, Tsimikas S. Oxidation-specific epitopes and immunological responses: translational biotheranostic implications for atherosclerosis. Curr Opin Pharmacol. 2013;13:168–79.
15. Lee S, Birukov KG, Romanoski CE, Springstead JR, Lusis AJ, Berliner JA. Role of phospholipid oxidation products in atherosclerosis. Circ Res. 2012;111:778–99.
16. Kadl A, Sharma PR, Chen W, Agrawal R, Meher AK, Rudraiah S, Grubbs N, Sharma R, Leitinger N. Oxidized phospholipid-induced inflammation is mediated by toll-like receptor 2. Free Rad Biol Med. 2011;51:1903–9.
17. Kadl A, Meher AK, Sharma PR, Lee MY, Doran AC, Johnstone SR, Elliott MR, Gruber F, Han J, Chen W, Kensler T, Ravichandran KS, Isakson BE, Wamhoff BR, Leitinger N. Identification of a novel macrophage phenotype that develops in response to atherogenic phospholipids via nrf2. Circ Res. 2010;107:737–46.

18. Miller YI, Choi SH, Fang L, Tsimikas S. Lipoprotein modification and macrophage uptake: role of pathologic cholesterol transport in atherogenesis. Subcell Biochem. 2010;51:229–51.
19. Lichtman AH, Binder CJ, Tsimikas S, Witztum JL. Adaptive immunity in atherogenesis: new insights and therapeutic approaches. J Clin Invest. 2013;123:27–36.
20. Lewis MJ, Malik TH, Ehrenstein MR, Boyle JJ, Botto M, Haskard DO. Immunoglobulin m is required for protection against atherosclerosis in low-density lipoprotein receptor-deficient mice. Circulation. 2009;120:417–26.
21. Kyaw T, Tay C, Krishnamurthi S, Kanellakis P, Agrotis A, Tipping P, Bobik A, Toh BH. B1a b lymphocytes are atheroprotective by secreting natural igm that increases igm deposits and reduces necrotic cores in atherosclerotic lesions. Circ Res. 2011;109:830–4.
22. Karvonen J, Paivansalo M, Kesaniemi YA, Horkko S. Immunoglobulin m type of autoantibodies to oxidized low-density lipoprotein has an inverse relation to carotid artery atherosclerosis. Circulation. 2003;108:2107–12.
23. Ravandi A, Boekholdt SM, Mallat Z, Talmud PJ, Kastelein JJ, Wareham NJ, Miller ER, Benessiano J, Tedgui A, Witztum JL, Khaw KT, Tsimikas S. Relationship of igg and igm autoantibodies and immune complexes to oxidized LDL with markers of oxidation and inflammation and cardiovascular events: results from the epic-norfolk study. J Lipid Res. 2011;52:1829–36.
24. Tsimikas S, Willeit P, Willeit J, Santer P, Mayr M, Xu Q, Mayr A, Witztum JL, Kiechl S. Oxidation-specific biomarkers, prospective 15-year cardiovascular and stroke outcomes, and net reclassification of cardiovascular events. J Am Coll Cardiol. 2012;60:2218–29.
25. Taleb A, Witztum JL, Tsimikas S. Oxidized phospholipids on apolipoprotein b-100 (oxpl/apoB) containing lipoproteins: a biomarker predicting cardiovascular disease and cardiovascular events. Biomarkers Med. 2011;5:673–94.
26. Kiechl S, Willeit J, Mayr M, Viehweider B, Oberhollenzer M, Kronenberg F, Wiedermann CJ, Oberthaler S, Xu Q, Witztum JL, Tsimikas S. Oxidized phospholipids, lipoprotein(a), lipoprotein-associated phospholipase a2 activity, and 10-year cardiovascular outcomes: prospective results from the bruneck study. Arterioscler Thromb Vasc Biol. 2007;27:1788–95.
27. Tsimikas S, Mallat Z, Talmud PJ, Kastelein JJ, Wareham NJ, Sandhu MS, Miller ER, Benessiano J, Tedgui A, Witztum JL, Khaw KT, Boekholdt SM. Oxidation-specific biomarkers, lipoprotein(a), and risk of fatal and nonfatal coronary events. J Am Coll Cardiol. 2010;56:946–55.
28. Kamstrup PR, Tybjaerg-Hansen A, Nordestgaard BG. Elevated lipoprotein(a) and risk of aortic valve stenosis in the general population. J Am Coll Cardiol. 2014;63:470–7.
29. Thanassoulis G, Campbell CY, Owens DS, Smith JG, Smith AV, Peloso GM, Kerr KF, Pechlivanis S, Budoff MJ, Harris TB, Malhotra R, O'Brien KD, Kamstrup PR, Nordestgaard BG, Tybjaerg-Hansen A, Allison MA, Aspelund T, Criqui MH, Heckbert SR, Hwang SJ, Liu Y, Sjogren M, van der Pals J, Kalsch H, Muhleisen TW, Nothen MM, Cupples LA, Caslake M, Di Angelantonio E, Danesh J, Rotter JI, Sigurdsson S, Wong Q, Erbel R, Kathiresan S, Melander O, Gudnason V, O'Donnell CJ, Post WS. Genetic associations with valvular calcification and aortic stenosis. N Engl J Med. 2013;368:503–12.
30. Kamstrup PR, Tybjaerg-Hansen A, Nordestgaard BG. Extreme lipoprotein(a) levels and improved cardiovascular risk prediction. J Am Coll Cardiol. 2013;61:1146–56.
31. Kamstrup PR, Tybjaerg-Hansen A, Steffensen R, Nordestgaard BG. Genetically elevated lipoprotein(a) and increased risk of myocardial infarction. JAMA. 2009;301:2331–9.
32. Hung MY, Witztum JL, Tsimikas S. New therapeutic targets for calcific aortic valve stenosis: the lipoprotein(a)-lipoprotein-associated phospholipase a_2-oxidized phospholipid axis. J Am Coll Cardiol. 2014;63:478–80.
33. Erqou S, Thompson A, Di Angelantonio E, Saleheen D, Kaptoge S, Marcovina S, Danesh J. Apolipoprotein(a) isoforms and the risk of vascular disease: systematic review of 40 studies involving 58,000 participants. J Am Coll Cardiol. 2010;55:2160–7.
34. Erqou S, Kaptoge S, Perry PL, Di Angelantonio E, Thompson A, White IR, Marcovina SM, Collins R, Thompson SG, Danesh J. Lipoprotein(a) concentration and the risk of coronary heart disease, stroke, and nonvascular mortality. JAMA. 2009;302:412–23.

35. Palinski W, Rosenfeld ME, Yla-Herttuala S, Gurtner GC, Socher SS, Butler SW, Parthasarathy S, Carew TE, Steinberg D, Witztum JL. Low density lipoprotein undergoes oxidative modification in vivo. Proc Natl Acad Sci U S A. 1989;86:1372–6.
36. Palinski W, Yla-Herttuala S, Rosenfeld ME, Butler SW, Socher SA, Parthasarathy S, Curtiss LK, Witztum JL. Antisera and monoclonal antibodies specific for epitopes generated during oxidative modification of low density lipoprotein. Arteriosclerosis. 1990;10:325–35.
37. Tsimikas S, Palinski W, Halpern SE, Yeung DW, Curtiss LK, Witztum JL. Radiolabeled MDA2, an oxidation-specific, monoclonal antibody, identifies native atherosclerotic lesions in vivo. J Nucl Cardiol. 1999;6:41–53.
38. Palinski W, Ord VA, Plump AS, Breslow JL, Steinberg D, Witztum JL. Apoe-deficient mice are a model of lipoprotein oxidation in atherogenesis. Demonstration of oxidation-specific epitopes in lesions and high titers of autoantibodies to malondialdehyde-lysine in serum. Arterioscler Thromb. 1994;14:605–16.
39. Palinski W, Horkko S, Miller E, Steinbrecher UP, Powell HC, Curtiss LK, Witztum JL. Cloning of monoclonal autoantibodies to epitopes of oxidized lipoproteins from apolipoprotein e-deficient mice. Demonstration of epitopes of oxidized low density lipoprotein in human plasma. J Clin Invest. 1996;98:800–14.
40. Friedman P, Horkko S, Steinberg D, Witztum JL, Dennis EA. Correlation of antiphospholipid antibody recognition with the structure of synthetic oxidized phospholipids. Importance of schiff base formation and aldol condensation. J Biol Chem. 2002;277:7010–20.
41. Horkko S, Bird DA, Miller E, Itabe H, Leitinger N, Subbanagounder G, Berliner JA, Friedman P, Dennis EA, Curtiss LK, Palinski W, Witztum JL. Monoclonal autoantibodies specific for oxidized phospholipids or oxidized phospholipid-protein adducts inhibit macrophage uptake of oxidized low-density lipoproteins. J Clin Invest. 1999;103:117–28.
42. Binder CJ, Horkko S, Dewan A, Chang MK, Kieu EP, Goodyear CS, Shaw PX, Palinski W, Witztum JL, Silverman GJ. Pneumococcal vaccination decreases atherosclerotic lesion formation: molecular mimicry between streptococcus pneumoniae and oxidized LDL. Nat Med. 2003;9:736–43.
43. Shaw PX, Horkko S, Chang MK, Curtiss LK, Palinski W, Silverman GJ, Witztum JL. Natural antibodies with the t15 idiotype may act in atherosclerosis, apoptotic clearance, and protective immunity. J Clin Invest. 2000;105:1731–40.
44. Shaw PX, Horkko S, Tsimikas S, Chang MK, Palinski W, Silverman GJ, Chen PP, Witztum JL. Human-derived anti-oxidized LDL autoantibody blocks uptake of oxidized LDL by macrophages and localizes to atherosclerotic lesions in vivo. Arterioscler Thromb Vasc Biol. 2001;21:1333–9.
45. Briley-Saebo KC, Cho YS, Shaw PX, Ryu SK, Mani V, Dickson S, Izadmehr E, Green S, Fayad ZA, Tsimikas S. Targeted iron oxide particles for in vivo magnetic resonance detection of atherosclerotic lesions with antibodies directed to oxidation-specific epitopes. J Am Coll Cardiol. 2011;57:337–47.
46. Briley-Saebo KC, Nguyen TH, Saeboe AM, Cho YS, Ryu SK, Volkava E, Dickson S, Leibundgut G, Weisner P, Green S, Casanada F, Miller YI, Shaw W, Witztum JL, Fayad ZA, Tsimikas S. In vivo detection of oxidation-specific epitopes in atherosclerotic lesions using biocompatible manganese molecular magnetic imaging probes. J Am Coll Cardiol. 2012;59:616–26.
47. Briley-Saebo KC, Shaw PX, Mulder WJ, Choi SH, Vucic E, Aguinaldo JG, Witztum JL, Fuster V, Tsimikas S, Fayad ZA. Targeted molecular probes for imaging atherosclerotic lesions with magnetic resonance using antibodies that recognize oxidation-specific epitopes. Circulation. 2008;117:3206–15.
48. Tsimikas S, Miyanohara A, Hartvigsen K, Merki E, Shaw PX, Chou MY, Pattison J, Torzewski M, Sollors J, Friedmann T, Lai NC, Hammond HK, Getz GS, Reardon CA, Li AC, Banka CL, Witztum JL. Human oxidation-specific antibodies reduce foam cell formation and atherosclerosis progression. J Am Coll Cardiol. 2011;58:1715–27.
49. Amir S, Hartvigsen K, Gonen A, Leibundgut G, Que X, Jensen-Jarolim E, Wagner O, Tsimikas S, Witztum JL, Binder CJ. Peptide mimotopes of malondialdehyde epitopes for clinical applications in cardiovascular disease. J Lipid Res. 2012;53:1316–26.

50. Miller YI, Tsimikas S. Oxidation-specific epitopes as targets for biotheranostic applications in humans: biomarkers, molecular imaging and therapeutics. Curr Opin Lipidol. 2013;24:426–37.
51. Tsimikas S, Shortal BP, Witztum JL, Palinski W. In vivo uptake of radiolabeled MDA2, an oxidation-specific monoclonal antibody, provides an accurate measure of atherosclerotic lesions rich in oxidized LDL and is highly sensitive to their regression. Arterioscler Thromb Vasc Biol. 2000;20:689–97.
52. Tsimikas S, Palinski W, Witztum JL. Circulating autoantibodies to oxidized LDL correlate with arterial accumulation and depletion of oxidized LDL in LDL receptor-deficient mice. Arterioscler Thromb Vasc Biol. 2001;21:95–100.
53. Torzewski M, Shaw PX, Han KR, Shortal B, Lackner KJ, Witztum JL, Palinski W, Tsimikas S. Reduced in vivo aortic uptake of radiolabeled oxidation-specific antibodies reflects changes in plaque composition consistent with plaque stabilization. Arterioscler Thromb Vasc Biol. 2004;24:2307–12.
54. Vucic E, Dickson SD, Calcagno C, Rudd JHF, Moshier E, Hayashi K, Mounessa JS, Roytman M, Moon MJ, Lin J, Tsimikas S, Fisher EA, Nicolay K, Fuster V, Fayad ZA. Pioglitazone modulates vascular inflammation in atherosclerotic rabbits: noninvasive assessment with fdg-pet-ct and dynamic contrast-enhanced mr imaging. J Am Coll Cardiol Img. 2011;4:1100–9.
55. Vucic E, Calcagno C, Dickson SD, Rudd JH, Hayashi K, Bucerius J, Moshier E, Mounessa JS, Roytman M, Moon MJ, Lin J, Ramachandran S, Tanimoto T, Brown K, Kotsuma M, Tsimikas S, Fisher EA, Nicolay K, Fuster V, Fayad ZA. Regression of inflammation in atherosclerosis by the lxr agonist r211945: a noninvasive assessment and comparison with atorvastatin. J Am Coll Cardiol Img. 2012;5:819–28.
56. Nguyen TH, Bryant H, Shapsa A, Street H, Mani V, Fayad ZA, Frank JA, Tsimikas S, Briley-Saebo KC. Manganese g8 dendrimers targeted to oxidation-specific epitopes: In vivo mr imaging of atherosclerosis. J Magn Reson Imaging. 2014. (in Press) doi:10.1002/jmri.24606.
57. Yla-Herttuala S, Palinski W, Rosenfeld ME, Parthasarathy S, Carew TE, Butler S, Witztum JL, Steinberg D. Evidence for the presence of oxidatively modified low density lipoprotein in atherosclerotic lesions of rabbit and man. J Clin Invest. 1989;84:1086–95.
58. Tsimikas S, Aikawa M, Miller Jr FJ, Miller ER, Torzewski M, Lentz SR, Bergmark C, Heistad DD, Libby P, Witztum JL. Increased plasma oxidized phospholipid: apolipoprotein b-100 ratio with concomitant depletion of oxidized phospholipids from atherosclerotic lesions after dietary lipid-lowering: a potential biomarker of early atherosclerosis regression. Arterioscler Thromb Vasc Biol. 2007;27:175–81.
59. Fang L, Green SR, Baek JS, Lee SH, Ellett F, Deer E, Lieschke GJ, Witztum JL, Tsimikas S, Miller YI. In vivo visualization and attenuation of oxidized lipid accumulation in hypercholesterolemic zebrafish. J Clin Invest. 2011;121:4861–9.
60. Purushothaman KR, Purushothaman M, Levy AP, Lento PA, Evrard S, Kovacic JC, Briley-Saebo KC, Tsimikas S, Witztum JL, Krishnan P, Kini A, Fayad ZA, Fuster V, Sharma SK, Moreno PR. Increased expression of oxidation-specific epitopes and apoptosis are associated with haptoglobin genotype: possible implications for plaque progression in human atherosclerosis. J Am Coll Cardiol. 2012;60:112–9.
61. Libby P, Aikawa M. Stabilization of atherosclerotic plaques: new mechanisms and clinical targets. Nat Med. 2002;8:1257–62.
62. Mintz GS, Pichard AD, Popma JJ, Kent KM, Satler LF, Bucher TA, Leon MB. Determinants and correlates of target lesion calcium in coronary artery disease: a clinical, angiographic and intravascular ultrasound study. J Am Coll Cardiol. 1997;29:268–74.
63. Scheuhammer AM, Cherian MG. Binding of manganese in human and rat plasma. Biochim Biophys Acta. 1985;840:163–9.
64. Briley-Saebo KC, Amirbekian V, Mani V, Aguinaldo JGS, Vucic E, Carpenter D, Amirbekian S, Fayad ZA. Gadolinium mixed-micelles: effect of the amphiphile on in vitro and in vivo efficacy in apolipoprotein e knockout mouse models of atherosclerosis. Magnet Reson Med. 2006;56:1336–46.
65. Briley-Saebo KC, Geninatti-Crich S, Cormode DP, Barazza A, Mulder WJ, Chen W, Giovenzana GB, Fisher EA, Aime S, Fayad ZA. High-relaxivity gadolinium-modified

high-density lipoproteins as magnetic resonance imaging contrast agents. J Phys Chem B. 2009;113:6283–9.

66. Kellar KE, Foster N. Determination of the relative amounts of free and complexed manganese ions in aqueous-solution by nuclear-magnetic-resonance. Anal Chem. 1991;63:2919–24.
67. Bryant Jr LH, Brechbiel MW, Wu C, Bulte JW, Herynek V, Frank JA. Synthesis and relaxometry of high-generation (g = 5, 7, 9, and 10) pamam dendrimer-dota-gadolinium chelates. J Magn Reson Imaging. 1999;9:348–52.

Live Cell Multiphoton Microscopy of Atherosclerotic Plaques in Mouse Aortas

7

Sara McArdle, Ekaterina Koltsova, Grzegorz Chodaczek, and Klaus Ley

Contents

Abstract

Atherosclerosis is a chronic inflammatory disease with both innate and adaptive immune components. Various static methods have been applied to investigate mechanisms of atherosclerosis development. However, they did not allow for monitoring dynamic changes in leukocyte behavior in normal and atherosclerotic

S. McArdle
Division of Inflammation Biology, La Jolla Institute for Allergy and Immunology, 9420 Athena Circle, La Jolla, CA 92037, USA

Department of Bioengineering, University of California, San Diego, La Jolla, CA, USA

E. Koltsova • G. Chodaczek • K. Ley, MD (✉)
Division of Inflammation Biology, La Jolla Institute for Allergy and Immunology, 9420 Athena Circle, La Jolla, CA 92037, USA
e-mail: Klaus@liai.org

E. Aikawa (ed.), *Cardiovascular Imaging: Arterial and Aortic Valve Inflammation and Calcification*, DOI 10.1007/978-3-319-09268-3_7

aortas. Live cell imaging is necessary to study dynamic or transient leukocyte functions relevant to disease pathology, such as antigen presentation, cell migration, and cell-cell interaction. We developed a protocol for ex vivo multiphoton microscopy of atherosclerotic aortas and used it to demonstrate that antigen presentation may occur within the arterial wall. Aortas are harvested from transgenic reporter mice with fluorescent myeloid cells and then incubated with labeled T cells. The cells are imaged with a multiphoton microscope, while a superfusion system maintains the explant in physiologic condition. Cells are tracked from the videos, and their motion is quantified. This system was used to demonstrate antigen presentation in the arterial wall in the context of atherosclerosis.

7.1 Introduction

7.1.1 Atherosclerosis

Atherosclerosis is an underlying cause of most heart attacks, strokes, and other forms of cardiovascular disease, which is one of the leading causes of death worldwide [1]. It is a chronic inflammatory disease, characterized by plaque buildup in large and medium arteries. Within plaques, leukocytes actively mediate both pro- and anti-inflammatory processes [2]. Disease progression and plaque content have traditionally been studied using static end-point methods, including histology, immunohistochemistry, immunofluorescence, and flow cytometry of aortas [3]. These methods provide qualitative and quantitative data on the numbers and phenotypes of cells in the plaque, but cannot evaluate dynamic cell functions, such as cell motion and cell-cell interaction. Live cell imaging is necessary to study these transient processes to better understand their contribution to disease progression.

One dynamic cell function that is integral to inflammation is antigen presentation. This is a process by which an antigen-presenting cell takes up antigen from its microenvironment and processes it to be recognizable by T cells in the context of MHC molecules. When a T cell receptor (TCR) recognizes an antigenic peptide on MHC on the surface of an antigen-presenting cell (APC) and coactivator signals are present, the T cell becomes activated, proliferates, and produces cytokines that influence plaque development [4]. During the typical immune response, dendritic cells, a type of APC, take up antigen from the area of inflammation and migrate to local lymph nodes, where they present this antigen to naïve T cells, leading to the T cells' initial activation. These antigen-experienced T cells acquire new homing properties (adhesion molecules and chemokine receptors), enabling them to traffic back to the original site of insult, and they polarize to characteristic functional subsets. Interactions between APCs and T cells have been observed in nonlymphoid tissues [5], and recent in vitro data suggests that antigen presentation to antigen-experienced T cells occurs in the arterial wall [6, 7]. Unlike static methods, live cell imaging can uniquely take advantage of changes in T cell behavior (slowing down) while interacting with an APC [8, 9] to demonstrate antigen presentation in the cells' native microenvironment. Here, we describe a technique to visualize leukocyte activity in the wall of healthy and atherosclerotic aorta explants using multiphoton microscopy [10].

7.1.2 Live Cell Microscopy

The choice of microscopy technique for imaging live cells in vivo or ex vivo depends on the optical properties of the target tissue and the spatial and temporal resolution needed to observe the phenomena in question. The four most common microscopy techniques for imaging ex vivo or in vivo are epifluorescence, spinning disk confocal, laser scanning confocal, and multiphoton [11, 12]. Each of these techniques has unique advantages and disadvantages for live cell fluorescence imaging (Table 7.1) [13, 14].

7.1.2.1 Epifluorescence Microscopy

Epifluorescence, or widefield, microscopy is frequently used for live imaging because of its high frame rate (up to 50 frames/s for a 512×512 pixel frame, depending on the camera [15]). Another advantage is that this technique can acquire transmitted light images, allowing for visualizing of tissue structure in combination with fluorescence. Unlike a confocal, all light that reaches the objective is collected, and therefore excitation intensity can be lowered to reduce photobleaching and phototoxicity. However, this leads to diminished lateral resolution due to out-of-focus light in thick tissues and explants. Epifluorescence microscopes cannot distinguish depth except via

Table 7.1 Advantages and disadvantages of common live cell imaging modalities

Method	Advantages	Disadvantages
Epifluorescence	Fast	Poor axial and lateral resolution
	Lower photobleaching than confocal	Limited to thin tissues Limited control of excitation wavelength
Spinning disk confocal (SDCM)	Fast	Low excitation tissue penetration
	Good axial and lateral resolution Less photobleaching than LSCM	Lower intensity and contrast than LSCM
Laser scanning confocal (LSCM)	Best resolution and contrast in XYZ	Slow Low excitation tissue penetration High photobleaching
Multiphoton	Deep tissue penetration	Slow
	Low photobleaching of out-of-focus planes	Poor axial resolution compared to LSCM and SDCM
	Good lateral resolution Single laser can excite broad range simultaneously	Difficult to sequentially excite different fluorophores

post-acquisition deconvolution [16] and so are inadequate for situations in which axial resolution is important. Epifluorescence microscopes use broad-spectrum lamps and control excitation wavelength through filter cubes. Filter wheels allow for rapid switching of excitation wavelength; however, different fluorophores must be analyzed sequentially, which decreases frame rate and may lead to poor registration between different colors in rapidly moving cells. Therefore, this technique is typically only used for samples with one or two fluorophores and only for thin tissues (<100 μm).

7.1.2.2 Confocal Microscopy

Confocal microscopy provides the best spatial resolution of the standard live cell techniques and so is often chosen for applications requiring resolution of subcellular structures. Spinning disk confocal systems can image at very high speeds (theoretically up to 2,000 fps [17], in practice highly limited by the CCD camera), making them ideal for imaging fast processes. If a very high speed is not necessary, laser scanning confocal systems can provide higher lateral and axial resolution with less noise (especially in weakly fluorescent samples), while still scanning up to 40 fps, depending on the image size. However, laser scanning confocal systems typically spend more time exciting each pixel, resulting in higher photobleaching and phototoxicity. Both types of confocal systems are limited by a small penetration depth (two to three times smaller than the maximum of a multiphoton microscope [18]) due to high scattering of visible excitation light by the sample. Unlike epifluorescence systems which use similar excitation wavelength, confocal microscopes retain high resolution in thick tissues by optically slicing with the confocal aperture. However, the aperture blocks a portion of the emitted light that reaches the detector, requiring more intense excitation and causing additional photobleaching than epifluorescence or multiphoton microscopy. The use of lasers of defined wavelengths makes it technically easier to image multiple fluorophores simultaneously, improving time resolution compared to epifluorescence microscopy. Typical imaging depths achieved by confocal microscopy are 100–200 μm.

7.1.2.3 Multiphoton Microscopy

Multiphoton microscopes excite the sample with a high-intensity, pulsed femtosecond laser with a long (infrared) wavelength to penetrate deeper into tissue with less scattering than confocal or epifluorescence microscopes (up to 500 μm) [19]. Thanks to the two-photon excitation, which only takes place in the objective's focal point, true optical slicing is achieved so only a small volume is excited at one time, minimizing the time each point in the sample is exposed to light while retaining good spatial resolution. Because there is no need for a confocal aperture, all of the emitted light that reaches the objective is collected, thus reducing the needed intensity of the excitation. Together, these phenomena reduce photobleaching and improve the signal intensity in thick tissues, making it a common choice for in vivo imaging. Most fluorophores have a broader two-photon excitation range than single-photon excitation [20], enabling the excitation of multiple fluorophores simultaneously. A disadvantage of this is that distinguishing fluorochromes by changing excitation wavelength is generally not feasible. Multiphoton microscopy has lower resolution in all three axes than laser scanning confocal, dictated by the long excitation wavelength (typically 800–1,000 nm). The use of low-noise, high-dynamic-range photomultipliers improves sensitivity but drastically reduces acquisition speed compared to spinning disk confocal and epifluorescence microscopy. Better acquisition speeds can be realized by using a resonant scanner.

7.1.3 Choice of Multiphoton Microscopy for Studying Atherosclerosis

Atherosclerotic plaques in mouse aortas can be more than 100 μm thick [21], making two-photon excitation necessary for viewing the depth of the plaque. A low frame rate is sufficient for visualizing leukocyte movement within the arterial wall, because migration speeds are less than 1 μm/s. The low photobleaching inherent in multiphoton microscopy enables acquisition of long (~1 h) movies, which is necessary for quantifying slow migration. Multiphoton microscopy also uniquely enables the visualization of unlabeled collagen in the wall through second-harmonic generation [22]. We used multiphoton microscopy to visualize antigen presentation in the context of atherosclerosis [10].

7.2 Materials and Methods

7.2.1 Aorta Harvest

7.2.1.1 Background

Aortas can be obtained from healthy or atherosclerotic mice that have transgenically labeled leukocytes. Mice deficient in apolipoprotein E ($Apoe^{-/-}$), a protein involved in lipoprotein transport, are a common model for atherosclerosis. They rapidly develop plaques when fed a high-fat western diet (WD) [23]. To study the interaction between antigen-presenting myeloid cells and T cells in atherosclerotic plaques, we used $CD11c^{YFP}$ mice, which express yellow fluorescent protein under the CD11c promoter [24]. This mouse has CD11b+ CD11c+ macrophages and dendritic cells in the plaque bright enough to be visualized with multiphoton microscopy. The precise relationship between YFP brightness and cell phenotype, including CD11c expression, needs to be established in each tissue and experimental setting. Non-atherosclerotic mice can be injected with 30 μg of CpG class B oligonucleotides (ODN 1826, Integrated DNA technologies), 2–3 h before sacrifice to induce myeloid cell recruitment to the aorta wall. Within atherosclerotic plaques, myeloid cells phagocytose lipids, scavenge dead cells, and secrete both pro- and anti-inflammatory cytokines [2].

7.2.1.2 Method

The mouse was killed by CO_2, and 0.5–1 mL of blood was withdrawn via cardiac puncture with a 25 G needle. The internal organs were removed, and then 10 mL of PBS (containing 20 U/mL heparin) were perfused through the aorta through the

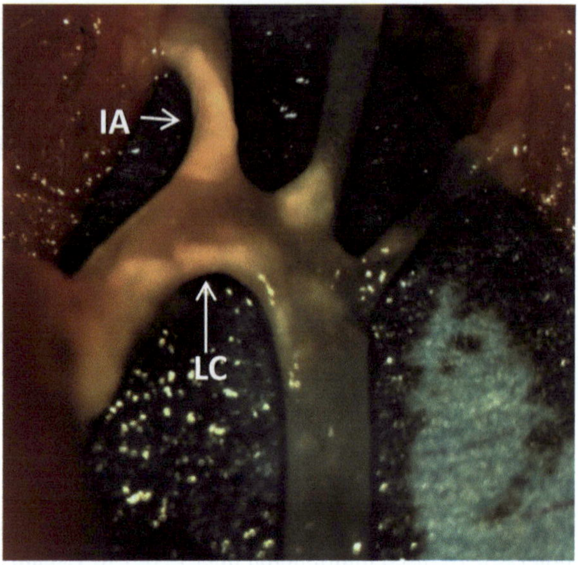

Fig. 7.1 The aorta of an *Apoe*$^{-/-}$ mouse that was fed WD for 12 weeks. After sacrifice, the aorta was perfused with PBS with 20 U/mL heparin and the artery was cleaned of fat (see Sect. 7.2.1.2) to reveal visible atherosclerotic plaque (opaque beige, *white arrows*). *IA* innominate artery, *LC* lesser curvature

heart. Using forceps and spring scissors, the fat and para-aortic lymph nodes were removed from around the artery. To maintain cell viability, it is important to disturb the wall of the aorta as little as possible, especially near the area that will be imaged, and to keep the tissue moist with PBS. The aorta was harvested, from its origin from the heart to above the renal arteries, including the branches to the innominate, left common carotid, and left subclavian arteries. Solid plaques develop first at the branch of the innominate artery from the aorta and also in the lesser curvature of the aorta. Both areas are suitable for imaging (Figs. 7.1 and 7.2). The artery was incubated overnight with T cells at 37 °C with 5 % CO_2 in complete RPMI 1640 media containing 10 % FBS, 1 % pen/strep, 2 mM L-Glu, 1 % NEAA, 1 mM HEPES, and 1 mM sodium pyruvate before imaging.

7.2.2 T Cell Harvest

7.2.2.1 Background

Theoretically, every T cell in a mouse may express a unique TCR that is specific for a different peptide. To investigate antigen-specific T cell activation, we used transgenic mice in which majority of CD4 T cells have a restricted TCR specificity to well-defined exogenous antigenic peptides. These mice are useful tools for studying antigen presentation because the presence of antigen can be easily controlled. We employed two different strains of mice with transgenic TCRs: OT-II, which have T cells specific for a peptide derived from ovalbumin [25], and SMARTA, which have T cells specific for a peptide derived from lymphocytic choriomeningitis virus (LCMV) [26] (see Table 7.2). Having two distinct TCR transgenic mice allowed us to image T cells with and without their cognate antigen in the same experimental setup to more accurately assess the specificity of antigen presentation in the aorta. Since neither antigen is present in a mouse, almost all T cells harvested from the

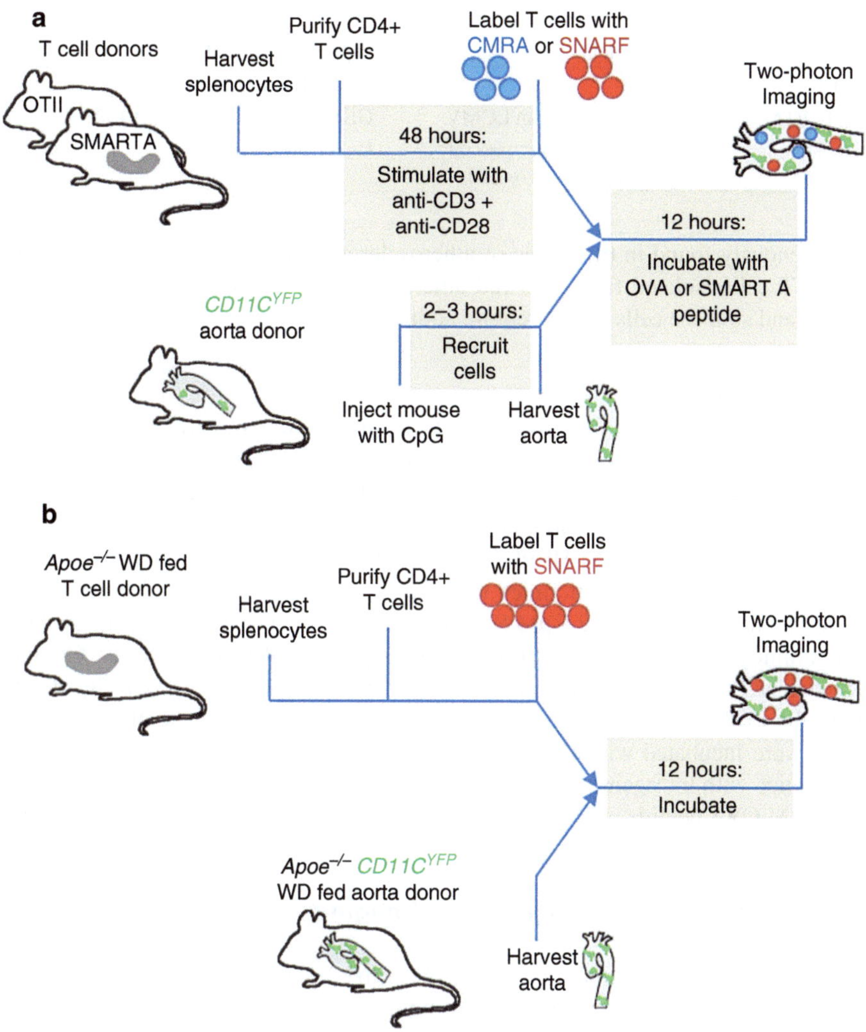

Fig. 7.2 Schematic timeline of procedure for imaging myeloid cells presenting antigen to T cells in the aorta wall. (**a**) To image antigen presentation with a known, exogenous antigen, CD4+ T cells with transgenic TCRs are harvested and purified from the spleen and restimulated in vitro. YFP+ myeloid cells are recruited to the aorta with an injection of CpG, and after 2–3 h the aorta is harvested. The T cells are labeled and incubated with the aorta in the presence of exogenously added antigenic peptide, and then the tissue is imaged using two-photon microscopy. (**b**) To image antigen presentation in the context of atherosclerosis, the aorta of an atherosclerotic mouse with YFP+ myeloid cells is harvested. CD4+ T cells are harvested and purified from an atherosclerotic mouse. The T cells are labeled and incubated with the aorta, and then the tissue is imaged using two-photon microscopy

transgenic mice are naïve. Naïve cells must be activated in vitro with anti-CD3 and anti-CD28 to maintain cell viability. To assay antigen presentation in the context of atherosclerosis, we also used polyclonal T cells from WD-fed *Apoe*$^{-/-}$ mice. The specific peptide that these cells recognize is unknown, but it is likely to be

Table 7.2 Sources of T cells and the peptides they recognize

Mouse strain	Antigen protein	Peptide recognized by TCR
OT-II	Ovalbumin	ISQAVHAAHAEINEAGR
SMARTA	Glycoprotein P13 from LCMV	GLNGPDIYKGVYQFKSVEFD
Apoe$^{-/-}$	Unknown endogenous, possibly ApoB100, HSP60, or oxLDL	Unknown

endogenously found in the aortas of atherosclerotic mice (see Table 7.2) [27–29]. Many T cells isolated from WD-fed atherosclerotic mice are endogenously activated, and so these cells do not require additional stimulation in vitro.

7.2.2.2 Method

CD4^{+} T cells were harvested from the spleens of atherosclerotic or TCR transgenic mice using a Robosep-negative selection kit (Stem Cell Technologies). These cells were stimulated for 48 h with 8 μg/mL anti-CD3 and 8 μg/mL anti-CD28 (eBioscience) in complete RPMI 1640 media containing 10 % FBS, 1 % pen/strep, 2 mM L-Glu, 1 % NEAA, 1 mM HEPES, and 1 mM sodium pyruvate. T cells isolated from WD-fed atherosclerotic mice were not restimulated in vitro. The cells were differentially labeled with 2.5 μM SNARF (red fluorescent carboxylic acid, acetate, succinimidyl ester, Molecular Probes) or 3 μM CMRA (CellTracker Orange, Molecular Probes) for 10 min at 37 °C. 0.5 million labeled cells were incubated with the explanted aorta in 750 μL media overnight. T cells from atherosclerotic mice were incubated with an aorta from an atherosclerotic mouse, while T cells from mice with transgenic TCRs were incubated with a healthy aorta with or without 1 μM OVA peptide or SMARTA peptide (Table 7.2).

7.2.3 Tissue Maintenance During Imaging

To visualize realistic cell motion, it is necessary to keep the tissue under physiological temperature, pH, oxygen tension, and osmolarity throughout imaging. Immediately before imaging, we secure the aorta to a coverslip by gluing the ends of the tissue with Histoacryl glue (TissueSeal LLC) or Vetbond (3 M). Tissue that touches the glue is unsuitable for imaging, so only the ends of the aorta should be glued down and only the middle used for imaging. A system (Fig. 7.3) was built to keep the tissue warm and superfused with recirculating, oxygenated media throughout the imaging procedure. A reservoir of oxygenated media was created by bubbling gas (95 % oxygen, 5 % CO_2) through ~25 mL of complete RPMI 1640 without phenol red, with 2 mM L-glutamine, 1 % pen/strep, and 1 % FBS, in a 50 mL conical tube. The sample glued to the coverslip was placed in a 60 mm dish with the same solution. A peristaltic pump (Harvard Apparatus, MPII) circulated media at approximately 10 mL/min from the reservoir through an in-line solution heater (Warner Instruments, SF-28) to the dish. The dish was heated by a warmer (Warner Instruments, QE-2 Quick Exchange Platform), and both this and the in-line heater were controlled by a dual feedback

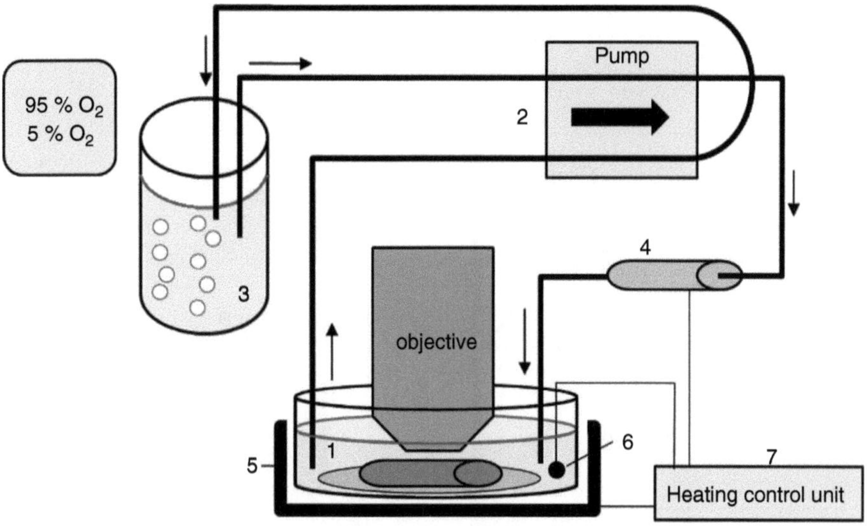

Fig. 7.3 Schematic diagram of recirculating superfusion and heating system to maintain aorta under physiological conditions during imaging. An aorta explant is incubated with T cells for 12 h to allow the T cells to migrate into the tissue. The artery is glued to a coverslip, and placed in a dish with complete RPMI 1,640 without phenol red, with 2 mM L-glutamine, 1 % pen/strep, and 1 % FBS. (*1*) A peristaltic pump (*2*) circulates the media from an oxygenated reservoir, (*3*) through an in-line solution heater (*4*), to the dish and back to the reservoir. The sample is warmed by a dish-warmer (*5*). The media temperature is monitored by a thermometer (*6*), and a control unit (*7*) regulates both heaters to maintain a solution temperature of 37 °C. *Arrows* show the direction of fluid flow

control unit (Warner Instruments, TC-334B) that maintained the liquid near the tissue at 37 °C. The peristaltic pump also returned the media from the dish to the reservoir so that the media constantly recirculate. The inlet and outlet to the dish must be as far as possible from the tissue to not disturb the imaging.

7.2.4 Microscopy and Hardware

Imaging was performed on a Leica TCS SP5 multiphoton system. This system utilizes a DM 6000 upright microscope with a 20× (NA=0.95) water-dipping objective (Olympus, XLUMPLFL), attached to a piezo-controlled objective holder (Piezosystem Jena, NV 40/1 CLE and MIPOS 500 SG) to set the focal plane. A Coherent Chameleon Ultra II Ti:sapphire-pulsed femtosecond laser excites the sample with wavelengths between 680 nm and 1,080 nm. Emitted light is split through a series of three dichroic mirrors and four filters up to four non-descanned photomultiplier tube detectors (PMT-NDD) (Fig. 7.4). The optical path to the detectors does not return through the scanning mirror, improving the sensitivity of detection. Laser scanning is accomplished with either a conventional or resonant scanner, depending on the needs of the experiment. The resonant scanner scans each line faster than the conventional scanner

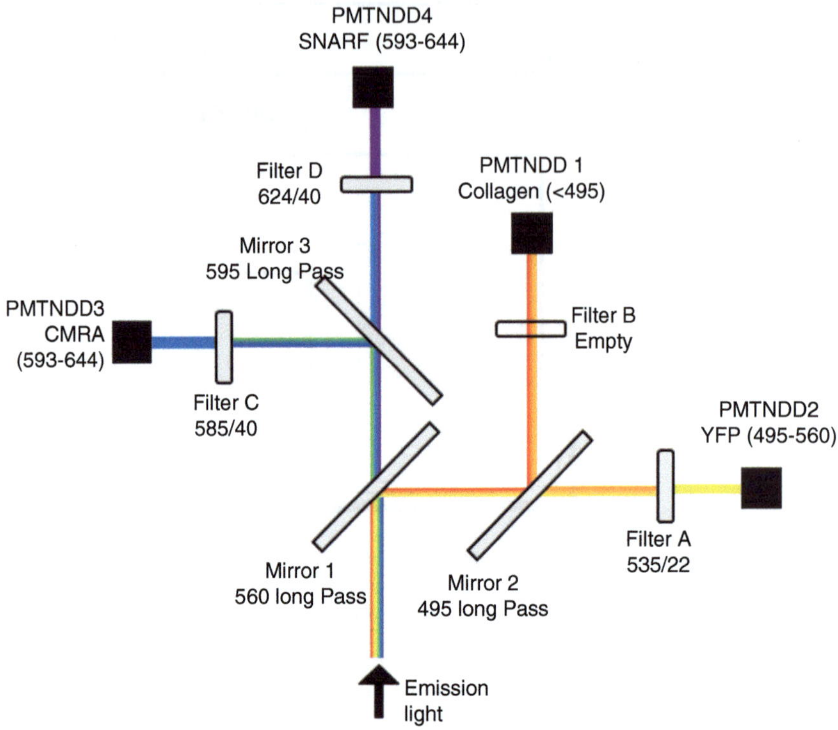

Fig. 7.4 Optical path with dichroic mirrors and filters to simultaneously detect emitted light from an aorta with YFP+ myeloid cells, CMRA-labeled T cells, and SNARF-labeled T cells as well as collagen via SHG. All dichroic mirrors are long-pass, and all filters are band-pass (width/middle). Each PMT is labeled with the fluorophore detected and the approximate wavelength range that reaches the detector

(8,000 lines/s compared to 200–1,400 lines/s). The speed can be effectively doubled in the bidirectional mode which allows for horizontal scanning in both directions, though this can lead to interlacing errors. The pixel dwell time of the resonant mode is shorter, which leads to a higher frame rate and less photobleaching, but more noise. Line or frame averaging can reduce this noise and may still allow for better time resolution than with a conventional scanner.

To observe interactions between YFP$^+$ antigen-presenting cells and SNARF- or CMRA-labeled T cells, the excitation laser was set to 920 nm. This wavelength allows for imaging of all three colors as well as collagen in the arterial wall via second-harmonic generation. The emitted light was split by three long-pass dichroic mirrors (495, 560, and 593 nm) into four bands and passed through three band-pass filters (535/22, 585/40, and 624/40 nm) (Semrock) (Fig. 7.4, Table 7.3). A large field of view (pixel size of ~1 μm) was chosen to capture as many cells as possible, although this does not allow for maximum spatial resolution as calculated by the Nyquist sampling frequency. The Nyquist frequency, which is the pixel size necessary to capture two points that are just optically resolved, is approximately 120 nm for two-photon excitation under our imaging conditions. Due to the inherent low axial resolution of two-photon excitation, 10–15 μm between *z*-planes was

Table 7.3 Typical hardware settings on Leica TCS SP5 multiphoton system with conventional scanner for imaging YFP + APCs, SNARF-labeled T cells, and CMRA-labeled T cells. See Fig. 7.4 for mirror and filter name explanations

Settings	Value	Comments
Dichroic 1	560 nm long pass	Optimized for simultaneous detection of YFP, SNARF, CMRA, and second-harmonic signal. Must be changed for any other color combination
Dichroic 2	495 nm long pass	
Dichroic 3	593 nm long pass	
Filter A	535/22	Detects YFP
Filter B	None	Detects second harmonic – no filter needed
Filter C	585/40	Detects CMRA
Filter D	624/40	Detects SNARF
PMT voltage	1,000–1,250 V	Set each PMT gain to almost the maximum and minimize laser power to reduce photobleaching
PMT offset	−10–0 %	Set such that tissue background is at or near 0
Excitation wavelength	900–920 nm	Optimized for combination of YFP, SNARF, and CMRA
Emitted laser power	2,200 mW	Determined by wavelength
Excitation neutral density filter	3 % [97 % blocked]	Highly dependent on individual laser and alignment. Blocking more reduces photobleaching
Laser gain	90–100 %	Keep as low as possible while detecting signal
Laser offset	50–60 %	Set such that there is no signal at 0 % laser gain
Frame size (pixels)	512×512	Higher for better spatial resolution, lower for faster scan speed and less photobleaching
Zoom	1×–2×	Zoom is a balance between improving spatial resolution by decreasing pixel size and increasing frame size to image more cells
Frame length (μm)	375–750 μm	
Pixel size (nm)	730–1,460 nm	
Scan speed	400 lines/s	Higher for faster frame rate, lower for less noise
Scan direction	1	Bidirectional scanning raises scan speed, but can lead to interlacing artifacts
Line/frame averaging	None	Averaging improves picture quality, but reduces frame rate and increases photobleaching
z-step	10–15 μm	Lower for better axial resolution but more photobleaching
Number of z-steps	8–20	From the adventitia to the deepest T cell
Stack frequency	1/min	Faster scan rates lead to more photobleaching and shorter movies, but better time resolution
Output format	LIF	Can be read by Imaris and ImageJ, or converted to TIF

sufficient for capturing cell location and shape while minimizing photobleaching. A full stack of 10–20 *z*-planes was acquired once per minute. Most of the exogenously added T cells were located in the adventitia, so typically only the outer layer of the artery was imaged. Taking advantage of the motorized stage, two to three locations were imaged concurrently by moving the sample between stacks. Aortas were imaged for roughly an hour, at which photobleaching became noticeable (Table 7.3).

These experimental settings were optimized for imaging with the conventional scanner. The spatial or temporal resolution of the movies could be improved with the resonant scanner by acquiring more *z*-planes or by acquiring stacks faster without a significant increase in photobleaching.

7.2.5 Image Processing

Autofluorescence signal was extracted from low-intensity pixels from YFP, CMRA, or SNARF channels, which were then combined and converted to a new channel. Autofluorescence comes mainly from the elastic lamina in the media layer [30] and can be used to distinguish the adventitia and intima. Collagen, visible through second-harmonic generation, is found in both the adventitia and media. Cell motion was quantified in three dimensions using an automated spot-tracking algorithm in Imaris (Bitplane) with occasional manual correction. The software detects cells based on difference in pixel intensity compared to background and then calculates the centroid of the cell. The cell centers are automatically tracked between frames using an auto-regressive motion algorithm, which assumes mostly random motion that tends towards the velocity and direction calculated in the previous frame. Dendritic projections of myeloid cells are often too thin (width <1 μm) or dim to be detected, so contact between T cells and APCs could not always be directly visualized. T cells were manually determined to be interacting with an APC when the T cell remained in the vicinity of a YFP+ cell for at least 5 min. Interaction times often ranged from 5 min to 1 h. Instantaneous velocity was calculated for each tracked cell between each pair of adjacent frames. Average velocity was calculated for interacting and noninteracting cells separately. Cells which did not move during the entire movie were presumed to be dead and not included in the statistics.

7.3 Results

Ex vivo multiphoton imaging of an explanted aorta allows for the visualization of live, active lymphocytes and myeloid cells within the intima and adventitia of the arterial wall. Collagen and elastin autofluorescence separates the intima from the adventitia. YFP+ myeloid cells were found in both the adventitia and intimal plaque of the aorta of atherosclerotic mice (Fig. 7.5). These cells move at approximately 1–3 μm/min, with significant deformation in cell shape as they travel.

Exogenously added T cells were typically only seen in the adventitial layer, although they can be found in intimal plaques when the plaque was exposed to the cells during the overnight incubation. These T cells migrate through the tissue at typical speeds of 10 μm/min (range 1–30 μm/min). When cognate antigen

Fig. 7.5 (**a**) Three different views of an aorta from an *Apoe*$^{-/-}$ *CD11cYFP* mouse fed WD to show localization of YFP+ cells to the intimal plaque and adventitia. *Green*, YFP+ cells; *Red*, SHG; *Blue*, autofluorescence from the internal elastic lamina (Adapted from Andor Technology [15]). (**b**) Cartoon depicting the anatomy of the aorta seen in (**a**)

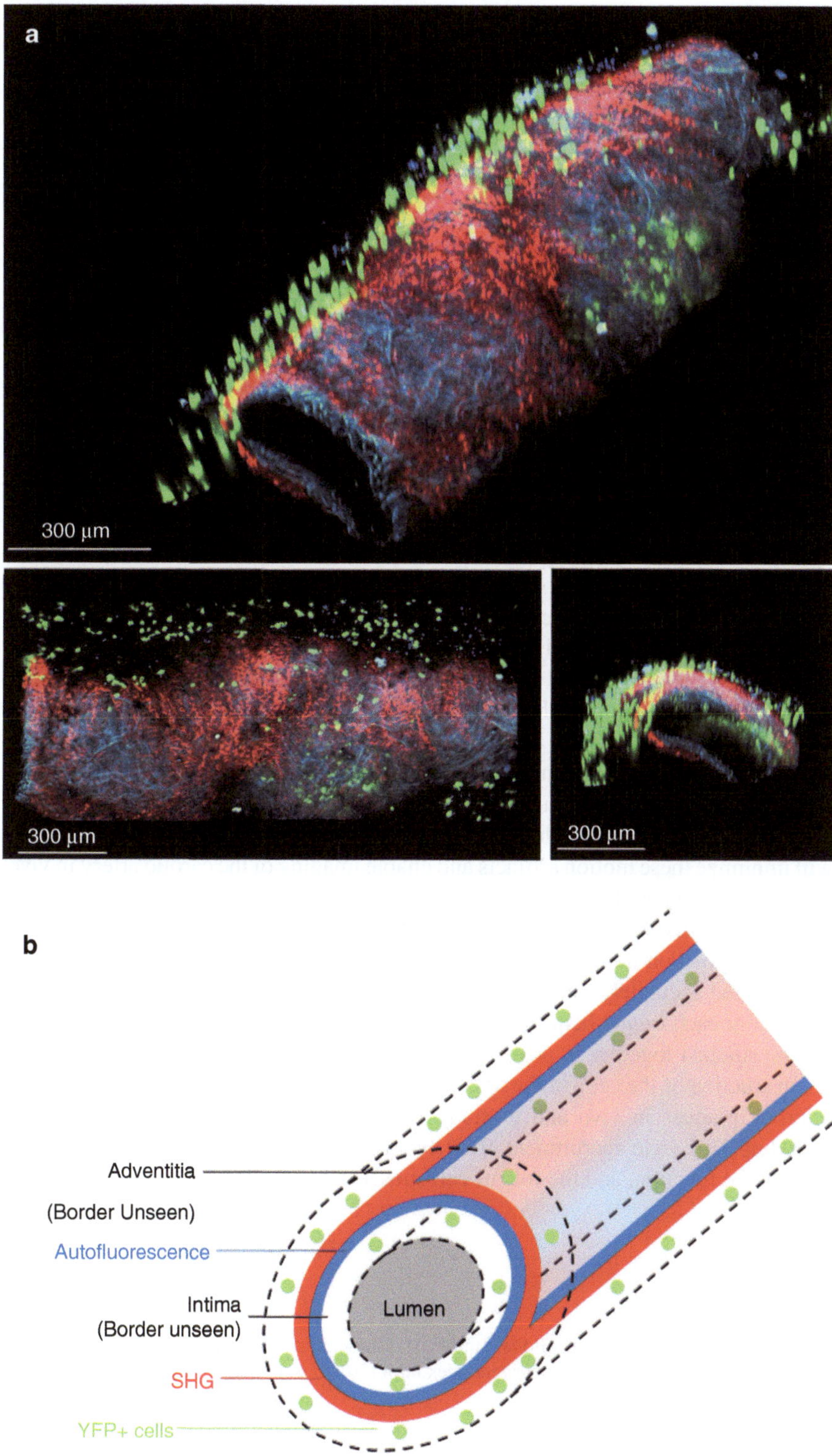
a
300 μm
300 μm
300 μm
b
Adventitia
(Border Unseen)
Autofluorescence
Intima
(Border unseen)
Lumen
SHG
YFP+ cells

(exogenous or endogenous) is present, more T cells interact with YFP+ APCs, and the average velocity of the T cells decreases to 1–3 μm/s [9], suggesting antigen presentation is occurring within the arterial wall.

7.4 Conclusion and Future Work

This novel approach provides new opportunities to study cell activity that cannot be investigated with traditional static methods. This protocol could be expanded to the study of other questions relevant to disease pathology through the use of other transgenic reporter mice with a variety of fluorescently labeled cells or proteins. For instance, imaging cell migration can reveal novel information about chemokine function or the mechanism of how leukocytes enter and leave the aortic wall. Currently, ex vivo multiphoton imaging is the most suitable tool for probing these dynamic processes in their native environment to elucidate inflammatory mechanisms in atherosclerosis.

However, explanted tissue cannot completely mimic the native microenvironment that the leukocytes experience in vivo. Specifically, the absence of pulsatile blood flow [31], the disruption of the extracellular matrix in the adventitia [32, 33], and the alteration of oxygen concentration [34] or other changes from physiological conditions can influence cell motion [8]. Certain questions can only be accurately studied by imaging live mice, such as recruitment of monocytes from the blood to the plaque. New technical challenges are introduced when imaging leukocytes in arteries in vivo, because the blood vessel pulses with each heartbeat. This motion leads to distortion of still images, misalignment of z-stacks, and inconsistency in time series. These artifacts make tracking cells infeasible.

To circumvent these problems, we are currently developing a new technique that will minimize these motion artifacts and enable imaging of the carotid artery in vivo. Custom circuitry will trigger image acquisition based on the cardiac cycle, measured noninvasively through pulse oximetry. This ensures that the artery is in a consistent position for each frame acquired, so that z-stacks and time series can be reassembled accurately. Imaging only a small field of view with a fast acquisition speed after each trigger helps minimize in-frame deformation. These small sections can be stitched together in post-processing to assemble a large three-dimensional reconstruction of the cells in the artery. This system will enable us to image atherosclerotic plaques in vivo and to study various questions involving cell motility, including leukocyte recruitment from blood, antigen presentation, phagocytosis, chemokine function, and the role of cell subsets in disease progression.

References

1. World Health Organization. Global burden of disease, http://www.who.int/healthinfo/global_burden_disease/estimates_country/en/index.html (2013). Accessed 7 May 2013.

2. Galkina E, Ley K. Immune and inflammatory mechanisms of atherosclerosis. Annu Rev Immunol. 2009;27:165–97. doi:10.1146/annurev.immunol.021908.132620.
3. Galkina E, Kadl A, Sanders J, Varughese D, Sarembock IJ, Ley K. Lymphocyte recruitment into the aortic wall before and during development of atherosclerosis is partially L-selectin dependent. The Journal of experimental medicine. 2006;203(5):1273–82. doi:10.1084/jem.20052205.
4. Schulte S, Sukhova GK, Libby P. Genetically programmed biases in Th1 and Th2 immune responses modulate atherogenesis. Am J Pathol. 2008;172(6):1500–8. doi:10.2353/ajpath.2008.070776.
5. Egen JG, Rothfuchs AG, Feng CG, Horwitz MA, Sher A, Germain RN. Intravital imaging reveals limited antigen presentation and T cell effector function in mycobacterial granulomas. Immunity. 2011;34(5):807–19. doi:10.1016/j.immuni.2011.03.022.
6. Han JW, Shimada K, Ma-Krupa W, Johnson TL, Nerem RM, Goronzy JJ, Weyand CM. Vessel wall-embedded dendritic cells induce T-cell autoreactivity and initiate vascular inflammation. Circ Res. 2008;102(5):546–53. doi:10.1161/CIRCRESAHA.107.161653.
7. Choi JH, Do Y, Cheong C, Koh H, Boscardin SB, Oh YS, Bozzacco L, Trumpfheller C, Park CG, Steinman RM. Identification of antigen-presenting dendritic cells in mouse aorta and cardiac valves. J Exp Med. 2009;206(3):497–505. doi:10.1084/jem.20082129.
8. Miller MJ, Wei SH, Parker I, Cahalan MD. Two-photon imaging of lymphocyte motility and antigen response in intact lymph node. Science. 2002;296(5574):1869–73. doi:10.1126/science.1070051.
9. Mempel TR, Henrickson SE, Von Andrian UH. T-cell priming by dendritic cells in lymph nodes occurs in three distinct phases. Nature. 2004;427(6970):154–9. doi:10.1038/nature02238.
10. Koltsova EK, Garcia Z, Chodaczek G, Landau M, McArdle S, Scott SR, von Vietinghoff S, Galkina E, Miller YI, Acton ST, Ley K. Dynamic T cell-APC interactions sustain chronic inflammation in atherosclerosis. J Clin Invest. 2012;122(9):3114–26. doi:10.1172/JCI61758.
11. Frigault MM, Lacoste J, Swift JL, Brown CM. Live-cell microscopy - tips and tools. J Cell Sci. 2009;122(Pt 6):753–67. doi:10.1242/jcs.033837.
12. Stephens DJ, Allan VJ. Light microscopy techniques for live cell imaging. Science. 2003;300(5616):82–6. doi:10.1126/science.1082160.
13. Nikon. MicroscopyU-introduction to live-cell imaging techniques. http://www.microscopyu.com/articles/livecellimaging/index.html (2013). Accessed 26 Apr 2013.
14. Zeiss. Live-cell imaging. http://zeiss-campus.magnet.fsu.edu/articles/livecellimaging/index.html (2013). Accessed 26 Apr 2013.
15. Andor Technology. iXon Ultra 897. http://www.andor.com/pdfs/specifications/Andor_iXon_Ultra_897_Specifications.pdf (2013). Accessed 3 May 2013.
16. McNally JG, Karpova T, Cooper J, Conchello JA. Three-dimensional imaging by deconvolution microscopy. Methods. 1999;19(3):373–85. doi:10.1006/meth.1999.0873.
17. Leica. Leica SD AF – the integrated confocal spinning disk solution. http://www.leica-microsystems.com/news-media/news/news-details/article/leica-sd-af-the-integrated-confocalspinning-disk-solution/.
18. Ntziachristos V. Going deeper than microscopy: the optical imaging frontier in biology. Nat Methods. 2010;7(8):603–14. doi:10.1038/nmeth.1483.
19. Zipfel WR, Williams RM, Webb WW. Nonlinear magic: multiphoton microscopy in the biosciences. Nat Biotechnol. 2003;21(11):1369–77. doi:10.1038/nbt899.
20. Drobizhev M, Makarov NS, Tillo SE, Hughes TE, Rebane A. Two-photon absorption properties of fluorescent proteins. Nat Methods. 2011;8(5):393–9. doi:10.1038/nmeth.1596.
21. Taatjes DJ, Wadsworth MP, Schneider DJ, Sobel BE. Improved quantitative characterization of atherosclerotic plaque composition with immunohistochemistry, confocal fluorescence microscopy, and computer-assisted image analysis. Histochem Cell Biol. 2000;113(3):161–73.
22. Zoumi A, Yeh A, Tromberg BJ. Imaging cells and extracellular matrix in vivo by using second-harmonic generation and two-photon excited fluorescence. Proc Natl Acad Sci USA. 2002;99(17):11014–9. doi:10.1073/pnas.172368799.

23. Zhang SH, Reddick RL, Piedrahita JA, Maeda N. Spontaneous hypercholesterolemia and arterial lesions in mice lacking apolipoprotein E. Science. 1992;258(5081):468–47.
24. Lindquist RL, Shakhar G, Dudziak D, Wardemann H, Eisenreich T, Dustin ML, Nussenzweig MC. Visualizing dendritic cell networks in vivo. Nat Immunol. 2004;5(12):1243–50. doi:10.1038/ni1139.
25. Barnden MJ, Allison J, Heath WR, Carbone FR. Defective TCR expression in transgenic mice constructed using cDNA-based alpha- and beta-chain genes under the control of heterologous regulatory elements. Immunol Cell Biol. 1998;76(1):34–40. doi:10.1046/j.1440-1711.1998.00709.x.
26. Oxenius A, Bachmann MF, Zinkernagel RM, Hengartner H. Virus-specific MHC-class II-restricted TCR-transgenic mice: effects on humoral and cellular immune responses after viral infection. Eur J Immunol. 1998;28(1):390–400.
27. Hermansson A, Ketelhuth DF, Strodthoff D, Wurm M, Hansson EM, Nicoletti A, Paulsson-Berne G, Hansson GK. Inhibition of T cell response to native low-density lipoprotein reduces atherosclerosis. J Exp Med. 2010;207(5):1081–93. doi:10.1084/jem.20092243.
28. Palinski W, Horkko S, Miller E, Steinbrecher UP, Powell HC, Curtiss LK, Witztum JL. Cloning of monoclonal autoantibodies to epitopes of oxidized lipoproteins from apolipoprotein E-deficient mice. Demonstration of epitopes of oxidized low density lipoprotein in human plasma. J Clin Invest. 1996;98(3):800–14. doi:10.1172/JCI118853.
29. Schett G, Xu Q, Amberger A, Van der Zee R, Recheis H, Willeit J, Wick G. Autoantibodies against heat shock protein 60 mediate endothelial cytotoxicity. J Clin Invest. 1995;96(6): 2569–77. doi:10.1172/JCI118320.
30. Zoumi A, Lu X, Kassab GS, Tromberg BJ. Imaging coronary artery microstructure using second-harmonic and two-photon fluorescence microscopy. Biophys J. 2004;87(4):2778–86. doi:10.1529/biophysj.104.042887.
31. Cinamon G, Shinder V, Alon R. Shear forces promote lymphocyte migration across vascular endothelium bearing apical chemokines. Nat Immunol. 2001;2(6):515–22. doi:10.1038/88710.
32. Megens RT, Reitsma S, Schiffers PH, Hilgers RH, De Mey JG, Slaaf DW, oude Egbrink MG, van Zandvoort MA. Two-photon microscopy of vital murine elastic and muscular arteries. Combined structural and functional imaging with subcellular resolution. J Vasc Res. 2007; 44(2):87–98. doi:10.1159/000098259.
33. Sorokin L. The impact of the extracellular matrix on inflammation. Nat Rev Immunol. 2010;10(10):712–23. doi:10.1038/nri2852.
34. Caldwell CC, Kojima H, Lukashev D, Armstrong J, Farber M, Apasov SG, Sitkovsky MV. Differential effects of physiologically relevant hypoxic conditions on T lymphocyte development and effector functions. J Immunol. 2001;167(11):6140–9.

Imaging of Complications in Atherosclerosis: Thrombosis and Platelet Aggregation

8

Satoshi Nishimura

Contents

Abstract

The thrombotic cellular mechanisms associated with cardiovascular events remain unclear, largely because of an inability to visualize thrombus formation in vivo. In this chapter, bio-imaging approach is introduced, mainly using in vivo imaging technique based on single-photon and multiphoton microscopy. Recent progress in optics enabled us to identify single-platelet behavior in the developing thrombus in living animals. In the physiological and pathological conditions, complex

S. Nishimura, MD, PhD
Department of Cardiovascular Medicine Translational Systems Biology and Medicine Initiative, The University of Tokyo, Tokyo, Japan

Center for Molecular Medicine, Jichi Medical University, Tochigi, Japan
e-mail: snishi-tky@umin.ac.jp

E. Aikawa (ed.), *Cardiovascular Imaging: Arterial and Aortic Valve Inflammation and Calcification*, DOI 10.1007/978-3-319-09268-3_8

cellular interplay takes place, and bio-imaging can directly elucidate cross talks among multiple cell types. We visualized that rapidly developing thrombi composed of discoid platelets were triggered by reactive oxygen species photochemically induced by laser irradiation, and developed thrombi occluded blood vessels. Inflammatory cytokine and adhesion molecules dynamically control these processes. Intravital imaging can be a powerful tool to analyze thrombus formation and evaluate the therapeutic strategies against thrombotic diseases.

8.1 Introduction

Cardiovascular disease contributes significantly to morbidity and mortality in developed countries. In addition to atherosclerosis in coronary and cerebral circulation, peripheral artery disease (PAD) is a major cause of disability [1]. The most common cause of PAD is atherosclerosis. In some cases, PAD may be caused by blood clots that restrict blood flow. Left untreated, PAD can ultimately lead to limb amputation. Each year, 1,000 new cases of limb ischemia are diagnosed per one million of the population, with an estimated cost of more than $200 million [2]. Despite this vast clinical significance, the methodological and imaging approaches to diagnose this disease early have not been successful due to various technical difficulties.

New evidence suggests a close etiological interrelationship between atherogenesis and thrombosis [3]. Thrombi can be incorporated within an adjacent plaque, thereby accelerating plaque development via cell proliferation and increasing extracellular matrix production [4]. This dynamic process of unstable plaque formation is often followed by arterial occlusion and plaque rupture. Recent findings indicate that inflammation contributes to these processes [5, 6]. Inflammatory processes play important roles from early plaque development to plaque rupture. Thus, understanding thrombotic events is a vital step for elucidation of the cellular mechanisms—not only for ischemic PAD but also for atherosclerosis in general.

Several imaging modalities beyond traditional angiography are currently available for PAD imaging, including ultrasonography, magnetic resonance angiography (MRA), computed tomographic angiography (CTA), digital subtraction angiography (DSA), and intravascular ultrasound (IVUS). Several approaches to the in vivo imaging of mice also are available, including magnetic resonance imaging (MRI), X-ray computed tomography, ultrasonography, and positron emission tomography (PET) [7]. These techniques have the advantages of deep imaging, but the time and spatial resolution involved are not enough to visualize dynamic cellular interplay in thrombotic events on a single-cell level, as compared to fluorescent-based intravital visualization methods.

Previously, the complex and dynamic multicellular interactions during thrombus formation were not understood due to a lack of available methods for direct visualization of thrombus in living animals. Platelets, the smallest cell in the body, cannot be visualized on a single-cell level by conventional imaging tools currently available in the clinic. In addition, human platelet composition can be evaluated only in aspirated thrombus obtained from patients with acute myocardial infarction or in autopsy samples. Both specimens, however, are susceptible to artifacts from sample preparation processes. Aspirated thrombus contains platelets, packed fibrin, von Willebrand factor, tissue factor, and inflammatory cells [8]. Large numbers of leukocytes (polymorphonuclear and mononuclear) indicate the contribution of white blood cells to thrombus formation [9]. The presence of multiple cell types in developing thrombus made it necessary to analyze multicellular interactions overtime and in real time. Thus, in vivo fluorescent imaging could serve as a powerful imaging tool to elucidate the kinetics of platelet activity, dynamic changes in cell shape, and the contribution of the coagulation system.

This chapter covers some of the evolving research-based molecular fluorescent imaging methods and their biological and technical aspects, particularly focusing on the in vivo imaging of platelets.

8.2 The Significance of Fluorescent Live Imaging

Recent advances in molecular biological techniques, especially high-throughput methodologies, have provided massive amounts of information about the (epi) genomes of mice and humans. But most physiological and pathological phenomena still cannot be explained or predicted due to their stochastic nature and dynamic behavior, and a large gap still exists between basic research and clinical application. There are also many differences between humans and mice at both the genetic and cellular function levels. Consequently, the application of molecular biological techniques—especially the use of "knockout mice"—is limited. Therefore, to gain further understanding of normal and disease conditions and to establish new specific therapies, we must reconsider current imaging approaches by using evolving technologies, including "imaging by light."

In vivo imaging has several technical limitations, one being spatial resolution. Fluorescent imaging has an advantage in spatial resolution compared to other methodologies (e.g., PET, MRI). In fact, our resolution approaches a "diffraction limit" with single-photon confocal microscopy in vivo [7]. Recently, new theoretical and technical improvements have enabled "super-resolution" imaging, over the diffraction limit. Theoretically, a super-resolution intravital imaging technique also is possible in vivo.

Another limitation is imaging depth. Single-photon techniques usually provide precise images only within 100 μm of depth from the tissue surface [10], but much deeper penetration is vital for in vivo imaging. The use of a nonlinear microscope, especially a "two-photon technique," is more powerful for in vivo deep imaging [11]. Briefly, in a femtopulse near-infrared microscope, two photons arrive almost simultaneously within ~0.5 fs, providing energy to the molecule to reach an excited state, which then proceeds along the fluorescence-emission reaction. Near-infrared wavelength of 700–1,000 nm range is usually used, whereas emission occurs in the visible spectrum. At this wavelength, light penetrates deeper into scattering tissue with less phototoxicity. In addition, the two-photon excitation occurs only in the focused area and provides better Z resolution. Recently, a more sensitive and dynamic GaAs (gallium arsenide)-based avalanche photodiode detector for multiphoton technique has been developed [12]. As a result of these multiple technical improvements, a two-photon microscope can visualize deeper layers inside the body—usually more than 200 μm from the organ surface.

8.3 Visualization of In Vivo Cell Kinetics with High Time Resolution and Spatial Resolution

Two major technical approaches are available for high-speed optics, which are vital for in vivo imaging. Spatial resolution and time resolution are key features given the rapid movement of in vivo cell kinetics. Previously, a spinning disk confocal system with multibeam excitations frequently was used for these purposes [13]. But the resonance scanning system, having recently become commercially available, now represents the alternative solution [14]. Noting definitively which system advantageous for specific visualization targets in living mice is difficult. The spinning disk system allows the performance of very rapid scanning; when this system is combined with high-speed C-MOS cameras, more than 1,000 frames per second (fps) can be obtained, but multicolor imaging is technically difficult. Multicolor imaging is easier to perform in resonance scanning systems, which are equipped with fast-scanning mirrors that enable four-color imaging at 30 fps at full frame (512 × 512 pixels). In addition, multiphoton scanning can be performed in the same setups, but the initial cost for the resonance setup is usually high.

There are two types of microscope systems: upright and inverted. For intravital observations, the upright microscope is used more often, even though the inverted system gives a more stabilized view. Except for the problems of motion artifact, the two types of microscope are essentially not different.

A broad spectrum of fluorescent dyes, probes, and proteins are used for intravital microscopy. Below, we show three major approaches to the design of fluorescent probes utilized for in vivo visualization.

8.3.1 Fluorescent Probes (Dyes)

(a) Nonspecific distribution is the most commonly used approach to create contrasts for observation. For example, injected fluorescent dextran visualizes small arteries and lymphatic vessels. Various fluorescent agents with several color choices could be employed for this method. The advantage of this method is that multicolor images can be obtained by combining several agents, allowing for simultaneous visualization of different structures.

(b) Fluorescent agents can be conjugated to antibodies or other targeting molecules. Fluorescent antibodies can be used to visualize specific cell populations and phenotypes. In addition, fluorescent isolectins can unmistakably visualize vessels in living mice.

(c) The most desirable imaging agent is a functional/activatable probe, which allows visualization of specific molecules or environments. Usually functional probes (e.g., calcium probe, proteolytic activity) stay in an "off" state but are turned into an "on" state of fluorescent signals when the targeted reaction occurs (e.g., increase of calcium level or proteolytic activity). These smart probes provide very high signal-to-noise ratios due to their specific nature (Fig. 8.1).

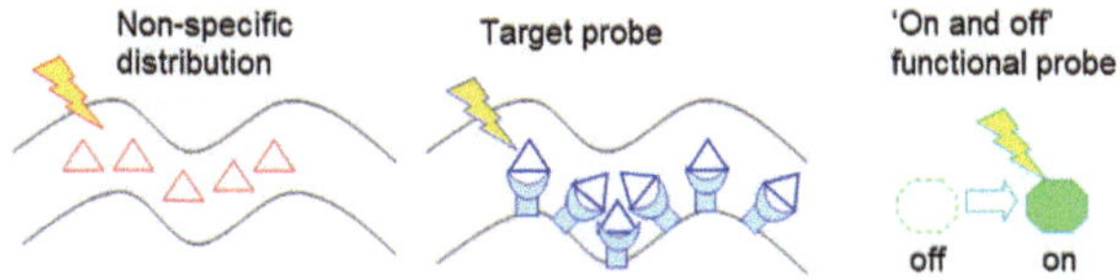

Fig. 8.1 Types of fluorescent imaging agents

8.3.2 Fluorescent Protein

Information about various biological processes and functions (e.g., specific cell types, enzymatic reactions, molecule distribution) can be directly obtained using transgenic mice labeled with fluorescent proteins. Recent progress in developmental biology techniques provides multiple choices for creating reporter mice, including conventional knock-in or transgenic approaches. Fluorescent protein expression can be induced in specific cell types and/or targeted organelles, using Cre/loxP systems. In addition, cell cycling can be directly monitored using "Fucci" mice [15]. Fluorescence resonance energy transfer (FRET) systems can visualize calcium signaling and intracellular enzymatic reactions. But while using these mice is very convenient, experiments need careful optimization and validation, as it is difficult to expect consistent signal specificity, quality, and intensity due to animal variations. In addition, there are technical difficulties related to protein excitation in red spectrum in living animals using a multiphoton setup, due to excitation problems in commercially available titan sapphire lasers with relatively low power for excitation in red-spectrum wavelength.

8.3.3 Nonstaining Approaches

Nonstaining methods include autofluorescence imaging and second harmonic generation observations [16]. Autofluorescence signals are often obtained from specific cytoplasmic organelles or tissue extracellular matrix (e.g., lysosomes, elastin). In some situations, autofluorescence signal is very useful, as it allows identification of specific cell types (e.g., macrophages) or serves as a helpful landmark for tissue orientation (e.g., elastin in the vessel wall).

Second harmonic generation is an optical process, in which photons with the same frequency interacting with a nonlinear material are effectively "combined" to generate new photons with twice the energy and therefore twice the frequency and half the wavelength of the initial photons. Combined second harmonic generation and two-photon excited fluorescence microscopy allows for visualization of collagen in living animals. These techniques are used to observe arterial adventitia, bone, and skin collagenous architecture without staining.

Combining these techniques, we can visualize the vessels, muscles, kidneys, liver, fat, and many other structures, as shown in Fig. 8.2. Imaging depth depends on tissues, but usually varies from 200 to 1,000 μm (Fig. 8.3).

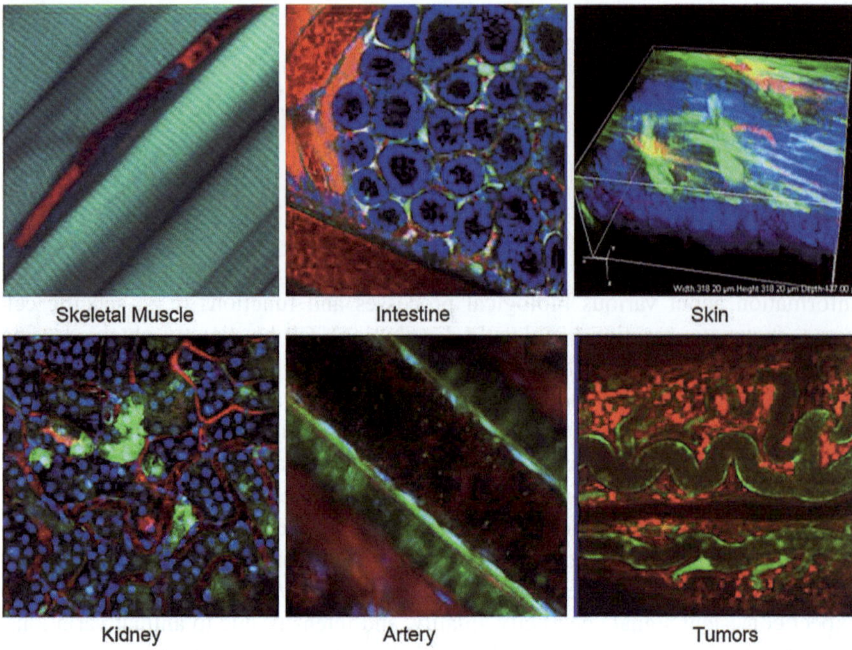

Fig. 8.2 Two-photon microscopy penetrates deep inside the body. CAG-eGFP transgenic mice with ubiquitous expression of eGFP in various tissues were used to visualize the muscle, intestine, skin, kidney, artery, and tumor. Texas Red dextran was injected to visualize vessels and blood cells (*red*), and Hoechst stain was used for nuclei contract (*blue*). Second harmonic generation signals were simultaneously obtained

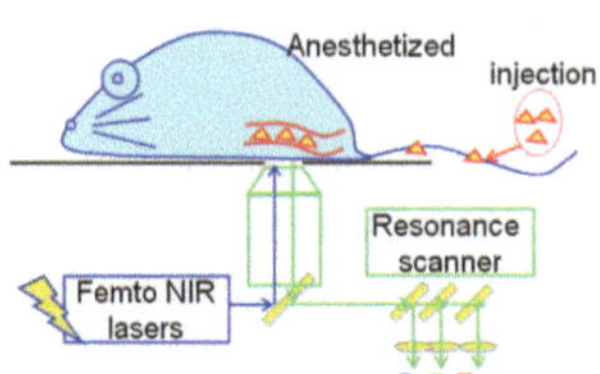

Fig. 8.3 Diagram of the confocal microscope for real-time in vivo imaging. CAG-eGFP transgenic mice with ubiquitous expression of eGFP in various tissues were used to visualize the muscle, intestine, skin, kidney, artery, and tumor. Texas Red dextran was injected to visualize vessels and blood cells (*red*), and Hoechst stain was used for nuclei contract (*blue*). Second harmonic generation signals were simultaneously obtained

8.4 Application of Fluorescence Imaging to Cardiovascular Diseases

To understand the molecular and cellular mechanisms underlying cardiovascular disease and its complications, including thrombosis, the fluorescence imaging approach could serve as a powerful tool. Recent progress in optical technologies

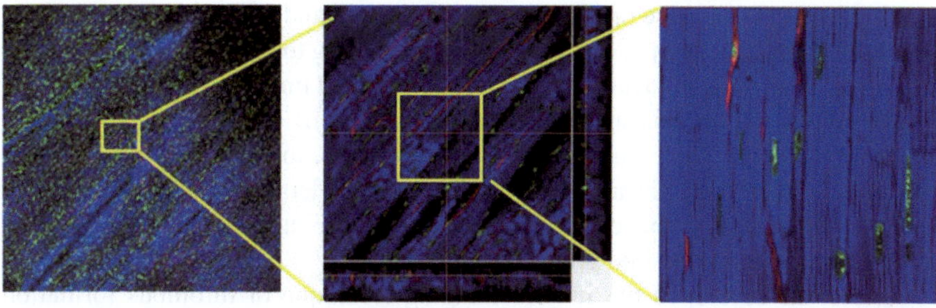

Fig. 8.4 Multi-scale heart tissue imaging. To visualize the heart tissue, endothelial cells were distinctively labeled using fluorescent isolectin dye (*red*), nuclei were stained with Hoechst 33342 (*green*), and cardiomyocytes were stained using mitochondria probe (*TMRE, blue*) in intact living heart tissue

and evolving knowledge in developmental biology enabled us to visualize biological processes in living animals with minimal invasiveness. Fluorescent imaging has advantages in temporal and spatial resolution, as discussed previously. As shown in Fig. 8.1, ex vivo multi-scale imaging can obtain information not only on specific heart structures, including cardiomyocytes and heart vessels, but also on single sarcomeres.

In contrast, the living tissue imaging method yields three-dimensional images, which enable the visualization of three-dimensional structures in the whole heart. A spinning disk or resonance confocal microscope could be used for living imaging. Lectin is a useful histochemical probe that specifically labels endothelial cells in many species [17]. Information regarding mitochondrial membrane potential, which reflects cardiomyocyte viability, also can be obtained. Lee et al. recently reported on intravital visualization techniques using synchronization and compensation for heartbeat movement [18], and we expect that in vivo observation will improve targeting for specific cell types or molecule behavior (Fig. 8.4).

8.5 Imaging of Thrombus

The intravital visualization technique of thrombus formation could serve as a powerful tool to analyze the complex cellular mechanisms underlying this cardiovascular complication, but due to technical difficulties, these techniques are not used broadly to image thrombotic events and their rapid phenomena. We discuss here the technical aspects of in vivo imaging and its application in thrombotic diseases.

$FeCl_3$-induced thrombus formation in carotid arteries is a frequently used animal model for thrombus imaging [19], but the reproducibility of results obtained using this experimental approach is low. In addition, the effects from direct vessel injuries by drug administration cannot be ruled out. Another major limitation is that this technique cannot identify and track single-platelet kinetic during thrombus formation.

With the recent advance of optical technologies, we and others have successfully visualized a single platelet in developing thrombus using the fluorescent microscope or confocal microscope. Jackson et al. recently reported imaging of a single platelet in a developing thrombus and elucidated the effect of shear stress for platelet activations [20, 21]. Their studies suggested a two-stage theory of in vivo thrombus formation. Under low shear stress conditions, platelets become activated and undergo a dynamic shape change; under high shear stress conditions, discoid platelets are incorporated into growing thrombi.

Furie et al. developed the in vivo imaging technique of thrombus formation using laser injuries to endothelial cell layers and following extracellular collagen exposure [22]. They reported that direct laser injuries increased tissue factor expression in the vessel wall, followed by platelet accumulation. After the fibrin network forms, the vessels become occluded by developed thrombus. This process contrasts with classical models in which clot formation is a vital step for thrombus stabilization. Von Willebrand factor (vWF) also plays a vital role in thrombus development after laser injuries, and vWF-deficient mice show decreased platelet attachment on endothelium after laser injuries. These results indicate the presence of both vWF-dependent and vWF-independent pathways for thrombus formation in this model [23].

Exposure of extracellular matrix, including collagen, takes place in platelet activation processes during hemostasis, induced by ferric chloride models [24] or direct laser injuries [22]. This platelet activation can be monitored by P-selectin expression on the platelet surface, using fluorescent antibodies. In addition, intracellular calcium mobilization occurs during platelet activation, and intracellular calcium concentration within platelets can be monitored by several fluorescent indicators (e.g., FLUO-8AM probes) or FRET animals.

8.6 Visualizing Platelets In Vivo

Three different approaches exist for direct platelet visualization in vivo. The first approach utilizes transgenic mice. For example, CAG-eGFP transgenic mice express strong green fluorescent protein that exhibits bright green fluorescence signal in platelets when exposed to light. The second approach is based on antibody binding to specific adhesion molecules detected in platelets, including CD41 and CD42b. These fluorescent antibodies could be injected into living animals. Two clones are commercially available for mouse injection (MWReg30 for CD41 and X488 CD42). But the antibody treatment can produce a "blocking effect," which should be monitored after injection. The third approach is platelet labeling ex vivo, followed by transfusion into mice. The platelets can be efficiently labeled with 5-TAMRA dye (5-carboxytetramethylrhodamine, succinimidyl ester) without platelet activation (Fig. 8.5).

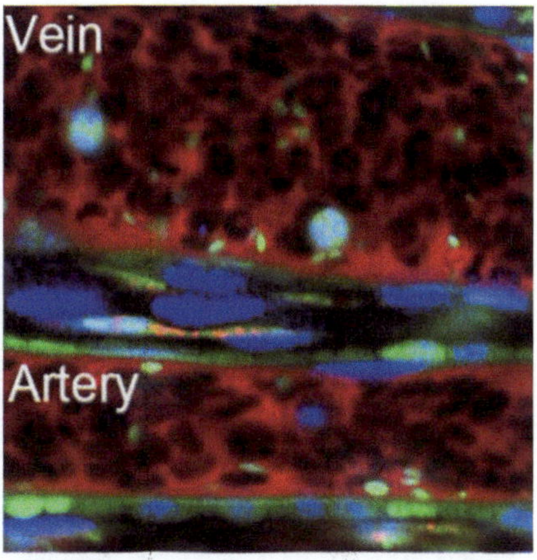

Fig. 8.5 Single platelet visualized by in vivo imaging technique. Multicolor visualization technique shows leukocytes (Hoechst, *blue*), erythrocytes (with the negative image for injected dextran, *red*), and platelets (eCAG-GFP signal, *green*) in both arteries and veins

8.7 Reactive Oxygen Species (ROS)-Induced Thrombosis Models

Can platelet aggregation be visualized in real time?

Several methods for platelet activation could be combined with fluorescent imaging in vivo. One of these approaches uses high-power laser irradiation, which completely disrupts the endothelial cell layer [22]. In this technique, after laser injuries, collagen extracellular matrix is exposed, platelets become activated, and thrombus formation is induced and accompanied by in vivo thrombus formation of activated and deformed P-selectin-positive platelets aggregate.

The other method uses photochemical reactions, visualizing single-platelet kinetics within aggregations of discoid platelets in thrombi in single-platelet levels [25, 26]. In contrast, based on the findings that reactive oxygen species (ROS) play a central role in atherosclerotic lesion formation and thrombotic diseases [27], we induced ROS production within the vessel. Porphyrin (hematoporphyrin) was used as a substrate. Thrombus formation could be observed with high reproducibility after ROS production by photochemical reactions. In these models, the platelet keeps its discoid shape, which is an important special feature of our method. We proposed that in our model, thrombus formation was initiated by the binding of platelet GPIb-alpha to endothelial vWF, followed by actin linker talin-dependent activation of alphaIIb-beta3 integrin, required for thrombus stability, in a later phase.

The most important technical advantage of this approach is that a photochemical reaction can be induced by the observation laser, and there is no need for two laser lines. For these purposes, the spinning disk confocal or resonance scanning system can be used.

Results can be quantified by software analysis, originally developed by modifying commercially available products [25]. The dynamic changes in platelet number

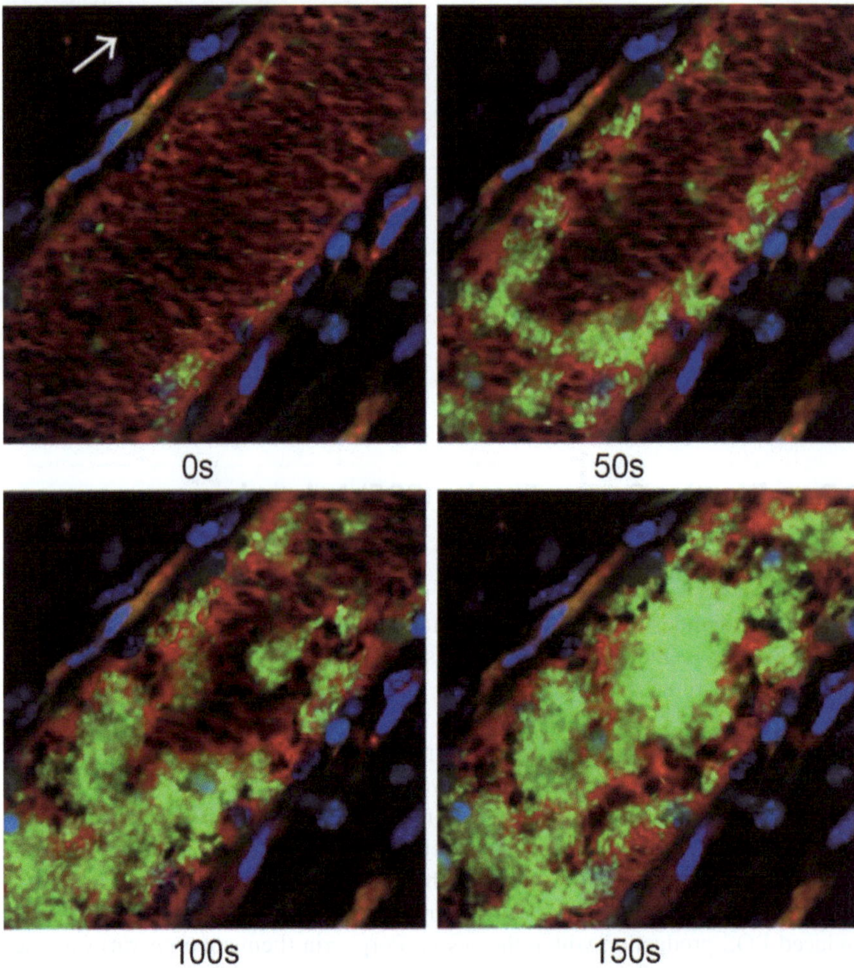

Fig. 8.6 ROS-induced thrombus models. Platelet aggregation was induced by laser irradiation and ROS production by photochemical reactions. CAG-eGFP mice were used for visualizing platelet (in *green*). Hoechst (*blue*) and Texas Red dextran (*red*) were also injected. *White arrow* indicated the direction of blood flow. Notice that the single platelet can be identified in the developing thrombus, and leukocyte was also incorporated

or thrombus area can be statistically analyzed with high reproducibility. By obtaining intravital images and analyzing the results objectively, the effect gene manipulation can be quantified, and a hypothesis can be obtained in combination with conventional in vitro analysis by molecular biology technique (Fig. 8.6).

8.8 Ex Vivo Imaging Techniques

In vitro platelet function analysis has several advantages. We can isolate platelet factors from other in vivo environmental factors (e.g., endothelial signals, humoral factors, shear stress). Analysis of gene or therapeutic interventions can be easily performed in vitro. Cytometry shows platelet activation status, and platelet aggregations can be performed using a flow cytometry method [28]. Platelet aggregometry showed dynamic reactions under agonist stimulations, but reproducibility is relatively low and clinical applications are limited.

Flow chamber assay is the gold standard for analysis of dynamic platelet attachment to collagen or vWF. Along with thrombus development, platelet morphological changes (i.e., lamelapodia formation) also can be visualized with high resolution [29]. Due to a small sample size, a microflow device must be used for tissue analysis. Previous results show that platelet activation status depends on shear stress rate, and thrombus formation in high shear stress conditions occurs via vWF or fibrinogen as a single ligand for alphaIIb-beta3.

8.9 Applications for Visualization Techniques for Metabolic Diseases

Fluorescent imaging techniques have many applications in metabolic diseases. Inflammation plays a pivotal role in the development of metabolic diseases, as well as atherosclerosis [30]. We previously showed that platelet activation via inflammation takes place in adipose tissue under metabolic conditions, by direct in vivo visualization [31]. In particular, in an obese environment, adipose tissue exhibits hallmarks of chronic inflammation, and cellular interplay occurs—including between macrophages, B cells, and CD8 T cells [32, 33]. Moreover, local and systemic inflammation directly alters adipose tissue function, leading to systemic insulin resistance. Because adipose tissue contains multiple cell types—including stromal cells, adipocytes, immune cells, and endothelial cells—it is tempting to speculate that their multicellular interactions are crucial to normal adipose tissue function and to dysfunction in pathological conditions, such as obesity.

Fluorescent imaging can directly visualize increased leukocyte–platelet–endothelial cell interactions in the microcirculation of visceral adipose tissue in obese mice, which is indicative of activation of the leukocyte adhesion cascade, a hallmark of inflammation [31]. The increased expression of adhesion molecules on stromal cells and platelet activation contributes to these cell dynamics, as shown in the experiments utilizing neutralizing antibodies or genetically modified mice. Thus, chronic inflammatory status might underlie metabolic diseases, and molecules involved in proinflammatory phases of platelet activation could serve as therapeutic targets for metabolic conditions (Fig. 8.7).

8.10 Summary and Conclusions

Cellular reactions in thrombotic diseases are particularly dynamic and involve multiple cell types. In vivo imaging represents a powerful tool for understanding the molecular and cellular basis of thrombotic diseases. Fluorescent imaging has several advantages and great potential to visualize biological processes on cellular and molecular levels simultaneously. Several recent technical advances, including the

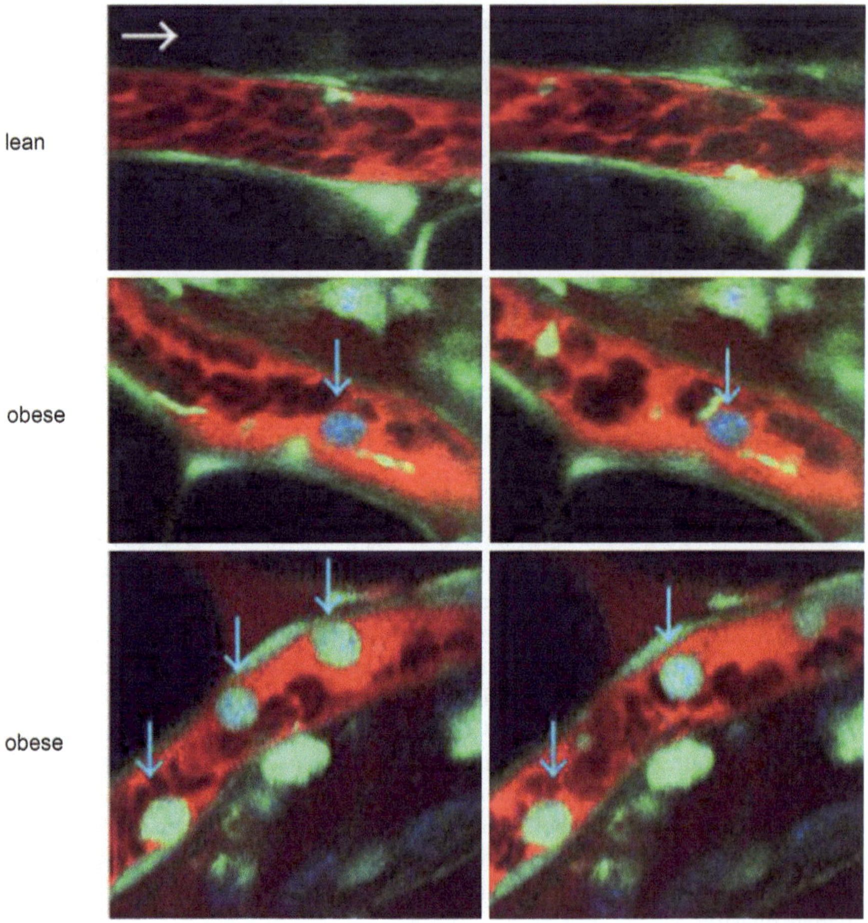

Fig. 8.7 Inflammatory cell dynamics in obese adipose tissue. Inflammatory cellular interrelationships were directly visualized by intravital imaging. CAG-eGFP mice (to visualize platelet in *green*) was injected with Hoechst (nucleus in *blue*) and Texas Red dextran (blood flow in *red*). Veins in the visceral adipose tissue were visualized. *Arrows* indicate rolling and adherent inflammatory leukocytes

availability of new light sources, high-resolution microscopy, development of confocal and two-photon systems, and advances in vascular biology, have enabled us to perform multiphoton and multicolor imaging with genetically modified or disease-induced animal models. The results can be quantified with high reproducibility using newly developed software and algorithms. Thus, we can not only "see" inside the animals but also better understand the dynamic changes in living organisms. In the future, imaging techniques combined with evolving molecular biology approaches will have broad applications for understanding common diseases and for the development of therapeutic approaches to combat them.

References

1. Diehm C, Schuster A, Allenberg JR, Darius H, Haberl R, Lange S, Pittrow D, von Stritzky B, Tepohl G, Trampisch HJ. High prevalence of peripheral arterial disease and co-morbidity in 6880 primary care patients: cross-sectional study. Atherosclerosis. 2004;172:95–105.
2. Peach G, Griffin M, Jones KG, Thompson MM, Hinchliffe RJ. Diagnosis and management of peripheral arterial disease. BMJ. 2012;345:e5208.
3. Libby P. Coronary artery injury and the biology of atherosclerosis: inflammation, thrombosis, and stabilization. Am J Cardiol. 2000;86:3J–8J; discussion 8J–9J.
4. Lendon CL, Davies MJ, Born GV, Richardson PD. Atherosclerotic plaque caps are locally weakened when macrophages density is increased. Atherosclerosis. 1991;87:87–90.
5. de Maat MP, Bladbjerg EM, Drivsholm T, Borch-Johnsen K, Moller L, Jespersen J. Inflammation, thrombosis and atherosclerosis: results of the glostrup study. J Thromb Haemost. 2003;1:950–7.
6. Carter AM. Inflammation, thrombosis and acute coronary syndromes. Diabet Vasc Dis Res. 2005;2:113–21.
7. Weissleder R. Scaling down imaging: molecular mapping of cancer in mice. Nat Rev Cancer. 2002;2:11–8.
8. Yamashita A, Sumi T, Goto S, Hoshiba Y, Nishihira K, Kawamoto R, Hatakeyama K, Date H, Imamura T, Ogawa H, Asada Y. Detection of von Willebrand factor and tissue factor in platelets-fibrin rich coronary thrombi in acute myocardial infarction. Am J Cardiol. 2006;97:26–8.
9. Freedman JE, Loscalzo J. Platelet-monocyte aggregates: bridging thrombosis and inflammation. Circulation. 2002;105:2130–2.
10. Helmchen F, Denk W. Deep tissue two-photon microscopy. Nat Methods. 2005;2:932–40.
11. Cahalan MD, Parker I, Wei SH, Miller MJ. Two-photon tissue imaging: seeing the immune system in a fresh light. Nat Rev Immunol. 2002;2:872–80.
12. Wu G, Jian Y, Wu E, Zeng H. Photon-number-resolving detection based on InGaAs/InP avalanche photodiode in the sub-saturated mode. Opt Express. 2009;17:18782–7.
13. Maddox PS, Moree B, Canman JC, Salmon ED. Spinning disk confocal microscope system for rapid high-resolution, multimode, fluorescence speckle microscopy and green fluorescent protein imaging in living cells. Methods Enzymol. 2003;360:597–617.
14. Hove JR, Craig MP. High-speed confocal imaging of zebrafish heart development. Methods Mol Biol. 2012;843:309–28.
15. Sakaue-Sawano A, Kurokawa H, Morimura T, Hanyu A, Hama H, Osawa H, Kashiwagi S, Fukami K, Miyata T, Miyoshi H, Imamura T, Ogawa M, Masai H, Miyawaki A. Visualizing spatiotemporal dynamics of multicellular cell-cycle progression. Cell. 2008;132:487–98.
16. Kim BM, Eichler J, Reiser KM, Rubenchik AM, Da Silva LB. Collagen structure and nonlinear susceptibility: effects of heat, glycation, and enzymatic cleavage on second harmonic signal intensity. Lasers Surg Med. 2000;27:329–35.
17. Nishimura S, Manabe I, Nagasaki M, Hosoya Y, Yamashita H, Fujita H, Ohsugi M, Tobe K, Kadowaki T, Nagai R, Sugiura S. Adipogenesis in obesity requires close interplay between differentiating adipocytes, stromal cells, and blood vessels. Diabetes. 2007;56:1517–26.
18. Lee S, Vinegoni C, Feruglio PF, Fexon L, Gorbatov R, Pivoravov M, Sbarbati A, Nahrendorf M, Weissleder R. Real-time in vivo imaging of the beating mouse heart at microscopic resolution. Nat Commun. 2012;3:1054.
19. Kurz KD, Main BW, Sandusky GE. Rat model of arterial thrombosis induced by ferric chloride. Thromb Res. 1990;60:269–80.
20. Jackson SP. The growing complexity of platelet aggregation. Blood. 2007;109:5087–95.
21. Nesbitt WS, Westein E, Tovar-Lopez FJ, Tolouei E, Mitchell A, Fu J, Carberry J, Fouras A, Jackson SP. A shear gradient-dependent platelet aggregation mechanism drives thrombus formation. Nat Med. 2009;15:665–73.

22. Furie B, Furie BC. In vivo thrombus formation. J Thromb Haemost. 2007;5 Suppl 1:12–7.
23. Varga-Szabo D, Pleines I, Nieswandt B. Cell adhesion mechanisms in platelets. Arterioscler Thromb Vasc Biol. 2008;28:403–12.
24. Watson SP. Platelet activation by extracellular matrix proteins in haemostasis and thrombosis. Curr Pharm Des. 2009;15:1358–72.
25. Nishimura S, Manabe I, Nagasaki M, Kakuta S, Iwakura Y, Takayama N, Ooehara J, Otsu M, Kamiya A, Petrich BG, Urano T, Kadono T, Sato S, Aiba A, Yamashita H, Sugiura S, Kadowaki T, Nakauchi H, Eto K, Nagai R. In vivo imaging visualizes discoid platelet aggregations without endothelium disruption and implicates contribution of inflammatory cytokine and integrin signaling. Blood. 2012;119:e45–56.
26. Takizawa H, Nishimura S, Takayama N, Oda A, Nishikii H, Morita Y, Kakinuma S, Yamazaki S, Okamura S, Tamura N, Goto S, Sawaguchi A, Manabe I, Takatsu K, Nakauchi H, Takaki S, Eto K. Lnk regulates integrin alphaIIbbeta3 outside-in signaling in mouse platelets, leading to stabilization of thrombus development in vivo. J Clin Invest. 2010;120:179–90.
27. Krotz F, Sohn HY, Pohl U. Reactive oxygen species: players in the platelet game. Arterioscler Thromb Vasc Biol. 2004;24:1988–96.
28. De Cuyper IM, Meinders M, van de Vijver E, de Korte D, Porcelijn L, de Haas M, Eble JA, Seeger K, Rutella S, Pagliara D, Kuijpers TW, Verhoeven AJ, van den Berg TK, Gutierrez L. A novel flow cytometry-based platelet aggregation assay. Blood. 2013;121:e70–80.
29. Moroi M, Jung SM, Shinmyozu K, Tomiyama Y, Ordinas A, Diaz-Ricart M. Analysis of platelet adhesion to a collagen-coated surface under flow conditions: the involvement of glycoprotein VI in the platelet adhesion. Blood. 1996;88:2081–92.
30. Weisberg SP, McCann D, Desai M, Rosenbaum M, Leibel RL, Ferrante Jr AW. Obesity is associated with macrophage accumulation in adipose tissue. J Clin Invest. 2003;112: 1796–808.
31. Nishimura S, Manabe I, Nagasaki M, Seo K, Yamashita H, Hosoya Y, Ohsugi M, Tobe K, Kadowaki T, Nagai R, Sugiura S. In vivo imaging in mice reveals local cell dynamics and inflammation in obese adipose tissue. J Clin Invest. 2008;118:710–21.
32. Nishimura S, Manabe I, Nagasaki M, Eto K, Yamashita H, Ohsugi M, Otsu M, Hara K, Ueki K, Sugiura S, Yoshimura K, Kadowaki T, Nagai R. CD8+ effector T cells contribute to macrophage recruitment and adipose tissue inflammation in obesity. Nat Med. 2009;15:914–20.
33. Nishimura S, Manabe I, Takaki S, Nagasaki M, Otsu M, Yamashita H, Sugita J, Yoshimura K, Eto K, Komuro I, Kadowaki T, Nagai R. Adipose natural regulatory B cells negatively control adipose tissue inflammation. Cell Metab. 2013;18:759–66.

Part II

Imaging Insights into Mechanisms of Calcific Aortic Valve Disease (CAVD) and Calcification

Pathobiology and Optical Molecular Imaging of Calcific Aortic Valve Disease

9

Joshua D. Hutcheson and Elena Aikawa

Contents

Abstract

Calcific aortic valve disease (CAVD) is a major contributor to cardiovascular morbidity and mortality, and given its association with age, the prevalence of CAVD is expected to rise with an increase in worldwide life expectancy. Currently, no therapies exist for the treatment or prevention of CAVD. Much of our understanding of the progression of CAVD has originated from preclinical data

J.D. Hutcheson, PhD
Division of Cardiovascular Medicine, Center for Interdisciplinary Cardiovascular Sciences, Brigham and Women's Hospital, Harvard Medical School, 3 Blackfan St., Room 1736, Boston, MA 02115, USA
e-mail: jhutcheson@partners.org

E. Aikawa, MD, PhD (✉)
Division of Cardiovascular Medicine, Center for Interdisciplinary Cardiovascular Sciences, Brigham and Women's Hospital, Harvard Medical School, 3 Blackfan St., Room 1736, Boston, MA 02115, USA

Division of Cardiovascular Medicine, Center for Excellence in Vascular Biology, Brigham and Women's Hospital, Harvard Medical School, Boston, MA 02114, USA
e-mail: eaikawa@partners.org

E. Aikawa (ed.), *Cardiovascular Imaging: Arterial and Aortic Valve Inflammation and Calcification*, DOI 10.1007/978-3-319-09268-3_9

using optical molecular imaging of animal models. Through these studies we now know that CAVD is an inflammatory disease with a fibrocalcific endpoint. In this chapter, we will review the preclinical molecular imaging data that have shaped our current understanding of CAVD, and we will discuss the future role that molecular imaging technologies may play in the clinical diagnosis and treatment of this disease.

9.1 Aortic Valve Structure, Function, and Disease

The aortic valve is a highly dynamic tissue that is situated between the left ventricle and the aorta and is responsible for maintaining unidirectional blood flow from the heart to the systemic circulation. This function is highly dependent on the structure of three thin leaflets attached to the base of the valve annulus. The action of the leaflets is governed largely by the pressure generated through the pumping action of the heart [1]. Pressure generated in the left ventricle during systolic contraction forces the leaflets to protrude into the aorta, opening the valve annulus such that blood can pass from the heart into systemic circulation (Fig. 9.1a). As the heart rests in diastole, the back pressure generated forces the leaflets back toward the ventricle, whereupon the adjacent leaflets meet to seal the valve and prevent retrograde blood flow (Fig. 9.1b).

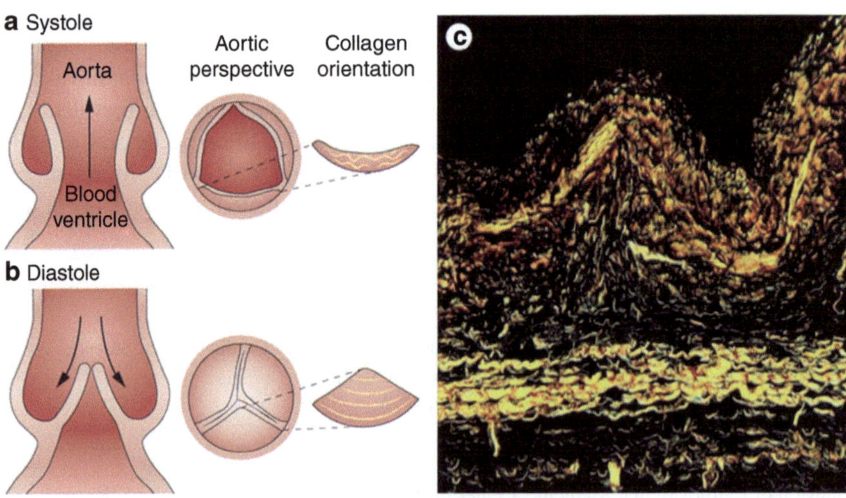

Fig. 9.1 Structure and function of the aortic valve. (**a**) Pressure generated in the left ventricle during systolic contraction forces the aortic valve leaflets into the aorta, allowing blood to be ejected from the heart. (**b**) As the heart rests during diastole, the leaflets strain radially to meet and close the valve, preventing retrograde blood flow into the ventricles. The circumferentially aligned collagen fibers give the leaflets strength to prevent prolapse. (**c**) The aligned collagen fibers are shown using polarized light imaging of picrosirius red staining. Original magnification ×200 (Figure adapted from Hutcheson et al. [14])

The leaflets must simultaneously exhibit the compliance necessary for opening during systole and the biomechanical strength to resist prolapse back into the left ventricle during diastole [2]. This is accomplished through a layered leaflet microarchitecture that is crucial to ensure proper valve function [3]. The aortic side of the leaflets, a region known as the fibrosa layer, is composed of circumferentially aligned collagen fibers that straighten during diastole and serve as the main tensile load bearing component of the leaflets (Fig. 9.1c) [4]. On the ventricular side of the leaflets, an elastin layer, known as the ventricularis, confers radial elasticity that allows the valve to open during systole and allows the leaflets to stretch radially and meet to close the valve during diastole [5]. An intermediary layer, known as the spongiosa, is enriched in glycosaminoglycans and is believed to serve as a lubricating layer between the fibrosa and ventricularis. This microarchitecture is maintained by two resident cell populations: the aortic valve endothelial cells (VECs) that sheath the leaflets and the aortic valve interstitial cells (VICs) that reside within the leaflets. Inflammation and pathological differentiation of these resident cells have been shown to lead to calcific aortic valve disease (CAVD). Histopathological analyses of CAVD reveal fibrotic collagen accumulation and the formation of calcific nodules on the aortic side of the leaflets [6]. These changes disrupt the microarchitecture of the leaflets and thereby compromise the biomechanical integrity of the aortic valve. The following sections detail the cellular and molecular changes observed in CAVD and the role that molecular imaging may play in both research and clinical intervention.

9.2 Imaging Criteria for Aortic Valve Disease

CAVD is a major contributor of cardiovascular morbidity and mortality. Of particular concern, the prevalence of CAVD is projected to increase dramatically due to the shift in age-related population demographics with an aging baby boomer generation. Moderate-to-severe symptoms of CAVD are observed in 2.8 % of patients over 75 years of age [7, 8]. Given this strong association with age, for many years, CAVD was presumed to be a passive, degenerative disease that occurs due to fatigue or a wearing out of the tissue caused by the stresses and strains of cardiac function as the aortic valve opens and closes more than three billion times over the course of an average life span [9]. Recently, however, the results of many studies on the molecular signaling processes associated with valvular homeostasis have led to a paradigm shift with CAVD now viewed as an active, cellular-driven disease [10]. This view offers some hope to patients as cellular processes may be targeted therapeutically; however, no clinically relevant therapeutic options for CAVD have been discovered.

The development of a therapeutic for CAVD dovetails with the need for detection strategies to identify early changes within the leaflets [11]. Once calcium deposits form within the valve, reversibility is unclear; however, inflammation and the early extracellular matrix remodeling responses that presage gross fibrosis and calcific nodule formation may fall within an appropriate therapeutic window

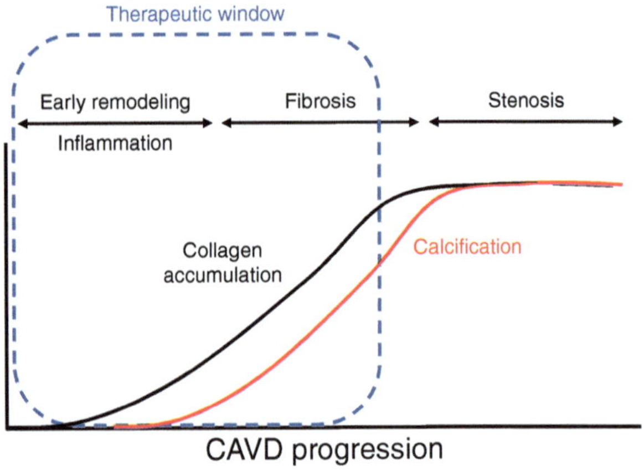

Fig. 9.2 Early tissue remodeling and inflammation is thought to precede gross fibrosis and calcification within CAVD leaflets. Calcification may be an irreversible endpoint; therefore, identifying patients in the early stages of CAVD may present the best opportunity for therapeutic intervention

(Fig. 9.2). Traditional detection of valvular insufficiency using echocardiography is unable to identify these early leaflet changes as regurgitant blood flow and leaflet thickening represent later stages of CAVD remodeling and calcification. Recently, PET/CT imaging modalities have emerged as a means to detect inflammation and mineralization within valve leaflets of human patients [12], and optical molecular imaging strategies have been successfully employed to visualize the progression of CAVD in mice [13]. These technologies are far more sensitive to small changes within the leaflets and may offer the resolution necessary to identify patients that fall within the appropriate therapeutic time frame. Utilizing these imaging strategies may also give better insight into the temporal aspects of CAVD and may lead to a better understanding of the required therapeutic strategy at each stage of CAVD.

The reader should note that many of the processes and techniques discussed in this chapter overlap with those discussed in Chap. 5. Many of the pathophysiological changes in CAVD and vascular calcification overlap; however, it should be noted that these diseases are now believed to have distinct etiologies [14]. Not every patient who presents prominent vascular calcification also exhibits signs of CAVD, suggesting that at least an extra set of variables are involved in CAVD initiation and progression. Further, valve cells are phenotypically different than their vascular counterparts, and therefore, different factors seem to be responsible for producing the fibrocalcific endpoint that is apparent in both diseases. The goal of molecular imaging for these two diseases is also different. In vascular calcification, a collagen-rich fibrous cap with a large calcification may serve to stabilize the atherosclerotic plaque [15, 16]; therefore, the first goal in imaging of atherosclerotic lesions is to identify regions of collagen disruption and the formation of spotty microcalcifications that lead to plaque instability. Conversely, in CAVD, aortic valve leaflet microarchitecture is essential to the appropriate biomechanical function of the valve. Therefore, molecular imaging tools should be designed around early identification of valve remodeling prior to the potentially irreversible endpoints of fibrosis and calcification. In this chapter, we will focus on the preclinical studies that have exhibited promise in imaging processes involved in CAVD and the novel findings that have resulted from these imaging modalities. We will also use our current understanding of the molecular underpinnings of CAVD to propose potential new targets for imaging that might distinguish CAVD from vascular calcification. Finally, we will discuss how molecular imaging techniques may be translated to clinical use to identify early markers of CAVD in patients.

9.3 Valve Endothelial Cell Activation and Migration

In other parts of the vascular system, endothelial cells have been observed to play a crucial role in the transduction of mechanical signals such as changes in shear stress [17]. Because these cells are the first to experience any changes in outside forces that affect valve dynamics, they have received growing attention in their potential roles in regulating valve homeostasis. VECs are phenotypically distinct from endothelial cells in the vasculature [18]. For instance, when subjected to the shear stresses of fluid flow, VECs align perpendicular to the flow [18]; whereas, endothelial cells from the aorta align parallel to the flow [17, 19]. This indicates that the VECs may play a distinct role in regulating the biomechanical properties of the valve through specially evolved mechanisms. Furthermore, VECs have been observed to exhibit genotypic heterogeneity along the surface of each leaflet. Simmons et al. found that 584 genes were differentially expressed between VECs from the aortic side and the ventricular side [20]. These genotypic differences may be important in regulating the differing biomechanical properties on each side of the valve, i.e., the collagen of the fibrosa and the elastin of the ventricularis, or conversely, the gene expression of these cells may be influenced by the differing shear stresses seen on each side of the leaflet.

VECs have also been shown to play a role in the etiology and progression of valve disease. In diseased or injured vascular tissues, endothelial cells direct the appropriate immune response through increased expression of cell adhesion molecules (CAMs) that mediate attachment and activation of leukocytes as well as by secreting cytokines that are recognized by specialized inflammatory cells [21–24]. Similarly, VECs have been observed to increase expression of ICAM-1 and VCAM-1 and secretion of inflammatory cytokines such as IL-8, IL-1β, and IFN-γ in response to oscillatory, turbulent fluid flows and pathological mechanical strains [25]. As discussed in the following section, the accumulation of leukocytes and related inflammatory cytokines is positively correlated with remodeling in CAVD leaflets and aortic stenosis in human patients. Ex vivo MRI and near-infrared fluorescence (NIRF) imaging of a VCAM-1-targeted agent demonstrated VEC activation localized in regions where the valve leaflets meet the aortic root [26] (Fig. 9.3). Correspondingly, this area of the leaflet—known as the commissure—experiences the greatest amount of mechanical stress and, therefore, is most likely to experience VEC damage that leads to CAM expression [27].

VECs may also play an important, though lesser known, function in CAVD, and the spatial heterogeneity of these cells could be responsible for the side-specific susceptibility to CAVD observed in histopathological analyses of diseased leaflets [20]. The VECs directly adjacent to the fibrosa have been found to express much lower levels of anti-calcification enzymes when compared to the VECs on the ventricular side of the leaflets [25]. This suggests that the VECs may also play an

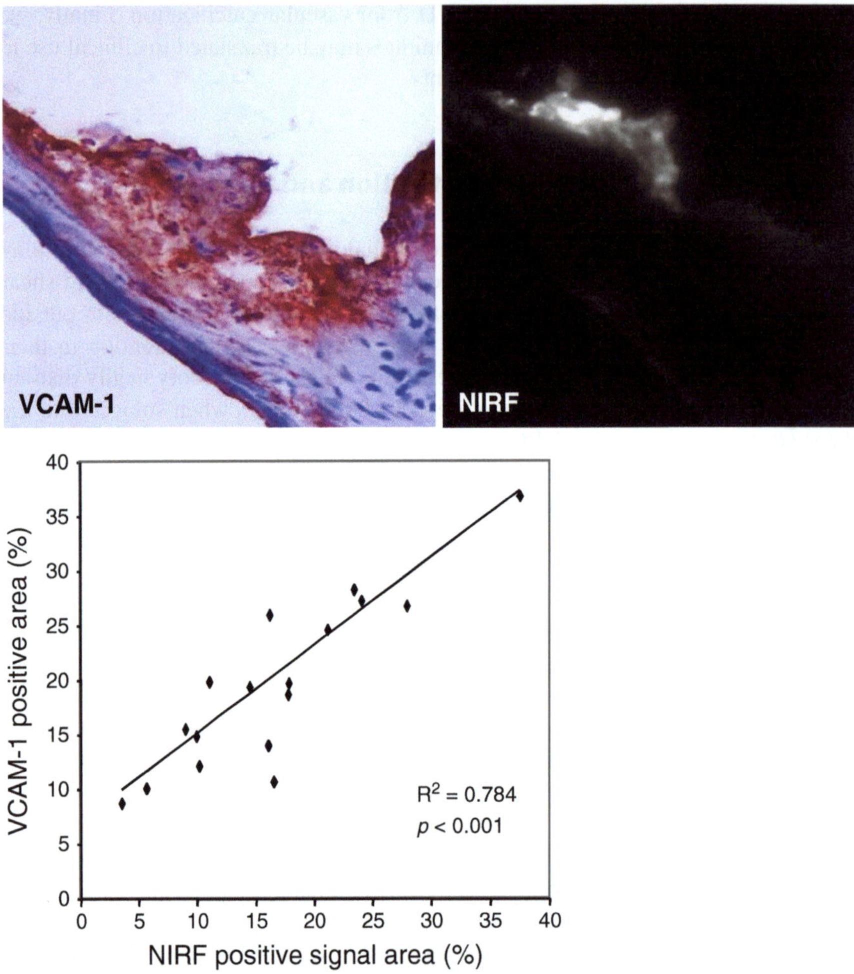

Fig. 9.3 A NIRF probe targeted to VCAM-1 was detected in the commissure region of apoE-deficient mouse aortic valves. The specificity of this probe was validated and quantified using traditional immunohistological staining and direct visualization of VCAM-1 activity using NIRF microscopy (Figure modified Aikawa et al. [13])

important role in sensing and responding to the various stresses on each side of the leaflets. Recent studies have suggested that VECs play an active role in valve remodeling during CAVD by invading the leaflet interstitium through endothelial-to-mesenchymal (EMT) processes that mirror those from development [28, 29]. The addition of mechanical strain to either valve leaflets in vivo or an in vitro culture system of VECs led to the expression of mesenchymal markers such as smooth muscle α-actin (α-SMA) within the VECs [28] (Fig. 9.4). VECs isolated from ovine mitral valve leaflets were shown to exhibit a propensity for osteogenic and chondrogenic differentiation that was not found in vascular endothelial cells [30]. Markers of differentiation were exacerbated by exposing leaflets to mechanical strain.

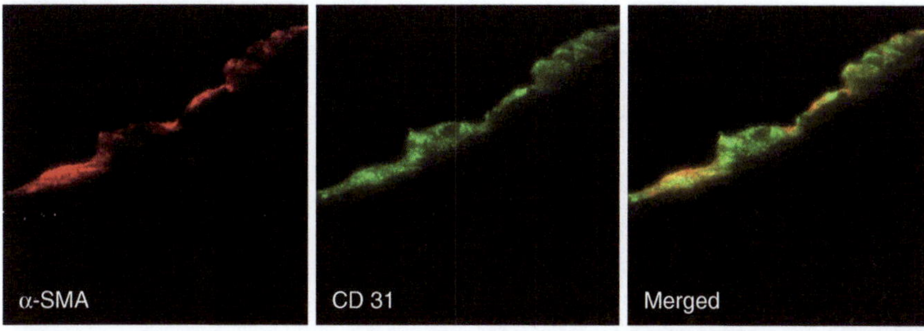

Fig. 9.4 The addition of mechanical strain to excised mitral valve leaflets showed an increase in mesenchymal markers such as **α**-SMA in the endothelium (identified by CD31 staining) (Images adapted from Wylie-Sears et al. [30])

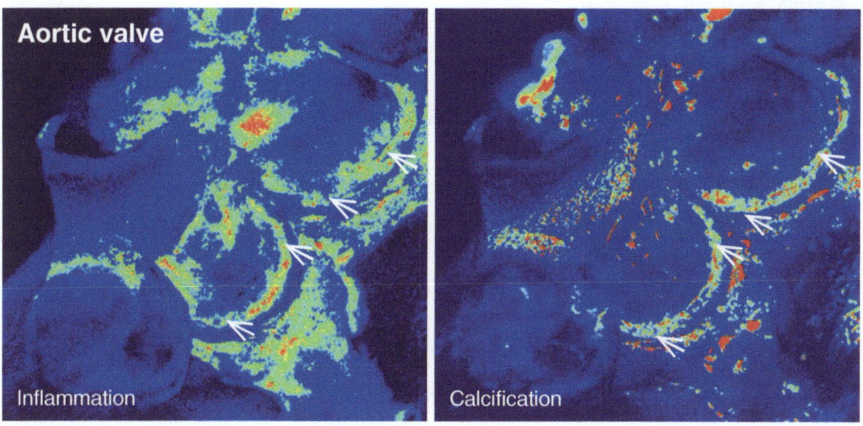

Fig. 9.5 Ex vivo NIRF imaging of the aortic valve of an apoE−/− mouse revealed a strong association between the presence of inflammation and calcification within the leaflets (Adapted from Aikawa et al. [34])

Therefore, future high-resolution imaging techniques may be able to search for localization of VEC marker proteins within the interstitial space or mesenchymal markers on the leaflet surface as early signs of CAVD.

9.4 Macrophages and Proteolytic Activity

Activation of VECs leads to the recruitment of monocytes and other leukocytes to the valve leaflets. As a result, CAVD (similar to calcification in atherosclerotic plaques) is hallmarked by the presence of inflammatory cells, such as macrophages and T cells, within and surrounding calcified regions of the tissue [12, 31–33]. Molecular imaging techniques using macrophage-targeted iron nanoparticles conjugated to a NIRF agent identified a strong correlation between macrophage accumulation and calcification in aortic valves of apolipoprotein E-deficient (apoE−/−) mice [34] (Fig. 9.5). These cells

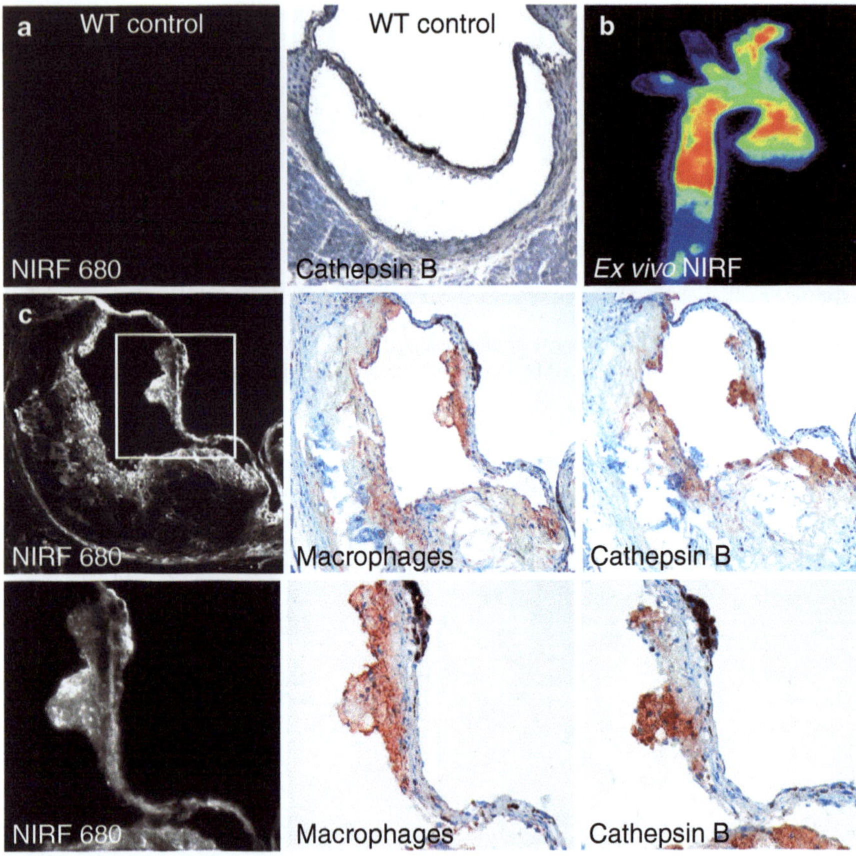

Fig. 9.6 Macrophage activity in the aortic valve. (**a**) Wild-type (WT) control mice did not exhibit detectable cathepsin B activity within the aortic valve. (**b**) ApoE–/– mice showed strong cardiovascular NIRF signal from a cathepsin B activatable probe. (**c**) Immunohistological analyses of the aortic valve showed a co-localization between the cathepsin NIRF signal and cathepsin B expression in macrophages within the valve (Modified from Aikawa et al. [13])

may play a role in initiating the remodeling processes that lead to calcification, as they actively release proteases that degrade extracellular matrix components, priming the tissue for new matrix secretion. Additionally, the accumulation of leukocytes and related inflammatory cytokines is positively correlated with remodeling in CAVD leaflets and aortic stenosis in human patients. Similarly, in an apoE–/– mouse model of atherosclerosis and CAVD, enzymatically activatable NIRF signal corresponding to a specific protease cathepsin B (as validated by immunohistological techniques) was shown to co-localize with macrophages within the valve leaflets (Fig. 9.6) [13].

Other members of the cathepsin family are involved in elastin degradation. As mentioned in the first section, the ventricularis layer of the aortic valve is composed mainly of elastin that allows the valve leaflets to exhibit a high radial strain response to diastolic loading. Disruption of this elastin layer has been shown to result in

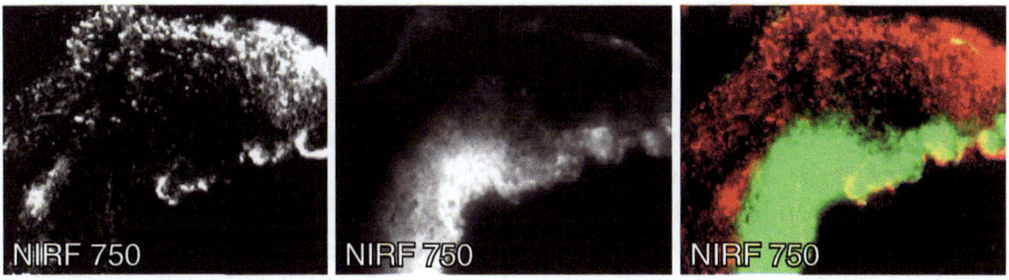

Fig. 9.7 The combination of a calcification NIRF probe with emission at 750 nm and an inflammation-targeted probe with emission at 680 nm allowed simultaneous imaging of both processes (Adapted from Aikawa et al. [13])

pathological remodeling associated with CAVD [34–36]. Chronic renal disease (CRD) is strongly correlated with CAVD in human patients, and CAVD processes in apoE−/− mice are accelerated by inducing CRD through resection of 5/6 of the total kidney volume (5/6 nephrectomy). Interestingly, induction of CRD in apoE−/− mice leads to a marked increase in activity of the elastolytic enzyme cathepsin S as shown by an enzymatically activatable NIRF agent. Deletion of cathepsin S in these mice mitigates CAVD progression [34]. Cathepsin S remodeling in this mouse model was found to be closely associated with the presence of inflammatory cell markers within the leaflets. In addition, elastin degradation peptides, also known as matrikines, highly biologically active molecules, may induce VIC osteogenic differentiation in aortic valves [34]. Application of pathological cyclic strain to aortic valve leaflets in an ex vivo bioreactor demonstrated significant increases in activity of cathepsin S and a similar protease, cathepsin K, within the leaflets.

9.5 Myofibroblast Activation, Osteogenic Differentiation, and Calcification

As noted in the vessel wall, molecular imaging of calcific mineral deposition has been achieved using bisphosphonates conjugated to NIRF molecules [37]. Bisphosphonates have a structure similar to the calcification inhibitor pyrophosphate [38] and is believed to bind to calcium and accumulate in mineralized crystals [39]. The accumulation of NIRF-bisphosphonates in calcific regions of CAVD leaflets yields detectable NIRF signal that is spectrally distinct from the protease agents discussed in the previous section, allowing for simultaneous imaging of these processes [40] (Fig. 9.7).

The mechanisms of mineralization are less clearly understood in CAVD compared to vascular calcification. As mentioned, VICs reside within the leaflet of the valve and directly remodel and maintain the microarchitecture of the leaflets by synthesis and degradation of extracellular matrix components [41, 42]. In the healthy adult valve, VICs remain in a quiescent state with characteristics similar to fibroblasts; however, these specialized cells exhibit a high degree of phenotypic plasticity with VIC differentiation observed during periods of valve development and disease [41]. Notably, activation of VICs to a myofibroblast phenotype—characterized by an increased expression of smooth muscle cell protein markers—is observed within developing valve leaflets and within fibrotic and calcific valve leaflets. This activated phenotype is believed to be responsible for the synthesis and remodeling of the extracellular matrix, and overactive VICs may be responsible for fibrotic accumulation of collagen during the initial stages of CAVD [43, 44]. Studies have also suggested that myofibroblastic VICs contribute to the formation of calcific nodules through cell death-mediated mechanisms [45, 46]. Additionally, markers of osteogenic differentiation of VICs have been observed in CAVD and may be responsible for the osteogenic nodules observed within CAVD leaflets [47]. The relationship between the activated myofibroblast and osteogenic phenotypes remains unknown. In addition to VICs, in pro-calcific environment, macrophages within the atherosclerotic plaque may actively participate in the deposition of calcium phosphate minerals [48], and similar processes may be relevant in CAVD. As we accrue more knowledge into the underlying mechanisms and roles of VECs, macrophages, and VIC phenotypes in the progression of CAVD, new imaging probes may be developed to target specific cellular processes of interest.

9.6 Future Perspectives

The molecular mechanisms of CAVD initiation and progression are less clear than those involved in the progression of vascular calcification. One reason for this is the lack of suitable in vitro models that adequately recapitulate the phenotypes observed in ex vivo analyses of CAVD tissues. The molecular imaging techniques outlined in this chapter have helped overcome these limitations by allowing detailed analysis of the cellular and molecular processes of CAVD in situ. The findings from these studies have provided valuable information concerning the temporal and endpoint aspects of CAVD. Moving forward, as these optical imaging techniques evolve, they may be incorporated into more traditional techniques of valve imaging that will be discussed in the following chapters. By combining these tools, researchers and clinicians would be able to connect gross changes in valve morphology and function to associated changes on the cellular and molecular level. These data may then be used to develop new benchtop models and paradigms of CAVD that would inform the ongoing search for CAVD therapies.

Sources of Funding Dr. Aikawa is supported by grants from the National Institute of Health (R01HL114805; R01HL109506) and Harvard Catalyst Reactor Program.

References

1. Yoganathan AP, He Z, Casey JS. Fluid mechanics of heart valves. Annu Rev Biomed Eng. 2004;6:331–62.
2. Sacks MS, Yoganathan AP. Heart valve function: a biomechanical perspective. Philos Trans R Soc Lond B Biol Sci. 2007;362:1369–91.
3. Sacks MS, Smith DB, Hiester ED. The aortic valve microstructure: effects of transvalvular pressure. J Biomed Mater Res. 1998;41:131–41.

4. Stella JA, Liao J, Sacks MS. Time-dependent biaxial mechanical behavior of the aortic heart valve leaflet. J Biomech. 2007;40:3169–77.
5. Schoen F. Aortic valve structure-function correlations: role of elastic fibers no longer a stretch of the imagination. J Heart Valve Dis. 1997;6:1–6.
6. Schoen FJ, Edwards WD. Valvular heart disease: general principles and stenosis. In: Silver MD, Gotlieb AI, Schoen FJ, editors. Cardiovascular pathology. New York: Churchill Livingstone; 2001. p. 402–42.
7. Go AS, Mozaffarian D, Roger VL, Benjamin EJ, Berry JD, Borden WB, Bravata DM, Dai S, Ford ES, Fox CS, Franco S, Fullerton HJ, Gillespie C, Hailpern SM, Heit JA, Howard VJ, Huffman MD, Kissela BM, Kittner SJ, Lackland DT, Lichtman JH, Lisabeth LD, Magid D, Marcus GM, Marelli A, Matchar DB, McGuire DK, Mohler ER, Moy CS, Mussolino ME, Nichol G, Paynter NP, Schreiner PJ, Sorlie PD, Stein J, Turan TN, Virani SS, Wong ND, Woo D, Turner MB. Heart disease and stroke statistics–2013 update: a report from the american heart association. Circulation. 2013;127:e6–245.
8. Nkomo VT, Gardin JM, Skelton TN, Gottdiener JS, Scott CG, Enriquez-Sarano M. Burden of valvular heart diseases: a population-based study. Lancet. 2006;368:1005–11.
9. Otto CM. Calcific aortic stenosis–time to look more closely at the valve. N Engl J Med. 2008;359:1395–8.
10. Rajamannan NM, Evans FJ, Aikawa E, Grande-Allen KJ, Demer LL, Heistad DD, Simmons CA, Masters KS, Mathieu P, O'Brien KD, Schoen FJ, Towler DA, Yoganathan AP, Otto CM. Calcific aortic valve disease: not simply a degenerative process: a review and agenda for research from the national heart and lung and blood institute aortic stenosis working group. Executive summary: calcific aortic valve disease-2011 update. Circulation. 2011;124: 1783–91.
11. New SE, Aikawa E. Molecular imaging insights into early inflammatory stages of arterial and aortic valve calcification. Circ Res. 2011;108:1381–91.
12. Dweck MR, Jones C, Joshi NV, Fletcher AM, Richardson H, White A, Marsden M, Pessotto R, Clark JC, Wallace WA, Salter DM, McKillop G, van Beek EJ, Boon NA, Rudd JH, Newby DE. Assessment of valvular calcification and inflammation by positron emission tomography in patients with aortic stenosis. Circulation. 2012;125:76–86.
13. Aikawa E, Nahrendorf M, Sosnovik D, Lok VM, Jaffer FA, Aikawa M, Weissleder R. Multimodality molecular imaging identifies proteolytic and osteogenic activities in early aortic valve disease. Circulation. 2007;115:377–86.
14. Hutcheson JD, Aikawa E, Merryman WD. Potential drug targets for calcific aortic valve disease. Nat Rev Cardiol. 2014;11:218–31.
15. Libby P, Sasiela W. Plaque stabilization: can we turn theory into evidence? Am J Cardiol. 2006;98:26P–33.
16. Lin TC, Tintut Y, Lyman A, Mack W, Demer LL, Hsiai TK. Mechanical response of a calcified plaque model to fluid shear force. Ann Biomed Eng. 2006;34:1535–41.
17. Stamatas GN, McIntire LV. Rapid flow-induced responses in endothelial cells. Biotechnol Prog. 2001;17:383–402.
18. Butcher JT, Penrod AM, Garcia AJ, Nerem RM. Unique morphology and focal adhesion development of valvular endothelial cells in static and fluid flow environments. Arterioscler Thromb Vasc Biol. 2004;24:1429–34.
19. Cucina A, Sterpetti AV, Pupelis G, Fragale A, Lepidi S, Cavallaro A, Giustiniani Q, Santoro DAL. Shear stress induces changes in the morphology and cytoskeleton organisation of arterial endothelial cells. Eur J Vasc Endovasc Surg. 1995;9:86–92.
20. Simmons CA, Grant GR, Manduchi E, Davies PF. Spatial heterogeneity of endothelial phenotypes correlates with side-specific vulnerability to calcification in normal porcine aortic valves. Circ Res. 2005;96:792–9.
21. Barakat AI, Davies PF. Mechanisms of shear stress transmission and transduction in endothelial cells. Chest. 1998;114:58S–63.
22. Davies PF, Tripathi SC. Mechanical stress mechanisms and the cell. An endothelial paradigm. Circ Res. 1993;72:239–45.
23. Ingber DE. Mechanobiology and diseases of mechanotransduction. Ann Med. 2003;35:564–77.

24. Jaalouk DE, Lammerding J. Mechanotransduction gone awry. Nat Rev Mol Cell Biol. 2009;10:63–73.
25. Butcher JT, Nerem RM. Valvular endothelial cells and the mechanoregulation of valvular pathology. Philos Trans R Soc Lond B Biol Sci. 2007;362:1445–57.
26. Nahrendorf M, Jaffer FA, Kelly KA, Sosnovik DE, Aikawa E, Libby P, Weissleder R. Noninvasive vascular cell adhesion molecule-1 imaging identifies inflammatory activation of cells in atherosclerosis. Circulation. 2006;114:1504–11.
27. Davies MJ, Treasure T, Parker DJ. Demographic characteristics of patients undergoing aortic valve replacement for stenosis: relation to valve morphology. Heart. 1996;75:174–8.
28. Balachandran K, Alford PW, Wylie-Sears J, Goss JA, Grosberg A, Bischoff J, Aikawa E, Levine RA, Parker KK. Cyclic strain induces dual-mode endothelial-mesenchymal transformation of the cardiac valve. Proc Natl Acad Sci U S A. 2011;108:19943–8.
29. Paruchuri S, Yang JH, Aikawa E, Melero-Martin JM, Khan ZA, Loukogeorgakis S, Schoen FJ, Bischoff J. Human pulmonary valve progenitor cells exhibit endothelial/mesenchymal plasticity in response to vascular endothelial growth factor-a and transforming growth factor-beta2. Circ Res. 2006;99:861–9.
30. Wylie-Sears J, Aikawa E, Levine RA, Yang JH, Bischoff J. Mitral valve endothelial cells with osteogenic differentiation potential. Arterioscler Thromb Vasc Biol. 2011;31:598–607.
31. Hjortnaes J, Butcher J, Figueiredo JL, Riccio M, Kohler RH, Kozloff KM, Weissleder R, Aikawa E. Arterial and aortic valve calcification inversely correlates with osteoporotic bone remodelling: a role for inflammation. Eur Heart J. 2010;31:1975–84.
32. Dweck MR, Chow MW, Joshi NV, Williams MC, Jones C, Fletcher AM, Richardson H, White A, McKillop G, van Beek EJ, Boon NA, Rudd JH, Newby DE. Coronary arterial 18f-sodium fluoride uptake: a novel marker of plaque biology. J Am Coll Cardiol. 2012;59:1539–48.
33. Giachelli CM. Vascular calcification mechanisms. J Am Soc Nephrol: JASN. 2004;15:2959–64.
34. Aikawa E, Aikawa M, Libby P, Figueiredo JL, Rusanescu G, Iwamoto Y, Fukuda D, Kohler RH, Shi GP, Jaffer FA, Weissleder R. Arterial and aortic valve calcification abolished by elastolytic cathepsin s deficiency in chronic renal disease. Circulation. 2009;119:1785–94.
35. Hinton RB, Adelman-Brown J, Witt S, Krishnamurthy VK, Osinska H, Sakthivel B, James JF, Li DY, Narmoneva DA, Mecham RP, Benson DW. Elastin haploinsufficiency results in progressive aortic valve malformation and latent valve disease in a mouse model. Circ Res. 2010;107:549–57.
36. Helske S, Syvaranta S, Lindstedt KA, Lappalainen J, Oorni K, Mayranpaa MI, Lommi J, Turto H, Werkkala K, Kupari M, Kovanen PT. Increased expression of elastolytic cathepsins s, k, and v and their inhibitor cystatin c in stenotic aortic valves. Arterioscler Thromb Vasc Biol. 2006;26: 1791–8.
37. Zaheer A, Murshed M, De Grand AM, Morgan TG, Karsenty G, Frangioni JV. Optical imaging of hydroxyapatite in the calcified vasculature of transgenic animals. Arterioscler Thromb Vasc Biol. 2006;26:1132–6.
38. Fleisch H. Development of bisphosphonates. Breast Cancer Res BCR. 2002;4:30–4.
39. Kozloff KM, Volakis LI, Marini JC, Caird MS. Near-infrared fluorescent probe traces bisphosphonate delivery and retention in vivo. J Bone Miner Res: Off J Am Soc Bone Miner Res. 2010;25:1748–58.
40. Aikawa E, Nahrendorf M, Figueiredo JL, Swirski FK, Shtatland T, Kohler RH, Jaffer FA, Aikawa M, Weissleder R. Osteogenesis associates with inflammation in early-stage atherosclerosis evaluated by molecular imaging in vivo. Circulation. 2007;116:2841–50.
41. Rabkin-Aikawa E, Farber M, Aikawa M, Schoen FJ. Dynamic and reversible changes of interstitial cell phenotype during remodeling of cardiac valves. J Heart Valve Dis. 2004;13:841–7.
42. Filip DA, Radu A, Simionescu M. Interstitial cells of the heart valves possess characteristics similar to smooth muscle cells. Circ Res. 1986;59:310–20.
43. Chester AH, Taylor PM. Molecular and functional characteristics of heart-valve interstitial cells. Philos Trans R Soc Lond B Biol Sci. 2007;362:1437–43.
44. Hinz B, Phan SH, Thannickal VJ, Galli A, Bochaton-Piallat ML, Gabbiani G. The myofibroblast: one function, multiple origins. Am J Pathol. 2007;170:1807–16.

45. Hutcheson JD, Chen J, Sewell-Loftin MK, Ryzhova LM, Fisher CI, Su YR, Merryman WD. Cadherin-11 regulates cell-cell tension necessary for calcific nodule formation by valvular myofibroblasts. Arterioscler Thromb Vasc Biol. 2013;33:114–20.
46. Hutcheson JD, Ryzhova LM, Setola V, Merryman WD. 5-ht (2b) antagonism arrests non-canonical tgf-beta1-induced valvular myofibroblast differentiation. J Mol Cell Cardiol. 2012;53:707–14.
47. Mohler 3rd ER, Gannon F, Reynolds C, Zimmerman R, Keane MG, Kaplan FS. Bone formation and inflammation in cardiac valves. Circulation. 2001;103:1522–8.
48. New SE, Goettsch C, Aikawa M, Marchini JF, Shibasaki M, Yabusaki K, Libby P, Shanahan CM, Croce K, Aikawa E. Macrophage-derived matrix vesicles: an alternative novel mechanism for microcalcification in atherosclerotic plaques. Circ Res. 2013;113:72–7.

PET/CT Imaging of Inflammation and Calcification in CAVD: Clinical Studies

10

Alex Thomas Vesey, Marc Richard Dweck, and David Ernest Newby

Contents

A.T. Vesey (✉) • M.R. Dweck, MD • D.E. Newby, MD
British Heart Foundation Centre for Cardiovascular Science,
Edinburgh University, Edinburgh, UK
e-mail: avesey@staffmail.ed.ac.uk; MDweck@staffmail.ed.ac.uk; d.e.newby@ed.ac.uk

E. Aikawa (ed.), *Cardiovascular Imaging: Arterial and Aortic Valve Inflammation and Calcification*, DOI 10.1007/978-3-319-09268-3_10

Abstract

Molecular imaging using positron-emission tomography combined with computed tomography (PET/CT) to demonstrate aortic valve inflammation (^{18}F-FDG) and calcification (^{18}F-NaF) in CAVD holds major promise. Several studies have now shown that these PET radiotracers are able to reproducibly quantify these two important intra-valvular pathological processes. This development represents an exciting opportunity not only to explore CAVD pathology in vivo and predict disease progression but also to provide the means of gaining early signal of efficacy in phase II trials of novel drug interventions.

10.1 Introduction

Aortic valve disease is a major and growing burden for patients and healthcare service providers. It is the commonest cause of valve replacement in Europe and North America, and the third leading cause of cardiovascular disease [1,2]. It has a general prevalence of 2 % that rises to 13 % in those patients aged between 75 and 85 years, such that, with the ageing demographic of the developed world, the future health economic impact of CAVD will be substantial.

There is no effective non-surgical treatment for CAVD. HMG-CoA reductase inhibitors have been the main agents tested formally in randomised trials and have proven ineffective [3–5]. As a consequence, echocardiographic surveillance with eventual aortic valve replacement (AVR) or transcatheter aortic valve implantation (TAVI) remains the only effective interventional strategy. Although highly efficacious, both procedures are nevertheless associated with significant cost and a high risk of morbidity and mortality and are often poorly suited to the elderly patients affected by this condition.

Clearly, what is required is an effective intervention to prevent disease progression. However, two problems are particularly germane when considering why this has not yet been achieved. First, the pathophysiology of CAVD has been difficult to clarify. The inevitable lack of human valvular tissue from early disease has hampered research, as have the many difficulties in developing robust and user-friendly animal models that truly recapitulate the human disease [6]. Second, the clinical end points in trials pose problems. Patients with CAVD commonly have coexistent atherosclerosis and other pathologies that frequently result in death not clearly attributable to CAVD. In addition, along with the slow and unpredictable nature of aortic stenosis progression, trials need to be long term and require large numbers to power and assess the clinical end points of death or cardiovascular death. This has major cost implications for drug and therapeutic developments. Valve replacement is a less hard end point with the thresholds for offering surgery or TAVI varying considerably. Finally, echocardiographic measures of disease progression are hampered by modest issues relating to scan-to-scan reproducibility.

What is needed are safe, repeatable and accurate biomarkers that reflect the activity of a variety of pathobiological pathways relevant to CAVD. Such biomarkers should simultaneously provide insight into early disease pathology and potential targets for intervention as well as permit the acquisition of early signals of efficacy in phase II clinical trials of novel pharmacological agents. They should also subsequently provide the means to monitor disease progression or response to treatment in the clinic.

Serum biomarkers have many potential advantages including low cost, rapidity and suitability for mass screening, but they lack anatomical resolution being systemic markers. Moreover, processes in small structures such as the aortic valve are unlikely to generate enough signal to become detectable in the blood. Attention has therefore shifted to molecular imaging techniques including positron-emission tomography combined with computed tomography (PET/CT). This approach allows the activity of a specific pathological process to be measured within even small structures in the body and for the first time has allowed us to investigate the pathological processes underlying aortic stenosis in a non-invasive manner as they occur in vivo.

The aim of this chapter is to introduce the basic concepts of PET/CT imaging, to describe how this imaging technique has been used to investigate the pathophysiology of CAVD and finally to explore the potential future role of this exciting approach in both the clinical and research arenas.

10.2 PET/CT

PET is a non-invasive molecular imaging technology that is able to resolve and quantitate in vivo a theoretically limitless number of biological processes by radiolabelling tuneable biomolecules and then detect them at picomolar concentrations using a scanning platform.

The modality takes advantage of the fact that it is now reasonably straightforward to generate 'proton-heavy' isotopes, usually by bombarding suitable targets with protons in a cyclotron. The most commonly used isotopes in PET imaging are ^{11}C, ^{13}N, ^{15}O and ^{18}F; others that are less commonly used include ^{64}Cu, ^{76}Br, ^{82}Rb, ^{68}Ga and ^{124}I. Using a hot cell, these reporters can then be chemically incorporated into a biomolecule, drug or peptide of interest before being administered to a patient as a radiotracer. One of the major challenges and expenses in PET science is the reliable, standardised and efficient production of bespoke complex radiotracers.

Once administered, the radiotracer localises to and interacts with the biological process of interest. At a given moment, the unstable reporter isotope will undergo β^+ decay; an excess proton is converted into a neutron thus restoring the optimal balance of protons and neutrons in the nucleus. This conversion also entails the generation of an electron neutrino and a positron. The emitted positron (with an energy of a few MeV) then travels for a distance in the tissue (the positron range) before thermalising and combining with an electron to form a positronium. The positronium then decays by annihilation and generates two 511 keV photons emitted at nearly 180° to each other (acollinearly). The photons go on to be detected by scintillators, coupled to photomultiplier tubes and arranged into a ring detector. They are then 'electronically collimated' in time by coincidence (i.e. only photons that strike the scintillator crystals within a 3–12 ns time window are counted as a true coincidences). It therefore becomes possible to localise the annihilation event along a line of coincidence (line of response). With enough events, the data acquired during scanning can be reconstructed using complex statistical software into an interpretable image. Although data on many millions of events is collected, this is still significantly less than CT, and as such, random coincidences, detector dead time, photon attenuation, photon scatter and other factors that increase the noise in PET significantly require correction by complex statistical algorithms. The spatial resolution of PET is also fundamentally limited by the positron distance (0.5 mm with ^{18}F) and acollinearity. As such, the resolution for most clinical PET systems is approximately 4–5 mm.

In order to aid image analysis, the PET scanner is usually employed as a hybrid system incorporating a CT scanner that allows for attenuation correction and for an anatomically detailed CT data set to be accurately registered with the functionally detailed PET data set. In order to then quantify radiotracer uptake in the tissues, the image data are analysed on commercially available software packages, and regions or volumes of interest (ROI/VOI) are drawn on the CT images and then translated to the PET images. Radiotracer uptake is normally quantified as tissue radioactivity normalised to the injected dose and body surface area by the following equation:

$$SUV(t) = \frac{c(t)}{a \div w}$$

where SUV is the standardised uptake value over *t*, *t is* the time of measurement, *c* is the radioactivity of the tissue within the region of interest, *a* is the decay corrected injected activity and *w* is either body weight, lean body weight or body surface area. All voxels in the volume of interest have a separate SUV, and most software packages will quote their mean, minimum, maximum and standard deviation. It has also become conventional to normalise tissue SUV to image-derived blood pool activity (normally from the caval or atrial lumen) to generate a tissue-to-background ratio:

$$TBR = \frac{Tissue\ VOI\ SUV(t)}{Blood\ pool\ SUV(t)}$$

This is of particular use in cardiovascular PET when the tissues of interest are often affected by overspill from the blood pool.

10.3 CAVD Pathology and PET Radiotracer Choice

Although still deficient, our current understanding of the pathophysiology of CAVD indicates that this process is triggered and then maintained by a complex interplay of multiple risk factors and noxious stimuli. These include hypertension, diabetes mellitus, hyperlipidaemia, systemic inflammation, oxidative stress and abnormal valvular mechanical stresses and reduced shear stresses (see Fig. 10.1). These factors combine to produce chronic endothelial injury and dysfunction that lead to the

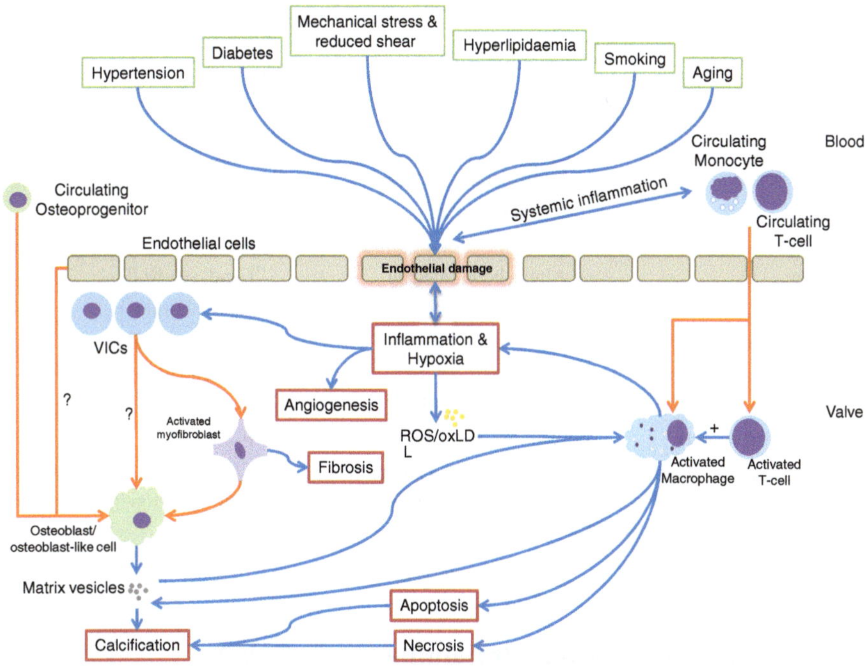

Fig. 10.1 Graphical representation of the key risk factors, triggers and pathological processes in CAVD. Processes and influences are represented by *blue arrows*, and cellular migration, differentiation or phenotypic switch by *orange arrows* (Adapted from Miller et al. [6] and Dweck et al. [7]). *ROS* reactive oxidant species, *oxLDL* oxidised low-density lipoprotein

initiation of certain key pathological processes within the valve itself: inflammation, angiogenesis, hypoxia, necrosis, apoptosis, fibrosis and calcification. These processes in turn interact with each other to drive valvular stiffening and narrowing with eventual ventricular hypertrophy, fibrosis and failure. A full review of the pathophysiology is beyond the scope of this chapter, but for further reading, see New et al. [8], Dweck et al. [9], New et al.[10] and Miller et al. [6].

All of these noxious stimuli and pathological process represent potential therapeutic and molecular imaging targets. This is indeed the reason that PET/CT provides such a rich source of potential avenues for research and development: disease biology, disease progression and response to novel therapy may all be explored simultaneously. However, whilst tracers targeting a wide range of pathological processes might potentially be of use in aortic stenosis (see Table 10.1), this review will concentrate on the two that have developed a track record in this condition: 2-deoxy-2-(^{18}F)fluro-D-glucose (^{18}F-FDG) and ^{18}F-fluoride (delivered as sodium fluoride; ^{18}F-NaF). These tracers are believed to demonstrate intra-valvular inflammation and active calcification, respectively, and aside from targeting two of the most important disease processes driving aortic stenosis, they also have the key advantage of being easy to manufacture and commercially available, facilitating their easy uptake and widespread use as novel research and future clinical tools.

Table 10.1 Potential relevant positron-emission tomography radiotracers in calcific aortic valve disease

Pathological process	Target example	PET ligand
Inflammation	Glycolysis	^{18}F-FDG
	Translocator protein	^{11}C-PK11195
	Somatostatin receptor	68Ga-DOTATATE
Hypoxia	Hypoxic tissue	^{18}F-MISO
		62Cu-ATSM
Fibrosis	Alpha$_V$beta$_3$ integrin	^{18}F-galacto-RGD
		^{18}F-fluciclatide
Angiogenesis	Alpha$_V$beta$_3$ integrin	^{18}F-galacto-RGD
		^{18}F-fluciclatide
Apoptosis	Phosphatidylserine	^{18}F-annexin V
Calcification activity	Apatite nanocrystals	^{18}F-fluoride

^{18}F-FDG, 2-deoxy-2-(^{18}F)fluro-D-glucose; 68Ga-DOTATATE, 68Ga-DOTA-octreotate; ^{18}F-MISO, ^{18}F-fluoromisonidazole; 62Cu-ATSM, 62Cu-diacetyl-bis(N 4-methylthiosemicarbazone); ^{18}F-galacto-RGD, ^{18}F-galacto-arginylglycylaspartic acid

10.4 PET/CT for Imaging Inflammation in CAVD

10.4.1 Background

As a result of its ubiquity, ^{18}F-FDG remains the only putative PET marker of inflammation to have been investigated in clinical studies of CAVD, although other markers, including 68Ga-DOTATATE and ^{11}C-PK11195, have been evaluated in atherosclerosis. ^{18}F-FDG was first administered to humans in 1976 [11] with the aim of demonstrating cerebral and total body glucose utilisation. Cells with high metabolic demand express large quantities of various GLUT transporter subtypes and metabolise glucose quickly thus generating a gradient across the cell membrane that causes a continuous large influx of glucose. ^{18}F-FDG directly competes with glucose for transportation by GLUT and then undergoes phosphorylation to ^{18}F-FDG-6-phosphate by hexokinase. Owing to the strict specificity of phosphoglucose isomerase for glucose-6-phosphate, ^{18}F-FDG-phosphate is not altered and is unable to progress down the glycolytic pathway. It thus becomes trapped within the cell and its continuing accumulation allows detection by the PET. ^{18}F-FDG is thus able to identify clusters of cells with very high rates of glucose uptake. Consequently, ^{18}F-FDG is not specific to one cell type but will accumulate in any cell with increased metabolic demand, e.g. neurons, active muscle cells, neoplastic cells and activated inflammatory cells. In PET imaging of atherosclerosis, pioneered by Rudd [12], Fayad [13] and Tawakol [14], it was hypothesised that macrophages, the key players in the inflammatory milieu of the high-risk plaque, were responsible for the observed signal. This was evidenced in Rudd's original paper using tritiated deoxyglucose autoradiography. Others have demonstrated a correlation between plaque SUV and

CD68 macrophage immunohistochemical staining in humans [15]. These data complement observations that macrophages have high baseline levels of glycolysis [16] that increase dramatically when the cell becomes activated [17]. This may be particularly germane in the hypoxic environment of the plaque where glycolysis may be the only pathway available for the generation of ATP [18]. Indeed recent preclinical and clinical data have suggested that hypoxia may be the most important factor governing the uptake of ^{18}F-FDG by macrophages [19,20]. Whether it is inflammation, hypoxia or a combination of both driving increased GLUT expression by macrophages, a growing body of clinical studies indicates that ^{18}F-FDG highlights a pathological, hypermetabolic state in the arterial wall that appears to improve with statin therapy [21]. Moreover, it seems highly likely that similar mechanisms should also govern ^{18}F-FDG uptake in the aortic valve.

10.4.2 Clinical Studies

To date, only two published studies have examined the use of ^{18}F-FDG in the imaging of valvular glycolytic activity [7,22]. The first published report of ^{18}F-FDG uptake in the aortic valve was produced by Marincheva-Savcheva and colleagues in 2011 [22]. This was a retrospective study of patients having whole body ^{18}F-FDG PET/CT for oncological staging. The group identified a cohort of 42 patients with a diagnosis of CAVD and age matched these patients to a second cohort of 42 cancer patients without CAVD. Patients with CAVD were stratified into echocardiographically mild, moderate and severe groups. A semi-quantitative assessment of CT valvular calcification was made. PET scans were manually registered with CT scans and ROIs were drawn in the centre of the aortic valves (to minimise overspill from myocardial uptake). Tissue-to-background ratios were computed by normalising valvular SUVs to blood pool uptake in the right atrium. Intra- and inter-observer reproducibility studies were undertaken, and in a subgroup, the authors addressed the ability of ^{18}F-FDG to predict disease progression.

To date, our group has performed the largest prospective study of PET/CT ^{18}F-FDG imaging in patients with CAVD [7]. A total of 121 patients were recruited and were representative of the full spectrum of CAVD severity including 20 subjects with aortic valve sclerosis and 20 age- and sex-matched controls with normal aortic valves. Baseline echocardiography was performed along with dedicated ^{18}F-FDG and ^{18}F-fluoride PET/CT imaging and CT calcium scoring of the aortic valve [23]. Patients were also asked to adhere to a carbohydrate-free diet prior to their ^{18}F-FDG scan in order to minimise myocardial uptake by encouraging the heart to switch from glucose to free fatty acid metabolism. PET/CT analysis was undertaken using dedicated PET/CT analysis software (OsiriX version 3.5.1 64 bit; OsiriX Imaging Software, Geneva, Switzerland). This permitted the automated registration and multiplanar reformatting of PET and CT imaging data, which in turn afforded the opportunity to explore and optimise the image analysis technique (see Fig. 10.2). In addition, extensive reproducibility studies were undertaken.

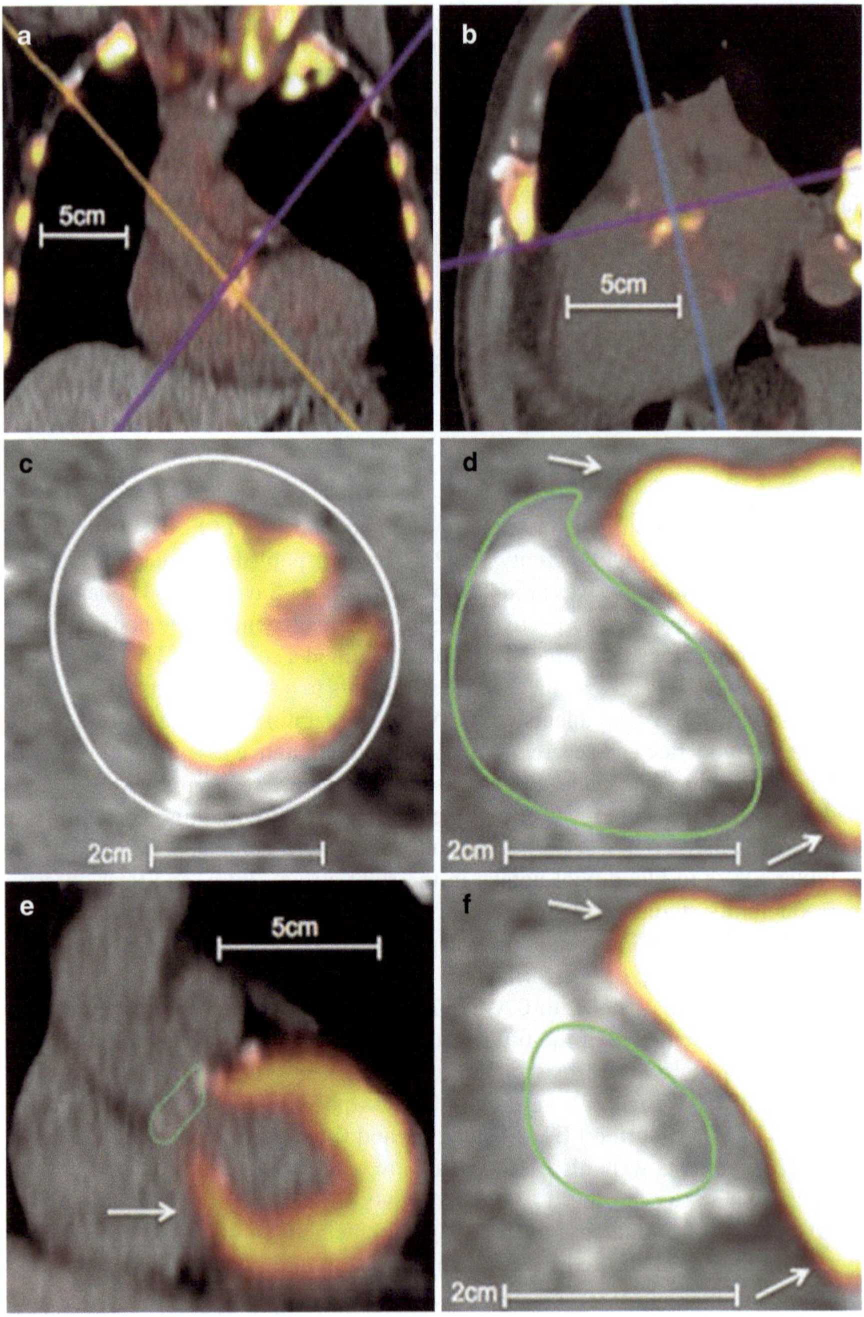
a
5cm
b
5cm
c
2cm
d
2cm
e
5cm
f
2cm

10.4.3 Relationship Between FDG Uptake and Lesion Severity

The key finding from Marincheva-Savcheva's study was that aortic valve ^{18}F-FDG uptake was significantly higher in CAVD patients compared to controls (median TBR 1.53 (1.42–1.76) vs. 1.34 (IQR: 1.20–1.55); $P<0.001$). There was also an apparent increase in ^{18}F-FDG uptake upon moving from mild to moderate aortic stenosis (1.50 [1.36–1.75] vs. 1.70 [1.52–1.94]). However, interestingly ^{18}F-FDG uptake reduced again in those with severe disease (1.51 [1.38–1.54]), leading the authors to conclude that CAVD occurs in two distinct stages: an early principally inflammatory stage followed by a second stage, decoupled from inflammation and dominated by a process of active calcification reminiscent of osteogenesis [24].

Our findings largely reproduced those of Marincheva-Savcheva, in that we observed a steady although modest positive correlation between ^{18}F-FDG uptake by all measures and aortic stenosis severity but did not see the fall in ^{18}F-FDG uptake in patients with the most severe lesions (Table 10.2). This discrepancy may be attributable to the small number of patients in the first study, the problems with reproducibility in one study or unaccounted differences in study populations such as cancer. The summary findings of both studies are shown in Fig. 10.3. It should be noted that in both trials large overlaps in TBR ranges between groups were observed, indicating that, although statistical differences were present, the ability of ^{18}F-FDG to distinguish between categories with confidence is limited.

10.4.4 Predicting Outcome and Disease Progression

In a subgroup of patients with serial echocardiographic data available ($n=19$), Marincheva-Savcheva showed that subjects with a valvular TBR greater than the median had a higher chance of progression: five of six patients with above median TBR progressed compared to two of nine patients with below median values. This result only just reached statistical significance ($P=0.04$), and the binary definition of progression was loose (any increase in severity class in any of the echocardiographic criteria). We have recently published a 1-year follow-up data [25] in a small subgroup of our original cohort. Disappointingly the baseline ^{18}F-FDG uptake failed

Fig. 10.2 Examples of ^{18}F-fluorodeoxyglucose and ^{18}F-fluoride uptake in the aortic valve. ^{18}F-fluoride (**a–c**). (**a**) Coronal view of the thorax. ^{18}F-NaF uptake is apparent in the aortic valve as well as visible bones and the aortic arch. (**b**) Modified sagittal view of the valve. (**c**) A coaxial short-axis view of the aortic valve (*purple axis*). The *white circle* is an example of a region of interest drawn on an ^{18}F-NaF scan. ^{18}F-flurodeoxyglucose (**d–f**). (**d**) A coaxial view of the aortic valve (*purple axis*) with significant myocardial overspill rendering quantification troublesome. A region of interest has been drawn using the short-axis technique (*green circle*). (**e**) Long-axis view of the heart and aortic valve (*blue axis*). A region of interest has been drawn using the long-axis technique (*green circle*). The myocardial uptake is obvious and the difficulties in quantifying valvular 18-fluorodeoxyglucose apparent. (**f**) Same image as (**d**) but employing the centre of valve technique for valvular SUV quantification with the region of interest drawn as a (*green circle*). All *white arrows* represent myocardial uptake of ^{18}F-FDG spilling over onto the valve

Table 10.2 Quantification of radiotracer uptake from Dweck 2012 and correlation against aortic stenosis severity

			Aortic stenosis			Correction with peak aortic jet velocity	
	Control	Aortic sclerosis	Mild	Moderate	Severe	r^2	P
^{18}F-NaF							
Mean SUV	1.20 (1.10–1.55)	1.35 (1.24–1.59)	1.59 (1.38–1.73)	1.82 (1.67–2.05)	2.10 (1.78–2.51)	0.461	<0.001
Mean TBR	1.23 (1.20–1.36)	1.53 (1.34–1.59)	1.73 (1.45–1.92)	2.03 (1.71–2.28)	2.17 (1.82–2.36)	0.534	<0.001
Maximum SUV	1.54 (1.33–1.86)	1.77 (1.58–2.09)	2.21 (1.84–2.45)	2.57 (2.27–2.99)	3.25 (2.47–4.42)	0.551	<0.001
Maximum TBR	1.56 (1.41–1.64)	1.96 (1.63–2.11)	2.45 (1.94–2.71)	2.89 (2.31–3.24)	3.25 (2.65–3.63)	0.540	<0.001
Patients with increased uptake %	0	45	76	95	100	–	–
^{18}F-FDG							
Mean SUV	1.49 (1.33–1.56)	1.73 (1.46–1.88)	1.66 (1.53–1.88)	1.71 (1.61–1.91)	1.76 (1.61–2.18)	0.142	<0.001
Mean TBR	1.18 (1.09–1.26)	1.35 (1.19–1.44)	1.29 (1.21–1.45)	1.33 (1.26–1.47)	1.42 (1.36–1.62)	0.203	<0.001
Maximum SUV	1.62 (1.47–1.68)	1.91 (1.64–2.07)	1.85 (1.72–2.07)	1.95 (1.81–2.18)	2.07 (1.88–2.25)	0.213	<0.001
Maximum TBR	1.27 (1.21–1.40)	1.47 (1.31–1.61)	1.44 (1.37–1.63)	1.58 (1.41–1.65)	1.65 (1.55–1.85)	0.218	<0.001
Patients with increased uptake, %	0	20	24	30	52	–	–

Values are median +/– interquartile range, with Pearson correlation

^{18}F-NaF ^{18}F-fluoride, *SUV* standardised uptake value, *TBR* tissue-to-background ratio

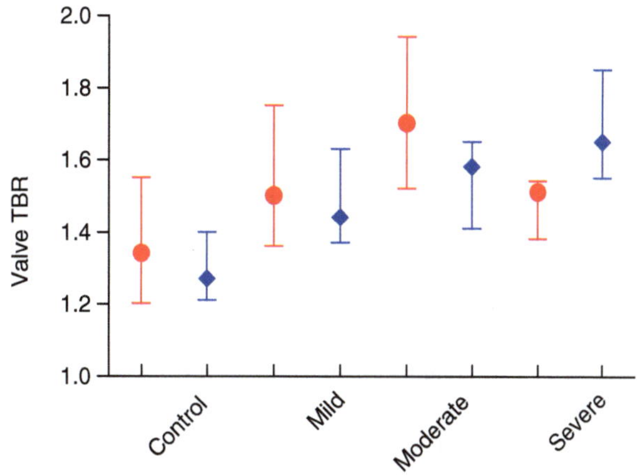

Fig. 10.3 Valvular ^{18}F-fluorodeoxyglucose maximum tissue-to-background ratios from Marincheva-Savcheva et al. [22] (*red*) and Dweck et al. [7] (*blue*). *Dots/diamonds* are median, and whiskers are interquartile range

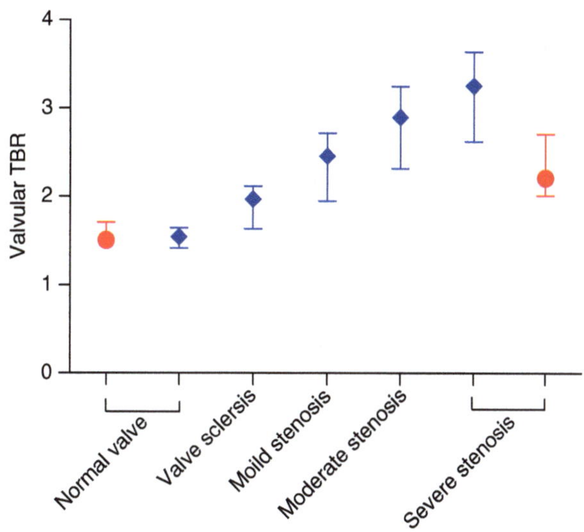

Fig. 10.4 Valvular ^{18}F-fluoride maximum tissue-to-background ratios from Hyafil et al. [55] (*red*) and Dweck et al. [7] (*blue*). *Dots/diamonds* are median, and whiskers are interquartile range

to predict disease progression adjudicated by the change in calcium score, although this may reflect the small patient numbers and the relatively short follow-up in this study [25].

10.4.5 Reproducibility and Methodological Strengths and Weaknesses

The Marincheva-Savcheva study is important in terms of proof of principle but is limited by several factors. The study was necessarily retrospective, and the patients were not primarily selected on the basis of their cardiac disease. Moreover, the PET/

CT protocols were neither standardised nor optimised for demonstrating intra-vascular or intra-valvular inflammation. The analysis was also limited by poor intra-observer reliability, with an intra-class correlation coefficient of 0.55 (95 % CI: 0.27–0.73), although, curiously, the inter-observer reliability was much better: intra-class correlation coefficient (ICC) = 0.97 (95 % CI: 0.96–0.98). Therefore, the results need to be interpreted with caution. Our group benefited from pre-specified and consistent PET/CT acquisition protocols, a prospectively recruited cohort and a standardised follow-up schedule. We explored multiple methods of analysing valvular ^{18}F-FDG uptake and concluded, like Marincheva-Savcheva, that the 'centre-valve' approach produced the best intra- and inter-observer reliability with narrow limits of agreement [7]. In keeping with Marincheva-Savcheva findings, we also found that our analysis was significantly hampered by overspill of signal from myocardial tissue near the aortic annulus (see Fig. 10.2). This occurred despite dietary modification and may have contaminated the valvular signal. Furthermore, as with any PET image analysis of relatively small volumes, the absolute measured activities may have been reduced by partial voluming artefact. Finally we did not employ ECG or respiratory gating of the PET data, which are of benefit when examining the PET signal in the coronary arteries [26].

10.4.6 Validation of Valvular ^{18}F-FDG Uptake

Our group has recently published work [25] that included some tissue validation experiments in 12 patients who had ^{18}F-FDG PET imaging of their valve shortly before proceeding to aortic valve replacement. Excised valvular tissue was decalcified and then immunostained with a variety of antibodies including anti-CD68. There was good inter-observer repeatability for the immunohistochemical measure of CD68 staining (ICC = 0.99 [0.99–1.00]). We were however unable to demonstrate correlation between any index of ^{18}F-FDG uptake and CD68 staining. This may reflect contamination of the valvular signal by myocardial activity. Alternatively, it is possible that valvular ^{18}F-FDG uptake might reflect the metabolic activity of cells other than macrophages in stenotic aortic valves. Indeed this is particularly likely in the latter stages of the disease, studied in these experiments, where valve osteoblasts and fibroblasts are likely to be especially active. Further work is required to investigate this interesting hypothesis.

10.4.7 Summary

When compared to normal controls, aortic valves affected by calcific stenosis show evidence of increased glucose utilisation with the more severe lesions showing a greater accumulation of ^{18}F-FDG. The exact mechanism underlying this observation in the aortic valve has not yet been demonstrated, but it seems likely that the ^{18}F-FDG signal reflects more than simply inflammatory activity within the valve. Nevertheless ^{18}F-FDG holds promise as a marker of metabolic activity and therefore disease activity in aortic stenosis, and whilst no apparent relationship was observed between its uptake and disease progression at 1 year, the 2-year follow-up from across the entire cohort is eagerly anticipated.

10.5 PET/CT for Imaging Calcification in CAVD

10.5.1 Background

^{18}F-fluoride (delivered as a solution of sodium fluoride; ^{18}F-NaF) was first mooted as a bone tracer in the seminal paper by Blau in 1972 [27]. It has since established a track record in PET imaging of bone metabolism and disease with an excellent safety record [28–43]. It has been used in humans to assess disease activity and indeed response to treatment in osteoporosis [29,33,35] and Paget's disease [30,37]. By virtue of its rapid elimination, high target specificity and availability for binding, it has pharmacokinetic and pharmacodynamic properties that are ideally suited to imaging, resulting in a high target-to-background ratio [27,44].

It is often contended that ^{18}F-NaF is a marker of bone deposition [43] or osteoblastic activity, but the reality is more complex [27,44,45]. Bone crystal is predominantly composed of calcium orthophosphate crystal that approaches mineral calcium hydroxylapatite. In purely physicochemical terms, the fluoride ion is incorporated onto the apatite surface by chemisorption and substituted for a hydroxyl group. In physiological conditions, this not a simple process with the original 4-step description by Blau still standing today. Fluoride must first be delivered to the bone by blood (1) and then leave the plasma to enter the extracellular fluid (ECF) (2). The fluoride will then enter the shell of bound water enveloping the crystal (3) before eventually undergoing full incorporation (4). Steps one and two are predominantly determined by blood flow. Steps three and four are however critically dependent upon the surface area of apatite available for incorporation. In bone, this relates to increased osteoblast and osteoclast activity. Osteoblasts generate matrix vesicles and the propagation of new regions of tiny nano-crystalline apatite particles, whilst osteoclasts promote the dissolution of solid blocks of established mineral. As a consequence ^{18}F-NaF uptake reflects a combination of increased osteoblastic and osteoclastic activity, thus acting predominantly as a marker of bone turnover. Indeed this hypothesis is now firmly supported by a large and expanding body of experimental and clinical PET data [34,39–42,44].

What then of ^{18}F-NaF uptake in the vasculature? Increased activity of this tracer in the aorta and carotid arteries was first published by Derlin [46,47] who made the key observation that some heavily calcified lesions did not demonstrate increased PET uptake and indeed that CT calcium scores in the aorta did not correlate well with ^{18}F-NaF uptake values. Subsequently studies have confirmed the disconnect between ^{18}F-NaF PET and CT calcium scoring, which, similar to bone, relates to calcification activity and the effects of surface area on ^{18}F-NaF binding.

In the early stage of aortic stenosis, calcification is, similar to atherosclerosis, likely to represent a complex cellularly and humorally regulated healing response to the injurious inflammatory and necrotic processes occurring within the valve. Aikawa et al. have published a series of elegant longitudinal experiments in mice that demonstrate the link between inflammation and calcification [48]. Briefly, they and others have shown that macrophage infiltration is very closely associated with osteogenic activity and that apoptotic bodies and matrix vesicles that contain calcium orthophosphate nanocrystals execute this early calcific process [49–51]. These early nanocrystals provide an extremely high surface area to which ^{18}F-NaF can bind, resulting in increased uptake of this tracer in regions of newly developing and active microcalcification. By contrast ^{18}F-NaF will bind with less affinity to regions of dormant macro-calcification where much of the hydroxyapatite will be internalised and not available for binding.

The latter stages of aortic stenosis are characterised by extensive valvular calcification that is coordinated by osteoblasts in a manner akin to skeletal bone formation, involving many of the same humoral factors. Indeed lamellar bone, microfractures and haemopoietic tissue have all been observed in the end stages of the disease. The mechanism of ^{18}F-NaF binding in these valves is therefore more likely to be similar to that of bone, reflecting the deposition of new micro-calcified deposits on the surface of the valve and the remodelling of existing calcium towards the end-stage bone phenotype.

In summary ^{18}F-NaF is believed to act as a marker of calcification activity in the valves of patients with aortic stenosis and, given its specificity, excellent kinetics and complete lack of myocardial spillover, holds major advantages over ^{18}F-FDG as an exciting novel biomarker of disease activity.

10.5.2 Validation of Valvular ^{18}F-Fluoride Uptake

We have recently published the first report validating the origin of the ^{18}F-NaF signal in the aortic valve [25]. In patients who underwent ^{18}F-NaF PET imaging shortly before aortic valve replacement, we undertook ^{18}F-NaF autoradiography and immunostaining for tissue non-specific alkaline phosphatase (a key executor of vascular mineralisation [52,53]) and osteocalcin (a protein secreted by osteoblasts and intimately related to biomineralisation [53]). We were able to show that ^{18}F-NaF co-localised with biomineral as demonstrated by Von Kossa staining (see Fig. 10.5) and that there was a good correlation between in vivo valvular ^{18}F-NaF uptake and both ex vivo alkaline phosphatase ($r=0.65$, $P=0.04$) and osteocalcin ($r=0.68$, $P=0.03$) staining. The histological variables were subjected to tests of inter-observer reliability and were characterised by an absence of fixed or proportional biases with relatively narrow limits of agreement (TNAP −13.4 to 9.3 %, osteocalcin −8.0 to 5.0 %) and ICC values of 0.90 (95 % CI 0.35–0.99) and 0.88 (95 % CI 0.60–0.97), respectively.

^{18}F-NaF uptake has been validated in atherosclerosis, with important implications for activity in the valve [26]. In excised symptomatic carotid tissue, we used ex vivo PET/CT and micro-CT to further demonstrate the co-localisation of ^{18}F-NaF to areas of microcalcification and were able to show that compared to

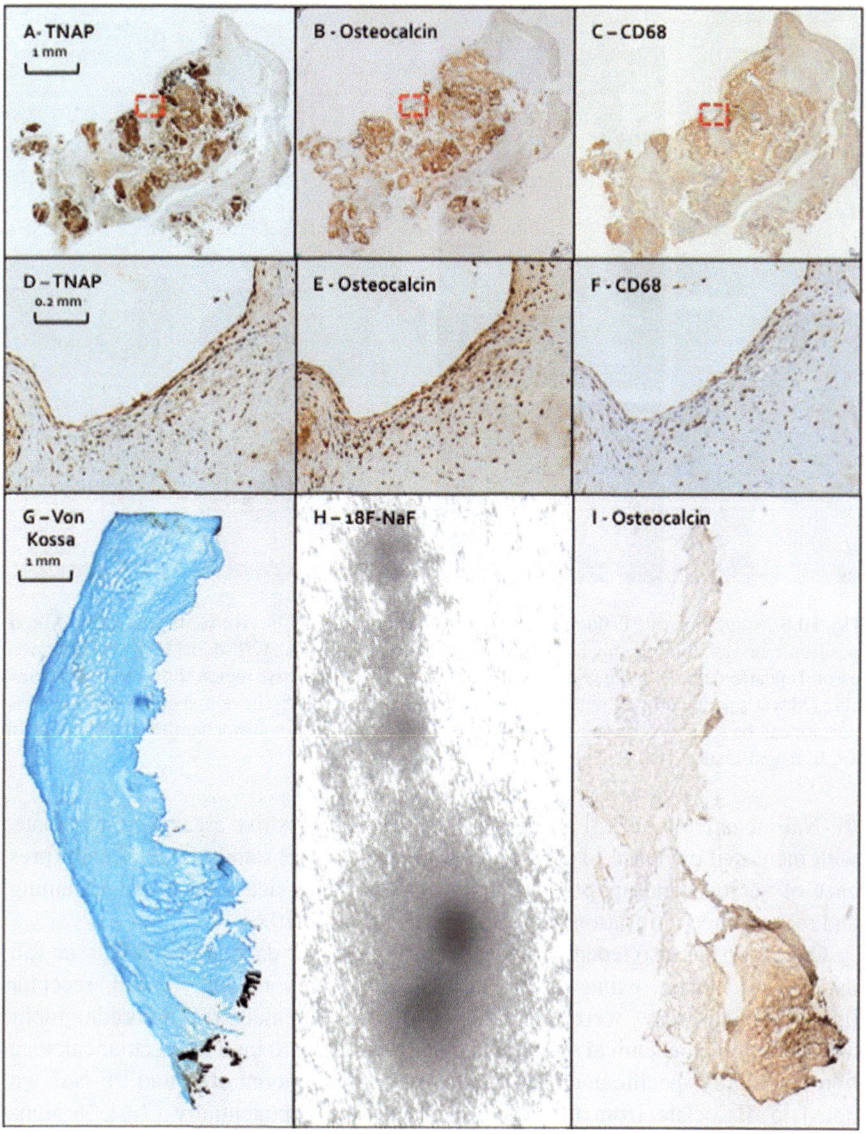

Fig. 10.5 Histological validation of ^{18}F-fluorodeoxyglucose and ^{18}F-fluoride uptake in the aortic valve. (**a**) Tissue non-specific alkaline phosphatase staining across the entire leaflet. (**b**) Osteocalcin staining across the entire leaflet. (**c**) CD68 staining across the entire leaflet. (**d**) Detail of (**a**) showing cellular staining. (**e**) Detail of (**b**). (**f**) Detail of (**c**) The *red* boxes in *A*, *B* and *C* are the areas magnified and shown in images *D*, *E* and *F* respectively. (**g**) Von Kossa stain of the leaflet (mineral stained black). (**h**) ^{18}F-fluoride autoradiography showing similar pattern of uptake as mineral staining in (**g**) and osteocalcin staining in (**i**). (**i**) Osteocalcin staining of the same leaflet as (**g**) and (**h**)

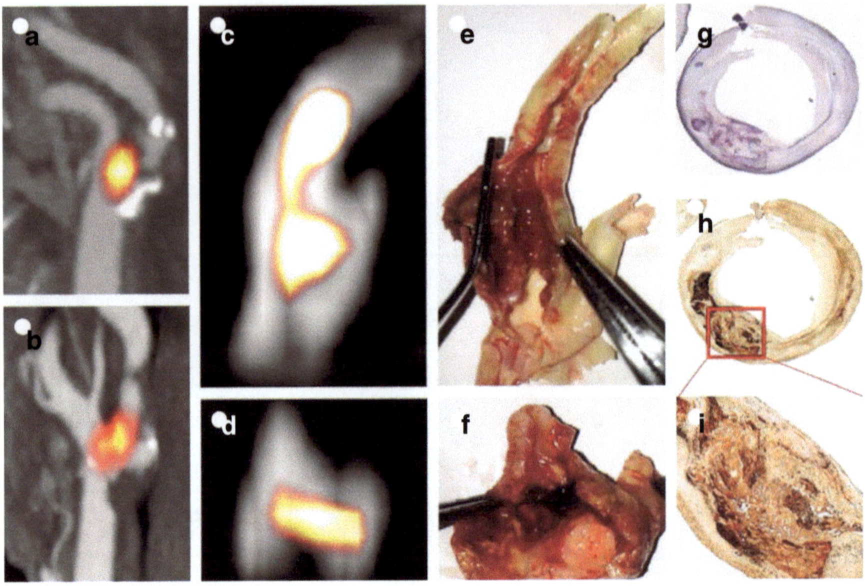

Fig. 10.6 Validation of ^{18}F-fluoride uptake in the carotid artery. In vivo (**a**, **b**) and ex vivo (**c**, **d**) positron-emission tomography and computed tomography images of ^{18}F-fluoride uptake in excised carotid endarterectomy tissue (**e**, **f**). Histology of the ^{18}F-NaF-positive region shows a large necrotic core (Movat's pentachrome) within which increased staining for tissue non-specific alkaline phosphatase can be seen as a marker of calcification activity on immunohistochemistry (magnification 4×, **h**; magnification 10×, **i**)

^{18}F-NaF-negative (control) areas of plaque, ^{18}F-NaF-positive areas were associated with increased evidence of calcification activity (TNAP staining), cell death (presence of necrosis and apoptotic activity as assayed by cleaved caspase-3 staining) and macrophage infiltration (CD68 staining) (see Fig. 10.6).

Our group has also recently presented further ex vivo data on ^{18}F-NaF tissue validation [54]. Again, using the carotid endarterectomy model, ^{18}F-NaF receptor-ligand binding assays were undertaken and complemented with autoradiographic and immunohistochemical studies. ^{18}F-NaF was shown to bind to vascular calcification in a highly specific and linear manner. A small amount of bound ^{18}F-NaF was noted to dissociate from the calcium and did so exponentially (7 ± 1 % signal decrease in 1 h, $t_{1/2}$ = 323 min). Immunohistochemistry and autoradiography showed that compared to large areas of field calcification, histological microcalcification (<5 μm; well beyond the resolution of CT) showed much greater ^{18}F-NaF binding. Indeed, only the outer surface of the blocks of field calcification showed ^{18}F-NaF binding, indicating that, as hypothesised, the interior of these large volume solid deposits is hidden from the fluoride ion. We also performed X-ray microanalysis to assay the ratio of calcium to fluoride following incubation with NaF; areas of microcalcification on electron microscopy showed significantly greater fluoride binding (Ca^{2+}/F^- = 2.4 ± 0.25 n = 10) than macro-calcification (Ca2+/F− 4.8 ± 0.33 n = 5). These results confirm that ^{18}F-NaF is a highly sensitive marker of tissue microcalcification (indicating active mineralisation) with very favourable pharmacodynamic characteristics for PET imaging.

10.5.3 Clinical Studies

To date, only two clinical studies have been published exploring the role of ^{18}F-NaF PET/CT imaging in CAVD [7,55]. Hyafil and colleagues employed a retrospective design looking at a small cohort ($n=5$) of oncological and rheumatological patients who happened to have a diagnosis of CAVD. A control cohort of ten patients without CAVD was randomly selected from the population who had undergone PET/CT. SUV_{max} and TBR_{max} values were obtained by drawing ROI around the aortic valve and within the right atrial lumen. Studies of intra- and inter-observer reliability were also undertaken. In our group's study, as described above, a cohort of 121 patients underwent ^{18}F-NaF PET/CT along with ^{18}F-FDG PET/CT and CT calcium scoring of the aortic valve.

10.5.4 Relationship Between ^{18}F-Fluoride and Lesion Severity

Both studies demonstrated that stenotic aortic valves showed considerably higher ^{18}F-NaF uptake than normal valves (see Fig. 10.4). Hyafil compared normal with severe: valvular TBR_{max} 1.5 (IQR 1.5–1.7) versus 2.2 (IQR 2.0–2.7), respectively. We recruited from across the CAVD severity spectrum, again demonstrating increased activity versus controls and a strong positive correlation (much stronger than for ^{18}F-FDG) between stenosis severity and all measures of ^{18}F-NaF uptake (see Table 10.2). This clear relationship remained if assessing severity by other echo parameters (time-velocity integral: $r^2=0.546$, $P<0.001$; aortic valve area: $r^2=0.387$, $P<0.001$; dimensionless index: $r^2=0.527$, $P<0.001$) or indeed by the aortic valve calcium score ($r^2=0.641$, $P<0.001$). However, as in the aorta, ^{18}F-NaF activity appeared to provide distinct and complementary information to CT calcium scoring, with regions of ^{18}F-NaF uptake frequently observed in the absence of underling calcium on CT and vice versa (Fig. 10.7).

10.5.5 Predicting Outcome and Disease Progression with ^{18}F-Fluoride

The critical determinant of whether ^{18}F-fluoride has a future role as a marker of aortic stenosis disease activity is whether it can predict disease progression and clinical outcomes.

We have recently published a 1-year outcome data [25] from a limited subgroup of our original cohort with exciting initial results. Eighteen patients with mild or moderate aortic stenosis were randomly selected to undergo repeat CT calcium scoring and clinical assessment at 1 year. Aortic valve calcium scores increased

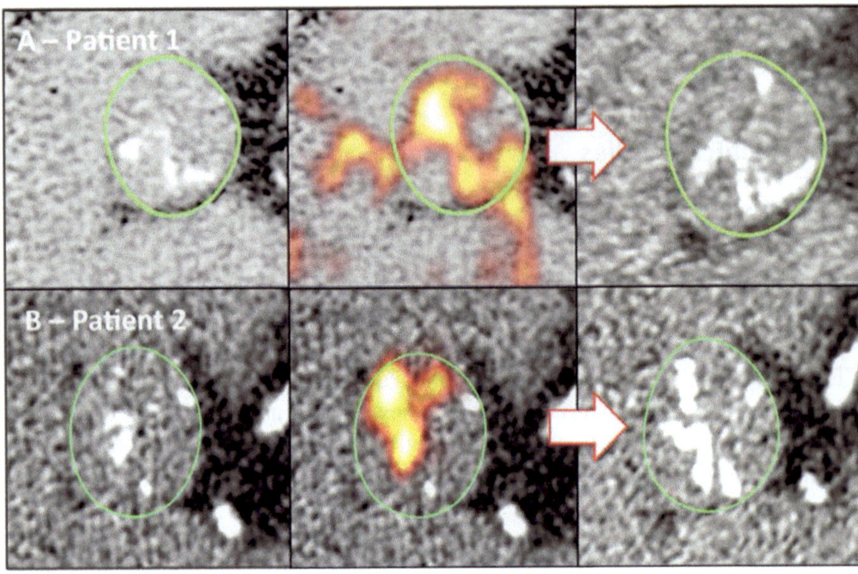

Fig. 10.7 Two examples (A and B) of baseline valvular computed tomography (*leftmost* panels) with positron-emission tomography data superimposed (*middle* panels) and 1 year valvular computed tomography (*rightmost* panels). The *green circles* are the regions of interest drawn around the aortic valve

from a median of 314 (IQR 193–540) to 365 (207–934) AU ($P<0.01$). Crucially, the distribution of new CT calcium matched that of the baseline ^{18}F-NaF uptake (Fig. 10.7), and accordingly, we observed an excellent correlation between baseline valvular ^{18}F-NaF PET uptake and the change in calcium score after 1 year ($r=0.66$, $P=0.003$). This was only slightly better than compared to the current gold standard, the baseline calcium score ($r=0.58$, $P=0.01$), but prediction improved further when only ^{18}F-NaF uptake in the absence of underlying CT calcium was assessed ($r=0.75$, $P=0.01$).

The longer-term follow-up from across our entire cohort will add to our knowledge as we shall also be able to assess the association between ^{18}F-NaF activity and changes in echocardiographic measures of disease severity.

10.5.6 Reproducibility and Methodological Strengths and Weaknesses

Hyafil's study reported on measurement reliability for both SUV_{max} and TBR_{max} and found these to be excellent: intra-observer ICC 0.99 (95 % CI 0.99–1.00) for SUV_{max}, 0.99 (95 % CI 0.93–0.99) for TBR_{max} and inter-observer 0.98 (95 % CI 0.96–0.99) for SUV_{max} and 0.97 (95 % CI 0.92–0.99) for TBR_{max}. These results closely match our own with all measures of ^{18}F-NaF uptake (SUV_{mean}, SUV_{max}, TBR_{mean} and TBR_{max}) demonstrating ICCs for intra- and inter-observer reproducibility >0.95. Furthermore, Bland-Altman analysis showed no fixed or proportional biases, with the majority of data points falling within narrow limits of agreement. These results were significantly better than those for ^{18}F-FDG, the discrepancy being explained by the lack of myocardial ^{18}F-NaF uptake.

Studies to date do have limitations. Hyafil's study provided proof of principle but was small and retrospective and involved patients having scans for indications other than cardiovascular disease. Furthermore, as with Marincheva-Savcheva's paper, PET/CT acquisition protocols were neither standardised nor optimised for cardiovascular imaging. Our study's limitations, as already discussed, pertain to a lack of ECG and respiratory gating as well as the difficulties in precisely measuring PET tracer uptake within small volumes of interest. The regions of interest for ^{18}F-fluoride were however significantly larger than for ^{18}F-FDG.

10.5.7 Summary

^{18}F-NaF PET/CT has considerable promise as a novel biomarker of disease activity in aortic stenosis. ^{18}F-NaF binds to calcium deposits in the aortic valve, and uptake is closely associated with histological markers of calcification activity. Moreover tracer uptake increases with disease severity and more importantly is able to predict disease progression at 1 year.

10.6 Conclusions and the Future

PET/CT imaging in CAVD is an exciting nascent research field with the results of early studies demonstrating clear promise. In particular, its ability to non-invasively quantify biological activity within the valve is likely to greatly enhance our understanding of the condition and our ability to test new therapies quickly. Ultimately therefore, it is hoped that this technique will accelerate our progress towards the development of an effective therapeutic intervention.

PET/CT is unlikely to replace echocardiography or CT calcium scoring, in the general assessment of patients with aortic stenosis given the clear advantages of these techniques with respect to cost, ionising radiation and ease of access. However, PET/CT provides complementary data to the anatomical information provided by these techniques acting as a useful marker of current disease activity in the valve. In particular, ^{18}F-NaF informs about calcification activity, which crucially appears to translate into novel areas of calcium in the valve at 1 year.

Large studies are required to confirm these findings but given that calcification appears to be the key process driving aortic stenosis progression, these early results would suggest that ^{18}F-NaF PET holds particular promise in two major areas: firstly, as a predictor of disease progression, (which is often highly variable and currently difficult to predict in the clinical arena) and, secondly, as a specific and early surrogate biomarker in trials of novel drug therapies. This approach has already been employed in the field of atherosclerosis [21,56–58], and it is our belief that similar studies could be used to detect an early treatment effect of therapies directed at calcification within the valve, informing the feasibility of larger and more expensive trials using clinical outcomes.

Why use ^{18}F-NaF and not ^{18}F-FDG given its greater track record in atherosclerosis? Although ^{18}F-FDG does correlate moderately with disease severity, the data on prediction of disease progression are less encouraging. Given that inflammation plays such a critical role in CAVD, its role should not yet be dismissed, but given the difficulties with lack of specificity and more importantly myocardial overspill, it may well be that, in the context of CAVD, an alternative PET marker of inflammation may prove more valuable. Certainly, for the time being, we believe that ^{18}F-NaF is better placed as the radioisotope to take forward; the data on outcome prediction and quantification reliability are undoubtedly stronger.

Acknowledgements We gratefully acknowledge the work of our group's collaborators in Cambridge University (Dr Anthony Davenport and Agnese Irkle) and thank them for sharing the data on the pharmacodynamics of ^{18}F-NaF binding in calcified vascular tissue.

References

1. Iung B, Baron G, Butchart EG, et al. A prospective survey of patients with valvular heart disease in Europe: the Euro heart survey on valvular heart disease. Eur Heart J. 2003;24:1231–43.
2. Nkomo VT, Gardin JM, Skelton TN, et al. Burden of valvular heart diseases: a population-based study. Lancet. 2006;368:1005–11. doi:10.1016/S0140-6736(06)69208-8.
3. Cowell SJ, Newby DE, Prescott RJ, et al. A randomized trial of intensive lipid-lowering therapy in calcific aortic stenosis. N Engl J Med. 2005;352:2389–97. doi:10.1056/NEJMoa043876.
4. Rossebø AB, Pedersen TR, Boman K, et al. Intensive lipid lowering with simvastatin and ezetimibe in aortic stenosis. N Engl J Med. 2008;359:1343–56. doi:10.1056/NEJMoa0804602.
5. Chan KL, Teo K, Dumesnil JG, et al. Effect of lipid lowering with rosuvastatin on progression of aortic stenosis: results of the Aortic Stenosis Progression Observation: Measuring Effects of Rosuvastatin (ASTRONOMER) trial. Circulation. 2010;121:306–14. doi:10.1161/CIRCULATIONAHA.109.900027.
6. Miller JD, Weiss RM, Heistad DD. Calcific aortic valve stenosis: methods, models, and mechanisms. Circ Res. 2011;108:1392–412. doi:10.1161/CIRCRESAHA.110.234138.
7. Dweck MR, Jones C, Joshi NV, et al. Assessment of valvular calcification and inflammation by positron emission tomography in patients with aortic stenosis. Circulation. 2012;125:76–86. doi:10.1161/CIRCULATIONAHA.111.051052.
8. New SEP, Aikawa E. Role of extracellular vesicles in de novo mineralization: an additional novel mechanism of cardiovascular calcification. Arterioscler Thromb Vasc Biol. 2013;33:1753–8. doi:10.1161/ATVBAHA.112.300128.
9. Dweck MR, Boon NA, Newby DE. Calcific aortic stenosis: a disease of the valve and the myocardium. J Am Coll Cardiol. 2012;60:1854–63. doi:10.1016/j.jacc.2012.02.093.
10. New SEP, Aikawa E. Cardiovascular calcification. Circ J. 2011;75:1305–13. doi:10.1253/circj.CJ-11-0395.
11. Reivich M, Kuhl D, Wolf A, et al. Measurement of local cerebral glucose metabolism in man with 18F-2-fluoro-2-deoxy-d-glucose. Acta Neurol Scand Suppl. 1977;64:190–1.
12. Rudd JHF. Imaging atherosclerotic plaque inflammation with [18F]-fluorodeoxyglucose positron emission tomography. Circulation. 2002;105:2708–11. doi:10.1161/01.CIR.0000020548.60110.76.
13. Fayad ZA, Mani V, Woodward M, et al. Safety and efficacy of dalcetrapib on atherosclerotic disease using novel non-invasive multimodality imaging (dal-PLAQUE): a randomised clinical trial. Lancet. 2011;378:1547–59. doi:10.1016/S0140-6736(11)61383-4.

14. Tawakol A, Migrino RQ, Hoffmann U, et al. Noninvasive in vivo measurement of vascular inflammation with F-18 fluorodeoxyglucose positron emission tomography. J Nucl Cardiol. 2005;12:294–301. doi:10.1016/j.nuclcard.2005.03.002.
15. Tawakol A, Migrino RQ, Bashian GG, et al. In vivo 18F-fluorodeoxyglucose positron emission tomography imaging provides a noninvasive measure of carotid plaque inflammation in patients. J Am Coll Cardiol. 2006;48:1818–24. doi:10.1016/j.jacc.2006.05.076.
16. Kaim AH, Weber B, Kurrer MO, et al. Autoradiographic quantification of 18F-FDG uptake in experimental soft-tissue abscesses in rats. Radiology. 2002;223:446–51. doi:10.1148/radiol.2232010914.
17. Babior BM. The respiratory burst of phagocytes. J Clin Invest. 1984;73:599–601. doi:10.1172/JCI111249.
18. Joshi F, Rosenbaum D, Bordes S, Rudd JHF. Vascular imaging with positron emission tomography. J Intern Med. 2011;270:99–109. doi:10.1111/j.1365-2796.2011.02392.x.
19. Folco EJ, Sheikine Y, Rocha VZ, et al. Hypoxia but not inflammation augments glucose uptake in human macrophages. J Am Coll Cardiol. 2011;58:603–14. doi:10.1016/j.jacc.2011.03.044.
20. Pedersen SF, Graebe M, Hag AMF, et al. 18F-FDG imaging of human atherosclerotic carotid plaques reflects gene expression of the key hypoxia marker HIF-1α. Am J Nucl Med Mol Imaging. 2013;3:384.
21. Tawakol A, Fayad ZA, Mogg R, et al. Intensification of statin therapy results in a rapid reduction in atherosclerotic inflammation: results of a multicenter fluorodeoxyglucose-positron emission tomography/computed tomography feasibility study. J Am Coll Cardiol. 2013;62:909–17. doi:10.1016/j.jacc.2013.04.066.
22. Marincheva-Savcheva G, Subramanian S, Qadir S, et al. Imaging of the aortic valve using fluorodeoxyglucose positron emission tomography increased valvular fluorodeoxyglucose uptake in aortic stenosis. J Am Coll Cardiol. 2011;57:2507–15. doi:10.1016/j.jacc.2010.12.046.
23. Agatston AS, Janowitz WR, Hildner FJ, et al. Quantification of coronary artery calcium using ultrafast computed tomography. J Am Coll Cardiol. 1990;15:827–32.
24. Aikawa E, Otto CM. Look more closely at the valve: imaging calcific aortic valve disease. Circulation. 2012;125:9–11. doi:10.1161/CIRCULATIONAHA.111.073452.
25. Dweck MR, Jenkins WSA, Vesey AT, et al. 18F-NaF uptake is a marker of active calcification and disease progression in patients with aortic stenosis. Circ Cardiovasc Imaging. 2014. doi:10.1161/CIRCIMAGING.113.001508.
26. Joshi NV, Vesey AT, Williams MC, et al. (18)F-fluoride positron emission tomography for identification of ruptured and high-risk coronary atherosclerotic plaques: a prospective clinical trial. Lancet. 2013. doi:10.1016/S0140-6736(13)61754-7.
27. Blau M, Ganatra R, Bender MA. 18F-fluoride for bone imaging. Semin Nucl Med. 1972;2:31–7.
28. Brenner W, Vernon C, Muzi M, et al. Comparison of different quantitative approaches to 18F-fluoride PET scans. J Nucl Med. 2004;45:1493–500.
29. Cook GJ, Lodge MA, Blake GM, et al. Differences in skeletal kinetics between vertebral and humeral bone measured by 18F-fluoride positron emission tomography in postmenopausal women. J Bone Miner Res. 2000;15:763–9. doi:10.1359/jbmr.2000.15.4.763.
30. Cook GJR, Blake GM, Marsden PK, et al. Quantification of skeletal kinetic indices in Paget's disease using Dynamic 18F-fluoride positron emission tomography. J Bone Miner Res. 2002;17:854–9. doi:10.1359/jbmr.2002.17.5.854.
31. Even-Sapir E, Mishani E, Flusser G, Metser U. 18F-fluoride positron emission tomography and positron emission tomography/computed tomography. Semin Nucl Med. 2007;37:462–9. doi:10.1053/j.semnuclmed.2007.07.002.
32. Frost ML, Blake GM, Park-Holohan SJ, et al. Long-term precision of 18F-fluoride PET skeletal kinetic studies in the assessment of bone metabolism. J Nucl Med. 2008;49:700–7. doi:10.2967/jnumed.107.046987.
33. Frost ML, Cook GJR, Blake GM, et al. A prospective study of risedronate on regional bone metabolism and blood flow at the lumbar spine measured by 18F-fluoride positron emission tomography. J Bone Miner Res. 2003;18:2215–22. doi:10.1359/jbmr.2003.18.12.2215.
34. Frost ML, Cook GJR, Blake GM, et al. The relationship between regional bone turnover measured using 18F-fluoride positron emission tomography and changes in BMD is equivalent to

that seen for biochemical markers of bone turnover. J Clin Densitom. 2007;10:46–54. doi:10.1016/j.jocd.2006.10.006.
35. Frost ML, Fogelman I, Blake GM, et al. Dissociation between global markers of bone formation and direct measurement of spinal bone formation in osteoporosis. J Bone Miner Res. 2004;19:1797–804. doi:10.1359/JBMR.040818.
36. Hawkins RA, Choi Y, Huang SC, et al. Evaluation of the skeletal kinetics of fluorine-18-fluoride ion with PET. J Nucl Med. 1992;33:633–42.
37. Installe J, Nzeusseu A, Bol A, et al. F-18-fluoride PET for monitoring therapeutic response in Paget's disease of bone. J Nucl Med. 2005;46:1650–8.
38. Messa C, Goodman WG, Hoh CK, et al. Bone metabolic activity measured with positron emission tomography and [18F]fluoride ion in renal osteodystrophy: correlation with bone histomorphometry. J Clin Endocrinol Metab. 1993;77:949–55. doi:10.1210/jcem.77.4.8408470.
39. Piert M, Zittel TT, Becker GA, et al. Assessment of porcine bone metabolism by dynamic [F-18] fluoride ion PET: Correlation with bone histomorphometry. J Nucl Med. 2001;42:1091–100.
40. Piert M, Zittel TT, Jahn M, et al. Increased sensitivity in detection of a porcine high-turnover osteopenia after total gastrectomy by dynamic 18F-fluoride ion PET and quantitative CT. J Nucl Med. 2003;44:117–24.
41. Schiepers C, Nuyts J, Bormans G, et al. Fluoride kinetics of the axial skeleton measured in vivo with fluorine-18-fluoride PET. J Nucl Med. 1997;38:1970–6.
42. Sörensen J, Ullmark G. PET scanning for evaluation of bone metabolism. Acta Orthop. 2009;80:738–9.
43. Ullmark G, Sörensen J, Nilsson O. Bone healing of severe acetabular defects after revision arthroplasty. Acta Orthop. 2009;80:179–83. doi:10.3109/17453670902947416.
44. Czernin J, Satyamurthy N, Schiepers C. Molecular mechanisms of bone 18F-NaF deposition. J Nucl Med. 2010;51:1826–9. doi:10.2967/jnumed.110.077933.
45. Foldager CB, Bendtsen M, Bünger C. PET scanning for evaluation of bone metabolism. Acta Orthop. 2009;80:737–8. doi:10.3109/17453670903487040; author reply 738–9.
46. Derlin T, Richter U, Bannas P, et al. Feasibility of 18F-sodium fluoride PET/CT for imaging of atherosclerotic plaque. J Nucl Med. 2010;51:862–5. doi:10.2967/jnumed.110.076471.
47. Derlin T, Wisotzki C, Richter U, et al. In vivo imaging of mineral deposition in carotid plaque using 18F-sodium fluoride PET/CT: correlation with atherogenic risk factors. J Nucl Med. 2011;52:362–8. doi:10.2967/jnumed.110.081208.
48. Aikawa E, Nahrendorf M, Figueiredo J-L, et al. Osteogenesis associates with inflammation in early-stage atherosclerosis evaluated by molecular imaging in vivo. Circulation. 2007;116:2841–50. doi:10.1161/CIRCULATIONAHA.107.732867.
49. Bobryshev YV, Killingsworth MC, Huynh TG, et al. Are calcifying matrix vesicles in atherosclerotic lesions of cellular origin? Basic Res Cardiol. 2006;102:133–43. doi:10.1007/s00395-006-0637-9.
50. Golub EE. Biomineralization and matrix vesicles in biology and pathology. Semin Immunopathol. 2010;33:409–17. doi:10.1007/s00281-010-0230-z.
51. Proudfoot D, Skepper JN, Hegyi L, et al. Apoptosis regulates human vascular calcification in vitro: evidence for initiation of vascular calcification by apoptotic bodies. Circ Res. 2000;87:1055–62.
52. Demer LL, Tintut Y. Vascular calcification: pathobiology of a multifaceted disease. Circulation. 2008;117:2938–48. doi:10.1161/CIRCULATIONAHA.107.743161.
53. Shanahan CM, Crouthamel MH, Kapustin A, Giachelli CM. Arterial calcification in chronic kidney disease: key roles for calcium and phosphate. Circ Res. 2011;109:697–711. doi:10.1161/CIRCRESAHA.110.234914.
54. Irkle A, Bird JL, Dweck MR, et al. 18F-NaF – a specific marker for vascular calcification in atherosclerosis. Paper presented at the American Heart Association Scientific Sessions, Dallas, 2013 p. 1–2.
55. Hyafil F, Messika-Zeitoun D, Burg S, et al. Detection of 18Fluoride sodium accumulation by positron emission tomography in calcified stenotic aortic valves. Am J Cardiol. 2012;109:1194–6. doi:10.1016/j.amjcard.2011.11.060.

56. Fayad ZA, Mani V, Woodward M, et al. Rationale and design of dal-PLAQUE: a study assessing efficacy and safety of dalcetrapib on progression or regression of atherosclerosis using magnetic resonance imaging and 18F-fluorodeoxyglucose positron emission tomography/computed tomography. Am Heart J. 2011;162:214–21.e2. doi:10.1016/j.ahj.2011.05.006.
57. Potter K, Lenzo N, Eikelboom JW, et al. Effect of long-term homocysteine reduction with B vitamins on arterial wall inflammation assessed by fluorodeoxyglucose positron emission tomography: a randomised double-blind, placebo-controlled trial. Cerebrovasc Dis. 2009;27:259–65. doi:10.1159/000199463.
58. Tahara N, Kai H, Ishibashi M, et al. Simvastatin attenuates plaque inflammation. J Am Coll Cardiol. 2006;48:1825–31. doi:10.1016/j.jacc.2006.03.069.

Ultrasound Imaging of Calcific Aortic Valve Disease

11

Jason P. Linefsky and Catherine M. Otto

Contents

Abstract

Echocardiography remains the primary diagnostic test in clinical practice for evaluation of CAVD and for entry criteria and end points in clinical research trials. The clinical paradigm is changing for earlier interventions in asymptomatic severe AS with the improvement in surgical care and the advent of transcutaneous aortic valve replacement. Novel echocardiographic methods hold

J.P. Linefsky, MD, MS
Division of Cardiology, Emory University School of Medicine, Atlanta, GA, USA
e-mail: jason.linefsky@emory.edu

C.M. Otto, MD (✉)
J. Ward Kennedy-Hamilton Endowed Chair in Cardiology,
University of Washington School of Medicine, Seattle, WA, USA
e-mail: cmotto@u.washington.edu

E. Aikawa (ed.), *Cardiovascular Imaging: Arterial and Aortic Valve Inflammation and Calcification*, DOI 10.1007/978-3-319-09268-3_11

promise to help identify those that will benefit from early intervention. Although current therapies are invasive, development of potential medical therapies for CAVD may be on the horizon and will rely on echocardiography to demonstrate efficacy.

11.1 Introduction

Ultrasound is the primary clinical imaging modality for evaluation of calcific aortic valve disease (CAVD). Cardiac ultrasound imaging, more commonly known as echocardiography, is widely available and portable and does not produce ionizing radiation allowing for safe serial evaluations. A real-time noninvasive assessment of aortic valve anatomy, hemodynamics, and prognosis can be obtained in most patients making echocardiography the principal tool for clinical decision-making. Similar to other imaging modalities, echocardiographic image quality continues to improve with advances in technology. New modalities such as three-dimensional (3D) echocardiography and speckle-tracking strain imaging provide additional diagnostic information.

11.2 Echocardiography Evaluation of CAVD Severity

11.2.1 Anatomy

Assessment of the aortic valve begins with two-dimensional (2D) transthoracic echocardiogram (TTE) of the aortic valve from parasternal long- and short-axis images. Parasternal images are obtained with the transducer at the left third or fourth intercostal space close to the sternum with the subject either supine or in a left lateral decubitus position. The long-axis plane is parallel to the left ventricular long axis intersecting the aortic valve at its center. From this view, the aortic root, right and noncoronary cusps, and attachment of the cusps to the annulus in the left ventricular outflow tract can be easily identified. Normal aortic valve leaflets are thin and open widely in systole, but in CAVD, thickening and calcification of the leaflets is readily seen and provides the first evidence of pathological changes (Fig. 11.1).

Rotating the transducer clockwise approximately 90° will image the parasternal short axis. The transducer angle should be adjusted to the aortic valve level to view the aortic cusps in the center of the image. From this view all three leaflets can be identified as well as congenital abnormalities such as a bicuspid valve. Normal valves should appear thin and open freely into a circular orifice during systole. In CAVD, calcification of the individual leaflets and annulus can be identified as well as valve thickening or reduced systolic opening. A bicuspid valve can be identified by demonstrating only two leaflets during systole; frequently a prominent raphe can make distinction of a bicuspid from tricuspid valve difficult during diastole when the valve is closed and calcified. Other distinctive features for a congenital bicuspid valve may include systolic doming, elliptical-shaped systolic orifice, and a central

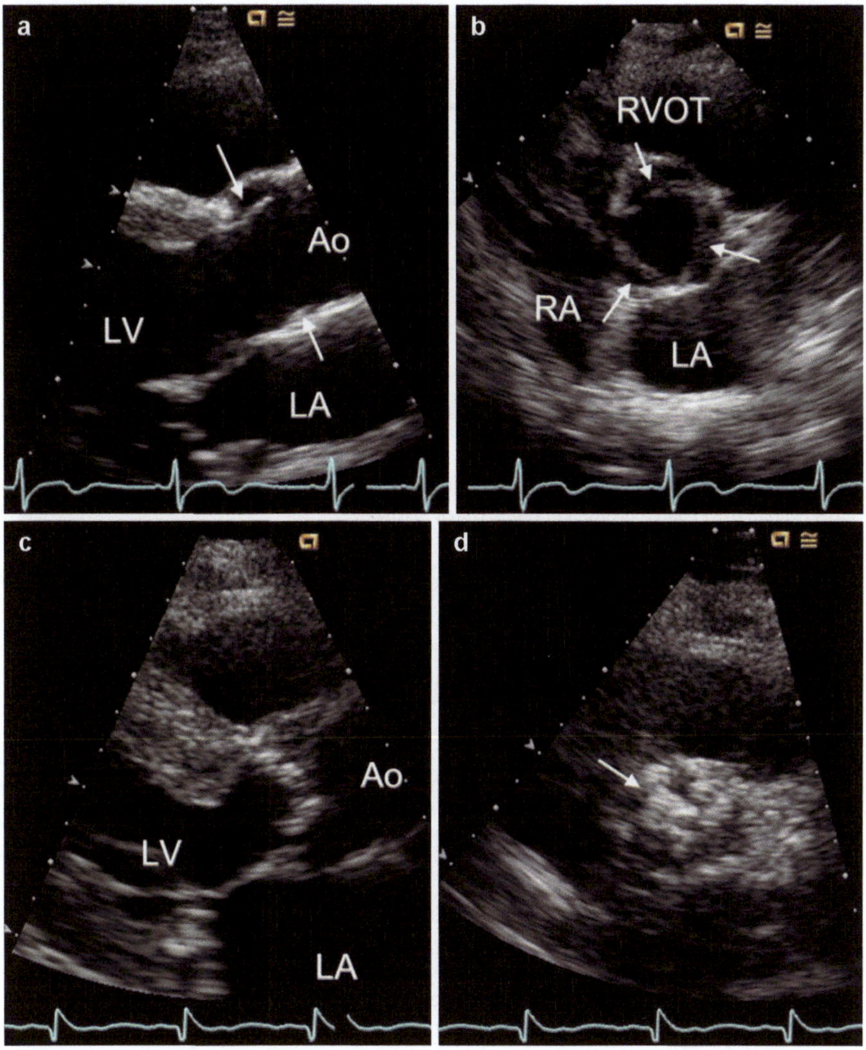

Fig. 11.1 Normal trileaflet aortic valve in parasternal long-axis view (**a**) and parasternal short-axis view (**b**). Severe calcific aortic valve disease is shown at the *bottom panels* (**c**, **d**) from the same views. *Arrows* point to aortic valve leaflets which are thin and have wide systolic opening in the normal valve but are heavily calcified with restricted systolic opening in advanced disease. Also evident is the increased left ventricular thickness in the parasternal view (**c**) compared to a patient with a normal aortic valve (**a**)

to commissural opening pattern. A bicuspid valve is found in approximately 1 % of the general population as reported in autopsy and echocardiographic series, but the prevalence is higher in those with other congenital abnormalities such as Turner syndrome or coarctation of the aorta. Rheumatic disease can lead to aortic stenosis

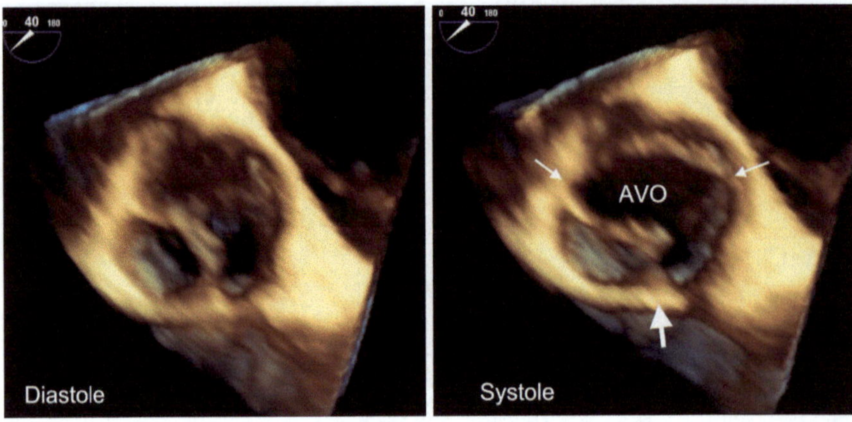

Fig. 11.2 A 3D TEE view from the aortic side of the valve appears tricuspid in diastole (**a**) but can be diagnosed as bicuspid in systole (**b**) with an oval aortic valve orifice (AVO) and two commissures (*thin arrows*) and a prominent raphe (*thick arrow*)

but is a distinct pathological process. Distinct echocardiographic features of rheumatic disease include commissural fusion and mitral valve involvement.

When transthoracic image quality is too poor to identify the etiology of the aortic valve disease, a transesophageal echocardiogram (TEE) can be performed. TEE provides higher resolution imaging than TTE, and images of the aortic valve can be obtained almost universally. However, TEE is a second-line choice for echocardiographic imaging in most situations as it carries procedural risk due to probe insertion into the esophagus and conscious sedation. The aortic valve can be imaged in long-axis and short-axis views from a high esophageal probe position at about 120° and 45° of rotation angle, respectively. The improved imaging resolution can help identify the correct number of aortic cusps, the anatomic orifice area at the leaflet tips, or any associated subvalvular or aortic root anomalies not identified by TTE. TEE imaging also allows 3D imaging of the valve which is helpful in distinguishing a bicuspid from a trileaflet valve (Fig. 11.2).

11.2.2 Velocity and Pressure Gradients

Doppler echocardiography allows measurement of various hemodynamic parameters that are important for the evaluation of CAVD severity (Table 11.1). By measuring backscatter ultrasound frequency changes due to movement of red blood cells, blood flow velocity can be accurately measured using the Doppler equation [1]. Normal aortic transvalvular blood flow is laminar and unobstructed with a peak aortic jet velocity (V_{max}) between 1 and 2 m/s. In CAVD, as the aortic valve orifice narrows, the peak aortic velocity increases. Measuring V_{max} requires a continuous-wave (CW) Doppler probe that is parallel to the direction of blood flow. Recorded velocities are displayed as a velocity curve with velocity on the vertical axis over

Table 11.1 Calcific aortic valve disease echocardiographic measurements

	Strengths	Weaknesses
Peak aortic jet velocity	Easy to measure	Underestimates severity in low-flow states
	Strongly associated with outcomes	Overestimate severity if significant pressure recovery
Mean gradient	Same as peak aortic jet velocity	Same as peak aortic jet velocity
Effective aortic valve area (continuity equation)	Well validated with catheter-based valve areas	Highly dependent on LVOT diameter measurements
	Less flow dependent than peak velocity or mean gradient	Severity can be overestimated in significantly impaired flow states
Anatomic aortic valve area (planimetry)	Does not require Doppler echocardiography	Calcification limits visualization of anatomic orifice
		Irregular 3D orifice areas can lead to over- or underestimation on 2D imaging
		Not as well studied as effective aortic valve area for CAVD outcomes
Velocity ratio	Simple to measure	Not validated with clinical outcomes
	Indirectly accounts for body size	May under- or overestimate severity with incorrect LVOT sample placement
	Does not require measurement of LVOT diameter	
Valvuloarterial impedance	Global assessment of ventricular load	Requires multiple measurements to calculate compounding potential measurement errors
	Accounts for hypertension and stroke volume	
Energy loss index	Accounts for pressure recovery	Requires multiple measurements
	Improved severity estimation with small body types	Indexing to body surface area can overestimate severity in large body types
	Less flow dependent than peak velocity and mean gradient	Severity can be overestimated in significantly impaired flow states
Valve calcification	Does not require Doppler	Mostly qualitative assessment
	Strongly associated with valvular outcomes	Weakly correlates with hemodynamics

LVOT left ventricular outflow tract

time on the horizontal axis. In CAVD, irregular opening of the valve can lead to an unpredictable direction of the maximum blood flow velocity; thus, a thorough TTE Doppler evaluation requires searching for the highest velocity in multiple acoustic windows from the apical, parasternal, subcostal, and suprasternal transducer positions. TEE probe positions are constrained, and thus measuring aortic velocities can be frequently underestimated from misalignment.

Under certain assumptions that are generally met in the clinical setting, instantaneous transvalvular pressure gradients (ΔP) can be estimated from measured aortic jet velocities (v) using the simplified Bernoulli equation, $\Delta P = 4v^2$. A mean gradient can be obtained easily with commercial echo packages by averaging the instantaneous gradients over the duration of the systolic ejection period. Mean gradients calculated by Doppler measurements have been shown to have strong correlation with mean gradients obtained during catheterization [2, 3].

Transaortic valve velocity and pressure gradients can determine the presence of hemodynamically important aortic stenosis and categorize the severity into mild, moderate, or severe [4]. Although these parameters are easily measured with good reproducibility, there are potential pitfalls with measurement and interpretation that need to be avoided. First, optimal Doppler measurements require the intercept angle of the ultrasound beam to be as parallel as possible to the direction of blood flow. Nonparallel alignment will lead to underestimation of the velocity and pressure gradient. Measurements should be averaged over at least 3 beats in sinus rhythm and more if in an irregular rhythm; care should be taken to avoid measurement of post-extrasystolic beats. Assumptions of the simplified Bernoulli equation may not be met if there are very high velocities present in the left ventricular outflow tract (>1.5 m/s) or abnormalities of blood viscosity from profound anemia or polycythemia. Finally, velocity and pressure gradients are heavily flow-dependent measures. To avoid erroneous CAVD severity assessment, a high or low transaortic flow state and aortic valve area (AVA) need to be assessed.

11.2.3 Aortic Valve Area

The AVA can be estimated using the continuity equation which states that stroke volume through the left ventricular outflow tract (LVOT) is the same as the stroke volume through the aortic valve, $SV_{LVOT} = SV_{AV}$. Proximal to the stenotic valve, blood flow is laminar which allows calculation of stroke volume as $SV = CSA \times VTI$, where CSA is the cross-sectional area of the flow and VTI is the velocity-time integral (area under the velocity curve). Substituting and rearranging the above equations provides the formula $AVA = (CSA_{LVOT} \times VTI_{LVOT})/VTI_{Ao}$. A simplified continuity equation substituting peak velocity (V) for VTI can be applied, $AVA = (CSA_{LVOT} \times V_{LVOT})/V_{max}$, because the shape and timing of the outflow tract and aortic jet velocity curves are similar. The cross-sectional area of the LVOT can be approximated from a zoomed in 2D TTE parasternal long-axis view. The diameter (D) of the LVOT is measured during mid-systole from the inner edge of the septal myocardium to the inner edge of the anterior mitral leaflet at the aortic cusp insertion points (Fig. 11.3a). By assuming a circular LVOT, the $CSA_{LVOT} = \pi(D/2)^2$. This is an adequate assumption for stroke volume calculation with numerous studies validating continuity equation valve area with catheter-based valve area [5–7]. However, the actual LVOT is frequently more oval than round, which is important to account for in transcatheter aortic valve replacement (TAVR) which relies on 3D

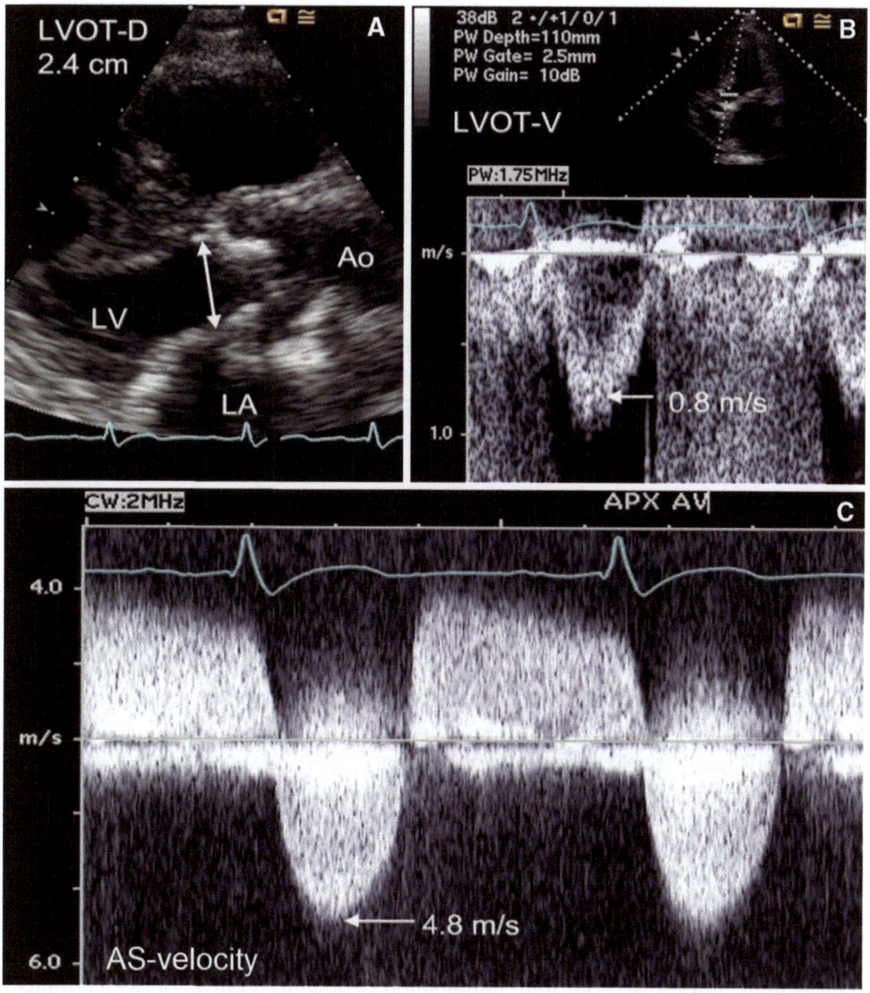

Fig. 11.3 Measurement of aortic valve area (*AVA*) in a patient with severe aortic stenosis. The left ventricular outflow tract (*LVOT*) dimension measuring 2.4 cm in a zoomed parasternal long-axis view (*Panel A*). Pulsed-wave Doppler shows a peak LVOT velocity of 0.8 m/s (*Panel B*), and continuous-wave Doppler through the aortic valve reveals a V_{max} of 4.8 m/s (*Panel C*). The aortic valve area is severely reduced at 0.75 cm^2 using the simplified continuity equation

imaging measurements, either by computed tomography (CT) or TEE, of area and eccentricity to minimize complications [8].

Measurement of the peak velocities and VTI requires that the Doppler beam have a parallel alignment with the blood flow. This is achieved with the transducer in the apical position. To obtain the velocity curve at a specific location such as the LVOT, a pulsed-wave (PW) Doppler signal is needed. The PW Doppler allows placement of a sample volume on the ventricular side of the aortic valve at the same location where the LVOT diameter is measured. Velocities are recorded over time at the location of the sample volume, and velocity curves are produced on the spectral Doppler display. The V_{LVOT} and VTI_{LVOT} are measured by tracing the modal velocity (brightest or most dense) portion of the spectral tracing (Fig. 11.3b) [1]. The V_{max} and VTI_{Ao} through the aortic valve are measured from tracing the outer edge of the velocity curve from the maximum aortic jet obtained from the CW Doppler (Fig. 11.3c). Gain should be adjusted to produce a dark envelope around the spectral velocity curve with careful attention to avoid measuring the faint signal broadening produced from the transit-time effect of the ultrasound signal.

Alternative echocardiographic approaches can be used to estimate valve area when the continuity equation AVA appears discrepant to clinical findings or the above parameters cannot be obtained due to poor image quality. Planimetry in a short-axis view to measure the anatomic (geometric) orifice area can be performed [9, 10]. This can be limited if using 2D TTE due to difficulty obtaining an accurate planar image of an irregular 3D valve orifice. Additionally, poor image resolution and calcification artifacts can lead to inaccurate tracing of the valve area. When TTE quality is suboptimal, a TEE can be used to measure the LVOT diameter from a high esophageal probe position angled between 120 and 150°. The high-resolution and multiplane imaging capability of TEE also allows for improved planimetry of the valve area [11] but can still suffer from similar difficult visualization problems in advanced CAVD [12]. The anatomic valve area when correctly measured from planimetry is expected to be slightly larger than the effective orifice area calculated from the continuity equation due to contraction of the flow stream through a narrowing orifice [13].

New advances in 3D echocardiography may improve valve area estimation by overcoming some inherent limitations of 2D imaging. Improved planimetry has been demonstrated by allowing accurate determination of the narrowest valve plane to measure and has shown good correlation with Doppler-derived and catheter-derived valve areas (Fig. 11.4) [14]. 3D echocardiography may also produce a more accurate estimation of stroke volume from either directly measuring LVOT area [15], using real-time 3D ventricular volumes [16], or calculating color Doppler flow-volume curves [17]. Despite initial studies showing promise of 3D techniques improving AVA estimation, 2D Doppler-based continuity equation remains the echo gold standard until further studies demonstrate that 3D techniques are clinically reproducible and are associated with outcomes.

11.2.4 Additional Measurements of Hemodynamic Severity

Traditional markers of hemodynamic severity (peak aortic jet velocity, mean gradient, and aortic valve area) may not always correlate with each other, clinical symptoms, left ventricular function, or outcomes. To resolve discrepancies, additional severity indices have been suggested that may help improve CAVD classification. A simple measure is the velocity ratio (or dimensionless index) defined as V_{LVOT}/V_{max}, where V_{LVOT} is the peak velocity obtained in the LVOT from the PW Doppler and V_{max} is the peak aortic jet velocity as described in the previous sections. The ratio avoids

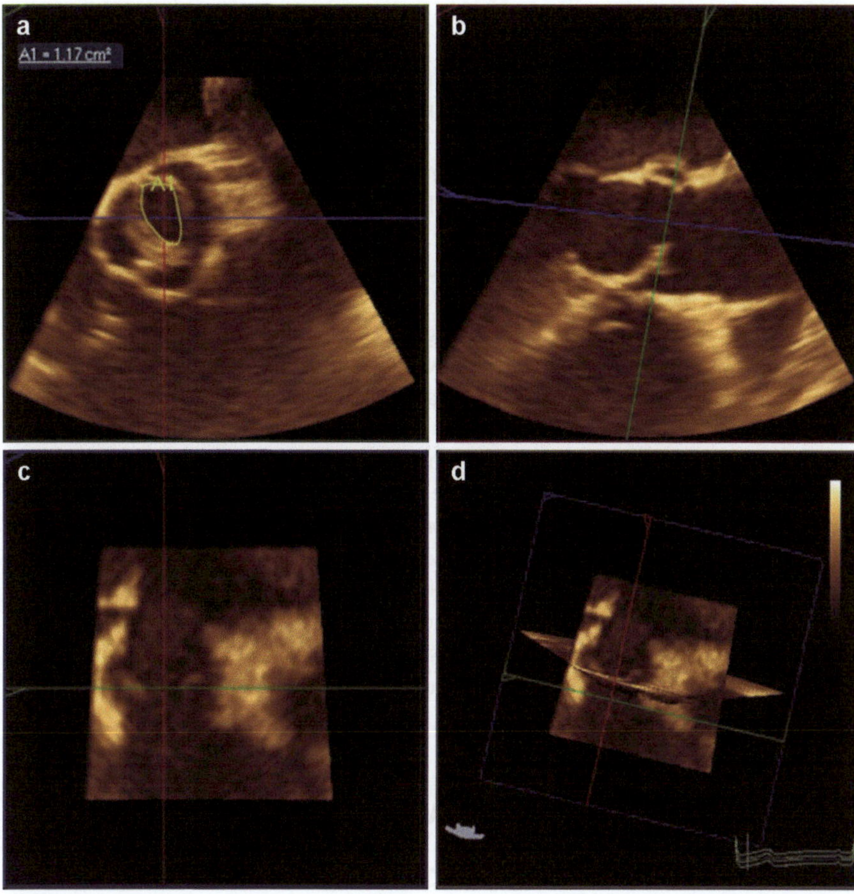

Fig. 11.4 Planimetry of the anatomic orifice valve area of a bicuspid valve using 3D echocardiography. Correct position at the leaflet tips in the transverse view (**a**) can be confirmed with 3D imaging by simultaneously viewing the perpendicular sagittal (**b**) and coronal (**c**) plane views. Note the systolic doming of the bicuspid valve in the long-axis (sagittal plane) view (**b**)

errors in the LVOT area estimation which may be significant due to the LVOT diameter measurement being squared in the area equation.

In small individuals, the indexed AVA may be appropriate to use, AVA/body surface area (BSA), as a person with a small body type (height <135 cm, BSA<1.5 m^2, body mass index (BMI) <22) may have a small but normal LVOT, AVA, and aorta. Indexing the valve area may reclassify smaller individuals from severe to moderate aortic stenosis (AS), but indexing all patients, particularly with extreme obesity, can lead to substantial overestimation of severity and should not be relied upon [18].

Another issue common to small body types and aortas is the concept of pressure recovery, the reconversion of kinetic energy into potential energy leading to an increase of pressure downstream from a stenosis. Doppler-derived pressure gradients represent the difference between left ventricular pressure and pressure in the vena contracta (lowest pressure in a stenosis), but do not measure the pressure recovery phenomena captured by a catheterization-based gradient (net pressure gradient). Pressure recovery accounts for differences between catheter- and Doppler-derived data [19, 20]. The net pressure gradient better reflects the hemodynamic significance and the amount of energy loss by the stenosis. To account for pressure recovery using echocardiography, Garcia and colleagues developed and validated the energy loss index $(\mathrm{ELI}) = [\mathrm{EOA} \times A_a/(A_a - \mathrm{EOA})]/\mathrm{BSA}$, where EOA is the effective orifice area using the Doppler-based continuity equation valve area and A_a represents the cross-sectional area of the aorta measured at 1 cm downstream of the sinotubular junction [21]. The ELI can be considered in situations when pressure recovery may be significant, such as individuals with aortic diameters <3 cm. The ELI has been shown to reclassify CAVD severity and provide independent and prognostic information above traditional severity measures [22, 23].

Hypertension is common in CAVD and can adversely affect hemodynamics, symptom burden, and traditional echo measure assessment [24–26]. To account for the "double load" of hypertension and aortic stenosis on the left ventricle, calculation of the valvuloarterial impedance (Z_{va}) can be obtained using the equation $Z_{va} = (\mathrm{SBP} + \mathrm{MG}_{net})/\mathrm{SVi}$, where SBP is the systolic blood pressure, MG_{net} is the mean net pressure gradient (taking into account pressure recovery), and SVi is the stroke volume indexed for BSA [27]. This global measure of vascular, valvular, and ventricular interplay may improve risk stratification in patients with asymptomatic moderate to severe CAVD [28].

11.3 Echocardiography and CAVD Outcomes

11.3.1 Aortic Valve Sclerosis and Cardiovascular Outcomes

Evidence of early CAVD, aortic valve sclerosis (AVS), can be detected by echocardiography as thickening and calcification of the aortic valve without obstruction to left ventricular outflow. The precise definition of AVS in clinical studies has varied using different qualitative descriptions of thickening, calcification, and cutoffs for hemodynamic significance. This lack of uniformity can lead to interobserver variability for diagnosing AVS between echocardiographers in the clinical setting [29]. Additionally, instrument settings can alter the interpretation of aortic valve thickening. The use of tissue harmonic over fundamental imaging has been demonstrated to significantly increase the diagnosis and severity of AVS [30]. Calcification of the aortic valve leaflets appears as bright focal echodensities and is most often qualitatively graded as mild (small isolated spots), moderate (multiple larger spots), or severe (extensive involving all cusps). In an effort to quantify valve thickening and calcification, measurement of ultrasound backscatter amplitude from aortic valves has demonstrated feasibility and reproducibility in animal models and small samples of elderly volunteers [31–33]. However, the value of backscatter quantification over qualitative assessment in longitudinal studies has yet to be evaluated and is not practiced in clinical settings.

Despite the potential heterogeneity of diagnosis, AVS has consistently been associated with cardiovascular outcomes. Whether the increased risk is due in part to a direct mechanistic effect from CAVD or only a marker of cardiovascular disease remains unresolved. CAVD is a progressive condition and longitudinal echocardiographic studies have shown AVS progression to hemodynamically significant AS. In a study of 400 subjects with AVS by Faggiano et al. [34], 33 % developed some degree of AS over a mean follow-up of 44 months. In the subgroup with over 5 years of follow-up, 22 % advanced to either moderate or severe AS. In a larger confirmatory study by Cosmi et al. [35], 2,131 patients diagnosed with valve thickening that had serial echocardiograms were evaluated for hemodynamic progression. These investigators found that 5.4 % of their AVS patients advanced to moderate or severe AS over a mean of 7.4 years; mitral annular calcification was the only identified risk factor for progression in multivariable modeling. Similarly, in an elderly population-based cohort in the Cardiovascular Health Study, 9 % of the 1,610 participants with baseline AVS developed AS over a 5-year period [36].

The association of early CAVD with the short-term risk of cardiovascular outcomes cannot be fully explained from the relatively slow progression to hemodynamically significant AS. Multiple echo studies have identified similar cardiovascular risk factors between coronary artery disease (CAD) and CAVD, including age, male sex, hypertension, diabetes, low-density lipoprotein cholesterol, and smoking [37–40]. In Cardiovascular Health Study participants with baseline AVS and no known CAD, cardiovascular death risk was increased by 52 % and myocardial infarction risk by 40 %, even after adjustment for traditional cardiovascular risk factors [41]. Subsequent studies have attributed some of the increased risk to concomitant CAD and inflammation [42, 43].

11.3.2 Aortic Stenosis and Valvular Outcomes

In patients with hemodynamically significant CAVD, progression to symptoms, aortic valve replacement (AVR), and death have been studied by several approaches. The natural history of aortic stenosis was first defined in autopsy series prior to the use of echocardiography [44]. These initial series described a long latent asymptomatic phase of disease that would eventually lead to symptoms (angina pectoris, syncope, and heart failure) which herald a poor prognosis. Over 75 years later, the prognosis of uncorrected symptomatic severe aortic stenosis remains dismal with a reported 68 % mortality over 2 years [45]. AVR is currently the only intervention known to reduce adverse clinical outcomes in symptomatic severe AS.

Echocardiographic studies have established predictors of clinical outcomes in patients with asymptomatic aortic stenosis (Table 11.2). Hemodynamic severity by TTE is the cornerstone of predicting valvular outcomes in AS. V_{max} is most

Table 11.2 Echocardiographic predictors of calcific aortic valve disease outcomes

Study	Year	*N*	Follow-up[a] (months)	Echo measurement	Outcome	Results
Pellikka [46]	1990	143	21	V_{max} ≥4.5 m/s	AVR or cardiac death	RR 4.9 (95 % CI, 1.64–14.6; $p=0.004$)
Otto [47]	1997	123	30	V_{max}	AVR or death	Categorized event rates at 2 years of 79 % (>4 m/s), 34 % (3–4 m/s), and 16 % (<3 m/s); $p<0.001$
Rosenhek [50]	2000	128	22	Calcification score (3 or 4)	AVR or death	RR 4.6 (95 % CI, 1.6–14; $p<0.01$)
Rosenhek [51]	2004	176	48	V_{max} ≥3 m/s calcification score (3 or 4)	AVR or death	RR 1.6 (95 % CI, 1.04–2.8; $p=0.034$)
						RR 2.0 (95 % CI, 1.3–3.3; $p=0.0012$)
Pellikka [48]	2005	622	65	AVA (per 0.2 cm^2)	Symptoms	RR 1.26 (95 % CI, 1.08–1.47; $p=0.004$)
				V_{max} (per 1 m/s)	AVR or cardiac death	RR 1.20 (95 % CI, 1.06–1.36; $p=0.006$)
					All-cause mortality	RR 1.46 (95 % CI, 1.03–2.08; $p=0.03$)
Hachicha [54]	2009	544	30	Z_{va} (per mmHg·ml/m^2)	Death	RR 1.36 (95 % CI, 1.03–5.75; $p=0.03$)
				LVH		RR 1.66 (95 % CI, 1.01–2.73; $p=0.05$)
Rosenhek [52]	2010	116	41	V_{max} ≥5.5 m/s	AVR or cardiac death	RR 1.88 (95 % CI, 1.19–2.96; $p=0.007$)
Lancellotti [28]	2010	163	20	V_{max} (per 1 m/s)	Symptoms, AVR, or death	RR 1.6 (95 % CI, 1.01–2.5; $p=0.04$)
				Z_{va} (per mmHg·ml/m^2)		RR 1.6 (95 % CI, 1.25–2.0; $p=0.001$)
				GLS (per 1 %)		RR 1.1 (95 % CI, 1.01–1.2; $p=0.03$)
Stewart [49]	2010	183	31	V_{max} (per 0.5 m/s)	Symptoms	RR 1.43 (95 % CI, 1.25–1.64; $p<0.0001$)
				AVA (per 0.1 cm^2)		RR 1.13 (95 % CI, 1.05–1.22; p 0.04)
Rieck [53]	2012	1418	43	Z_{va} >5 mmHg·ml/m^2	AVR, CHF hospitalization, or death	RR 1.41 (95 % CI, 1.12–1.78; $p=0.004$)
Bahlmann [23]	2013	1563	51	ELI (per cm^2/m^2)	AVR, CHF hospitalization, or death	RR 2.05 (95 % CI, 1.48–2.85; $p<0.001$)

AVA aortic valve area, *AVR* aortic valve replacement, *CI* confidence interval, *CHF* congestive heart failure, *ELI* energy loss index, *GLS* global longitudinal strain, *LVH* left ventricular hypertrophy, *RR* relative risk, V_{max} peak aortic jet velocity, Z_{va} valvuloarterial impedance

[a]Mean follow-up in months; if mean was not provided, the median is reported

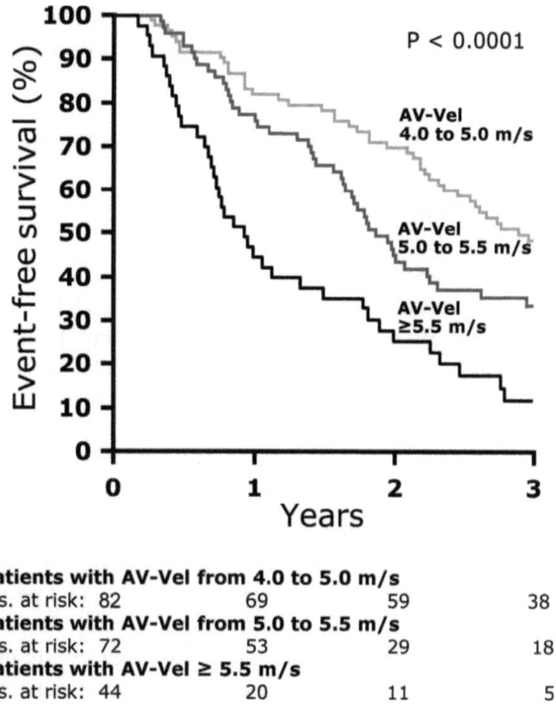

Fig. 11.5 Event-free survival in patients with severe aortic stenosis stratified by peak aortic jet velocity (V_{max}) (Rosenhek et al. [52])

consistently associated with outcomes across longitudinal studies after adjusting for clinical and echocardiographic parameters, including mean gradient and valve area [28, 46–49]. Those with V_{max} >4 m/s have up to 80 % likelihood of AVR or death over the next 2 years [47]. Additionally, moderate to severe calcification of the aortic valve by TTE has been shown to be a strong predictor of AVR and death in mild, moderate, and severe AS [50, 51]. The prognostic value of calcification becomes attenuated in hemodynamically very severe AS (V_{max} ≥5 m/s) as it almost universally presents and because progression to symptom onset is rapid in all patients with this degree of valve obstruction (Fig. 11.5) [52]. The combination of rapid hemodynamic progression (increase in V_{max} ≥0.3 m/s/year) and significant valve calcification can identify a very high-risk cohort.

Newer echocardiographic measures of hemodynamic severity, ELI and Z_{va}, also have been evaluated in longitudinal outcome studies [23, 28, 53, 54]. In a large subcohort of the Simvastatin and Ezetimibe in Aortic Stenosis (SEAS) study, ELI provided independent prognostic information beyond V_{max} and mean gradients [23]. However the discriminatory ability of ELI for aortic valve events was similar to AVA, and both perform less well than the V_{max}. In the same SEAS study population, a high Z_{va} was found to be predictive for aortic valve events independent of V_{max} and mean gradient, but was no longer significant when adjusting for AVA [53]. Despite the logical hemodynamic basis for these measures, their ability to associate with CAVD outcomes independent of traditional measures has yet to be proven. Future studies validating these measures with outcomes when traditional measures and clinical findings are discrepant may prove useful [55].

11.4 CAVD Pathophysiology and Echocardiography

11.4.1 Ventricular Changes

11.4.1.1 Hypertrophy

In advancing CAVD, valvular obstruction to left ventricular (LV) outflow leads to significant afterload excess. In most patients, pumping function is preserved and wall stress remains normal with a ventricular "response" to pressure overload of hypertrophy and concentric remodeling. These changes have been thought to be "compensatory" in the past but may instead be part of the disease process leading to myocardial fibrosis and persistent diastolic dysfunction even after AVR. Changes in ventricular size and geometry can be assessed with standard parasternal 2D TTE and M-mode imaging, although 3D ventricular volumes are more accurate and reproducible and are likely to replace linear and 2D measurements in the near future.

The most utilized measurements are end-diastolic minor-axis linear dimensions of septal (SWTd) and posterior wall thickness (PWTd) and LV cavity (LVIDd). Measurements should be obtained by 2D directed M-mode perpendicular to the LV long axis at the tips of the mitral leaflets [56]. If the M-mode beam cannot be aligned appropriately, 2D measurements may be used although the lower frame rate limits identification of the endocardial border. From these measurements, LV mass can be estimated from the following validated formula: LV $\text{mass} = 0.8 \times \{1.04[(\text{LVIDd} + \text{PWTd} + \text{SWTd})^3 - \text{LVIDd}^3]\} + 0.6\,\text{g}$ [57]. Cutoff values for hypertrophy are gender specific and indexed by BSA, 95 g/m^2 for women and 115 g/m^2 for men. Changes in LV geometry can be described as concentric when regional wall thickness (RWT) exceeds 0.42, using the formula $\text{RWT} = (2 \times \text{PWTd})/\text{LVIDd}$.

Recent data suggests that the hypertrophic and concentric remodeling response to pressure overload in CAVD may be maladaptive and is associated with fibrosis, ventricular dysfunction, and worse clinical outcomes [54, 58–61]. Relief of the pressure overload with aortic valve replacement commonly results in significant reduction in the hypertrophy, but it rarely normalizes [62]. The hypertrophic and remodeling response to pressure overload is variable due to combination of genetics and gender. Consistently females have been shown to develop higher RWT due to both smaller LV cavities and thicker ventricular walls [63, 64]. Although hypertrophy may be associated with adverse prognosis, it has limited ability to predict outcomes in asymptomatic patients after accounting for traditional echocardiographic severity measures such as V_{max} and AVA [49].

11.4.1.2 Diastolic Dysfunction

Diastolic dysfunction is common in CAVD with LV hypertrophy and can be evaluated with the use of echocardiography. Decreased myocardial relaxation and

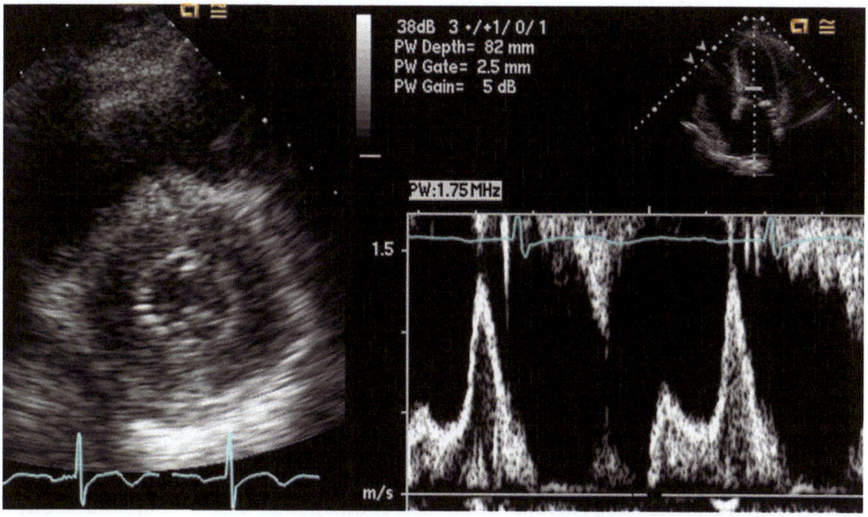

Fig. 11.6 A short-axis view of significant concentric hypertrophy and small left ventricular cavity in a patient with severe aortic stenosis (*left panel*). The patient has evidence of diastolic dysfunction with an impaired relaxation pattern of mitral inflow using PW Doppler from the apical view (*right panel*)

increased LV stiffness frequently precede changes in systolic function and are associated with fibrosis and increased LV filling pressures [60, 65]. Evaluation of LV filling patterns and mitral annular velocities and estimation of filling pressures can be routinely performed by 2D TTE Doppler methods [66].

LV filling is evaluated with PW Doppler parallel to mitral inflow from the apical (4-chamber) view. The sample volume is placed between the mitral valve leaflet tips, and a typical early diastolic peak velocity (E) and a late diastolic peak velocity from atrial contraction (A) can be measured (Fig. 11.6). The E/A ratio can categorize filling pattern severity into normal, impaired relaxation, pseudonormal, and restrictive. However, LV filling parameters alone are not sufficient to distinguish myocardial diastolic dysfunction in CAVD as they are dependent on loading conditions, heart rate, and age, and when compared to age-matched controls, no significant differences can be detected [67].

To overcome these limitations, PW tissue Doppler imaging (TDI) of the mitral annulus can provide information about myocardial relaxation and estimated filling pressures. TDI allows measurement of large-amplitude, low-frequency signals produced from myocardial motion of the septal or lateral mitral annulus. The early peak diastolic mitral annular velocity (e′) has been studied in patients with CAVD [49, 68, 69]. The e′ is a relatively preload independent index of myocardial relaxation when not limited by mitral valve disease. In patients with AS, the E/e′ ratio has been shown to correlate with LV end-diastolic pressure, pulmonary pressure, and prognosis [70–72]. An E/e′ ≥15 reasonably predicts LV end-diastolic pressures >15 mmHg in AS. Similar to echo findings of hypertrophy, echo parameters of diastolic dysfunction provide only limited predictive information above stenosis severity measures and may not fully normalize after AVR [49, 73].

11.4.1.3 Speckle-Tracking Strain

Subclinical systolic dysfunction in patients with normal ejection fraction (EF) can be detected in CAVD. Longitudinal fibers in the subendocardium are the most susceptible to myocardial ischemia and fibrosis in pressure overload states, and impaired longitudinal contractility is present before a decline in the EF. Initial echocardiographic studies demonstrated reduced longitudinal systolic function with M-mode or TDI showing reduced mitral annular longitudinal displacement or velocity (S′) in patients with AS and normal EF [74, 75]. However, measurements of displacement and velocity are inherently limited by translational motion of the heart and angle dependency of Doppler ultrasound.

Recent advances in technology allow for 2D speckle-tracking echocardiography (STE) which can measure regional strain that is independent of translational motion and ultrasound angle [76]. Speckles are the result of the constructive and destructive interference of ultrasound backscatter from a structure smaller than the length of the ultrasound signal. Small segments of myocardium produce unique speckle patterns, sometimes referred to as blocks or kernels, which can be tracked frame to frame. Offline measurement of displacement, velocity, stain, and strain rates can be made between any two kernels, allowing for measurement in any direction. Accurate STE depends on excellent image quality and high frame rates to provide the temporal resolution required to track speckles.

Strain is the fractional change in the length of a myocardial segment, expressed as a percentage. By convention, positive and negative values reflect lengthening and shortening, respectively. Although STE allows for strain evaluation in any direction, radial and circumferential strain has not been as strongly associated in CAVD as longitudinal strain [77, 78]. Peak longitudinal strain values are calculated for multiple LV segments and in CAVD are commonly expressed as an average of either global (GLS) or basal (BLS) segments (Fig. 11.7). GLS and BLS have been associated with hemodynamic severity, symptomatic status, exercise parameters, and event-free survival in patients with CAVD [28, 78, 79]. Exact cutoffs for severity of GLS or BLS require further validation, as current studies are limited by small sample size and nonuniform strain evaluation by different ultrasound vendors and researchers. Currently, clinical use of GLS or BLS is limited by significant overlap of values between hemodynamic severity and symptomatic status of CAVD patients that approach the inter- and intraobserver variability in measurements [80].

11.4.2 Stress Testing

Management of AS can be challenging when hemodynamic severity and symptom status are discordant. Symptomatic status is variable and subjective between patients with AS and cannot be predicted by echocardiographic measures alone. Patients

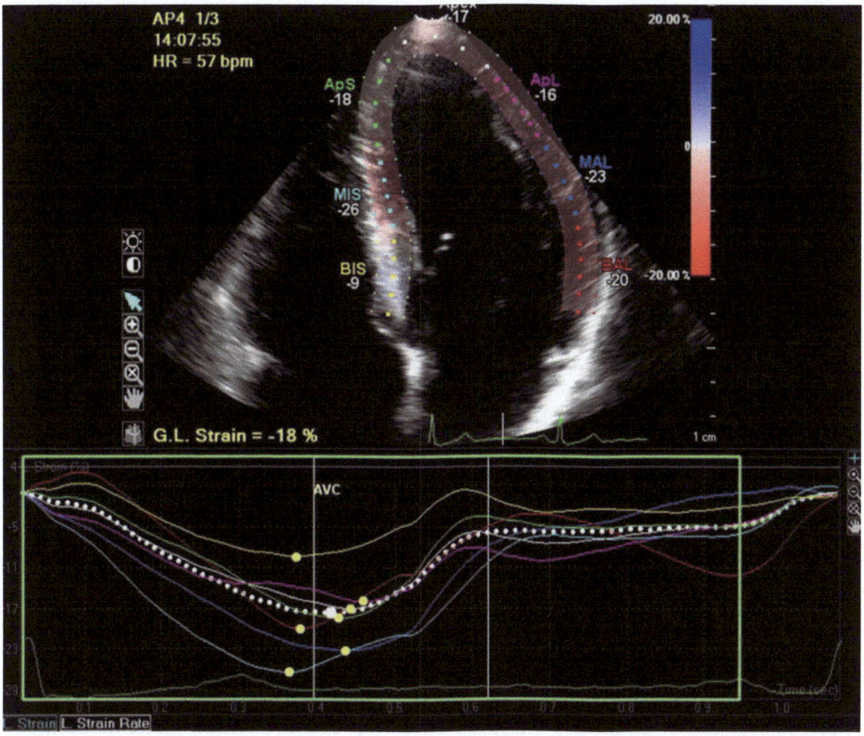

Fig. 11.7 Example of speckle-tracking global longitudinal strain (*GLS*) measured by echocardiography in an apical four-chamber view. Myocardial speckles are tracked during the cardiac cycle for each segment, shown by *colored dots* on the 2D image corresponding to the graph of strain versus time for each segment shown at the *bottom* of the image. Although there is some asynchrony in the timing of strain in this patient with moderate AS, overall maximum GLS is within normal limits at −18 %, shown by the *white dotted line*

considered asymptomatic with normal ejection fractions may have adverse outcomes such as sudden cardiac death or irreversible subclinical myocardial dysfunction, and further risk stratification with exercise testing may be helpful to identify those that will benefit from early AVR. Conversely, symptomatic patients may have confounding comorbidities as etiologies for symptoms, such as coronary artery disease or systolic heart failure, and may not benefit from AVR.

11.4.2.1 Normal EF

Exercise stress testing can provide important information for clinical decision-making when the functional capacity and asymptomatic nature of a patient with severe AS is in doubt (Fig. 11.8). Exercise testing alone has been shown to risk stratify self-reported asymptomatic patients with severe AS and normal EF, but exercise testing in clearly symptomatic patients should be avoided. Asymptomatic severe AS patients with a positive exercise test, defined by symptoms (chest pain or dizziness), ST depressions, complex ventricular arrhythmias, or failure of systolic blood pressure to rise with

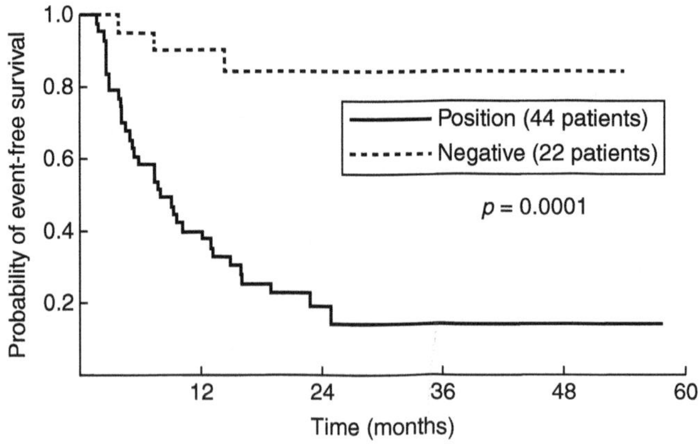

Fig. 11.8 Kaplan-Meier life table analysis for probability of event-free survival over 60 months for patients with asymptomatic severe aortic stenosis, according to positive or negative results of exercise testing (Amato et al. [81])

exercise, have a sevenfold increase risk of future symptoms or sudden death [81]. The use of echocardiography can provide further prognostic information during exercise testing. The change in mean transaortic pressure gradients during peak exercise can be measured, and an increase of 18 mmHg during semisupine bicycle exercise was independently associated with cardiac valve events in asymptomatic severe AS patients [82]. An increase of 20 mmHg was predictive of events in asymptomatic moderate to severe disease in those with normal exercise testing [83]. Furthermore, asymptomatic severe AS patients with exercise-induced systolic pulmonary pressure >60 mmHg have a twofold increase risk of cardiovascular death or AVR after adjusting for demographics, baseline echocardiographic ventricular and valvular severity, and exercise parameters [84]. The peak pulmonary systolic pressure was derived from the tricuspid regurgitation Doppler velocity using the Bernoulli equation and adding a constant of 10 mmHg to estimate right atrial pressure.

11.4.2.2 Reduced EF

Significant systolic dysfunction with reduced EF is a very late finding in severe AS and is associated with a very poor prognosis. The evaluation of AS is complicated in low-flow states due to the flow dependency of AS severity measures including V_{max}, mean gradient, and AVA. Patients with severely reduced systolic function and small valve areas can be further risk stratified with the use of low-dose dobutamine stress echocardiography (DSE). Dobutamine up to 20 mcg/kg/min can be used to evaluate for contractile reserve, increase in SV by 20 % or more, and change in valve area and velocity with increase in flow (Fig. 11.9). A DSE starts at a low dose (typically 2.5 or 5 mg/kg/min) and increases by 5 mg/kg/min every 3–5 min to a max dose of 20 mcg/kg/min. Termination of the study occurs when target dose is reached, a positive test for severe AS is achieved, or an adverse reaction occurs (ventricular arrhythmias, hypotension, or significant symptoms).

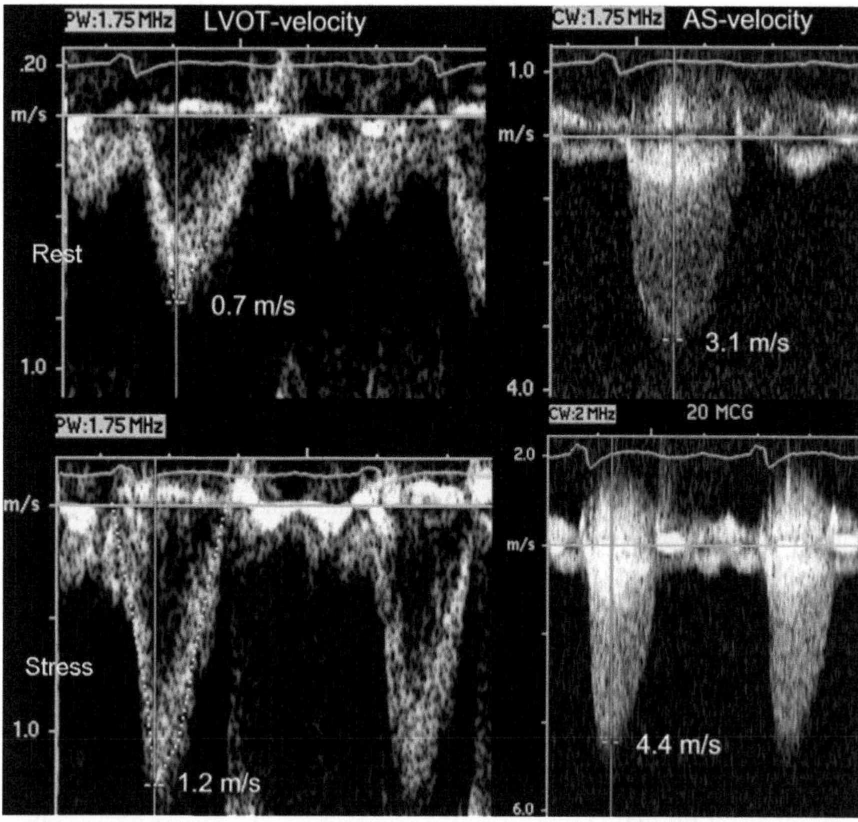

Fig. 11.9 Peak velocities in the left ventricular outflow tract (*LVOT*) and aortic jet (V_{max}) measured during rest (*top*) and with dobutamine stress in a patient with reduced systolic function and a moderate severity range V_{max} at rest. Augmentation of flow is seen at stress with a normalized LVOT velocity and a severe V_{max} of 4.4 m/s; an LVOT diameter of 2 cm^2 would lead to a calculated AVA of 0.85 cm^2 indicating true severe AS in this patient

Individuals at peak stress with intact contractile reserve and an AVA above 1 cm^2 or an increase in AVA of at least 0.2 cm^2 are categorized as having relative or pseudosevere AS. People with pseudosevere AS are not likely to benefit from a high-risk AVR operation as their prognosis is determined by their underlying cardiomyopathy and not from the afterload excess of the aortic valve. A positive test occurs with true severe AS patients that develop a Vmax >4 or mean gradient >40 mmHg with a valve area ≤1.0 cm^2 during DSE. These patients have the most benefit from AVR [85]. However, many patients may not have contractile reserve, and the lack of flow augmentation limits differentiation between true and pseudosevere AS. Despite a lack of ventricular response to inotropic stimulation, observational studies have shown that patients selected for surgery with low-flow AS and reduced systolic function have better outcomes; thus, DSE should not be solely relied upon to exclude a patient from AVR [85–87].

11.4.3 Low-Flow, Low-Gradient AS with Normal EF

Up to a quarter of CAVD patients with valve area in the severe range (≤1.0 cm2) have a preserved EF ≥50 % with evidence of low flow (SV index <35 ml/m^2) as measured by echocardiography, a situation frequently termed "paradoxical" [88]. A low SV is due to a combination of impaired LV filling from diastolic dysfunction, reduced LV cavity size from concentric remodeling, high global afterload, and decreased longitudinal systolic function. Hachicha et al. first described patients with low-flow severe AS despite normal LV EFs to be treated more conservatively and have a worse prognosis compared to those patients with normal-flow severe AS [89]. A later analysis by Jander et al. evaluated participants in the Simvastatin and Ezetimibe in Aortic Stenosis clinical trial with valve areas in the severe range but mean gradients ≤40 mmHg [90]. Outcomes were comparable to those with moderate AS severity. These two studies however are difficult to directly compare due to differences in study population and in the categorization of either "low-flow" or "low-gradient" patients; highlighted by Lancellotti et al., four categories of flow-gradient patterns exist with different prognosis: normal flow/low gradient, normal flow/high gradient, low flow/high gradient, and low flow/low gradient [91]. Those patients with a normal flow/low gradient had the best prognosis in the study, patients with low flow/high gradient and normal flow/high gradient had similar event rates, and low-flow/low-gradient patients had the worst prognosis with a nearly 90 % event rate for cardiovascular death or AVR at 3 years. Treatment with AVR has been shown to be a predictor of lower mortality in patients with severe AS (AVA ≤1.0 cm^2) but with low gradients (≤30 mmHg) and preserved EF [92]. An important caveat in the evaluation of flow-gradient patterns is to avoid misclassification of severe AS by paying careful attention to technical factors such as measurement errors (the LVOT diameter or Doppler LVOT VTI), severe mitral regurgitation, and small body size. Additionally, "paradoxical" low-flow AS should be considered only with severely calcified aortic valves with reduced opening when the patient is normotensive (systolic blood pressure <140 mmHg) [93].

References

1. Quiñones MA, Otto CM, Stoddard M, Waggoner A, Zoghbi WA. A report from the Doppler quantification task force of the nomenclature and standards committee of the American Society of Echocardiography. J Am Soc Echocardiogr. 2002;15:167–84.
2. Currie PJ, Seward JB, Reeder GS, Vlietstra RE, Bresnahan DR, Bresnahan JF, Smith HC, Hagler DJ, Tajik AJ. Continuous-wave Doppler echocardiographic assessment of severity of calcific aortic stenosis: a simultaneous Doppler-catheter correlative study in 100 adult patients. Circulation. 1985;71:1162–9.
3. Burwash IG, Forbes AD, Sadahiro M, Verrier ED, Pearlman AS, Thomas R, Kraft C, Otto CM. Echocardiographic volume flow and stenosis severity measures with changing flow rate in aortic stenosis. Am J Physiol. 1993;265:H1734–43.
4. Baumgartner H, Hung J, Bermejo J, Chambers JB, Evangelista A, Griffin BP, Iung B, Otto CM, Pellikka PA, Quiñones M, Echocardiography ASo, Echocardiography EAo. Echocardiographic

assessment of valve stenosis: EAE/ASE recommendations for clinical practice. J Am Soc Echocardiogr. 2009;22:1–23. Quiz 101–2.
5. Otto CM, Pearlman AS, Comess KA, Reamer RP, Janko CL, Huntsman LL. Determination of the stenotic aortic valve area in adults using Doppler echocardiography. J Am Coll Cardiol. 1986;7:509–17.
6. Oh JK, Taliercio CP, Holmes DR, Reeder GS, Bailey KR, Seward JB, Tajik AJ. Prediction of the severity of aortic stenosis by Doppler aortic valve area determination: prospective Doppler-catheterization correlation in 100 patients. J Am Coll Cardiol. 1988;11:1227–34.
7. Zoghbi WA, Farmer KL, Soto JG, Nelson JG, Quinones MA. Accurate noninvasive quantification of stenotic aortic valve area by Doppler echocardiography. Circulation. 1986;73:452–9.
8. Binder RK, Webb JG, Willson AB, Urena M, Hansson NC, Norgaard BL, Pibarot P, Barbanti M, Larose E, Freeman M, Dumont E, Thompson C, Wheeler M, Moss RR, Yang TH, Pasian S, Hague CJ, Nguyen G, Raju R, Toggweiler S, Min JK, Wood DA, Rodés-Cabau J, Leipsic J. The impact of integration of a multidetector computed tomography annulus area sizing algorithm on outcomes of transcatheter aortic valve replacement: a prospective, multicenter, controlled trial. J Am Coll Cardiol. 2013;62:431–8.
9. Okura H, Yoshida K, Hozumi T, Akasaka T, Yoshikawa J. Planimetry and transthoracic two-dimensional echocardiography in noninvasive assessment of aortic valve area in patients with valvular aortic stenosis. J Am Coll Cardiol. 1997;30:753–9.
10. DeMaria AN, Bommer W, Joye J, Lee G, Bouteller J, Mason DT. Value and limitations of cross-sectional echocardiography of the aortic valve in the diagnosis and quantification of valvular aortic stenosis. Circulation. 1980;62:304–12.
11. Cormier B, Iung B, Porte JM, Barbant S, Vahanian A. Value of multiplane transesophageal echocardiography in determining aortic valve area in aortic stenosis. Am J Cardiol. 1996;77:882–5.
12. Bernard Y, Meneveau N, Vuillemenot A, Magnin D, Anguenot T, Schiele F, Bassand JP. Planimetry of aortic valve area using multiplane transoesophageal echocardiography is not a reliable method for assessing severity of aortic stenosis. Heart. 1997;78:68–73.
13. Gilon D, Cape EG, Handschumacher MD, Song JK, Solheim J, VanAuker M, King ME, Levine RA. Effect of three-dimensional valve shape on the hemodynamics of aortic stenosis: three-dimensional echocardiographic stereolithography and patient studies. J Am Coll Cardiol. 2002;40:1479–86.
14. Goland S, Trento A, Iida K, Czer LS, De Robertis M, Naqvi TZ, Tolstrup K, Akima T, Luo H, Siegel RJ. Assessment of aortic stenosis by three-dimensional echocardiography: an accurate and novel approach. Heart. 2007;93:801–7.
15. Gaspar T, Adawi S, Sachner R, Asmer I, Ganaeem M, Rubinshtein R, Shiran A. Three-dimensional imaging of the left ventricular outflow tract: impact on aortic valve area estimation by the continuity equation. J Am Soc Echocardiogr. 2012;25:749–57.
16. Gutiérrez-Chico JL, Zamorano JL, Prieto-Moriche E, Hernández-Antolín RA, Bravo-Amaro M, Pérez de Isla L, Sanmartín-Fernández M, Baz-Alonso JA, Iñiguez-Romo A. Real-time three-dimensional echocardiography in aortic stenosis: a novel, simple, and reliable method to improve accuracy in area calculation. Eur Heart J. 2008;29:1296–306.
17. Poh KK, Levine RA, Solis J, Shen L, Flaherty M, Kang YJ, Guerrero JL, Hung J. Assessing aortic valve area in aortic stenosis by continuity equation: a novel approach using real-time three-dimensional echocardiography. Eur Heart J. 2008;29:2526–35.
18. Jander N, Gohlke-Bärwolf C, Bahlmann E, Gerdts E, Boman K, Chambers JB, Egstrup K, Nienaber CA, Pedersen TR, Ray S, Rossebø AB, Willenheimer R, Kienzle RP, Wachtell K, Neumann FJ, Minners J. Indexing aortic valve area by body surface area increases the prevalence of severe aortic stenosis. Heart. 2014;100:28–33.
19. Garcia D, Dumesnil JG, Durand LG, Kadem L, Pibarot P. Discrepancies between catheter and Doppler estimates of valve effective orifice area can be predicted from the pressure recovery phenomenon: practical implications with regard to quantification of aortic stenosis severity. J Am Coll Cardiol. 2003;41:435–42.
20. Baumgartner H, Stefenelli T, Niederberger J, Schima H, Maurer G. "Overestimation" of catheter gradients by Doppler ultrasound in patients with aortic stenosis: a predictable manifestation of pressure recovery. J Am Coll Cardiol. 1999;33:1655–61.

21. Garcia D, Pibarot P, Dumesnil JG, Sakr F, Durand LG. Assessment of aortic valve stenosis severity: a new index based on the energy loss concept. Circulation. 2000;101:765–71.
22. Bahlmann E, Cramariuc D, Gerdts E, Gohlke-Baerwolf C, Nienaber CA, Eriksen E, Wachtell K, Chambers J, Kuck KH, Ray S. Impact of pressure recovery on echocardiographic assessment of asymptomatic aortic stenosis: a seas substudy. JACC Cardiovasc Imaging. 2010;3:555–62.
23. Bahlmann E, Gerdts E, Cramariuc D, Gohlke-Baerwolf C, Nienaber CA, Wachtell K, Seifert R, Chambers JB, Kuck KH, Ray S. Prognostic value of energy loss index in asymptomatic aortic stenosis. Circulation. 2013;127:1149–56.
24. Kadem L, Dumesnil JG, Rieu R, Durand LG, Garcia D, Pibarot P. Impact of systemic hypertension on the assessment of aortic stenosis. Heart. 2005;91:354–61.
25. Little SH, Chan KL, Burwash IG. Impact of blood pressure on the Doppler echocardiographic assessment of severity of aortic stenosis. Heart. 2007;93:848–55.
26. Antonini-Canterin F, Huang G, Cervesato E, Faggiano P, Pavan D, Piazza R, Nicolosi GL. Symptomatic aortic stenosis: does systemic hypertension play an additional role? Hypertension. 2003;41:1268–72.
27. Briand M, Dumesnil JG, Kadem L, Tongue AG, Rieu R, Garcia D, Pibarot P. Reduced systemic arterial compliance impacts significantly on left ventricular afterload and function in aortic stenosis: implications for diagnosis and treatment. J Am Coll Cardiol. 2005;46:291–8.
28. Lancellotti P, Donal E, Magne J, Moonen M, O'Connor K, Daubert JC, Pierard LA. Risk stratification in asymptomatic moderate to severe aortic stenosis: the importance of the valvular, arterial and ventricular interplay. Heart. 2010;96:1364–71.
29. Gharacholou SM, Karon BL, Shub C, Pellikka PA. Aortic valve sclerosis and clinical outcomes: moving toward a definition. Am J Med. 2011;124:103–10.
30. Hawkins K, Henry JS, Krasuski RA. Tissue harmonic imaging in echocardiography: better valve imaging, but at what cost? Echocardiography. 2008;25:119–23.
31. Ngo DT, Wuttke RD, Turner S, Marwick TH, Horowitz JD. Quantitative assessment of aortic sclerosis using ultrasonic backscatter. J Am Soc Echocardiogr. 2004;17:1123–30.
32. Nightingale AK, Sverdlov AL, Rajendran S, Mishra K, Heresztyn T, Ngo DT, Horowitz JD. Lack of association between aortic sclerosis and left ventricular hypertrophy in elderly subjects. Int J Cardiol. 2011;150:33–8.
33. Roosens B, Bala G, Gillis K, Remory I, Droogmans S, Somja J, Delvenne E, De Nayer J, Schiettecatte J, Delvenne P, Lancellotti P, Van Camp G, Cosyns B. Echocardiographic integrated backscatter for detecting progression and regression of aortic valve calcifications in rats. Cardiovasc Ultrasound. 2013;11:4.
34. Faggiano P, Antonini-Canterin F, Erlicher A, Romeo C, Cervesato E, Pavan D, Piazza R, Huang G, Nicolosi GL. Progression of aortic valve sclerosis to aortic stenosis. Am J Cardiol. 2003;91:99–101.
35. Cosmi JE, Kort S, Tunick PA, Rosenzweig BP, Freedberg RS, Katz ES, Applebaum RM, Kronzon I. The risk of the development of aortic stenosis in patients with "benign" aortic valve thickening. Arch Intern Med. 2002;162:2345–7.
36. Novaro G, Katz R, Aviles R, Gottdiener J, Cushman M, Psaty B, Otto C, Griffin B. Clinical factors, but not c-reactive protein, predict progression of calcific aortic-valve disease: the cardiovascular health study. J Am Coll Cardiol. 2007;50:1992–8.
37. Stewart BF, Siscovick D, Lind BK, Gardin JM, Gottdiener JS, Smith VE, Kitzman DW, Otto CM. Clinical factors associated with calcific aortic valve disease. Cardiovascular health study. J Am Coll Cardiol. 1997;29:630–4.
38. Fox CS, Guo CY, Larson MG, Vasan RS, Parise H, O'Donnell CJ, D'Agostino RB, Keaney JF, Benjamin EJ. Relations of inflammation and novel risk factors to valvular calcification. Am J Cardiol. 2006;97:1502–5.
39. Stritzke J, Linsel-Nitschke P, Markus MR, Mayer B, Lieb W, Luchner A, Döring A, Koenig W, Keil U, Hense HW, Schunkert H, Investigators MK. Association between degenerative aortic valve disease and long-term exposure to cardiovascular risk factors: results of the longitudinal population-based KORA/MONICA survey. Eur Heart J. 2009;30:2044–53.
40. Olsen MH, Wachtell K, Bella JN, Palmieri V, Gerdts E, Smith G, Nieminen MS, Dahlöf B, Ibsen H, Devereux RB. Aortic valve sclerosis and albuminuria predict cardiovascular events

independently in hypertension: a losartan intervention for endpoint-reduction in hypertension (life) substudy. Am J Hypertens. 2005;18:1430–6.

41. Otto CM, Lind BK, Kitzman DW, Gersh BJ, Siscovick DS. Association of aortic-valve sclerosis with cardiovascular mortality and morbidity in the elderly. N Engl J Med. 1999;341: 142–7.
42. Chandra HR, Goldstein JA, Choudhary N, O'Neill CS, George PB, Gangasani SR, Cronin L, Marcovitz PA, Hauser AM, O'Neill WW. Adverse outcome in aortic sclerosis is associated with coronary artery disease and inflammation. J Am Coll Cardiol. 2004;43: 169–75.
43. Barasch E, Gottdiener J, Marino Larsen E, Chaves P, Newman A. Cardiovascular morbidity and mortality in community-dwelling elderly individuals with calcification of the fibrous skeleton of the base of the heart and aortosclerosis (the cardiovascular health study). Am J Cardiol. 2006;97:1281–6.
44. Braunwald E. On the natural history of severe aortic stenosis. J Am Coll Cardiol. 1990;15: 1018–20.
45. Makkar RR, Fontana GP, Jilaihawi H, Kapadia S, Pichard AD, Douglas PS, Thourani VH, Babaliaros VC, Webb JG, Herrmann HC, Bavaria JE, Kodali S, Brown DL, Bowers B, Dewey TM, Svensson LG, Tuzcu M, Moses JW, Williams MR, Siegel RJ, Akin JJ, Anderson WN, Pocock S, Smith CR, Leon MB, Investigators PT. Transcatheter aortic-valve replacement for inoperable severe aortic stenosis. N Engl J Med. 2012;366:1696–704.
46. Pellikka PA, Nishimura RA, Bailey KR, Tajik AJ. The natural history of adults with asymptomatic, hemodynamically significant aortic stenosis. J Am Coll Cardiol. 1990;15:1012–7.
47. Otto CM, Burwash IG, Legget ME, Munt BI, Fujioka M, Healy NL, Kraft CD, Miyake-Hull CY, Schwaegler RG. Prospective study of asymptomatic valvular aortic stenosis. Clinical, echocardiographic, and exercise predictors of outcome. Circulation. 1997;95:2262–70.
48. Pellikka PA, Sarano ME, Nishimura RA, Malouf JF, Bailey KR, Scott CG, Barnes ME, Tajik AJ. Outcome of 622 adults with asymptomatic, hemodynamically significant aortic stenosis during prolonged follow-up. Circulation. 2005;111:3290–5.
49. Stewart RA, Kerr AJ, Whalley GA, Legget ME, Zeng I, Williams MJ, Lainchbury J, Hamer A, Doughty R, Richards MA, White HD, Investigators NZHVS. Left ventricular systolic and diastolic function assessed by tissue Doppler imaging and outcome in asymptomatic aortic stenosis. Eur Heart J. 2010;31:2216–22.
50. Rosenhek R, Binder T, Porenta G, Lang I, Christ G, Schemper M, Maurer G, Baumgartner H. Predictors of outcome in severe, asymptomatic aortic stenosis. N Engl J Med. 2000;343:611–7.
51. Rosenhek R, Klaar U, Schemper M, Scholten C, Heger M, Gabriel H, Binder T, Maurer G, Baumgartner H. Mild and moderate aortic stenosis. Natural history and risk stratification by echocardiography. Eur Heart J. 2004;25:199–205.
52. Rosenhek R, Zilberszac R, Schemper M, Czerny M, Mundigler G, Graf S, Bergler-Klein J, Grimm M, Gabriel H, Maurer G. Natural history of very severe aortic stenosis. Circulation. 2010;121:151–6.
53. Rieck AE, Gerdts E, Lønnebakken MT, Bahlmann E, Cioffi G, Gohlke-Bärwolf C, Ray S, Cramariuc D. Global left ventricular load in asymptomatic aortic stenosis: covariates and prognostic implication (the seas trial). Cardiovasc Ultrasound. 2012;10:43.
54. Hachicha Z, Dumesnil JG, Pibarot P. Usefulness of the valvuloarterial impedance to predict adverse outcome in asymptomatic aortic stenosis. J Am Coll Cardiol. 2009;54:1003–11.
55. Pibarot P, Dumesnil JG. Improving assessment of aortic stenosis. J Am Coll Cardiol. 2012;60:169–80.
56. Lang RM, Bierig M, Devereux RB, Flachskampf FA, Foster E, Pellikka PA, Picard MH, Roman MJ, Seward J, Shanewise JS, Solomon SD, Spencer KT, Sutton MS, Stewart WJ, Group CQW, Committee ASoEsGaS, Echocardiography EAo. Recommendations for chamber quantification: a report from the American Society of Echocardiography's guidelines and standards committee and the chamber quantification writing group, developed in conjunction with the European Association of echocardiography, a branch of the European Society of Cardiology. J Am Soc Echocardiogr. 2005;18:1440–63.

57. Devereux RB, Alonso DR, Lutas EM, Gottlieb GJ, Campo E, Sachs I, Reichek N. Echocardiographic assessment of left ventricular hypertrophy: comparison to necropsy findings. Am J Cardiol. 1986;57:450–8.
58. Kupari M, Turto H, Lommi J. Left ventricular hypertrophy in aortic valve stenosis: preventive or promotive of systolic dysfunction and heart failure? Eur Heart J. 2005;26:1790–6.
59. Duncan AI, Lowe BS, Garcia MJ, Xu M, Gillinov AM, Mihaljevic T, Koch CG. Influence of concentric left ventricular remodeling on early mortality after aortic valve replacement. Ann Thorac Surg. 2008;85:2030–9.
60. Villari B, Hess OM, Kaufmann P, Krogmann ON, Grimm J, Krayenbuehl HP. Effect of aortic valve stenosis (pressure overload) and regurgitation (volume overload) on left ventricular systolic and diastolic function. Am J Cardiol. 1992;69:927–34.
61. Villari B, Campbell SE, Hess OM, Mall G, Vassalli G, Weber KT, Krayenbuehl HP. Influence of collagen network on left ventricular systolic and diastolic function in aortic valve disease. J Am Coll Cardiol. 1993;22:1477–84.
62. Lund O, Erlandsen M. Changes in left ventricular function and mass during serial investigations after valve replacement for aortic stenosis. J Heart Valve Dis. 2000;9:583–93.
63. Douglas PS, Otto CM, Mickel MC, Labovitz A, Reid CL, Davis KB. Gender differences in left ventricle geometry and function in patients undergoing balloon dilatation of the aortic valve for isolated aortic stenosis. NHLBI balloon valvuloplasty registry. Br Heart J. 1995;73:548–54.
64. Villari B, Campbell SE, Schneider J, Vassalli G, Chiariello M, Hess OM. Sex-dependent differences in left ventricular function and structure in chronic pressure overload. Eur Heart J. 1995;16:1410–9.
65. Hess OM, Villari B, Krayenbuehl HP. Diastolic dysfunction in aortic stenosis. Circulation. 1993;87:IV73–6.
66. Nagueh SF, Appleton CP, Gillebert TC, Marino PN, Oh JK, Smiseth OA, Waggoner AD, Flachskampf FA, Pellikka PA, Evangelista A. Recommendations for the evaluation of left ventricular diastolic function by echocardiography. J Am Soc Echocardiogr. 2009;22:107–33.
67. Otto CM, Pearlman AS, Amsler LC. Doppler echocardiographic evaluation of left ventricular diastolic filling in isolated valvular aortic stenosis. Am J Cardiol. 1989;63:313–6.
68. Steine K, Rossebø AB, Stugaard M, Pedersen TR. Left ventricular systolic and diastolic function in asymptomatic patients with moderate aortic stenosis. Am J Cardiol. 2008;102:897–901.
69. Jassal DS, Tam JW, Dumesnil JG, Giannoccaro PJ, Jue J, Pandey AS, Joyner CD, Teo KK, Chan KL. Clinical usefulness of tissue Doppler imaging in patients with mild to moderate aortic stenosis: a substudy of the aortic stenosis progression observation measuring effects of rosuvastatin study. J Am Soc Echocardiogr. 2008;21:1023–7.
70. Bruch C, Stypmann J, Grude M, Gradaus R, Breithardt G, Wichter T. Tissue Doppler imaging in patients with moderate to severe aortic valve stenosis: clinical usefulness and diagnostic accuracy. Am Heart J. 2004;148:696–702.
71. Biner S, Rafique AM, Goykhman P, Morrissey RP, Naghi J, Siegel RJ. Prognostic value of e/e′ ratio in patients with unoperated severe aortic stenosis. JACC Cardiovasc Imaging. 2010;3:899–907.
72. Casaclang-Verzosa G, Nkomo VT, Sarano ME, Malouf JF, Miller FA, Oh JK. E/Ea is the major determinant of pulmonary artery pressure in moderate to severe aortic stenosis. J Am Soc Echocardiogr. 2008;21:824–7.
73. Brown J, Shah P, Stanton T, Marwick TH. Interaction and prognostic effects of left ventricular diastolic dysfunction and patient-prosthesis mismatch as determinants of outcome after isolated aortic valve replacement. Am J Cardiol. 2009;104:707–12.
74. Takeda S, Rimington H, Smeeton N, Chambers J. Long axis excursion in aortic stenosis. Heart. 2001;86:52–6.
75. Dumesnil JG, Shoucri RM, Laurenceau JL, Turcot J. A mathematical model of the dynamic geometry of the intact left ventricle and its application to clinical data. Circulation. 1979;59:1024–34.
76. Mor-Avi V, Lang RM, Badano LP, Belohlavek M, Cardim NM, Derumeaux G, Galderisi M, Marwick T, Nagueh SF, Sengupta PP, Sicari R, Smiseth OA, Smulevitz B, Takeuchi M, Thomas JD, Vannan M, Voigt JU, Zamorano JL. Current and evolving echocardiographic techniques for the quantitative evaluation of cardiac mechanics: ASE/EAE consensus statement on methodology and indications endorsed by the Japanese Society of Echocardiography. J Am Soc Echocardiogr. 2011;24:277–313.

77. Cramariuc D, Gerdts E, Davidsen ES, Segadal L, Matre K. Myocardial deformation in aortic valve stenosis: relation to left ventricular geometry. Heart. 2010;96:106–12.
78. Ng AC, Delgado V, Bertini M, Antoni ML, van Bommel RJ, van Rijnsoever EP, van der Kley F, Ewe SH, Witkowski T, Auger D, Nucifora G, Schuijf JD, Poldermans D, Leung DY, Schalij MJ, Bax JJ. Alterations in multidirectional myocardial functions in patients with aortic stenosis and preserved ejection fraction: a two-dimensional speckle tracking analysis. Eur Heart J. 2011;32:1542–50.
79. Lafitte S, Perlant M, Reant P, Serri K, Douard H, DeMaria A, Roudaut R. Impact of impaired myocardial deformations on exercise tolerance and prognosis in patients with asymptomatic aortic stenosis. Eur J Echocardiogr. 2009;10:414–9.
80. Attias D, Macron L, Dreyfus J, Monin JL, Brochet E, Lepage L, Hekimian G, Iung B, Vahanian A, Messika-Zeitoun D. Relationship between longitudinal strain and symptomatic status in aortic stenosis. J Am Soc Echocardiogr. 2013;26:868–74.
81. Amato MC, Moffa PJ, Werner KE, Ramires JA. Treatment decision in asymptomatic aortic valve stenosis: role of exercise testing. Heart. 2001;86:381–6.
82. Lancellotti P, Lebois F, Simon M, Tombeux C, Chauvel C, Pierard LA. Prognostic importance of quantitative exercise Doppler echocardiography in asymptomatic valvular aortic stenosis. Circulation. 2005;112:I377–82.
83. Maréchaux S, Hachicha Z, Bellouin A, Dumesnil JG, Meimoun P, Pasquet A, Bergeron S, Arsenault M, Le Tourneau T, Ennezat PV, Pibarot P. Usefulness of exercise-stress echocardiography for risk stratification of true asymptomatic patients with aortic valve stenosis. Eur Heart J. 2010;31:1390–7.
84. Lancellotti P, Magne J, Donal E, O'Connor K, Dulgheru R, Rosca M, Pierard LA. Determinants and prognostic significance of exercise pulmonary hypertension in asymptomatic severe aortic stenosis. Circulation. 2012;126:851–9.
85. Monin JL, Quéré JP, Monchi M, Petit H, Baleynaud S, Chauvel C, Pop C, Ohlmann P, Lelguen C, Dehant P, Tribouilloy C, Guéret P. Low-gradient aortic stenosis: operative risk stratification and predictors for long-term outcome: a multicenter study using dobutamine stress hemodynamics. Circulation. 2003;108:319–24.
86. Pereira JJ, Lauer MS, Bashir M, Afridi I, Blackstone EH, Stewart WJ, McCarthy PM, Thomas JD, Asher CR. Survival after aortic valve replacement for severe aortic stenosis with low transvalvular gradients and severe left ventricular dysfunction. J Am Coll Cardiol. 2002;39:1356–63.
87. Quere JP, Monin JL, Levy F, Petit H, Baleynaud S, Chauvel C, Pop C, Ohlmann P, Lelguen C, Dehant P, Gueret P, Tribouilloy C. Influence of preoperative left ventricular contractile reserve on postoperative ejection fraction in low-gradient aortic stenosis. Circulation. 2006;113:1738–44.
88. Pibarot P, Dumesnil JG. Low-flow, low-gradient aortic stenosis with normal and depressed left ventricular ejection fraction. J Am Coll Cardiol. 2012;60:1845–53.
89. Hachicha Z, Dumesnil JG, Bogaty P, Pibarot P. Paradoxical low-flow, low-gradient severe aortic stenosis despite preserved ejection fraction is associated with higher afterload and reduced survival. Circulation. 2007;115:2856–64.
90. Jander N, Minners J, Holme I, Gerdts E, Boman K, Brudi P, Chambers JB, Egstrup K, Kesäniemi YA, Malbecq W, Nienaber CA, Ray S, Rossebø A, Pedersen TR, Skjærpe T, Willenheimer R, Wachtell K, Neumann FJ, Gohlke-Bärwolf C. Outcome of patients with low-gradient "severe" aortic stenosis and preserved ejection fraction. Circulation. 2011;123:887–95.
91. Lancellotti P, Magne J, Donal E, Davin L, O'Connor K, Rosca M, Szymanski C, Cosyns B, Piérard LA. Clinical outcome in asymptomatic severe aortic stenosis: insights from the new proposed aortic stenosis grading classification. J Am Coll Cardiol. 2012;59:235–43.
92. Tarantini G, Covolo E, Razzolini R, Bilato C, Frigo AC, Napodano M, Favaretto E, Fraccaro C, Isabella G, Gerosa G, Iliceto S, Cribier A. Valve replacement for severe aortic stenosis with low transvalvular gradient and left ventricular ejection fraction exceeding 0.50. Ann Thorac Surg. 2011;91:1808–15.
93. Nishimura RA, Otto CM, Bonow RO, Carabello BA, Erwin JP, Guyton RA, O'Gara PT, Ruiz CE, Skubas NJ, Sorajja P, Sundt TM, Thomas JD. 2014 AHA/ACC guideline for the management of patients with valvular heart disease: a report of the American College of Cardiology/American Heart Association Task Force on practice guidelines. Circulation. 2014; 129:e521–e643.

Innovations in Microscopic Imaging of Atherosclerosis and Valvular Disease

12

Yu Nomura, Kengyeh K. Chu, Joseph A. Gardecki, Chen-hsin Sun, Linbo Liu, Eduardo Martinez-Martinez, Elena Aikawa, and Guillermo J. Tearney

Contents

Y. Nomura • K.K. Chu • J.A. Gardecki • C.-h. Sun • L. Liu • E. Martinez-Martinez
Wellman Center for Photomedicine,
Massachusetts General Hospital, Boston, MA 02114, USA

G.J. Tearney, MD, PhD (✉)
Department of Pathology and Wellman Center for Photomedicine,
Massachusetts General Hospital, BHX604A,
Boston, MA 02114, USA
e-mail: gtearney@partners.org

E. Aikawa, MD
Division of Cardiovascular Medicine,
Brigham and Women's Hospital, Harvard Medical School,
Boston, MA 02115, USA
e-mail: eaikawa@partners.org; eaikawa@rics.bwh.harvard.edu

E. Aikawa (ed.), *Cardiovascular Imaging: Arterial and Aortic Valve Inflammation and Calcification*, DOI 10.1007/978-3-319-09268-3_12

Abstract

Calcific aortic valve disease (CAVD) is still an unsolved medical problem, because the pathogenesis of CAVD is poorly understood and early calcification is hard to identify. The lack of high-resolution imaging tools to study early stage disease further hampers the search for therapeutic targets.

Micro-optical coherence tomography (μOCT), which is a new form of OCT, is the highest-resolution cross-sectional OCT technology available today with 1 μm resolution. We used μOCT to visualize detailed cellular and subcellular structure associated with early calcific changes in diseased human and murine aortic valves. The results suggest that μOCT imaging has the potential to provide new insights into underlying mechanisms of CAVD.

12.1 Introduction

Atherosclerosis, which is a putative cause of both coronary artery disease and aortic valve stenosis, is one of the critical medical problems in the United States and other industrialized countries. According to FDA statistics, 815,000 Americans die from cardiovascular disease every year [1].

Accumulating evidence supports a key role of inflammation in the progression of atherosclerosis, including macrophage activation and microcalcifications. Unfortunately, few methods exist that are suitable for directly visualizing these microscopic contributors to cardiovascular atherosclerosis; much of our current understanding emanates from indirect methods or ex vivo studies. Histology, which has long been accepted as the gold standard method to analyze microscopic anatomy of cells and tissues, is susceptible to artifacts such as shrinkage, tissue loss during processing, color changes for different tissue types, and alterations of the tissue structure. Furthermore, histological sections by nature represent very thin slices of the artery, requiring hundreds of slides to obtain a complete sampling of the volume of interest, or to find specific cellular features. Electron microscopy techniques, including scanning electron microscopy (SEM) or transmission electron microscopy (TEM), are similarly limited in addition to their high cost. Other imaging modalities, such as intravascular ultrasound (IVUS), x-ray computed tomography (CT), or magnetic resonance imaging (MRI), do provide volumetric imaging of whole samples, but do not provide sufficient resolution to identify cellular structures. The development of new therapeutic strategies would be greatly aided by tools that can reveal early microscopic changes of disease to precisely identify mechanisms that contribute to atherosclerosis.

Optical imaging technology, specifically optical coherence tomography (OCT), has been implemented with small-diameter fiber-optic catheters to allow simultaneous measurements of the multiple types of plaque features at the microscopic architectural level, shedding new light into the fundamental problems underlying cardiovascular medicine. OCT combines the advantages of in vivo access and volumetric sampling with the inherent high resolution of optical imaging. Until recently, technical constraints have limited the maximum resolution obtainable with OCT be approximately 10 μm, which represents an order of magnitude improvement over comparable alternatives, but remaining too coarse to resolve the macrophages, cholesterol crystals, and microcalcifications that drive current interest in the field.

In this chapter, we will summarize the contributions and limitations of modern OCT in present cardiovascular biomedical sciences and clinical practice. We will further overview the progression of next-generation forms of OCT, such as micro-OCT (μOCT), toward true cellular-level microscopic imaging. We further evaluate the potential for this technology especially for visualizing the pathological features associated with the early initiation and progression of facets of cardiovascular disease that are characterized by microscopic defects and infiltrates. We will specifically examine the diagnostic potential of μOCT in the context of calcific aortic valve disease (CAVD) and coronary atherosclerosis.

12.2 OCT

Optical coherence tomography (OCT) is an optical imaging technique that generates high-resolution cross-sectional images of tissue microstructure. OCT produces cross-sectional images by measuring the depth of reflecting objects in a sample. OCT can thus be thought of as ultrasound with light, or microscopic radar, except that infrared light waves are used rather than acoustic pulses or microwaves. OCT measures the echo time delay of light reflected or backscattered from the tissue at different depths by using interferometry.

In its original and most basic implementation [2], OCT images are constructed point by point. Infrared light is focused into a column in the sample, and a reference mirror scans through each imaging depth. The presence or absence of optical interference at each reference arm position corresponds to the presence or absence of a scattering object at that depth. Once a single column is scanned through depth, the beam is moved, and a new column is scanned. This original form is now known as time-domain OCT (TD-OCT). In 2003, several laboratories concurrently discovered that an alternative configuration of OCT yields substantial improvements in imaging speed and sensitivity [3–5]. In this new configuration, it is not necessary to take a separate measurement for each imaging depth. The optical spectrum of the interference between a fixed reference mirror and sample light is transformed to generate an entire column's worth of image data. This second-generation form of OCT is known broadly as frequency-domain OCT (FD-OCT). The spectral data can be generated using a laser that sweeps through a range of optical wavelengths through time, known as swept-source OCT (SS-OCT) or optical frequency-domain imaging (OFDI) [6]. Alternatively, all wavelengths may be utilized simultaneously but segregated with a spectrometer, which is known as spectral-domain OCT (SD-OCT). These newer generation forms of OCT have mostly consigned the slower TD-OCT to obsolescence for the purposes of in vivo imaging.

The axial resolution of OCT is determined primarily by the bandwidth of its illumination, with broader spectra generating finer resolutions. In a typical OFDI system, the resolution is approximately 10 μm, up to ten times higher than any clinically available diagnostic imaging modality including intravascular ultrasound [7]. Fiber-optic probes have been incorporated into coronary catheters and provide high-resolution images of internal coronary microstructure, which has developed quite rapidly and ascended to clinical use [8, 9]. This intravascular optical coherence tomography (IVOCT) has the potential to guide therapeutic interventions and diagnose atherosclerosis and can be used to study the causes of coronary artery disease. In order to acquire high-quality images, earlier generation TD-OCT systems required an occlusive saline flush to remove blood from the field of view. The rise of second-generation FD-OCT systems enabled much faster 3D pullback imaging during the non-occlusive administration of optical transparent media such as contrast media or Lactated Ringer's solution, greatly increasing the convenience of IVOCT imaging in the cardiac catheterization lab [10].

Histopathological studies have shown that OCT can provide information about the microstructure of the coronary artery and detailed tissue characterization, correlated by histopathological comparison data [11–13]. Despite limited penetration depth through the necrotic core, the greatly improved resolution compared to intravascular ultrasound reveals superficial endothelium intima defects, coronary artery dissection, stent malposition, and edge dissection, among others [9]. Additionally, intracoronary OCT has been utilized to improve our understanding of inflammatory characters of atherosclerosis, such as necrotic core, thin fibrous cap, and macrophage accumulations [11, 12, 14, 15].

However, a resolution of 10 μm remains too coarse to resolve many of the most interesting and important features of atherosclerosis, including inflammatory cells such monocytes and macrophages, as well as subcellular features including platelets, fibrin, microcalcifications, and crystalline cholesterol deposits. To address this limitation, micro-OCT (μOCT) has recently been developed, with approximately 1 μm resolution in the axial dimension and 2 μm resolution in the transverse dimensions [16]. Early data suggests that μOCT holds promise for providing a greater understanding of the cellular and subcellular pathophysiology of coronary artery disease in patients.

12.3 μOCT Technology

The principal limits of resolution in OCT are twofold. First, axial resolution is determined by the bandwidth of the illumination, and the limited spectral widths of typical OCT sources such as swept-source lasers and superluminescent diodes have kept resolutions in the 10 μm range. Second, lateral resolution is determined by classical microscopy considerations, which dictate that high numerical aperture (NA) lenses are required to focus a beam to the small sizes that correspond to high resolution. Unfortunately, these same high NA beams exhibit very shallow depths of focus (DOF), which would result in OCT images that maintain its desired resolution over an insignificant depth range. Because of these limitations, the resolution attainable by OCT has remained approximately an order of magnitude below that of other light microscopy techniques. Micro-OCT (μOCT) is a new implementation of OCT that addresses both axial and lateral resolution limitations in conventional OCT [16]. Recent advances in commercially available ultra-wideband sources known as supercontinuum lasers have provided extraordinary bandwidth and acceptable levels of noise for high-sensitivity OCT, enabling very high axial resolution. Additionally, a special annular beam geometry is used to strike a balance between lateral resolution and depth of focus, resulting in lateral resolution of approximately 2 μm sustained over an imaging depth of ~300 μm [16].

12.4 Calcific Aortic Valve Disease (CAVD)

12.4.1 Current Status: A Still Unsolved Medical Problem

Calcific aortic valve disease (CAVD) is characterized by a buildup of calcium deposits within the aortic valve leaflets. When CAVD progresses to symptomatic aortic stenosis, morbidity and mortality are already very high (20 % 5-year mortality) [17]. The only effective therapy is valve replacement, which is expensive and has a small but finite risk. Hyperlipidemia is hypothesized to contribute to CAVD, though intensive lipid lowering therapy has failed to demonstrate clinical efficiency in preventing the progression of aortic valve stenosis between the patients with mild to moderate asymptomatic aortic valve stenosis in the prospective SALTIRE, SEAS, and ASTRONOMER clinical trials [18–21]. A possible reason that the outcome of such trials has been negative is the late onset of treatments. Patients selected for trials may already have formed irreversible macrocalcifications that are intractable to pharmacologic treatment. Identification of CAVD at an earlier stage would be clearly advantageous to the investigation of potential drug therapies [22]. Additionally, the pathogenesis of CAVD is poorly understood, further obscuring the search for therapeutic targets. One key barrier for understanding CAVD is the lack of a high-resolution imaging tool to study early stage disease in vivo [23, 24].

12.4.2 Mechanism of Aortic Valve Calcification

The aortic valve is stratified into three major extracellular matrix (ECM) layers: the fibrosa, spongiosa, and ventricularis, including valve interstitial cells (VICs) and valve endothelial cells (VECs) at the blood-containing surfaces. The fibrosa layer, which is close to the outflow surface, is mainly composed of dense collagens and provides mechanical strength to the valve. The spongiosa layer, the central core of loose connective tissue, contains rich glycosaminoglycans (GAG). The ventricularis layer is rich in elastin below the inflow surface to diminish radial strain (Fig. 12.1) [23, 25–27]. Although these layers interact to maintain homeostasis of the valve environment, various environmental factors, such as shear stress, hypertension, hyperlipidemia, metabolic syndromes, or chronic renal failure, can incite the inflammatory signal cascade of aortic valve calcification [23, 28]. Endothelial cell injury amplified by these atherosclerotic risk factors may provoke an injury-repair cycle

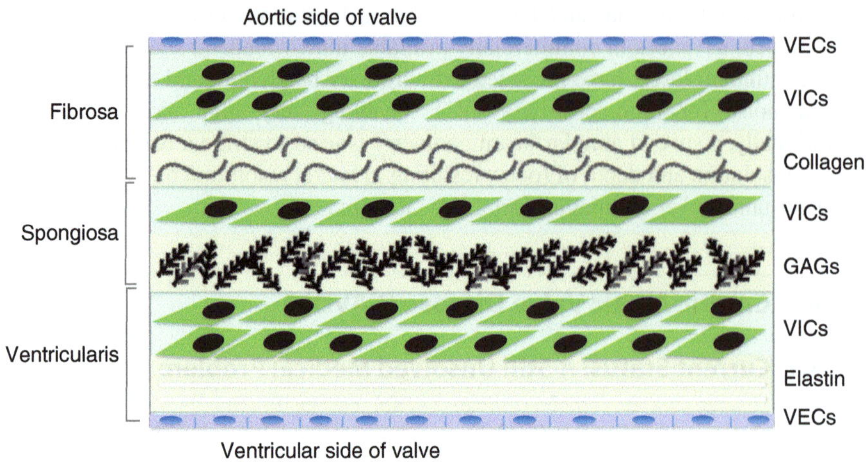

Fig. 12.1 Cellular and architectural microscopic morphology of the normal aortic valve (Adapted from Rajamannan et al. [23])

that increases inflammatory cytokines and adhesive molecules. Activated macrophages, differentiated from monocytes, follow with the release of proteolytic enzymes, which affects the extracellular matrix causing cell apoptosis and transforming VICs to osteoblast-like cells. A series of activated osteogenic processes contribute to valvular calcification. The early stages of proliferated mineralization are identified as microcalcification. These processes are amplified and propagated, leading to bone formation with neovascularization in the skeleton and ECM degradation, and finally result in prominent macrocalcification [23–25].

12.4.3 μOCT Imaging of Aortic Valves

Investigation of heart valve calcification has lagged that of coronary artery calcification. However, based on the concept that calcific aortic valve disease may represent one direction of the end stages of atherosclerosis, as coronary artery disease does, our laboratory has explored the use of μOCT in visualizing the pathological features associated with the early initiation and progression of calcific aortic valve disease [29].

We imaged human and murine aortic valve leaflets ex vivo [**2011P000970**]. Human valves were harvested from autopsy heart explants and surgical fragments obtained from aortic valve replacement surgeries. Each human aortic valve was dissected from the root of an aorta and placed in a sample chamber. The aortic valve leaf was partially submerged in phosphate-buffered saline to prevent tissue dehydration during image acquisition. The valve tissue was further sectioned into 2 mm stripes to match the μOCT system image acquisition range and to enable localization of the scanned area for histopathological validation. We chose regions of interest after gross visual inspection of the tissue and applied conventional OCT

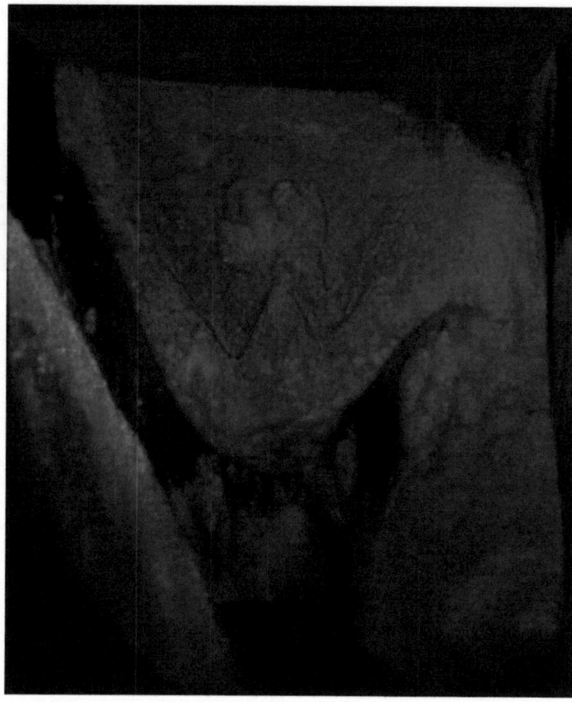

Fig. 12.2 3D reconstruction of a murine aortic valve cusp

examination at room temperature. After imaging, we placed ink dots at the beginning of the scan volume to be able to identify the initial scan plane. Acquired images were processed with MATLAB and Image J [41]. We used H&E, Masson's trichrome, and von Kossa stains for the histological study. Each μOCT image was correlated with histology.

We also imaged aortic valves from wild-type and ApoE knockout mice ex vivo to identify pathological features of early aortic valve calcification. Mice received a high-cholesterol diet for 20 weeks. The aortic root was dissected after the mice were euthanized. The valves were placed in the sample chamber with care not to destroy the tissue and were immersed in PBS during imaging at room temperature. Because the murine valves were too small to place registration ink dots, we matched histology by comparing each slide to two-dimensional recuts of the 3D μOCT dataset. Three-dimensional renderings of the μOCT images also provided information pertaining to gross valve morphology (Fig. 12.2). Histology was stained with von Kossa for detecting calcium deposition and alkaline phosphatase for visualizing early osteogenesis.

12.4.4 Extracellular Matrix

The role of the ECM is to maintain valve homeostasis against mechanical forces of the aortic valve. Previous in vitro work suggested disarrayed or decreased collagen

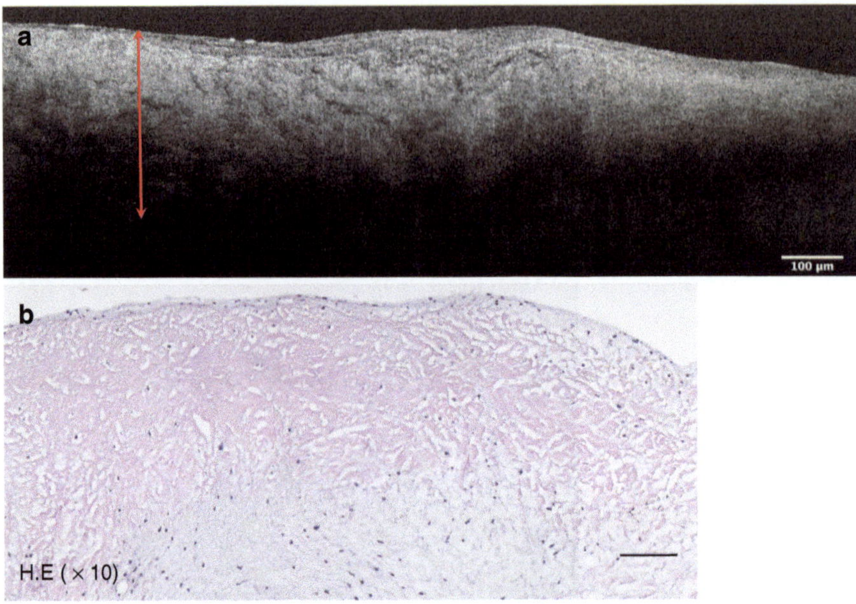

Fig. 12.3 µOCT image of the disorganized ECM (bidirectional *arrow*) of the diseased valve (**a**). Correlated histology shows thickened fibrosa layer and decreased VICs (**b**)

layer contributed to increased proliferation of valvular interstitial cells (VICs), apoptosis, and valve calcification [30]. The unique aortic valve structure contributes to valve pliability, enabling ~100,000 open/close cycles a day and withstanding lifelong exposure to high aortic pressure. Normal valves exhibit organized ECM layers and compartmentalization of VICs, while diseased valves are marked by increased thickness, ECM disorganization, and VIC disarray [26, 27].

In our µOCT datasets, we were also able to identify similar disorganized structure in the diseased human valve. Correlated H&E histology demonstrated thickened fibrosa layers and decreased VICs (Fig. 12.3). Disorganized collagen fibrils are visible with Masson's trichrome stain, which labels collagen as blue [23] (Fig. 12.4). Other µOCT images show a comparison between murine aortic valves of wild-type mice and ApoE-deficient mice given a high-fat diet. The organized ECM layers and compartmentalization of VICs can be seen in cross-sectional µOCT images of the mid-level cusps (right). A thickened, disorganized ECM is visible in the diseased valve (Fig. 12.5).

12.4.5 Cells

As in arterial atherosclerosis, various inflammatory cells such as activated macrophages, foam cells, and lymphocytes are involved in the mechanisms that underlie the development of CAVD. Once endothelial cells become inflamed, adhesion

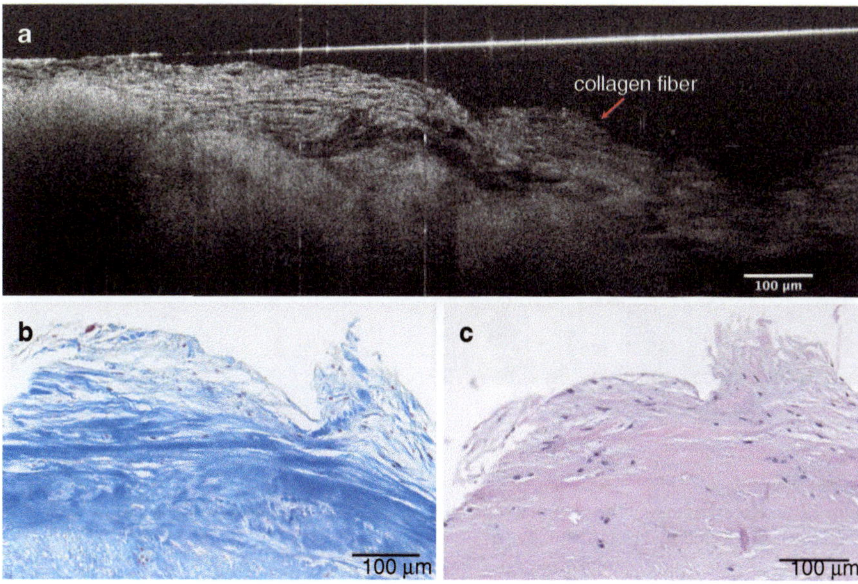

Fig. 12.4 μOCT image of disorganized collagen fibers (*red arrow*) (**a**). Correlated histology stained by Masson's trichrome (**b**) and H&E (**c**)

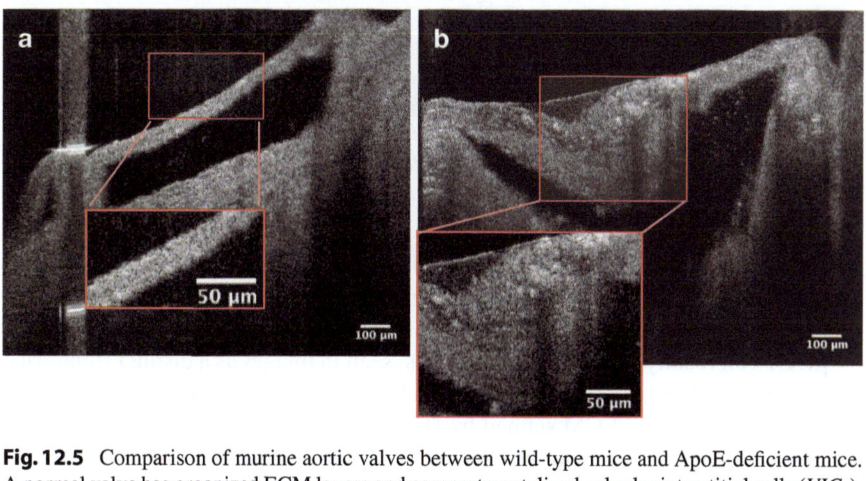

Fig. 12.5 Comparison of murine aortic valves between wild-type mice and ApoE-deficient mice. A normal valve has organized ECM layers and compartmentalized valvular interstitial cells (*VICs*), as shown in a wild-type leaflet (**a**, *red box*). Valve thickness is on the order of 50 μm and organized elastin fibers are clearly visible in the aortic root. A diseased valve exhibits thickened (>100 μm) and disorganized ECM (**b**, *red box*)

molecules not found in normal valves are expressed. Monocytes adhere to the adhesion molecules, migrate into the subendothelial space in the valve, and differentiate into activated macrophages [31]. Activated macrophages are thought to play a central role in the proteolytic action of early valve calcification by producing a

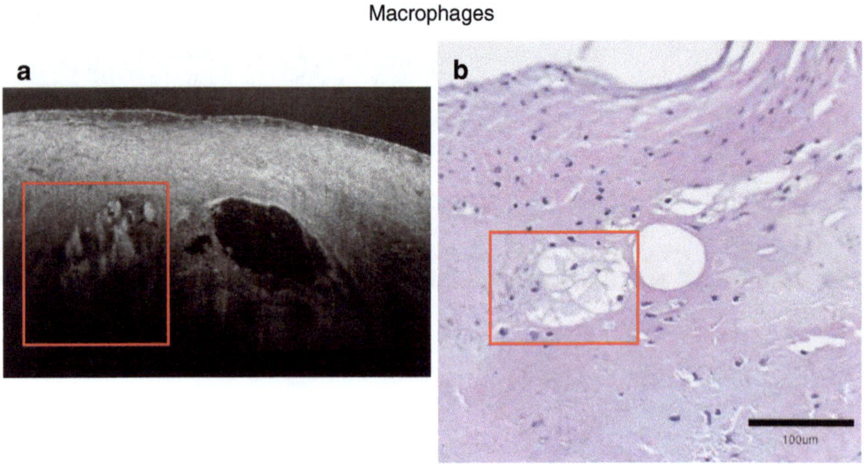

Fig. 12.6 Representative image of macrophages (**a**). Macrophages (*red boxes*) accumulate within the voids, supported by H&E histology (**b**)

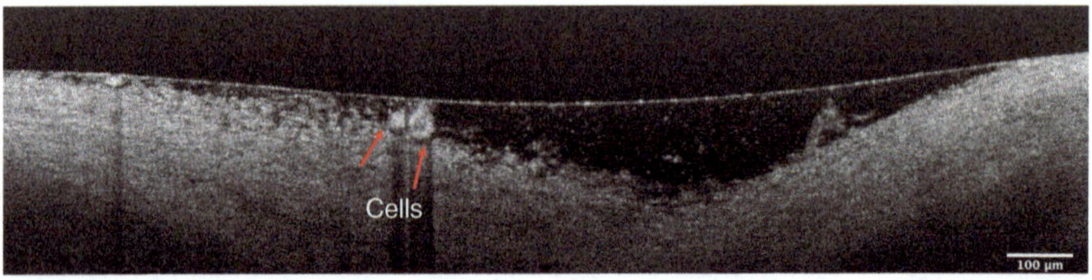

Fig. 12.7 Cells adherent to the endothelium (*red arrows*). 30 µm large cells are considered to be macrophages judging from the size and shape

variety of cytokines that cause ECM remodeling and consequently increasing valve stiffness and thickening. Aikawa et al. demonstrated the accumulation of macrophages in early aortic valve lesions using fluorescence reflectance imaging [32].

µOCT can readily visualize macrophages, seen in images as a distinct signal-rich region of oval shape. Correlated histology showed numerous macrophage accumulations in disorganized ECM stained by H&E (Fig. 12.6). In another representative image, a 30 µm large cell can be seen adherent to the endothelium, likely to be a monocyte based on size and shape (Fig. 12.7).

12.4.6 Cholesterol

Cholesterol facilitates the vicious cycle of cardiovascular inflammation [29]. The initiation is saturated lipoprotein entry and accumulation in the arterial wall or subendothelium within the aortic valve, and oxidation, which invites the entry of

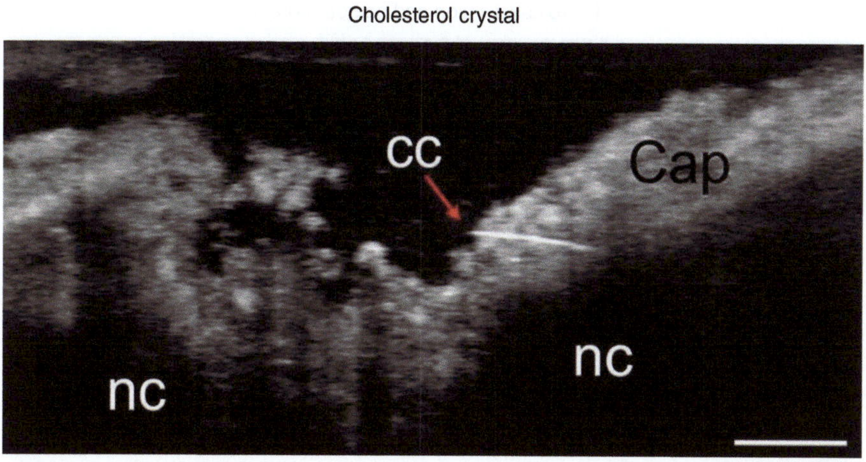

Fig. 12.8 Representative image of cholesterol crystal (*red arrow*), which penetrates into the cap of a necrotic core within a human coronary artery. Scale bar, 30 μm. *CC* cholesterol crystal, *NC* necrotic core (Reproduced from Linbo et al. [16])

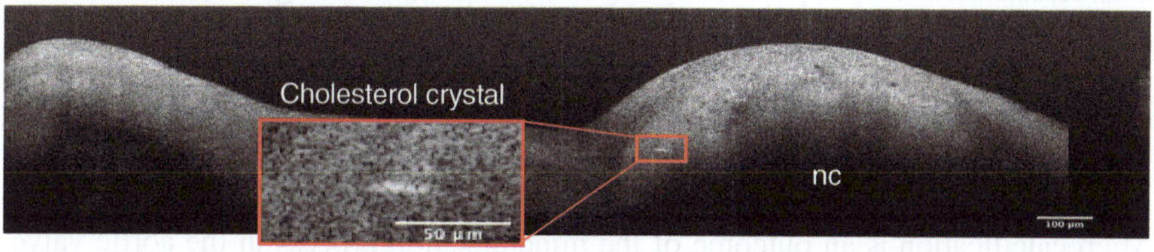

Fig. 12.9 A linear structure consistent with a cholesterol crystal identified in a human aortic valve

macrophages. Accumulation of macrophage-derived foam cells leads to the formation of cholesterol crystals, finally resulting in foam cell apoptosis and extracellular lipid deposit [33]. Previous study suggested products of oxidized cholesterol may facilitate aortic valve calcification [34, 35]. Duewell et al. demonstrated cholesterol crystal appearance in early atherosclerotic lesions and that the NLRP3 inflammasome cytokine pathway is triggered by cholesterol crystals and results in acute inflammation [36]. On μOCT images, cholesterol crystals are seen as signal-rich needlelike structures. A single cholesterol crystal penetrating the cap of the necrotic core is resolvable by μOCT [16] (Fig. 12.8). The high resolution of μOCT appears to lower the threshold of detection for cholesterol crystals, which have been inconsistently visualized by previous lower resolution OCT technologies [9]. Similar to coronary artery atherosclerosis, lipid accumulation is found in early lesions of calcified valves and may accelerate valve calcification [29, 31, 37, 38]. Cholesterol crystals may be seen as fine linear structure adjacent to huge necrotic core in our μOCT images (Fig. 12.9). It is potentially useful to detect cholesterol deposition in an early stage of CAVD, which could enable the discrimination of high-risk patients that may undergo subsequent disease progression.

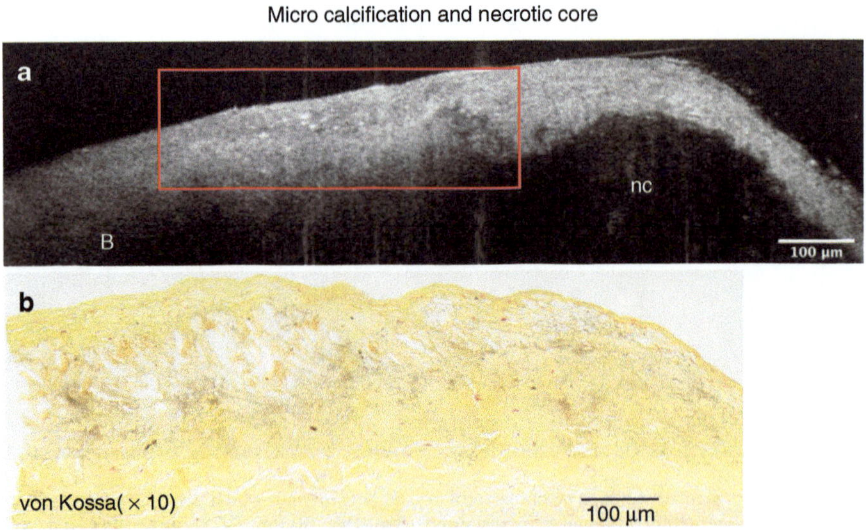

Fig. 12.10 Microcalcification adjacent to necrotic core (**a**). Microcalcification (*red box*) appears as an accumulation of small, punctate high signal densities in μOCT images, supported by corresponding von Kossa stain (**b**)

12.4.7 Microcalcification

Microcalcification is an outcome of the mineralization process in the aortic valve. Microcalcifications may enhance inflammation and contribute to more abundant deposition of calcium and increased valve stiffness [23, 39]. Vengrenyuk et al. hypothesized that microcalcification in a fibrous cap may cause stress concentration and contribute to rupture based on finite element analysis (FEM) and high-resolution imaging, including confocal microscopy and micro-computed tomography, which confirmed the existence of microcalcifications in autopsy samples ex vivo [40].

μOCT can identify microcalcifications as accumulations of small, punctate high signal densities adjacent to a large necrotic core (Fig. 12.10). Correlated histology shows microcalcifications stained by von Kossa and a large necrotic core (Fig. 12.10). Figure 12.11 shows an aortic valve of ApoE-deficient mice subject to a high-fat diet, imaged by μOCT. Microcalcification is visualized as distinct punctate densities in the thickened diseased valve, supported by correlated histology with von Kossa staining (Fig. 12.11).

12.5 Limitations of μOCT

Compared to conventional OCT, μOCT provides an order of magnitude improvement in resolution, though two main compromises were necessary to achieve this gain. First, shorter wavelengths are used in μOCT to attain high axial resolution.

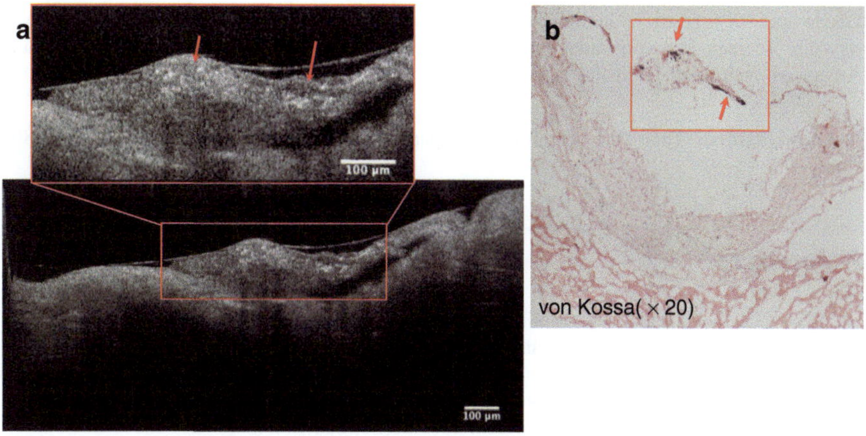

Fig. 12.11 Microcalcification (*red arrows*) of the murine aortic valves (**a**) and corresponding histology stained by von Kossa (**b**)

The center wavelength of μOCT is approximately 800 nm compared to ~1,300 nm in typical intravascular OCT. The shorter center wavelength results in poorer penetration into tissue. Second, though loss of focal depth is mitigated in μOCT using its annular beam geometry, the overall depth of focus in μOCT remains shallower than conventional OCT. Like conventional OCT, the penetration depth of μOCT images also depends on how well light transmits through the tissue. As the light passes through the specimen, it is attenuated by scattering and absorption. For example, the light is highly attenuated by macrophages and necrotic core and so not much is seen by μOCT below these tissues. On the other hand, when light passes through collagen or calcium that has lower attenuation, μOCT image data can be visualized much deeper in the tissue. It is also sometimes difficult to correlate μOCT with histology due to the presence of histology processing artifacts and the possibility of tissue deformation.

12.6 Conclusion and Future Perspective

In this study, μOCT enabled visualization of detailed cellular and subcellular structure associated with early calcific changes in diseased human and murine aortic valves. This data suggests that μOCT imaging has the potential to provide new insights into underlying mechanisms of CAVD. Currently, our μOCT system is limited to experiments conducted ex vivo. Catheter-based μOCT will allow us to visualize these cellular and subcellular constituents of atherosclerosis and CAVD in vivo. The advent of catheter-based μOCT will be very exciting indeed, as it will give us new insight into the microscopic mechanisms that underlie atherosclerosis and valvular disease.

Disclosures Drs. Tearney, Gardecki, Liu, and Chu have applied for patents on the μOCT technology. Dr. Tearney is a consultant for and receives sponsored research funding from Samsung Advanced Institute of Technology.

Acknowledgment This work was funded in part by NIH R01HL076398 and R01HL114805 (to EA).

References

1. FDA U.S. Food and Drug Administration. http://www.fda.gov/ForConsumers/ByAudience/ForPatientAdvocates/CardiovascularInfo/default.htm.
2. Huang D, et al. Optical coherence tomography. Science. 1991;254(5035):1178–81.
3. de Boer JF, et al. Improved signal-to-noise ratio in spectral-domain compared with time-domain optical coherence tomography. Opt Lett. 2003;28(21):2067–9.
4. Leitgeb R, Hitzenberger CF, Fercher AF. Performance of fourier domain vs. time domain optical coherence tomography. Opt Express. 2003;11(8):889–94.
5. Choma MA, et al. Sensitivity advantage of swept source and Fourier domain optical coherence tomography. Opt Express. 2003;11(18):2183–9.
6. Yun S, et al. High-speed optical frequency-domain imaging. Opt Express. 2003;11(22):2953–63.
7. Suter MJ, et al. Intravascular optical imaging technology for investigating the coronary artery. JACC Cardiovasc Imaging. 2011;4(9):1022–39.
8. Tearney GJ, et al. In vivo endoscopic optical biopsy with optical coherence tomography. Science. 1997;276(5321):2037–9.
9. Tearney GJ, et al. Consensus standards for acquisition, measurement, and reporting of intravascular optical coherence tomography studies: a report from the International Working Group for Intravascular Optical Coherence Tomography Standardization and Validation. J Am Coll Cardiol. 2012;59(12):1058–72.
10. Tearney GJ, et al. Three-dimensional coronary artery microscopy by intracoronary optical frequency domain imaging. J Am Coll Cardiol Img. 2008;1(6):752–61.
11. Yabushita H, et al. Characterization of human atherosclerosis by optical coherence tomography. Circulation. 2002;106:1640–5.
12. Tanaka A, Tearney GJ, Bouma BE. Challenges on the frontier of intracoronary imaging: atherosclerotic plaque macrophage measurement by optical coherence tomography. J Biomed Opt. 2010;15(1):011104.
13. Tearney GJ, Jang IK, Bouma BE. Optical coherence tomography for imaging the vulnerable plaque. J Biomed Opt. 2013;11(2):021002.
14. Tanaka A, et al. Morphology of exertion-triggered plaque rupture in patients with acute coronary syndrome: an optical coherence tomography study. Circulation. 2008;118(23):2368–73.
15. Virmani R, et al. Lessons from sudden coronary death: a comprehensive morphological classification scheme for atherosclerotic lesions. Arterioscler Thromb Vasc Biol. 2000;20(5):1262–75.
16. Liu L, et al. Imaging the subcellular structure of human coronary atherosclerosis using micro-optical coherence tomography. Nat Med. 2011;17(8):1010–4.
17. Horstkotte D, Loogen F. The natural history of aortic valve stenosis. Eur Heart J. 1988;9(Suppl E):57–64.
18. Otto CM. Calcific aortic stenosis–time to look more closely at the valve. N Engl J Med. 2008;359(13):1395–8.
19. Chan KL, et al. Effect of lipid lowering with rosuvastatin on progression of aortic stenosis: results of the aortic stenosis progression observation: measuring effects of rosuvastatin (ASTRONOMER) trial. Circulation. 2010;121(2):306–14.
20. Cowell SJ, et al. A randomized trial of intensive lipid-lowering therapy in calcific aortic stenosis. N Engl J Med. 2005;352(23):2389–97.

21. Farmer JA. Intensive lipid lowering with simvastatin and ezetimibe in aortic stenosis (the SEAS trial). Curr Atheroscler Rep. 2009;11(2):82–3.
22. Bonow RO, et al. Guidelines for the management of patients with valvular heart disease: executive summary. A report of the American College of Cardiology/American Heart Association Task Force on Practice Guidelines (Committee on Management of Patients with Valvular Heart Disease). Circulation. 1998;98(18):1949–84.
23. Rajamannan NM, et al. Calcific aortic valve disease: not simply a degenerative process: a review and agenda for research from the National Heart and Lung and Blood Institute Aortic Stenosis Working Group. Executive summary: calcific aortic valve disease-2011 update. Circulation. 2011;124(16):1783–91.
24. New SE, Aikawa E. Molecular imaging insights into early inflammatory stages of arterial and aortic valve calcification. Circ Res. 2011;108((11):1381–91.
25. Leopold J, et al. Cellular mechanisms of aortic valve calcification. Circ Cardiovasc Interv. 2012;5(4):605–14.
26. Hinton Jr RB, et al. Extracellular matrix remodeling and organization in developing and diseased aortic valves. Circ Res. 2006;98(11):1431–8.
27. Schoen FJ. Evolving concepts of cardiac valve dynamics: the continuum of development, functional structure, pathobiology, and tissue engineering. Circulation. 2008;118(18):1864–80.
28. Stewart BF, et al. Clinical factors associated with calcific aortic valve disease. J Am Coll Cardiol. 1997;29((3):630—4.
29. Demer LL. Cholesterol in vascular and valvular calcification. Circulation. 2001;104(16):1881–3.
30. Rodriguez KJ, et al. Manipulation of valve composition to elucidate the role of collagen in aortic valve calcification. BMC Cardiovasc Disord. 2014;14(1):29.
31. Mohler 3rd ER. Mechanisms of aortic valve calcification. Am J Cardiol. 2004;94(11):1396–402.
32. Aikawa E, et al. Multimodality molecular imaging identifies proteolytic and osteogenic activities in early aortic valve disease. Circulation. 2007;115(3):377–86.
33. Tangirala RK, et al. Formation of cholesterol monohydrate crystals in macrophage-derived foam cells. J Lipid Res. 1994;35(1):93–104.
34. Olsson M, Thyberg J, Nilsson J. Presence of oxidized low density lipoprotein in nonrheumatic stenotic aortic valves. Arterioscler Thromb Vasc Biol. 1999;19(5):1218–22.
35. Mohler ER, et al. Identification and characterization of calcifying valve cells from human and canine aortic valves. J Heart Valve Dis. 1999;8:254–60.
36. Duewell P, et al. NLRP3 inflammasomes are required for atherogenesis and activated by cholesterol crystals. Nature. 2010;464(7293):1357–61.
37. Elmariah S, Mohler ER. The pathogenesis and treatment of the valvulopathy of aortic stenosis: beyond the SEAS. Curr Cardiol Rep. 2010;12(2):125–32.
38. O'Brien KD. Pathogenesis of calcific aortic valve disease: a disease process comes of age (and a good deal more). Arterioscler Thromb Vasc Biol. 2006;26(8):1721–8.
39. Aikawa E, et al. Osteogenesis associates with inflammation in early-stage atherosclerosis evaluated by molecular imaging in vivo. Circulation. 2007;116(24):2841–50.
40. Vengrenyuk Y, et al. A hypothesis for vulnerable plaque rupture due to stress-induced debonding around cellular microcalcifications in thin fibrous caps. Proc Natl Acad Sci U S A. 2006;103(40):14678–83.
41. Rasband, W.S., ImageJ, U. S. National Institutes of Health, Bethesda, Maryland, USA, http://imagej.nih.gov/ij/, 1997–14.

Part III

Clinical Imaging of Cardiovascular Inflammation and Calcification

Molecular MR Imaging of Atherosclerosis

13

Rik P.M. Moonen, Gustav J. Strijkers, Zahi A. Fayad, Mat J.A.P. Daemen, and Klaas Nicolay

Contents

R.P.M. Moonen, PhD • K. Nicolay, PhD (✉)
Biomedical NMR, Department of Biomedical Engineering,
Eindhoven University of Technology, HTC 11 1.247,
High Tech Campus 11, 5656 AE Eindhoven, The Netherlands

Center for Imaging Research and Education (CIRE), Eindhoven, The Netherlands
e-mail: r.p.m.moonen@tue.nl; rikmoonen@gmail.com; k.nicolay@tue.nl

G.J. Strijkers, PhD
Biomedical NMR, Department of Biomedical Engineering,
Eindhoven University of Technology, HTC 11 1.247,
High Tech Campus 11, 5656 AE Eindhoven, The Netherlands

Center for Imaging Research and Education (CIRE), Eindhoven, The Netherlands

Department of Biomedical Engineering and Physics,
Academic Medical Center, University of Amsterdam, Amsterdam, The Netherlands
e-mail: g.j.strijkers@tue.nl

Z.A. Fayad, PhD
Translational and Molecular Imaging Institute,
Icahn School of Medicine at Mount Sinai, New York, NY, USA
e-mail: zahi.fayad@mssm.edu; zahi.fayad@gmail.com

M.J.A.P. Daemen, MD
Department of Pathology, Academic Medical Center,
University of Amsterdam, Amsterdam, The Netherlands
e-mail: m.j.daemen@amc.uva.nl

E. Aikawa (ed.), *Cardiovascular Imaging: Arterial and Aortic Valve Inflammation and Calcification*, DOI 10.1007/978-3-319-09268-3_13

Abstract

In recent years, extensive research in atherosclerosis disease has elucidated many of the biological and molecular mechanisms and pathways involved in plaque development and progression. This has identified dozens of novel targets for diagnosis, therapy, and treatment evaluation. In vivo molecular imaging techniques, and in particular molecular magnetic resonance imaging (MRI), facilitate studies on the etiology of atherosclerosis and the evaluation of emerging therapies. In this chapter, we review contrast agents and (quantitative) MRI pulse sequences and strategies that have been developed for molecular MRI of atherosclerosis. We focus on targeted and nontargeted MRI contrast agents for specific imaging of inflammation (and especially macrophages), lipids, fibrous cap, thrombus, intra-plaque hemorrhage, apoptosis, and neovascularization. Contrast agents that are discussed include iron oxide-based agents (USPIO, MPIO), gadolinium-based materials (low molecular weight agents, micelles, liposomes, HDL-like particles) for ^{1}H MRI, as well as perfluorocarbon (PFC) emulsions for ^{19}F MRI. The most promising strategies for diagnosis (vulnerable, rupture-prone plaque detection), for determining therapeutic pathways, for monitoring of therapy, and for treatment personalization will be reviewed in more detail, discussing their value for preclinical research and clinical translation.

13.1 Introduction

In recent years, atherosclerosis research has elucidated many of the biological and molecular mechanisms and pathways involved in development and progression of the disease. This research has identified dozens of new potential targets for diagnosis, therapy, and treatment evaluation. Molecular imaging plays a vital role in unraveling these mechanisms and also provides a broad range of valuable diagnostic and monitoring tools. Molecular magnetic resonance imaging (MRI) possesses some advantageous properties that make it a highly useful tool at all levels, ranging from fundamental research and drug development to clinical diagnosis and readout of therapy response.

The multitude of identified imaging and therapeutic targets have variable potential for clinical translation. However, even when an imaging agent has been found unsuitable for human application, it may still serve an important role as a preclinical tool for monitoring treatment effects and unveiling the therapeutic pathways in animal models. In this chapter, we will discuss how molecular imaging in general, and molecular MRI in particular, can improve our current understanding of atherosclerotic disease and how it can be treated.

13.1.1 Application Areas for Molecular Imaging

In preclinical atherosclerosis research, molecular imaging finds its main application in identifying treatment options and providing both early and long-term readouts of treatment effects. This requires standardized methods for assessing various plaque properties, e.g., the composition of the extracellular matrix or the activity and subtypes of inflammatory cells. Standardization of methods is required to enable the comparison of results between different research centers and, perhaps more important, comparison of different therapies targeting similar pathways.

During the clinical stage of developing a new therapy, molecular imaging can fulfill a similar role. It can be used to confirm the relevance of the pathway that is targeted. Obviously, there exist important differences between humans and animal models in terms of atherosclerotic plaque composition and development. Consequently, translation may not always be straightforward and mechanisms of therapy may be quite different [1]. Standardized molecular imaging methods for various plaque components and pathways are therefore important for clinical translation. Another important role for molecular imaging in clinical research is in monitoring treatment effect and dose finding. Once the relevance of a therapeutic pathway has been confirmed, the same target may be used for molecular imaging of treatment response. This monitoring role extends to the final clinical application of new therapies and as such may help to personalize treatment. Monitoring the effects of treatment in the clinic could help to identify nonresponding patients at an early stage after which an alternative treatment regime can be started. Furthermore, molecular imaging may aid in determining surrogate treatment end points. Not only does this improve patient care it also saves costs by preventing continuation of ineffective treatment.

Ultimately, molecular imaging could fulfill a diagnostic role in standard cardiovascular clinical care. Currently, treatment decisions are mostly based on the degree of arterial stenosis although this measure is not a good predictor of clinical events [2]. On the contrary, in the early stages of plaque development outward remodeling of plaque often leaves the vessel lumen diameter largely unchanged [3]. Yet, nonstenotic plaques with a thin fibrous cap and a large lipid core may present a high risk of rupture, while highly stenosed plaques may be stable [4]. Molecular imaging may be capable of assessing the risk factors of plaque rupture and could therefore provide a much better diagnostic readout than traditional imaging approaches.

To be able to appreciate the different molecular MR imaging strategies and to what extent they may address the demands of atherosclerosis research and clinical care, a brief overview of the pathophysiology of atherosclerosis, the commonly used animal models, and the basic principles of MRI is presented below.

13.1.2 Molecular and Cellular Processes in Atherogenesis

Below we provide a brief overview of the processes involved in initiation, progression, and rupture of the atherosclerotic plaque necessary for understanding the molecular imaging strategies discussed in the remainder of this chapter. For a more detailed discussion, we refer to a number of excellent reviews on this topic [1, 3, 5] and the contribution on the pathophysiology of atherosclerosis in Chap. 1 of this book. During the different stages of plaque development, various processes are active, each characterized by different cellular and molecular markers as schematically illustrated in Fig. 13.1. It is the current understanding that atherogenesis

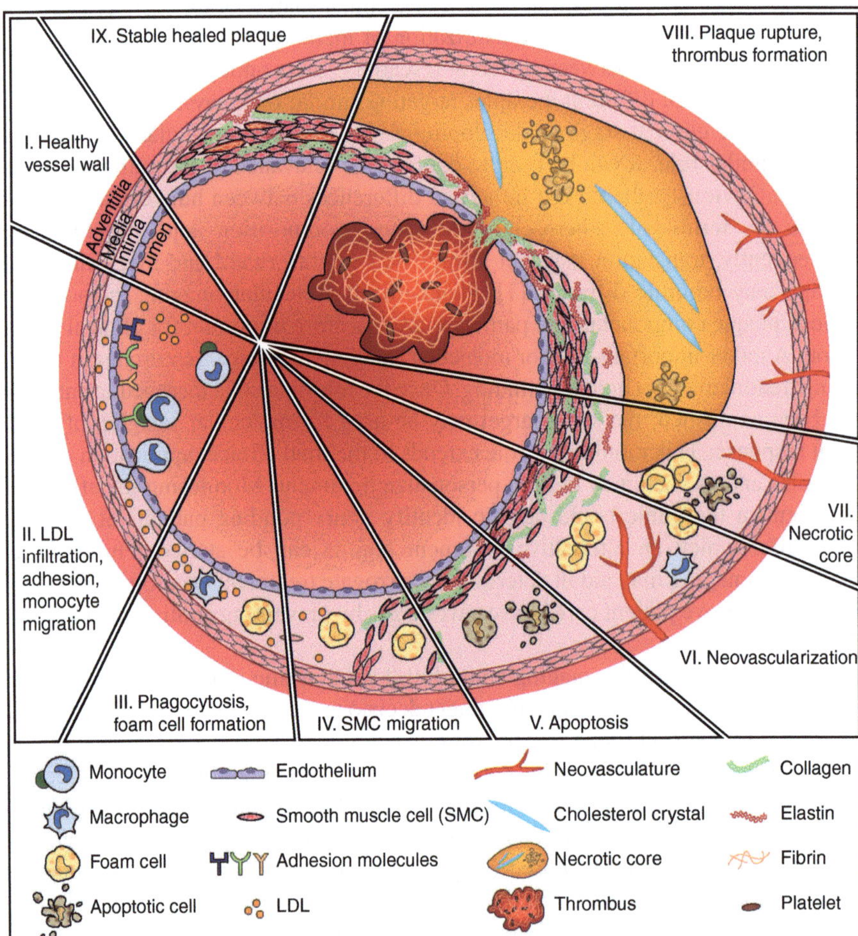

Fig. 13.1 Schematic overview of plaque development. Starting from the *upper left panel (I)* with a healthy vessel wall, in counterclockwise direction, each panel shows the major molecular and cellular processes during different stages of plaque progression

starts with a dysfunctional endothelium initiated by various factors including hypertension, low nitric oxide (NO) level, or low wall shear stress. The endothelium becomes permeable to cholesterol-rich low-density lipoprotein (LDL), which subsequently infiltrates the intima (the inner layer of the artery) (Fig. 13.1II). At the same time, endothelial cells start recruiting monocytes by expressing adhesion molecules (VCAM-1, ICAM-1, E-selectin, P-selectin) (Fig. 13.1II). This stimulates migration of monocytes from the blood to the intima (Fig. 13.1II), where the monocytes become phagocytic and turn into macrophages. Scavenger receptors allow the macrophages to phagocytize oxidized LDL (oxLDL) particles, turning the macrophages into lipid-laden foam cells (Fig. 13.1III). Macrophages can possess either pro- or anti-atherogenic properties, and the balance between the different macrophage phenotypes ultimately determines the fate of the plaque. Pro-atherogenic macrophages and foam cells play an important role throughout disease progression and regulation by expressing pro-inflammatory cytokines, growth factors, and proteinases. Smooth muscle cells (SMCs), which are already sparsely present in a healthy human intima, are stimulated to migrate into the intima in large numbers (Fig. 13.1IV). SMCs produce extracellular matrix (ECM) components such as collagen and elastin, providing stability to the growing plaque by covering it with a fibrous cap. As the plaque grows, its internal milieu may become hypoxic, triggering angiogenesis from the vasa vasorum into the intima (Fig. 13.1VI). This not only allows transport of nutrients and oxygen but also provides new access routes to inflammatory cells into the plaque. At this stage, cells in the plaque may become apoptotic (Fig. 13.1V). Dying foam cells release lipids and cholesterol, which together with cellular debris may accumulate to form a necrotic core (Fig. 13.1VII). A thick fibrous cap consisting of SMCs and ECM on top of the necrotic core can stabilize the plaque, keeping its thrombogenic contents separated from the circulation. Proteinases such as matrix metalloproteinases (MMP) excreted by macrophages, however, may degrade the ECM and destabilize the plaque. Finally, the fibrous cap may rupture, exposing the plaque content to the blood and triggering thrombosis (Fig. 13.1VIII). After rupture, there is a high risk of downstream arterial occlusion and acute clinical events such as myocardial infarction, stroke, or limb ischemia. Small thrombotic events may, however, go unnoticed and result in fibrin deposition at the site of healing. SMCs may proliferate at these locations, covering them with a new fibrous cap (Fig. 13.1IX). Endothelial erosion is another factor that may induce this type of fibrin deposition. Thrombotic events may also occur inside the plaque, as the neovasculature is often leaky, leading to intra-plaque hemorrhage and associated fibrin deposition.

The degree of luminal stenosis is currently regarded as the key indicator for treatment [2]. Highly stenosed vessels, however, often have thick fibrous caps, making them stable and less prone to rupture and thrombotic events [4]. During plaque formation outward remodeling may occur, leading to plaque progression with little effect on lumen diameter [3]. Although stenosed vessels may cause ischemia, the majority of acute clinical events are initiated by rupture of plaques without flow-limiting stenosis [3].

13.1.3 Animal Models of Atherosclerosis

Genetically modified mice are commonly used as a model of atherosclerosis. Of these the apolipoprotein E-knockout (ApoE –/–) mouse is the most widely used, followed by the LDL-receptor knockout (LDL-R –/–) mouse [6]. ApoE –/– mice have elevated cholesterol levels and spontaneously develop atherosclerosis throughout the major arteries. Often this process is accelerated by a high-fat/high-cholesterol diet. The LDL-R –/– mouse on a regular diet more slowly develops atherosclerosis than the ApoE –/–mouse. Also in this model, plaque development is significantly accelerated by a high-fat/high-cholesterol diet. Both mouse models eventually develop advanced plaques with a lipid-rich necrotic core, a fibrous cap, calcifications, and active inflammation. In contrast to humans, plaques in these mice will not rupture spontaneously. The Watanabe heritable hyperlipidemic (WHHL) rabbit and the New Zealand white (NZW) rabbit are also commonly used in atherosclerosis research [7]. WHHL rabbits have a natural mutation in the LDL-R gene and form unprompted atherosclerotic lesions, while other rabbit models such as the NZW need an atherogenic diet to initiate plaque formation. Additionally, atherosclerosis can be triggered by mechanical injuring of the endothelium, e.g., by balloon denudation. Models of plaque rupture may be generated by mechanical disruption of the atherosclerotic plaque. A large animal model of atherosclerosis is the swine. The pig has characteristics that are more similar to humans than small animal models, not only because of a similar body size. They also possess similar dietary preferences, metabolism, and a similar predisposition for developing atherosclerosis [7]. Nevertheless, small animals are easier to house and breed, are easier to handle, and, because of the smaller body size, require lower amounts of therapeutic compound or contrast agent. This makes the use of small animal models less costly. A difficulty of small animals may be to gather enough blood or tissue for ex vivo analysis.

13.1.4 Magnetic Resonance Imaging

Protons (^{1}H) possess a property called spin, associated with a nuclear magnetic moment, which aligns in parallel or antiparallel direction to an applied magnetic field. Due to a small imbalance in the number of parallel and antiparallel aligned proton spins, a net magnetization oriented parallel to the magnetic field will arise. In MRI, an electromagnetic induction signal is generated from this net magnetization by radiofrequency (RF) excitation. After excitation, the proton magnetization will relax back to equilibrium. The rate of this process is governed by the longitudinal or spin-lattice (T_1) and transversal or spin-spin (T_2) relaxation times. Relaxation rates are defined as $R_1 = 1/T_1$ and $R_2 = 1/T_2$. T_2 may be shortened by local field inhomogeneities, and the effective spin-spin relaxation time is then called T_2*. Specifically designed RF pulse sequences are used to generate images with contrast between tissues based on differences in proton density, T_1, T_2, or T_2*. MR contrast agents interact with water protons in their environment and lower the T_1 and T_2 relaxation times. This ability of a contrast agent to lower T_1 and T_2 is expressed in its relaxivities r_1 and r_2, in units of per millimolar per second ($mM^{-1} s^{-1}$). The ratio r_2/r_1 determines whether an agent is most efficient as a T_1 or T_2 contrast agent. T_1 contrast agents are typically based on the lanthanide gadolinium in the form of the Gd^{3+} ion and are characterized by a low r_2/r_1 ratio. By shortening the T_1 of surrounding water protons, a local signal increase in the T_1-weighted MR image is observed, and therefore these agents are also known as positive contrast agents. Contrast agents which shorten T_2 and T_2*, such as iron oxide nanoparticles, have high r_2/r_1 ratios and lead to signal decrease or darkening of T_2- or T_2*-weighted MR images. Hence, they are called negative contrast agents. In molecular MRI, contrast agents are exploited to report on molecular and cellular processes. Typically, this involves binding to a specific molecular marker by a compatible ligand, which is attached to a carrier containing the contrast agent. This concept is also used to enhance detection sensitivity by increasing the number of contrast agent moieties per carrier and thus ultimately per successfully targeted biomarker.

An essential MRI parameter is the field strength. In the clinical setting, 1.5 T and 3 T are most commonly used, but the number of 7 T scanners utilized for clinical research is steadily growing. Dedicated preclinical small animal scanners usually have a higher magnetic field strength ranging from 4.7 T to 17.6 T. High-field MRI scanners benefit from a higher signal-to-noise ratio (SNR) and higher spatial resolution. However, contrast agent relaxivities are field strength dependent. The r_1 of Gd-containing agents strongly decreases at high field strength [8]. In contrast, iron oxide nanoparticles may benefit from higher field strengths because of increasing r_2 and r_2/r_1 ratio.

Not all MRI applications require the use of a contrast agent, though. Figure 13.2 shows some examples of endogenous contrast MRI relevant to atherosclerosis imaging. Time-of-flight (TOF) MRI exploits the inflow of blood for luminal imaging by saturating all static tissues and can thus be used to detect arterial stenosis (Fig. 13.2a). Multi-contrast MRI protocols (TOF, T_1-weighted, T_2-weighted, proton density-weighted, diffusion-weighted) enable identification of various plaque features such as fibrous matrix, necrotic core, calcification, and hemorrhage or thrombus. Classification of these features is based on their hypo-, hyper- or isointense appearance on the various weighted images and allows for coarse plaque staging (Fig. 13.2B) [10]. Calcifications appear as regions of hypointense signal on these traditional weightings due to a low water content and low T_2, and detection is thus based on the absence of signal making unambiguous detection of calcification difficult. Recent developments in ultrashort echo time (UTE) MRI allow for hyperintense imaging of tissue components with very low T_2 values, enabling assessment of calcification density and providing a valuable addition to the multi-contrast MRI protocols [12–14]. Fresh thrombi and intra-plaque hemorrhage appear as hyperintense areas on T_1-weighted images because they contain methemoglobin which shortens T_1 (Fig. 13.2C) [11, 15]. These are examples of the clinical application of non-contrast-enhanced MRI, and the preclinical use of such methods has also been explored [16]. Another example of non-contrast-enhanced MRI is the use of flow-sensitive MRI techniques to distinguish areas with low shear stress [17], which is believed to be an early inducer of atherosclerosis [18]. Furthermore, nontargeted

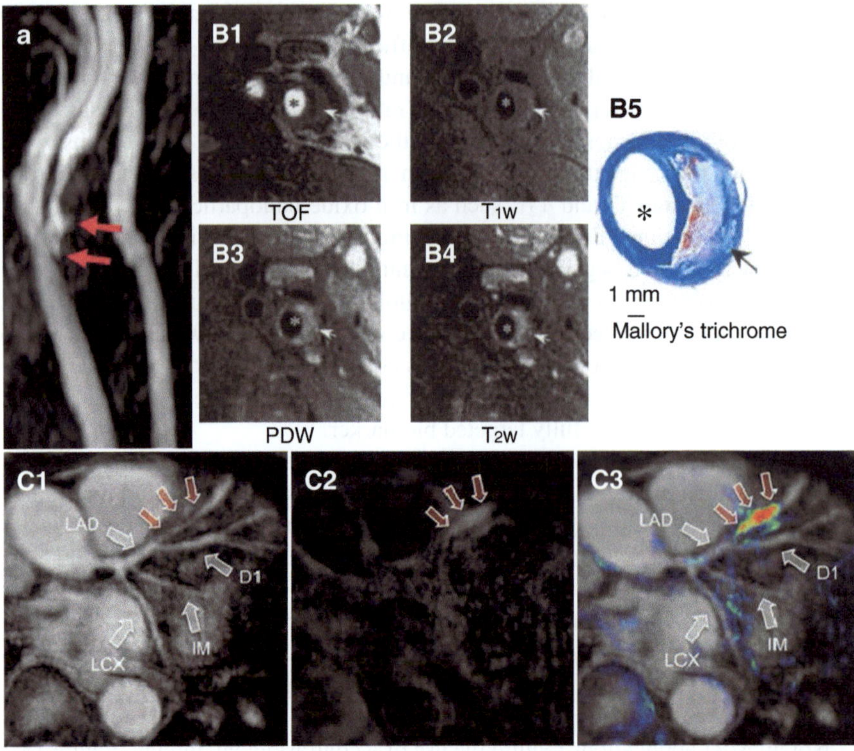

Fig. 13.2 Three types of non-contrast-enhanced MRI, which are relevant to atherosclerosis imaging. (*a*) Time-of-flight (*TOF*) MR angiogram of a patient with stenosis in the right internal carotid artery. *Arrows* point at plaque ulceration. (*B1*) TOF, (*B2*) T_1-weighted, (*B3*) proton density-weighted (*PDW*), and (*B4*) T_2-weighted MR images of a carotid artery atherosclerotic plaque in a patient scheduled for endarterectomy compared to (*B5*) Mallory's trichrome histology showing a lipid-rich necrotic core (*arrow*) and lumen (*). (*C1*) TOF, (*C2*) T_1-weighted, and (*C3*) false-color overlay of T_1 signal intensity on TOF MR images show evidence of a thrombus in the left anterior descending (*LAD*) coronary artery of a patient (*red arrows*). *LCX* left circumflex artery, *IM* ramus intermedius (Images were adapted with permission from (*a*) Josephs et al. [9], (*B*) Cai et al. [10], and (*C*) Jansen et al. [11])

dynamic contrast-enhanced (DCE) imaging approaches are used for evaluating endothelial permeability [19] or neovascularization [20]. DCE-MRI comprises the measurement of T_1-weighted images with a high temporal resolution during the intravenous injection of a low molecular weight Gd-based contrast agent. Microvessel density and permeability may be derived by pharmacokinetic modeling of dynamic signal enhancement. Low molecular weight Gd-based contrast agents are clinically available, and DCE-MRI has therefore become an important method in clinical research. Typical doses of low molecular weight Gd-based contrast agents are in the order of 0.1 mmol per kilogram bodyweight.

Next, major biological characteristics of atherosclerotic plaques are discussed in relation to the relevant biomarkers and molecular imaging strategies. These characteristics include inflammation, the lipid core, the fibrous cap, thrombus formation, intra-plaque hemorrhage, apoptosis, and neovascularization.

13.2 Inflammation

Plaque inflammation plays an important role in the development and progression of atherosclerosis, and active inflammation is believed to be one of the major hallmarks of high rupture risk [5]. Inflammation is characterized by infiltration of macrophages and T-cells. Macrophages have the tendency to phagocytize foreign bodies – a trait which has been exploited for passive targeting of contrast materials. Furthermore, active targeting strategies have been developed for plaque inflammation imaging.

13.2.1 Active Targeting

Active targeting can be defined by the use of a ligand to achieve selective binding of the contrast agent to a molecular target of interest. For imaging of plaque inflammation several targets are available. The first stage of inflammation is the recruitment of blood-borne pro-inflammatory cells by the expression of adhesion molecules on endothelial cells. These cell-surface receptors can therefore be exploited for molecular imaging during the first stage of inflammation. Examples include VCAM-1 targeting with ultrasmall superparamagnetic iron oxide particles (USPIO) [21, 22] and Gd-based contrast agents [23], ICAM-1 targeting with micron-sized particles of iron oxide (MPIO) and Gd-liposomes [24], as well as CD44-specific imaging with superparamagnetic iron oxide nanoparticles (SPION) [25]. McAteer et al. showed that simultaneous targeting of MPIO to two types of adhesion molecules, VCAM-1 and P-selectin, yields greater binding affinity in vitro and more effective and more rapid homing to activated endothelium in vivo (Fig. 13.3) [26]. This latter aspect of targeting kinetics is important for clinical application, where injection of the agent and imaging should be feasible within a single clinical examination for reasons of efficiency.

The location of the target restricts or dictates the useable size of the targeted contrast agent. Large particles such as MPIO and Gd-liposomes have a high relaxivity per particle, making them ideal contrast agents for intravascular targets like adhesion molecules. Since larger particles have more difficulty to extravasate, smaller contrast agents, such as USPIO, Gd-micelles, and low molecular weight Gd-based contrast agents, are more suitable for intra-plaque targeting. Apart from extravasation, retention of the agent in the plaque should be considered. Van Bochove et al. compared the passive accumulation of three differently sized Gd-based contrast agents, i.e., Gd-HP-DO3A, micelles, and liposomes, in mouse atherosclerotic carotid plaques [27]. It was concluded that Gd-micelles of ~15 nm are able to permeate the plaque abundantly, whereas Gd-liposomes with a diameter of ~125 nm remain mostly intravascular and therefore would be more suitable for intravascular targets.

Other strategies for plaque inflammation target the macrophages and foam cells directly. Proteins, such as scavenger receptors, expressed on the cell surface have been targeted using USPIO [28], Gd-micelles [29, 30], and Gd-metallofullerene-containing liposomes [31]. LOX-1, which is involved in oxLDL binding and

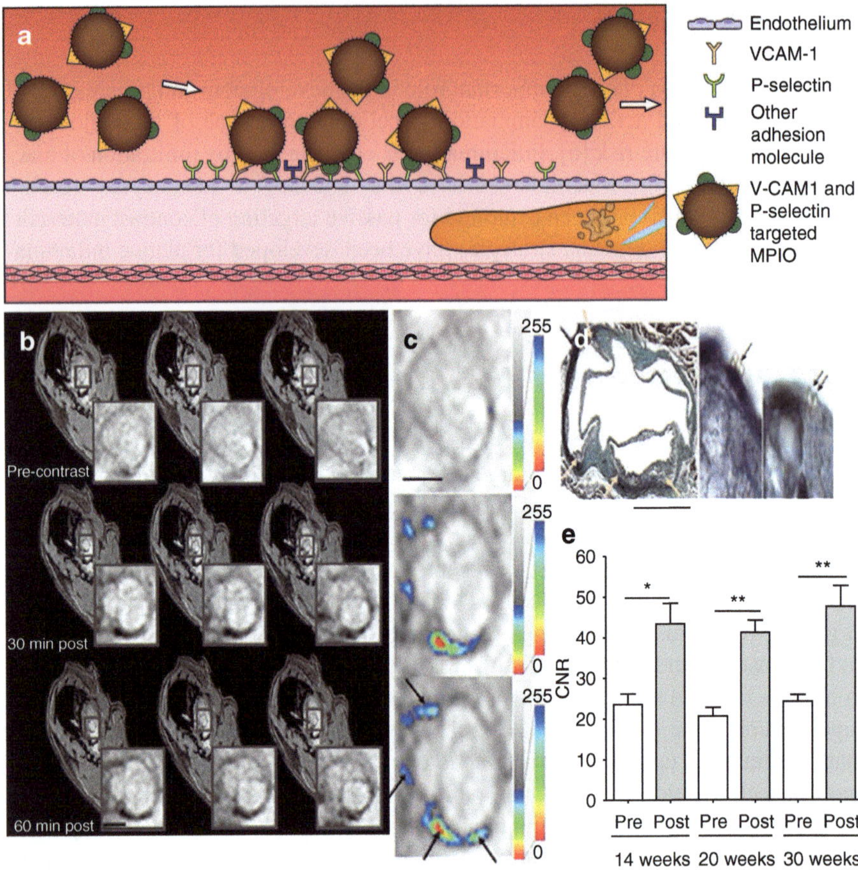

Fig. 13.3 (**a**) Targeted inflammation imaging, in which micron-sized particles of iron oxide (*MPIO*) conjugated with ligands for adhesion molecules VCAM-1 and P-selectin home rapidly to activated endothelium. (**b**) T_2*-weighted images of the aortic root of ApoE –/– mice after 14 weeks on regular chow diet show signal decrease at 30 and 60 min postinjection compared to preinjection. (**c**) T_2* signal intensity maps show the distribution of MPIO indicated by false color-coded overlay. (**d**) Histology (Masson trichrome and elastin stain) confirms that MPIO adhesion is confined to atherosclerotic foam cell lesions. (**e**) Contrast-to-noise ratio (*CNR*) of atherosclerotic lesions was significantly increased after injection of dual-targeted MPIO with no significant difference between time points. (**b–d**) Scale bars = 1 mm (Images (**b–e**) were adapted with permission from McAteer et al. [26])

expressed on macrophages and other cell types involved in inflammation, has been targeted with USPIO [32]. The most common way to directly target plaque-associated macrophages is, however, by passive targeting exploiting the natural phagocytic property of this inflammatory cell type.

13.2.2 Passive Targeting

Macrophages readily phagocytize foreign bodies, and this behavior is widely exploited for passive targeting of MRI contrast materials. Nontargeted USPIOs were shown to accumulate in macrophage-rich plaques upon intravenous

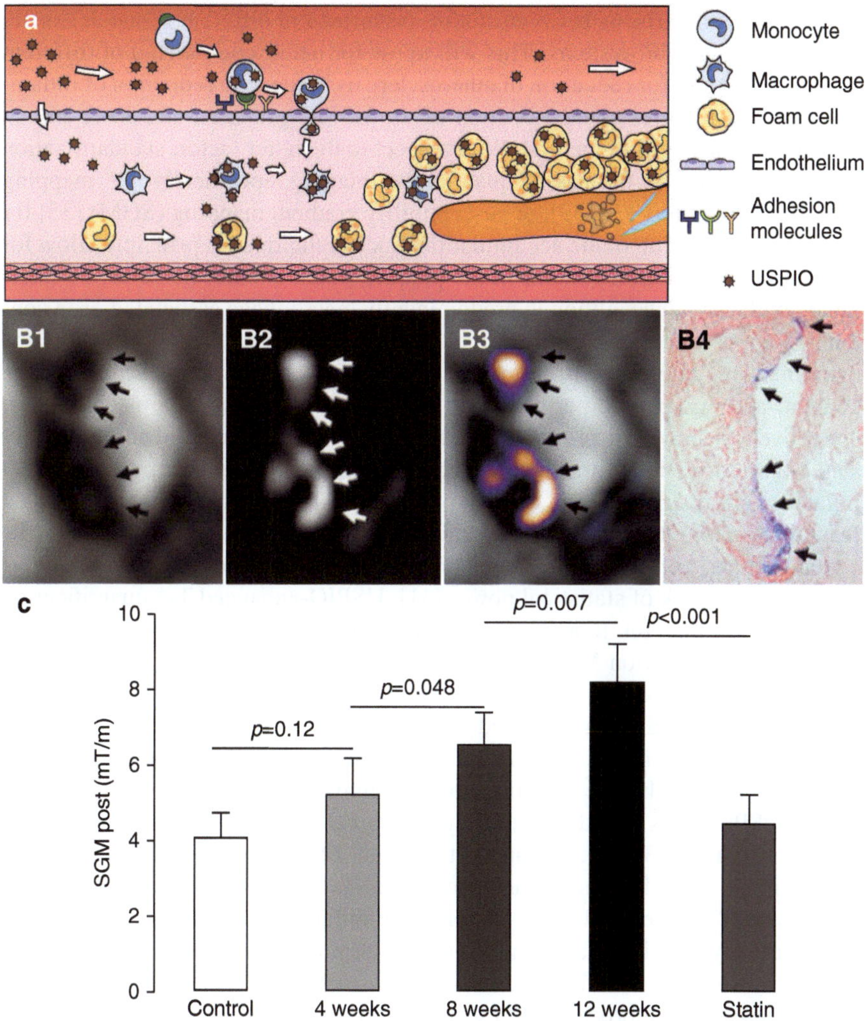

Fig. 13.4 (**a**) Passive targeting of plaque inflammation with ultrasmall superparamagnetic iron oxide (*USPIO*) nanoparticles. USPIO are taken up via phagocytosis by blood monocytes, plaque macrophages, and foam cells. (**b**) In vivo imaging of plaque in the brachiocephalic artery of ApoE –/– mice on a 12 week high-fat diet 48 h post USPIO injection: (*B1*) dark spots on T_2*-weighted image, (*B2*) bright signal on susceptibility gradient mapping (*SGM*), (*B3*) SGM overlay, and (*B4*) Perls' iron stain histology. (**c**) SGM values increased with plaque progression and decreased to control levels in the statin-treated group (Images (**b**, **c**) were adapted with permission from Makowski et al. [35])

injection in rabbits [33] as well as in symptomatic patients [34]. Experimental studies in ApoE –/– mice showed the ability of the technique to image both age-related plaque progression and the effects of treatment with anti-inflammatory drugs (Fig. 13.4) [35–37]. Passive macrophage targeting using USPIOs has thus become a useful preclinical tool for readout of the plaque inflammatory status. We believe that standardization of the technique should be improved to allow more direct comparisons between studies performed in different research centers and on different MR systems. This will allow for better comparison of different therapies that aim for reduction of atherosclerosis burden via reduction of inflammation. This requires standardization of the USPIO preparations, dose, animal models, and acquisition method. With respect to the latter factor, standardization can be improved by the use of quantitative imaging, specifically T_2* mapping [36, 37], T_2 mapping [38, 39], or susceptibility gradient mapping (SGM) [35] for the evaluation of iron oxide accumulation. Such techniques in principle allow for a quantification of iron content in the plaque, which should, however, be interpreted with care since, although predominantly macrophage associated, iron content is not a direct measure of the number of macrophages. Although the quantified imaging readout is a result of the cumulative effect of macrophage content, activity, plaque permeability, and contrast material pharmacokinetics, collectively it may still provide a quantifiable readout of overall inflammatory status that correlates with plaque progression and treatment response. USPIO inflammation imaging shows clinical potential. Gillard et al. have demonstrated feasibility in long-term follow-up studies [40], and although USPIO-induced MR signal changes were not proven to be predictive for clinical events, this was most likely due to a lack of statistical power [41]. USPIO-enhanced T_2* quantification was demonstrated for treatment monitoring in a clinical setting [42]. It was shown that preinjection MRI scans were not needed for assessing differences in USPIO uptake. Most of the early studies have been performed with Sinerem (ferumoxtran-10), a dextran-coated USPIO of approximately 30 nm. However, currently Sinerem is not commercially available anymore, as production has been discontinued by the manufacturer. Ferumoxytol, a ~30 nm carbohydrate-coated USPIO, was found to induce larger signal changes than Sinerem in preclinical studies [43, 44]. Ferumoxytol is an FDA-approved supplement for treatment of iron deficiency but also serves as an MRI contrast agent [45]. Ferumoxytol is investigated for imaging the inflammatory response in patients with acute myocardial infarction [46] and is currently evaluated in a clinical trial for monitoring inflammation in carotid atherosclerosis [47].

Nontargeted perfluorocarbon (PFC) nanoparticles are also phagocytized by macrophages and thus can be exploited for molecular imaging of inflammation, with the additional advantage that PFC can be imaged by ^{19}F MRI separately from the proton anatomical image. PFC inflammation imaging has been explored in various pathologies [48, 49] and holds promise for plaque inflammation as well. ^{19}F MRI of PFC-containing nanoparticles has several advantages over traditional (T_1 and T_2) proton-detected contrast agents. The ^{19}F MR signal is directly proportional to the PFC concentration, and background fluorine signal is absent resulting in a high detection specificity. Furthermore, some PFC-containing nanoparticles suitable for MRI purposes are FDA approved as blood substitutes [50]. Nevertheless, detection of low numbers of macrophages using the fluorine approach may remain challenging because of sensitivity issues [51, 52].

13.3 Lipids

Atherosclerotic plaques with a large core containing lipids and cellular debris are considered at risk of rupture. Plaque-borne lipids are involved in the early stages of plaque formation, when LDL enters the intima where it is oxidized and taken up by macrophages to form foam cells. This process continues throughout plaque progression, and a large plaque core is a strong predictor of rupture. Improved visualization of the lipid-rich core was achieved using lipophilic contrast agents such as Gd-based gadofluorine M, which accumulates in lipid-rich areas of the plaque [53]. USPIO [54, 55] and Gd-micelles [56] were targeted to oxLDL. Alternatively, manganese (Mn(II))-containing micelles were used [56]. While in the blood, these micelles have low relaxivity; once bound to oxLDL, however, the micelles become internalized by macrophages and release their manganese payload in the intracellular compartment, resulting in a strongly increased relaxivity. This renders the observed signal enhancement on T_1-weighted MRI specific to macrophage and foam cell phagocytic activity.

Native or synthetically produced LDL and HDL can be modified to include MRI contrast agent facilitating imaging of plaque uptake. Injection of Gd-containing LDL-like nanoparticles led to increased signal intensity in atherosclerotic plaque by macrophage uptake [57]. HDL is responsible for reverse cholesterol transport from macrophages and thus may serve both imaging as well as therapeutic purposes [58]. For that purpose, several versions of HDL-like particles were designed for molecular imaging with various imaging modalities [58]. Recently, it was revealed that the effective plaque enhancement from Gd-containing HDL-like particles is mediated by transfer of Gd-phospholipids to LDL which in turn are taken up by macrophages [59]. HDL can be designed to incorporate contrast-generating nanoparticles in the HDL core, including USPIO, for T_2-weighted MRI, and gold nanoparticles for CT [60]. The delivery method of these particles is important. Intraperitoneal injection of USPIO-containing HDL-like particles yields a constant blood concentration over several hours allowing for higher uptake compared to intravenous injection [61]. In vivo particle accumulation in the plaque was not sufficient to induce significant signal changes in T_2*-weighted MRI. Nevertheless, ex vivo T_2* mapping showed a significant difference between native and postinjection T_2* relaxation times (Fig. 13.5) [61]. Advanced T_2 or T_2* mapping methods may facilitate more robust in vivo detection and quantification of nanoparticle uptake [38, 39].

13.4 Fibrous Cap and ECM Components

A thick fibrous cap is considered a feature of plaque stability. The fibrous cap contains SMC and ECM components such as collagen and elastin. Pro-inflammatory macrophages may excrete proteinases such as matrix metalloproteinases (MMP), breaking down the ECM components, destabilizing the plaque, and increasing the

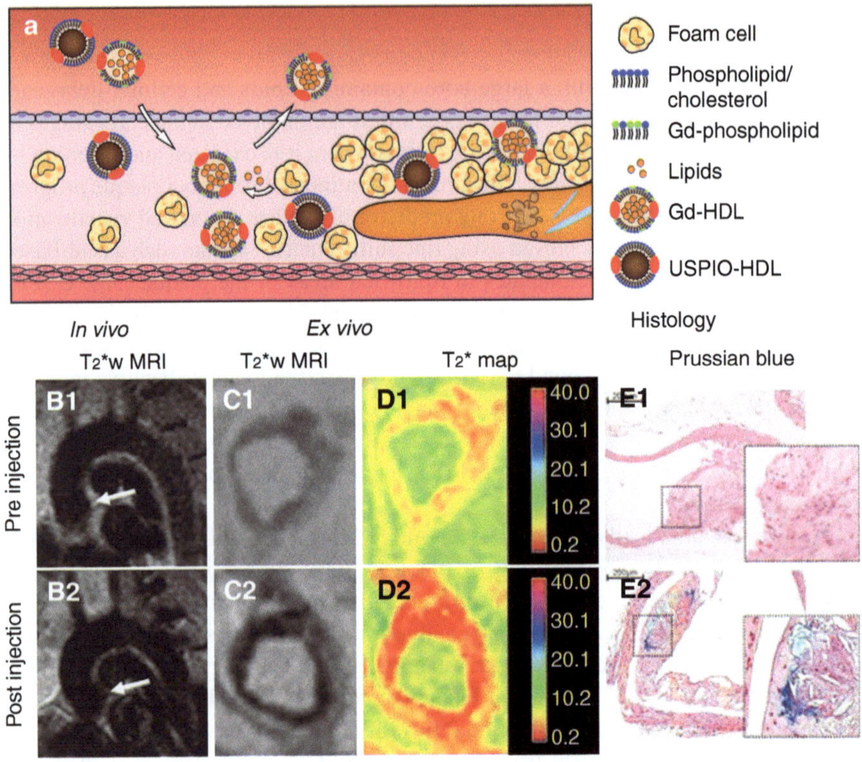

Fig. 13.5 (**a**) High-density lipoprotein (*HDL*) homes to sites with high macrophage/foam cell content and is involved in reverse cholesterol transport. HDL-like particles can be functionalized, e.g., with Gd-phospholipids in the phospholipid layer or USPIO particles in their core and subsequently can individually be used for molecular MR of plaque inflammation. (**b**) In vivo T_2*-weighted MRI of the aortic arch of ApoE −/− mice (*B1*) before and (*B2*) 24 h after USPIO-HDL injection shows signal decrease upon USPIO-HDL uptake. (*C1, 2*) Ex vivo T_2*-weighted MRI shows a similar decrease in signal in the aortic root which was quantified with (*D1, 2*) T_2* mapping. (**e**) Prussian blue iron staining confirmed the uptake of iron particles in (*E2*) the plaque of injected mice but not (*E1*) in non-injected mice (Images (**b**–**e**) were adapted with permission from Jung et al. [61])

chance of rupture. Both the ECM and the presence of proteinases, such as MMP, therefore have been explored as molecular imaging targets.

The most abundant component of the fibrous cap is collagen. In a mouse model of plaque regression, Gd-containing HDL-like particles functionalized with a collagen-binding peptide (EP3533) were used to image collagen content during the change from a phenotype with many macrophages and little collagen into a phenotype with few macrophages and increased collagen content (Fig. 13.6) [62]. Collagen-functionalized particles generated significant signal enhancement in the regressed phenotype with high collagen content, while their nonfunctionalized counterparts did this in the vulnerable, high macrophage content phenotype. Since both HDL-like particles are equipped with Gd for MRI detection, they provided positive and therefore easier detectable contrast. Because both agents provided

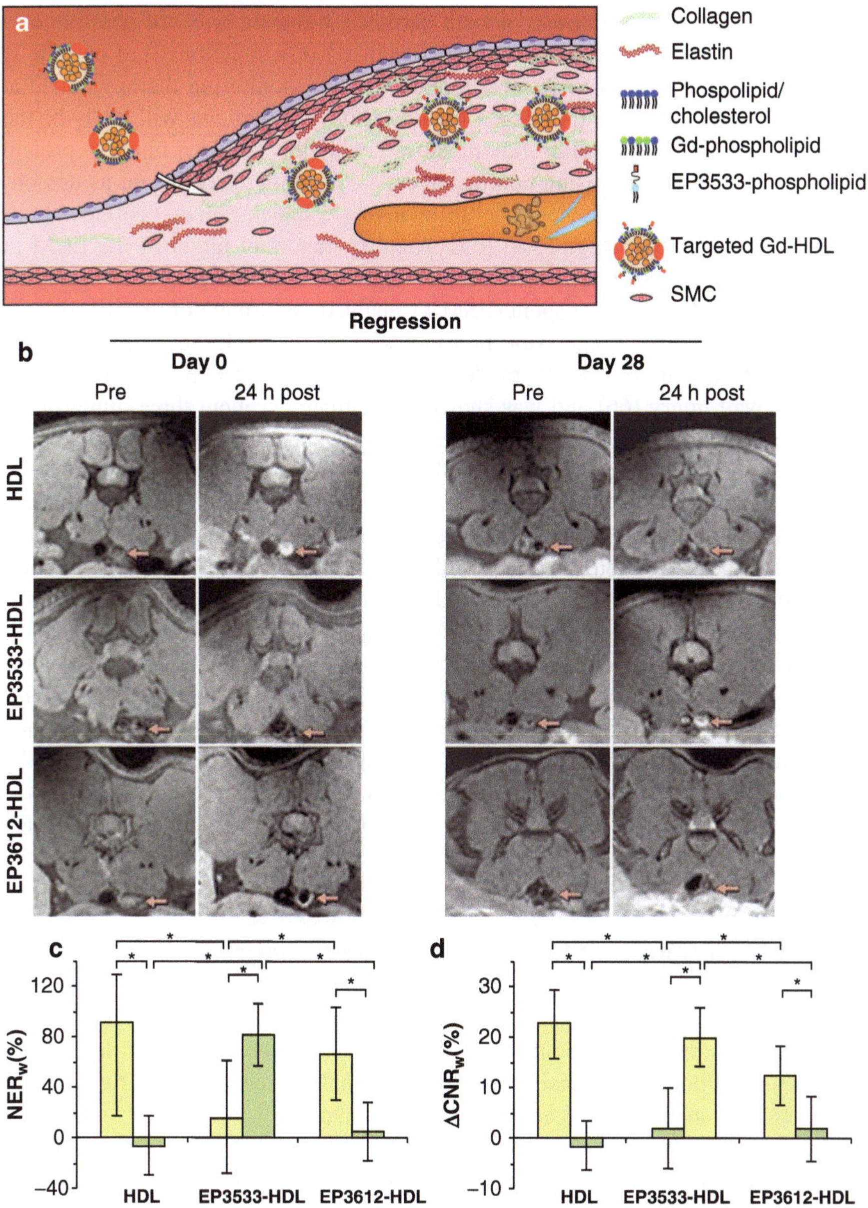

Fig. 13.6 (**a**) Gd-HDL particles functionalized with the EP3533 peptide bind to collagen in the atherosclerotic plaque. (**b**) MR images before and 24 h after injection of nontargeted HDL-like particles, collagen-targeted EP3533-HDL, and EP3612-HDL as a nonfunctional control at day 0 and day 28 of plaque regression in the abdominal aorta in a mice (*arrows* point to the aorta). (**c**) Normalized enhancement ratio (NER_w) and (**d**) the difference between pre- and postinjection contrast-to-noise ratios (ΔCNR_w) of the aortic wall show a significant increase for EP3533-HDL and significant decrease for HDL and EP3612-HDL between day 28 (*green bars*) and day 0 (*yellow bars*) (Images (**b–d**) were adapted with permission from Chen et al. [62])

similar contrast, concurrent use of both particles, however, was not possible in a single subject. The choice for a nonfunctionalized or a functionalized particle is dependent on the kind of target and application. For monitoring therapy aimed at increasing collagen content, collagen-binding HDL-like particles will likely be the preferred choice. Gd-micelles functionalized with the collagen-binding protein CNA35 are another promising contrast agent for imaging of collagen, as demonstrated in an ApoE −/− mouse model of relatively collagen-rich and collagen-poor carotid atherosclerosis (Fig. 13.7) [63]. Another important target of the ECM in atherosclerosis is elastin. A low molecular weight Gd-containing contrast agent, the elastin-specific MR contrast agent (ESMA), enabled assessment of plaque progression and statin-induced regression in a mouse model (Fig. 13.8b, c) [64]. ESMA was subsequently used in swine models for detection of vascular remodeling after coronary wall injury [66] and was shown to facilitate excellent three-dimensional aortic vessel wall imaging (Fig. 13.8d1–2) [65].

MMPs can be imaged by exploiting their proteolytic activity or by binding to a specific ligand [67]. One recent and promising example is the Gd-based contrast agent P947 based on an MMP-inhibiting peptide. P947 was shown to accumulate in vivo in ApoE −/− mouse plaques with high MMP content [68, 69]. In a rabbit model of atherosclerosis, P947 was used to detect diet-induced differences in atherosclerotic MMP-related enzymatic activity (Fig. 13.9) [70]. P947 not only enables visualization of MMP activity but also of other vulnerable plaque-related proteinases [71]. Other enzymes have also served as molecular MRI target, such as myeloperoxidase (MPO), an inflammatory protein playing an important role in plaque destabilization partly mediated by MMP activation. A Gd-based MPO sensor, MPO (Gd), enabled detection of inflammatory activity in rabbit atherosclerotic plaques in a manner that is less sensitive to macrophage numbers but rather to macrophage subtype and activity [72].

13.5 Thrombus and Intra-plaque Hemorrhage

Thrombi are not only generated during plaque rupture, they can also develop by plaque erosion and inside the plaque by intra-plaque hemorrhage from leaky neovasculature. Often, such smaller thrombotic events precede plaque rupture and therefore they are considered an important risk factor.

Fibrin is one of the major constituents of thrombus and hence a favorable target for molecular MRI. The abundance of fibrin in thrombi allows for binding of large quantities of contrast agent, and this aids to overcome sensitivity issues. The most successful fibrin-targeting MR contrast agent known to date is EP-2104R, which consists of a fibrin-binding peptide conjugated to four Gd-chelate complexes. EP-2104R is efficient at low dose due to its high relaxivity, especially when bound to fibrin. The compound has already been used successfully for thrombus imaging in patients in phase II clinical trials [73, 74]. Makowski et al. recently showed applicability of EP-2104R for non-luminal thrombus-associated fibrin in a mouse model of atherosclerosis with low doses of the contrast agent (10 μmol/kg compared to a typical dose of 0.1 mmol/kg for nontargeted Gd-based contrast agents) [75].

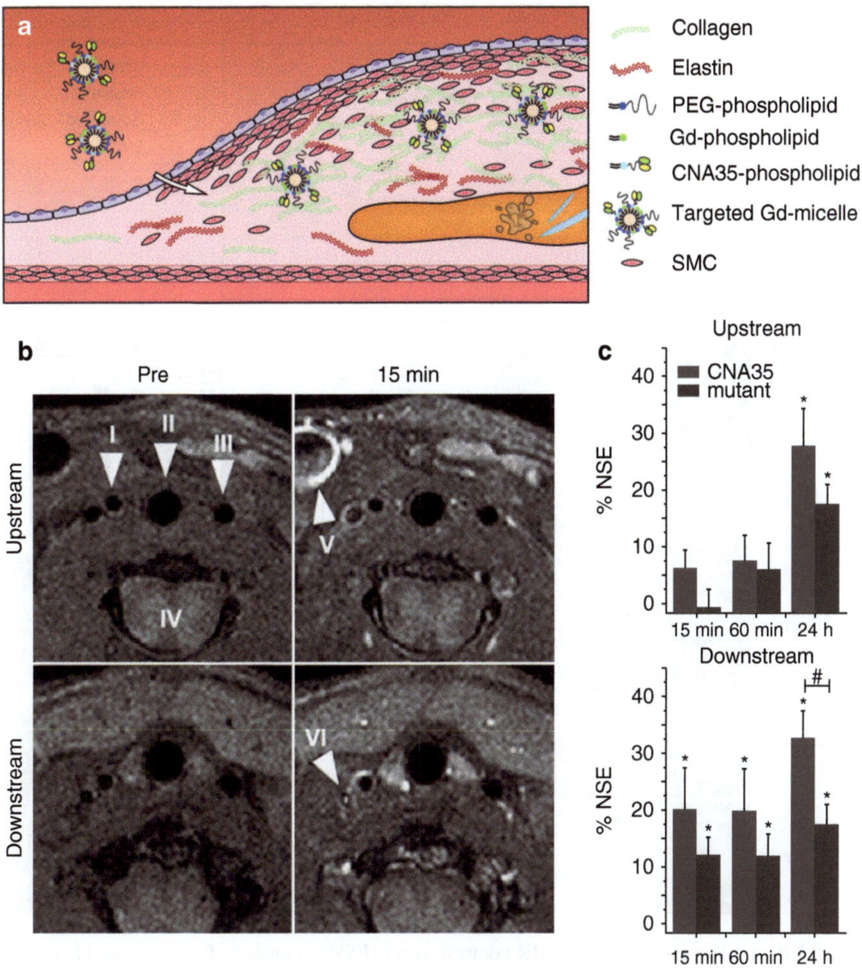

Fig. 13.7 (**a**) Gd-micelles functionalized with CNA35 protein and protected from detection by the immune system with polyethylene glycol (*PEG*)-phospholipids bind to collagen in the atherosclerotic plaque. (**b**, **c**) In ApoE –/– mice a cast was placed in the right carotid artery, leading to induction of plaques with a difference in collagen content upstream and downstream (more collagen) from the cast. (**b**) T1-weighted imaging shows enhancement of the plaque richer in collagen already 15 min after injection of CNA35 micelles. *Arrowheads* indicate the right carotid artery (*I*), trachea (*II*), left carotid artery (*III*), spinal cord (*IV*), external jugular vein (*V*), and internal jugular vein (*VI*). (**c**) The calculated percentage normalized signal enhancement (*% NSE*) upon CNA35-micelle injection shows significant enhancement (* = $p < 0.05$) in the downstream collagen-rich plaque at all time points, yet only significantly different compared to mutant (*dysfunctional*) CNA35 micelles (# = $p < 0.05$) at 24 h after injection. In the upstream plaque, significant enhancement is only reached after 24 h (Images (**b**, **c**) were adapted with permission from van Bochove et al. [63])

This non-luminal thrombus-associated fibrin might enter the plaque via leaky neovasculature or form at locations of eroded endothelium and was hypothesized to mark the transition to a vulnerable plaque type [76]. In their study, Makowski et al.

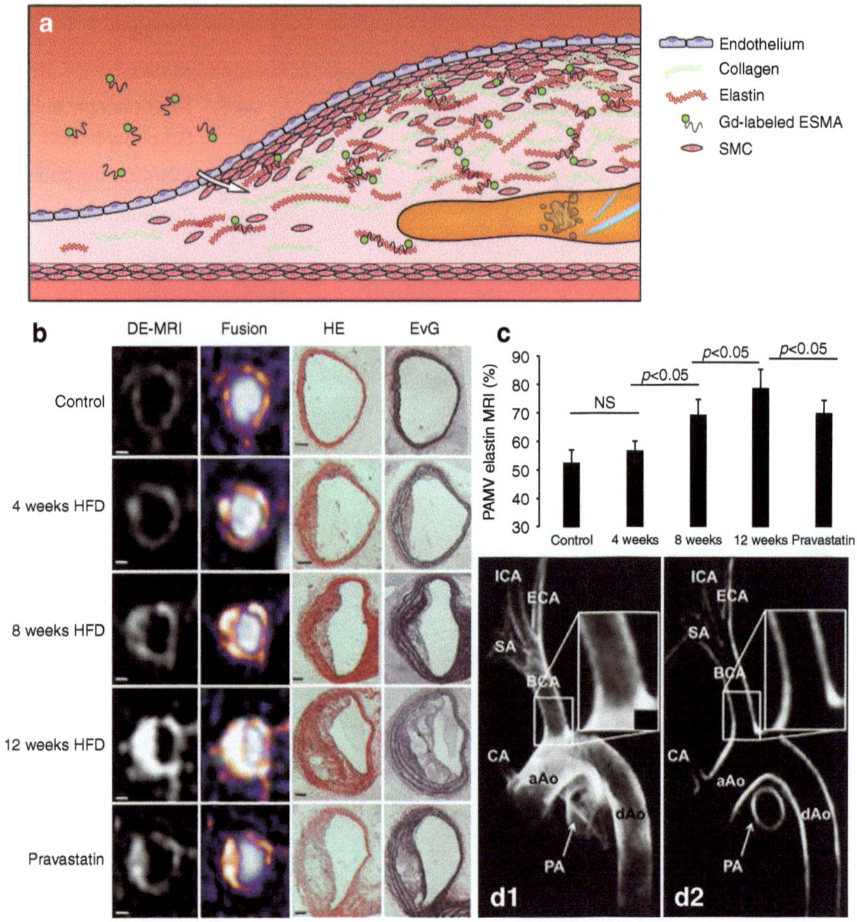

Fig. 13.8 (**a**) The elastin-specific MR contrast agent (*ESMA*) consists of a small peptide conjugated to a Gd-chelate and can bind to elastin in the atherosclerotic plaque. (**b**) Delayed-enhancement (*DE*) MRI and fusion images with DE-MRI overlaid on time-of-flight (*TOF*) images show that ESMA-induced MRI signal increases with plaque progression in the brachiocephalic artery of ApoE –/– mice on a high-fat diet, except for pravastatin-treated animals. Plaque progression and increased elastin content were confirmed with histology using hematoxylin and eosin (*HE*) and Elastica van Gieson (*EvG*) staining. Scale bars 250 μm. (**c**) The MR images allow estimation of the percentage atheroma/media volume (PAMV) which increases with plaque progression, but significantly less in the pravastatin-treated group. (**d**) Excellent 3D vessel wall imaging with ESMA was demonstrated in the porcine aortic arch: (*D1*) maximum intensity projection and (*D2*) multi-planar reconstructed images 90–100 min after injection. *aAo* ascending aorta, *BCA* brachiocephalic artery, *CA* proximal coronary artery, *dAo* descending aorta, *ECA* external carotid artery, *ICA* internal carotid artery, *PA* pulmonary artery, *SA* subclavian artery (Images (**b**, **c**) were adapted with permission from Makowski et al. [64] (**d**) [65])

obtained late gadolinium enhancement images with excellent contrast as well as pre- and postinjection T_1 maps to generate data that can be quantitatively analyzed (Fig. 13.10) [75]. R_1 was observed to be significantly higher in mice with more advanced plaques after 3 months of high-fat diet as opposed to statin-treated and

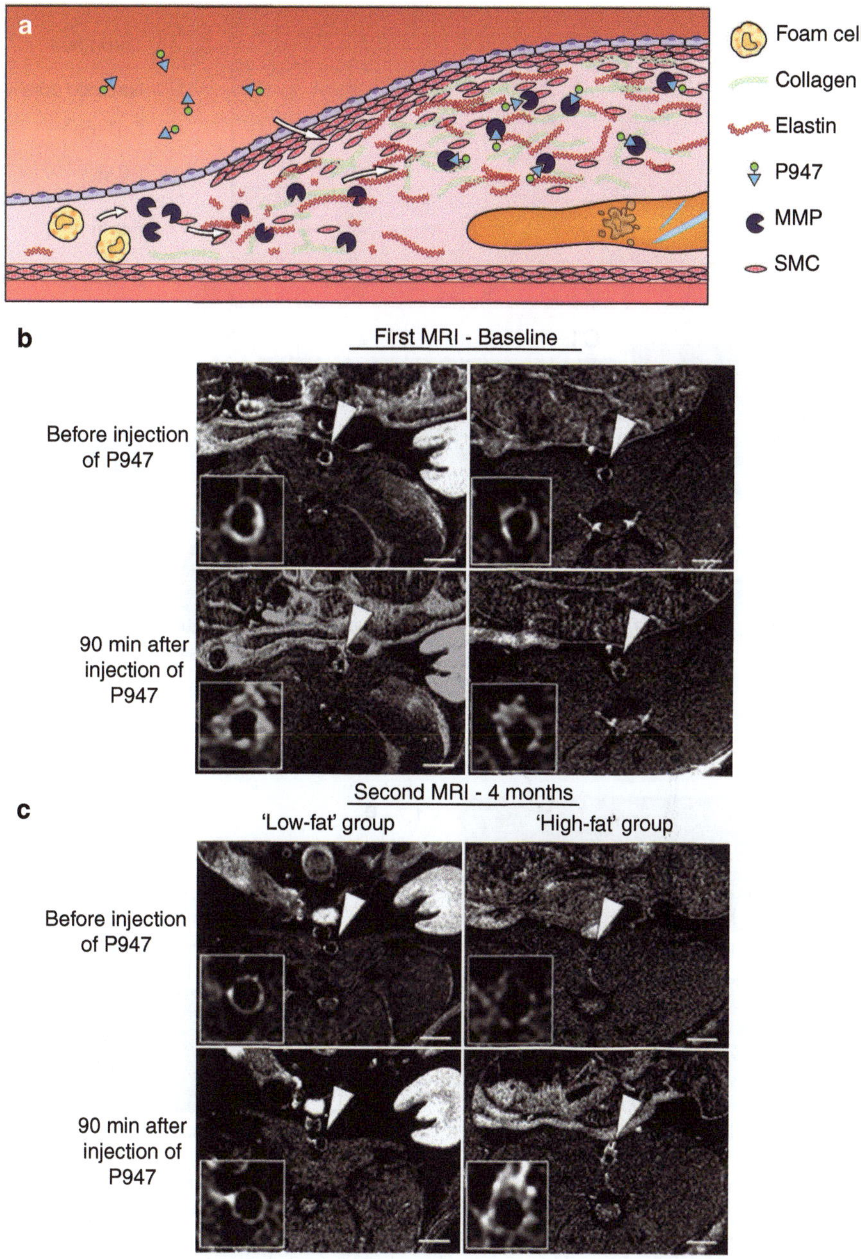

Fig. 13.9 (**a**) Macrophages and foam cells can excrete matrix metalloproteinases (*MMP*), which degrade extracellular matrix (*ECM*) proteins such as collagen and elastin. P947 is a contrast agent based on an MMP inhibitor conjugated to a Gd-chelate. (**b**) P947 was used to image plaque burden in the abdominal aorta of rabbits induced by 4 months of high-fat diet and balloon injury (*baseline*) and (**c**) plaque regression after another 4 months of low-fat diet as compared to continued high-fat diet. *Insets* in (**b**) and (**c**) show enlarged images of the aorta (Images (**b**, **c**) were adapted with permission from Hyafil et al. [70])

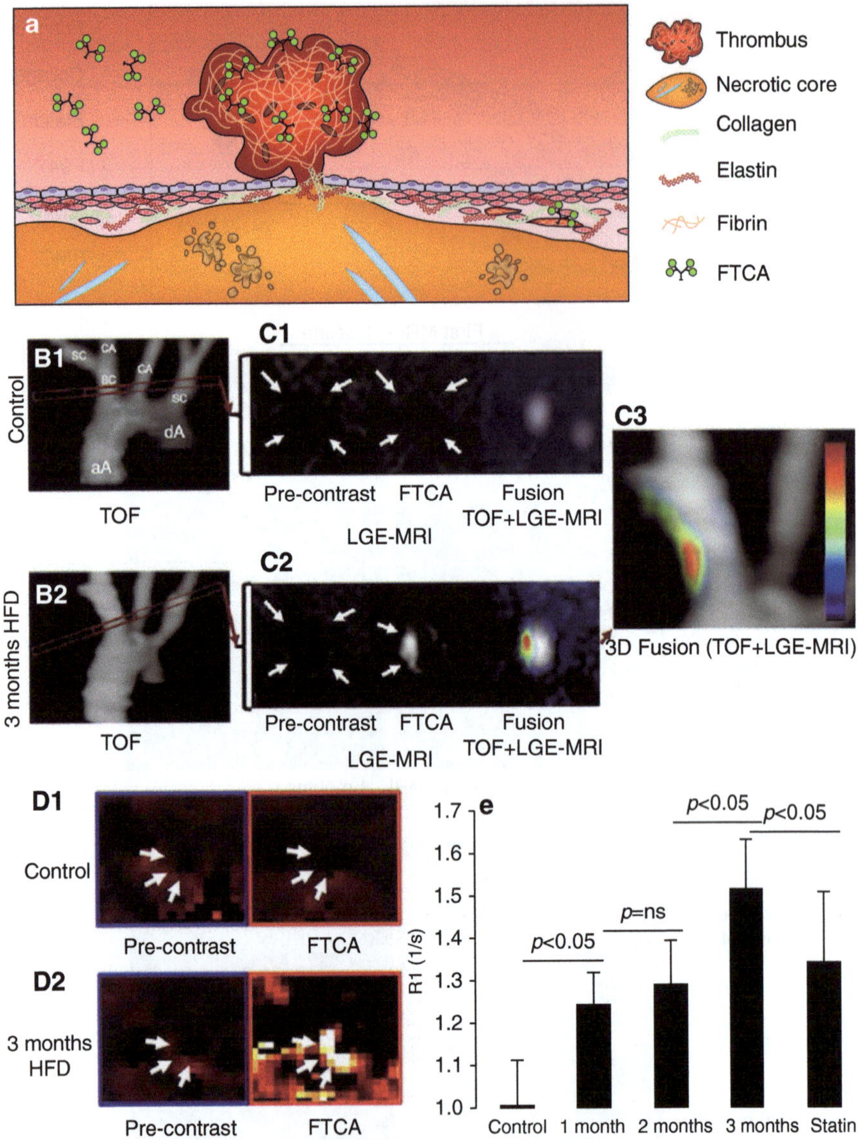

Fig. 13.10 (**a**) The fibrin-targeted contrast agent (*FTCA*) (EP-2104R) consists of a fibrin-binding peptide conjugated to four Gd-chelates and is capable of binding fibrin in thrombi and atherosclerotic plaques. (**b–e**) FTCA was tested in the brachiocephalic artery of ApoE –/– mice on a high-fat diet (*HFD*) and compared to wild-type controls and statin-treated mice to test affinity for intraplaque and endothelial fibrin. (*B1, 2*) Time-of-flight (*TOF*) images reveal the lumen of the aortic arch and branches and allow for accurate slice planning. (*C2*) FTCA yields signal enhancement in late gadolinium enhancement (*LGE*) images 90 min after injection in mice on 3 month HFD, but not (*C1*) in controls. Fusion of LGE-MRI over TOF images shows the localization of FTCA binding with anatomical reference in (*C1, 2*) 2D and (*C3*) 3D images. (**d**) Additionally, T_1 maps were acquired to quantify signal enhancement, and (**e**) R_1 significantly increased compared to control mice and at 3 months versus shorter diet and statin treatment. *aA* ascending aorta, *dA* descending aorta, *BC* brachiocephalic artery, *SC* subclavian artery, *CA* carotid artery (Images (**b–e**) were adapted with permission from Makowski et al. [75])

shorter-time diet groups [75]. In principle, the difference between pre- and postinjection R_1 could be directly correlated to local contrast agent concentration. However, these values were not reported in this study. In another relevant fibrin-targeting study, PFC nanoparticles were functionalized with monoclonal antibodies for ^{19}F MRI quantification of local fibrin content ex vivo in a human carotid endarterectomy sample [77].

There are other thrombus-related targets besides fibrin. Activated platelets can be targeted via the $\alpha_{IIb}\beta_3$-integrin. This has been done with a ligand-induced binding sites (LIBS) antibody coupled to MPIO, yielding significant signal decrease in induced atherothrombosis in a mouse model [78]. Since activated platelets are only involved in the developing thrombus, this method allows for detection of early thrombi and thereby can be used for thrombus staging. A potential pitfall for this technique could be nonspecific inclusion of particles in the developing thrombus. The administration of nontargeted MPIO did, however, not lead to signal decrease, ruling out nonspecific inclusion as the main targeting mechanism. An alternative method for imaging of early thrombi is the Gd-labeled α_2-antiplasmin-based peptide, as demonstrated in a model of induced thrombosis [79]. During thrombus formation the α_2-antiplasmin is covalently cross-linked to fibrin, and this approach thus reports on active thrombus formation.

13.6 Apoptosis

Nutrient-deprived hypoxic conditions in the intima of the progressing plaque as well as endoplasmic reticulum stress are factors which can lead to foam cell death and formation of the necrotic core. During cell death by apoptosis, phosphatidylserine, a phospholipid normally only present in the internal leaflet of the cell membrane, is exposed at the outer cell membrane. The phosphatidylserine can be targeted from the extracellular space with the annexin A5 protein. Functionalization of Gd-micelles by conjugation to annexin A5 yielded enhanced contrast agent uptake in atherosclerotic plaques in the abdominal aorta of ApoE −/− mice [80]. This was demonstrated with in vivo T_1-weighted MRI and confirmed with ex vivo near-infrared fluorescence imaging. Alternatively a phosphatidylserine-targeting peptide conjugated to a Gd-chelate may be used [81].

13.7 Neovascularization

Angiogenesis can occur in more advanced plaques, and leaky neovasculature may lead to intra-plaque hemorrhage. Neovascularization is therefore also considered a risk factor indicating plaque vulnerability. Molecular imaging of plaque neovascularization has focused on the $\alpha\nu\beta_3$-integrin, which is abundantly expressed on the endothelium of newly formed blood vessels. The $\alpha\nu\beta_3$-integrin can be targeted with the Arg-Gly-Asp (RGD) peptide or peptide mimetic, e.g., by direct conjugation to a Gd-chelate [82]. Winter et al. conjugated a RGD-mimetic to PFC emulsion nanoparticles with gadolinium in the phospholipid monolayer coating to image neovascularization in rabbit atherosclerotic plaques [83]. In later studies, these nanoparticles

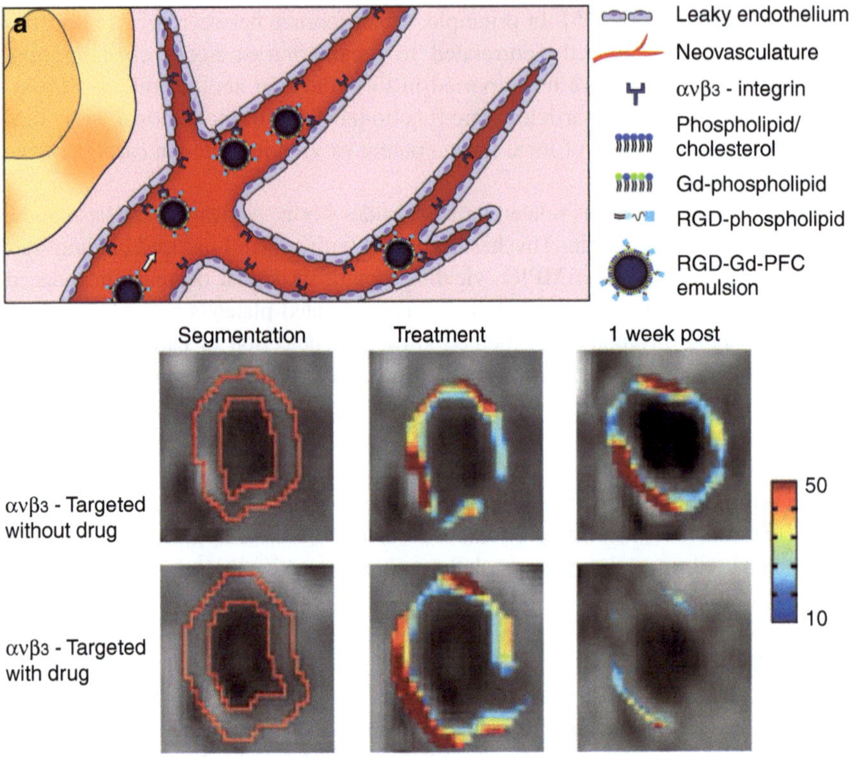

Fig. 13.11 (**a**) The endothelium of intra-plaque neovasculature expresses $\alpha\nu\beta_3$-integrins which can be targeted with RGD-peptides and RGD-mimics, e.g., with targeted paramagnetic perfluorocarbon (*PFC*) emulsions. (**c**, **d**) In the abdominal aorta of atherosclerotic rabbits, reduction of angiogenesis was observed as decreased signal enhancement 1 week after treatment with (*D2* vs. *C2*) fumagillin-containing $\alpha\nu\beta_3$-targeted contrast agent and (*D1* vs. *C1*) not after injection with $\alpha\nu\beta_3$-targeted contrast agent without drug. False color maps of the enhancement were made within (*B1, 2*) a segmented region of interest, and a threshold of 10 % enhancement was applied (Images (**b**–**d**) were adapted with permission from Winter et al. [84])

were adapted by incorporation of fumagillin, an anti-angiogenic agent, allowing for simultaneous targeted therapy and imaging (Fig. 13.11) [84]. The incorporation of a therapeutic agent and an imaging agent in the same targeted particle allows for direct monitoring of drug delivery, which is predictive of therapeutic effect. This makes it a valuable tool for preclinical drug development, which, however, requires adaptations for each new application and careful evaluation of the possible influence of the imaging agent on the treatment effect.

13.8 Conclusions and Future Perspective

As the molecular and cellular pathways involved in the development, progression, and clinical manifestation of atherosclerosis are being revealed, new molecular imaging strategies are developed to visualize these processes in vivo. For molecular

MR imaging this involves many different contrast agent types, most of which are based on iron oxides, low molecular weight Gd compounds, lipid-based Gd carriers, and PFC emulsions, each with specific benefits and drawbacks as detailed in this review. Along with the development of novel contrast agents comes the need to develop effective MRI acquisition and analysis techniques to maximize detection sensitivity. In this chapter, several of these molecular MR imaging strategies were highlighted and discussed with respect to specific applications in molecular imaging of atherosclerosis.

Most molecular MR imaging strategies discussed here primarily have proven valuable in a preclinical setting. Preclinical research has tremendously improved our understanding of the biological mechanisms of atherosclerosis at the molecular and cellular level. Moreover, molecular MRI can play a significant role in preclinical development of new drugs for treatment of atherosclerosis. Examples include studies on the effects of statin therapy, which has been shown to reduce fibrin [75] and elastin [64] content as well as the number and inflammatory activity of plaque macrophages [35]. The latter was also demonstrated in the clinical setting [42].

Molecular MRI provides us with a versatile toolkit for assessing atherosclerosis. Standardization of the tools to facilitate assessments of animal models and emerging therapies with comparable reproducibility and robustness between different sites, however, remains challenging. The development of quantitative MRI techniques, such as T_1 and T_2 mapping, is an important first step to improve standardization, alleviating some of the drawbacks of image-intensity-based MRI methods. Also, ^{19}F MRI for direct visualization of the molecular imaging probe improves quantification and furthermore eliminates the need for a pre- and post-scan MRI, as the ^{19}F signal can be detected independently from the proton anatomical image. ^{19}F MRI, however, requires dedicated hardware and pulse sequences and is therefore not (yet) widely available.

We find that the development of a molecular MR toolkit for evaluation of therapy should principally focus on the major plaque characteristics that are considered important for vulnerability, including inflammation, the thickness of the fibrous cap, the size of the necrotic core, and presence of plaque erosion, in order to obtain early readouts of therapeutic efficacy [5]. For some of these features, molecular imaging methods are currently evaluated in humans, including inflammation imaging by passive targeting macrophages with USPIO [40–42] and fibrin imaging with Gd-conjugated peptides [73, 74].

At the time of writing, there are several ongoing clinical trials aimed at evaluating the value of specific molecular MRI methods for imaging atherosclerosis. ^{19}F MRI is under investigation for imaging of carotid neovasculature with Gd-containing PFC nanoparticles functionalized with the $\alpha_\nu\beta_3$-targeted RGD-peptide [85], and ferumoxytol is undergoing clinical testing as passive macrophage-targeting MRI contrast agent for carotid atherosclerosis [47]. Although these are promising developments, overall there has been little progress in translating molecular MR imaging into the clinic. This is in part due to the high costs involved in the transition from preclinical to clinical stage. Large-scale production according to good manufacturing practice (GMP) standards is expensive [86]. There are few research sites with sufficient financial resources to take a diagnostic agent through the expensive process of phases I, II, and III clinical testing. Furthermore, from an economical point of view, cost over potential benefit may be unfavorable for a screening diagnostic agent. The situation may be much better when the main application of the agent and molecular MRI is to serve as surrogate readout of therapeutic efficacy during drug development.

In conclusion, the last decade has witnessed major developments in the use of targeted nanoparticles as signal beacons for cardiovascular molecular MR imaging. The probes hold great promise for the facilitation of more specific patient diagnosis and treatment follow-up in the clinical management of atherosclerosis. Nevertheless, more work needs to be done to translate promising preclinical ideas into scientifically and economically viable clinical applications.

Acknowledgments Part of the research on the topic of this contribution in the authors' laboratories was performed within the framework of CTMM, the Center for Translational Molecular Medicine (www.ctmm.nl), project PARISk is park of the CTMM (grant 01C-202), which is supported by the Dutch Heart Foundation. Further funding was provided by the Besluit Subsidies Investeringen Kennisinfrastructuur (BSIK) program entitled Molecular Imaging of Ischemic Heart Disease (project number BSIK03033), the European Community EC-FP6-project Diagnostic Molecular Imaging (DiMI; LSHB-CT-2005-512146), and by the Dutch Heart Foundation (project number 2006 T106).

References

1. Libby P, Ridker PM, Hansson GK. Progress and challenges in translating the biology of atherosclerosis. Nature. 2011;473:317–25.
2. Quillard T, Libby P. Molecular imaging of atherosclerosis for improving diagnostic and therapeutic development. Circ Res. 2012;111:231–44.
3. Virmani R, Burke AP, Farb A, Kolodgie FD. Pathology of the vulnerable plaque. J Am Coll Cardiol. 2006;47:C13–8.
4. Pasterkamp G, Schoneveld AH, van der Wal AC, Haudenschild CC, Clarijs RJ, Becker AE, et al. Relation of arterial geometry to luminal narrowing and histologic markers for plaque vulnerability: the remodeling paradox. J Am Coll Cardiol. 1998;32:655–62.
5. Naghavi M, Libby P, Falk E, Casscells SW, Litovsky S, Rumberger J, et al. From vulnerable plaque to vulnerable patient: a call for new definitions and risk assessment strategies: Part I. Circulation. 2003;108:1664–72.
6. Heeneman S, Lutgens E, Schapira KB, Daemen MJAP, Biessen EAL. Control of atherosclerotic plaque vulnerability: insights from transgenic mice. Front Biosci. 2008;13:6289–313.
7. Russell JC, Proctor SD. Small animal models of cardiovascular disease: tools for the study of the roles of metabolic syndrome, dyslipidemia, and atherosclerosis. Cardiovasc Pathol. 2006;15:318–30.
8. Caravan P, Farrar CT, Frullano L, Uppal R. Influence of molecular parameters and increasing magnetic field strength on relaxivity of gadolinium- and manganese-based T1 contrast agents. Contrast Media Mol Imaging. 2009;4:89–100.
9. Josephs S, Rowley H, Rubin G. Atherosclerotic peripheral vascular disease symposium II: vascular magnetic resonance and computed tomographic imaging. Circulation. 2008;118:2837–44.
10. Cai J-M. Classification of human carotid atherosclerotic lesions with in vivo multicontrast magnetic resonance imaging. Circulation. 2002;106:1368–73.
11. Jansen CHP, Perera D, Makowski MR, Wiethoff AJ, Phinikaridou A, Razavi RM, et al. Detection of intracoronary thrombus by magnetic resonance imaging in patients with acute myocardial infarction. Circulation. 2011;124:416–24.

12. Chan CF, Keenan NG, Nielles-Vallespin S, Gatehouse P, Sheppard MN, Boyle JJ, et al. Ultra-short echo time cardiovascular magnetic resonance of atherosclerotic carotid plaque. J Cardiovasc Magn Reson. 2010;12:17.
13. Sharma S, Boujraf S, Bornstedt A, Hombach V, Ignatius A, Oberhuber A, et al. Quantification of Calcifications in Endarterectomy Samples by Means of High-Resolution Ultra-Short Echo Time Imaging. Invest Radiol. 2010;45:109–13.
14. Károlyi M, Seifarth H, Liew G, Schlett CL, Maurovich-Horvat P, Stolzmann P, et al. Classification of coronary atherosclerotic plaques ex vivo with T1, T2, and ultrashort echo time CMR. JACC Cardiovasc Imaging. 2013;6:466–74.
15. Singh N, Moody AR, Rochon-Terry G, Kiss A, Zavodni A. Identifying a high risk cardiovascular phenotype by carotid MRI-depicted intraplaque hemorrhage. Int J Cardiovasc Imaging. 2013;29:1477–83.
16. Fayad ZA, Fallon JT, Shinnar M, Wehrli S, Dansky HM, Poon M, et al. Noninvasive in vivo high-resolution magnetic resonance imaging of atherosclerotic lesions in genetically engineered mice. Circulation. 1998;98:1541–7.
17. Galizia MS, Barker A, Liao Y, Collins J, Carr J, McDermott MM, et al. Wall morphology, blood flow and wall shear stress: MR findings in patients with peripheral artery disease. Eur Radiol. 2013.
18. Chiu J, Chien S. Effects of disturbed flow on vascular endothelium: pathophysiological basis and clinical perspectives. Physiol Rev. 2011;327–87.
19. Phinikaridou A, Andia ME, Passacquale G, Ferro A, Botnar RM. Noninvasive MRI monitoring of the effect of interventions on endothelial permeability in murine atherosclerosis using an albumin-binding contrast agent. J Am Heart Assoc. 2013;2:e000402.
20. Gaens ME, Backes WH, Rozel S, Lipperts M, Sanders SN, Jaspers K, et al. Dynamic contrast-enhanced MR imaging of carotid atherosclerotic plaque: model selection, reproducibility, and validation. Radiology. 2013;266:271–9.
21. Michalska M, Machtoub L, Manthey HD, Bauer E, Herold V, Krohne G, et al. Visualization of vascular inflammation in the atherosclerotic mouse by ultrasmall superparamagnetic iron oxide vascular cell adhesion molecule-1-specific nanoparticles. Arterioscler Thromb Vasc Biol. 2012;32:2350–7.
22. Burtea C, Ballet S, Laurent S, Rousseaux O, Dencausse A, Gonzalez W, et al. Development of a magnetic resonance imaging protocol for the characterization of atherosclerotic plaque by using vascular cell adhesion molecule-1 and apoptosis-targeted ultrasmall superparamagnetic iron oxide derivatives. Arterioscler Thromb Vasc Biol. 2012;32:e36–48.
23. Burtea C, Laurent S, Port M, Lancelot E, Ballet S, Rousseaux O, et al. Magnetic resonance molecular imaging of vascular cell adhesion molecule-1 expression in inflammatory lesions using a peptide-vectorized paramagnetic imaging probe. J Med Chem. 2009;52:4725–42.
24. Deddens LH, van Tilborg GAF, van der Toorn A, van der Marel K, Paulis LEM, van Bloois L, et al. MRI of ICAM-1 upregulation after stroke: the importance of choosing the appropriate target-specific particulate contrast agent. Mol Imaging Biol. 2013;15:411–22.
25. El-Dakdouki MH, El-Boubbou K, Kamat M, Huang R, Abela GS, Kiupel M, et al. CD44 targeting magnetic glyconanoparticles for atherosclerotic plaque imaging. Pharm Res. 2013.
26. McAteer MA, Mankia K, Ruparelia N, Jefferson A, Nugent HB, Stork L-A, et al. A leukocyte-mimetic magnetic resonance imaging contrast agent homes rapidly to activated endothelium and tracks with atherosclerotic lesion macrophage content. Arterioscler Thromb Vasc Biol. 2012;32:1427–35.
27. Van Bochove GS, Paulis LEM, Segers D, Mulder WJM, Krams R, Nicolay K, et al. Contrast enhancement by differently sized paramagnetic MRI contrast agents in mice with two phenotypes of atherosclerotic plaque. Contrast Media Mol Imaging. 2011;6:35–45.
28. Segers FME, den Adel B, Bot I, van der Graaf LM, van der Veer EP, Gonzalez W, et al. Scavenger receptor-AI-targeted iron oxide nanoparticles for in vivo MRI detection of atherosclerotic lesions. Arterioscler Thromb Vasc Biol. 2013;33:1812–9.
29. Amirbekian V, Lipinski MJ, Briley-Saebo KC, Amirbekian S, Aguinaldo JGS, Weinreb DB, et al. Detecting and assessing macrophages in vivo to evaluate atherosclerosis noninvasively using molecular MRI. Proc Natl Acad Sci U S A. 2007;104:961–6.

30. Mulder WJM, Strijkers GJ, Briley-Saboe KC, Frias JC, Aguinaldo JGS, Vucic E, et al. Molecular imaging of macrophages in atherosclerotic plaques using bimodal PEG-micelles. Magn Reson Med. 2007;58:1164–70.
31. Dellinger A, Olson J, Link K, Vance S, Sandros MG, Yang J, et al. Functionalization of gadolinium metallofullerenes for detecting atherosclerotic plaque lesions by cardiovascular magnetic resonance. J Cardiovasc Magn Reson. 2013;15:7.
32. Wen S, Liu D-F, Cui Y, Harris SS, Chen Y-C, Li KC, et al. In vivo MRI detection of carotid atherosclerotic lesions and kidney inflammation in ApoE-deficient mice by using LOX-1 targeted iron nanoparticles. Nanomedicine. 2013.
33. Ruehm SG, Corot C, Vogt P, Kolb S, Debatin JF. Magnetic resonance imaging of atherosclerotic plaque with ultrasmall superparamagnetic particles of iron oxide in hyperlipidemic rabbits. Circulation. 2001;103:415–22.
34. Kooi ME, Cappendijk VC, Cleutjens KB, Kessels AG, Kitslaar PJ, Borgers M, et al. Accumulation of ultrasmall superparamagnetic particles of iron oxide in human atherosclerotic plaques can be detected by in vivo magnetic resonance imaging. Circulation. 2003;107:2453–8.
35. Makowski MR, Varma G, Wiethoff AJ, Smith A, Mattock K, Jansen CHP, et al. Noninvasive assessment of atherosclerotic plaque progression in ApoE–/– mice using susceptibility gradient mapping. Circ Cardiovasc Imaging. 2011;4:295–303.
36. Sigovan M, Bessaad A, Alsaid H, Lancelot E, Corot C, Neyran B, et al. Assessment of age modulated vascular inflammation in ApoE–/– mice by USPIO-enhanced magnetic resonance imaging. Invest Radiol. 2010;45:702–7.
37. Sigovan M, Kaye E, Lancelot E, Corot C, Provost N, Majd Z, et al. Anti-inflammatory drug evaluation in ApoE–/– mice by ultrasmall superparamagnetic iron oxide-enhanced magnetic resonance imaging. Invest Radiol. 2012;47:546–52.
38. Moonen RPM, Nicolay K, Strijkers GJ. Quantification of USPIO uptake in mouse atherosclerotic plaque by T2 mapping MRI. MAGMA, ESMRMB 2012, 29th annual scientific meeting, Lisbon, 4–6 Oct. Abstr. 2012;25:1 Suppl; 73 p. 55–6.
39. Coolen BF, Simonis FFJ, Geelen T, Moonen RPM, Arslan F, Paulis LEM, et al. Quantitative T2 mapping of the mouse heart by segmented MLEV phase-cycled T2 preparation. Magn Reson Med. 2013.
40. Sadat U, Howarth SPS, Usman A, Tang TY, Graves MJ, Gillard JH. Sequential imaging of asymptomatic carotid atheroma using ultrasmall superparamagnetic iron oxide-enhanced magnetic resonance imaging: a feasibility study. J Stroke Cerebrovasc Dis. 2013;22:e271–6.
41. Degnan AJ, Patterson AJ, Tang TY, Howarth SPS, Gillard JH. Evaluation of ultrasmall superparamagnetic iron oxide-enhanced MRI of carotid atherosclerosis to assess risk of cerebrovascular and cardiovascular events: follow-up of the ATHEROMA trial. Cerebrovasc Dis. 2012;34:169–73.
42. Patterson AJ, Tang TY, Graves MJ, Müller KH, Gillard JH. In vivo carotid plaque MRI using quantitative T2* measurements with ultrasmall superparamagnetic iron oxide particles: a dose-response study to statin therapy. NMR Biomed. 2011;24:89–95.
43. Yancy AD, Olzinski AR, Hu TC-C, Lenhard SC, Aravindhan K, Gruver SM, et al. Differential uptake of ferumoxtran-10 and ferumoxytol, ultrasmall superparamagnetic iron oxide contrast agents in rabbit: critical determinants of atherosclerotic plaque labeling. J Magn Reson Imaging. 2005;21:432–42.
44. Herborn CU, Vogt FM, Lauenstein TC, Dirsch O, Corot C, Robert P, et al. Magnetic resonance imaging of experimental atherosclerotic plaque: comparison of two ultrasmall superparamagnetic particles of iron oxide. J Magn Reson Imaging. 2006;24:388–93.
45. Coyne DW. Ferumoxytol for treatment of iron deficiency anemia in patients with chronic kidney disease. Expert Opin Pharmacother. 2009;10:2563–8.
46. Alam SR, Shah ASV, Richards J, Lang NN, Barnes G, Joshi N, et al. Ultrasmall superparamagnetic particles of iron oxide in patients with acute myocardial infarction: early clinical experience. Circ Cardiovasc Imaging. 2012;5:559–65.
47. Metabolic Imaging in Carotid Atherosclerosis (MICA) (Internet). Clinical trials.gov. 2013 (cited 7 Feb 2014). Available from: http://clinicaltrials.gov/show/NCT01674257.

48. Temme S, Bönner F, Schrader J, Flögel U. 19F magnetic resonance imaging of endogenous macrophages in inflammation. Wiley Interdiscip Rev Nanomed Nanobiotechnol. 2012;4:329–43.
49. Stoll G, Basse-Lüsebrink T, Weise G, Jakob P. Visualization of inflammation using (19) F-magnetic resonance imaging and perfluorocarbons. Wiley Interdiscip Rev Nanomed Nanobiotechnol. 2012;4:438–47.
50. Spahn DR. Blood substitutes. Artificial oxygen carriers: perfluorocarbon emulsions. Crit Care. 1999;3:R93–7.
51. Kok MB, de Vries A, Abdurrachim D, Prompers JJ, Grüll H, Nicolay K, et al. Quantitative (1) H MRI, (19)F MRI, and (19)F MRS of cell-internalized perfluorocarbon paramagnetic nanoparticles. Contrast Media Mol Imaging. 2011;6:19–27.
52. De Vries A, Moonen R, Yildirim M, Langereis S, Lamerichs R, Pikkemaat JA, et al. Relaxometric studies of gadolinium-functionalized perfluorocarbon nanoparticles for MR imaging. Contrast Media Mol Imaging. 2014;9:83–91.
53. Sirol M, Itskovich VV, Mani V, Aguinaldo JGS, Fallon JT, Misselwitz B, et al. Lipid-rich atherosclerotic plaques detected by gadofluorine-enhanced in vivo magnetic resonance imaging. Circulation. 2004;109:2890–6.
54. Wen S, Liu D-F, Liu Z, Harris S, Yao Y-Y, Ding Q, et al. OxLDL-targeted iron oxide nanoparticles for in vivo MRI detection of perivascular carotid collar induced atherosclerotic lesions in ApoE-deficient mice. J Lipid Res. 2012;53:829–38.
55. Briley-Saebo KC, Cho YS, Shaw PX, Ryu SK, Mani V, Dickson S, et al. Targeted iron oxide particles for in vivo magnetic resonance detection of atherosclerotic lesions with antibodies directed to oxidation-specific epitopes. J Am Coll Cardiol. 2011;57:337–47.
56. Briley-Saebo KC, Nguyen TH, Saeboe AM, Cho Y-S, Ryu SK, Volkova ER, et al. In vivo detection of oxidation-specific epitopes in atherosclerotic lesions using biocompatible manganese molecular magnetic imaging probes. J Am Coll Cardiol. 2012;59:616–26.
57. Lowell AN, Qiao H, Liu T, Ishikawa T, Zhang H, Oriana S, et al. Functionalized low-density lipoprotein nanoparticles for in vivo enhancement of atherosclerosis on magnetic resonance images. Bioconjug Chem. 2012;23:2313–9.
58. Cormode D, Frias J, Ma Y, Chen W. HDL as a contrast agent for medical imaging. Clin Lipidol. 2009;4:493–500.
59. Barazza A, Blachford C, Even-Or O, Joaquin VA, Briley-Saebo KC, Chen W, et al. The complex fate in plasma of gadolinium incorporated into high-density lipoproteins used for magnetic imaging of atherosclerotic plaques. Bioconjug Chem. 2013;24:1039–48.
60. Cormode DP, Skajaa T, van Schooneveld MM, Koole R, Jarzyna P, Lobatto ME, et al. Nanocrystal core high-density lipoproteins: a multimodality contrast agent platform. Nano Lett. 2008;8:3715–23.
61. Jung C, Kaul MG, Bruns OT, Ducic T, Freund B, Heine M, et al. Intraperitoneal injection improves the uptake of nanoparticle labeled HDL to atherosclerotic plaques compared to intravenous injection: a multimodal imaging study in ApoE−/− mice. Circ Cardiovasc Imaging. 2013.
62. Chen W, Cormode DP, Vengrenyuk Y, Herranz B, Feig JE, Klink A, et al. Collagen-specific peptide conjugated HDL nanoparticles as MRI contrast agent to evaluate compositional changes in atherosclerotic plaque regression. JACC Cardiovasc Imaging. 2013;6:373–84.
63. Van Bochove GS, Sanders HMHF, de Smet M, Keizer HM, Mulder WJM, Krams R, et al. Molecular MR imaging of collagen in mouse atherosclerosis by using paramagnetic CNA35 micelles. Eur J Inorg Chem. 2012;2012:2115–25.
64. Makowski MR, Wiethoff AJ, Blume U, Cuello F, Warley A, Jansen CHP, et al. Assessment of atherosclerotic plaque burden with an elastin-specific magnetic resonance contrast agent. Nat Med. 2011;17:383–8.
65. Makowski MR, Preissel A, von Bary C, Warley A, Schachoff S, Keithan A, et al. Three-dimensional imaging of the aortic vessel wall using an elastin-specific magnetic resonance contrast agent. Invest Radiol. 2012;47:438–44.
66. Von Bary C, Makowski M, Preissel A, Keithahn A, Warley A, Spuentrup E, et al. MRI of coronary wall remodeling in a swine model of coronary injury using an elastin-binding contrast agent. Circ Cardiovasc Imaging. 2011;4:147–55.

67. Quillard T, Croce K, Jaffer F, Weissleder R, Libby P. Molecular imaging of macrophage protease activity in cardiovascular inflammation in vivo. Thromb Haemost. 2011;105:828–36.
68. Lancelot E, Amirbekian V, Brigger I, Raynaud J-S, Ballet S, David C, et al. Evaluation of matrix metalloproteinases in atherosclerosis using a novel noninvasive imaging approach. Arterioscler Thromb Vasc Biol. 2008;28:425–32.
69. Amirbekian V, Aguinaldo J, Amirbekian S. Atherosclerosis and matrix metalloproteinases: experimental molecular MR imaging in vivo. Radiology. 2009;251:429–38.
70. Hyafil F, Vucic E, Cornily J-C, Sharma R, Amirbekian V, Blackwell F, et al. Monitoring of arterial wall remodelling in atherosclerotic rabbits with a magnetic resonance imaging contrast agent binding to matrix metalloproteinases. Eur Heart J. 2011;32:1561–71.
71. Ouimet T, Lancelot E, Hyafil F, Rienzo M, Deux F, Lemaître M, et al. Molecular and cellular targets of the MRI contrast agent P947 for atherosclerosis imaging. Mol Pharm. 2012;9:850–61.
72. Ronald JA, Chen JW, Chen Y, Hamilton AM, Rodriguez E, Reynolds F, et al. Enzyme-sensitive magnetic resonance imaging targeting myeloperoxidase identifies active inflammation in experimental rabbit atherosclerotic plaques. Circulation. 2009;120:592–9.
73. Vymazal J, Spuentrup E, Cardenas-Molina G, Wiethoff AJ, Hartmann MG, Caravan P, et al. Thrombus imaging with fibrin-specific gadolinium-based MR contrast agent EP-2104R. Invest Radiol. 2009;44:697–704.
74. Spuentrup E, Botnar RM, Wiethoff AJ, Ibrahim T, Kelle S, Katoh M, et al. MR imaging of thrombi using EP-2104R, a fibrin-specific contrast agent: initial results in patients. Eur Radiol. 2008;18:1995–2005.
75. Makowski MR, Forbes SC, Blume U, Warley A, Jansen CHP, Schuster A, et al. In vivo assessment of intraplaque and endothelial fibrin in ApoE(−/−) mice by molecular MRI. Atherosclerosis. 2012;222:43–9.
76. Tavora F, Cresswell N, Li L, Ripple M, Burke A. Immunolocalisation of fibrin in coronary atherosclerosis: implications for necrotic core development. Pathology. 2010;42:15–22.
77. Morawski AM, Winter PM, Yu X, Fuhrhop RW, Scott MJ, Hockett F, et al. Quantitative "magnetic resonance immunohistochemistry" with ligand-targeted (19)F nanoparticles. Magn Reson Med. 2004;52:1255–62.
78. Von Elverfeldt D, von zur Muhlen C, Wiens K, Neudorfer I, Zirlik A, Meissner M, et al. In vivo detection of activated platelets allows characterizing rupture of atherosclerotic plaques with molecular magnetic resonance imaging in mice. PLoS One. 2012;7:e45008.
79. Miserus R-JJHM, Herías MV, Prinzen L, Lobbes MBI, Van Suylen R-J, Dirksen A, et al. Molecular MRI of early thrombus formation using a bimodal alpha2-antiplasmin-based contrast agent. JACC Cardiovasc Imaging. 2009;2:987–96.
80. Van Tilborg GAF, Vucic E, Strijkers GJ, Cormode DP, Mani V, Skajaa T, et al. Annexin A5-functionalized bimodal nanoparticles for MRI and fluorescence imaging of atherosclerotic plaques. Bioconjug Chem. 2010;21:1794–803.
81. Burtea C, Laurent S, Lancelot E. Peptidic targeting of phosphatidylserine for the MRI detection of apoptosis in atherosclerotic plaques. Mol Pharm. 2009;6:1903–19.
82. Burtea C, Laurent S, Murariu O, Rattat D, Toubeau G, Verbruggen A, et al. Molecular imaging of alpha v beta3 integrin expression in atherosclerotic plaques with a mimetic of RGD peptide grafted to Gd-DTPA. Cardiovasc Res. 2008;78:148–57.
83. Winter PM, Morawski AM, Caruthers SD, Fuhrhop RW, Zhang H, Williams TA, et al. Molecular imaging of angiogenesis in early-stage atherosclerosis with alpha(v)beta3-integrin-targeted nanoparticles. Circulation. 2003;108:2270–4.
84. Winter PM, Neubauer AM, Caruthers SD, Harris TD, Robertson JD, Williams TA, et al. Endothelial alpha(v)beta3 integrin-targeted fumagillin nanoparticles inhibit angiogenesis in atherosclerosis. Arterioscler Thromb Vasc Biol. 2006;26:2103–9.
85. Perrone-Filardi P, Dellegrottaglie S, Rudd JHF, Costanzo P, Marciano C, Vassallo E, et al. Molecular imaging of atherosclerosis in translational medicine. Eur J Nucl Med Mol Imaging. 2011;38:969–75.
86. Buxton DB, Antman M, Danthi N, Dilsizian V, Fayad ZA, Garcia MJ, et al. Report of the national heart, lung, and blood institute working group on the translation of cardiovascular molecular imaging. Circulation. 2011;123:2157–63.

Cardiac PET Imaging in Coronary Artery Disease

14

Marcelo F. Di Carli

Contents

Abstract

PET is a powerful tool for translational research that offers unique quantitative insights into physiologic and molecular processes in vivo. PET/CT is rapidly advancing our ability to image in great detail the structure and function in the heart and vasculature. By providing concurrent quantitative information about myocardial blood flow and metabolism with coronary and cardiac anatomy,

M.F. Di Carli, MD
Noninvasive Cardiovascular Imaging Program,
Departments of Radiology and Medicine;
Division of Nuclear Medicine and Molecular Imaging,
Department of Radiology; and Division of Cardiovascular Medicine,
Department of Medicine, Brigham and Women's Hospital,
ASB-L1 037C, 75 Francis St, Boston, MA 02115, USA
e-mail: mdicarli@partners.org

E. Aikawa (ed.), *Cardiovascular Imaging: Arterial and Aortic Valve Inflammation and Calcification*, DOI 10.1007/978-3-319-09268-3_14

PET/CT offers the opportunity for a comprehensive noninvasive evaluation of the consequences of atherosclerosis in the coronary arteries and the myocardium. Indeed, the quantification of myocardial blood flow (in mL/min/g) and coronary flow reserve provides increased sensitivity for identifying and excluding significant coronary artery stenoses. In addition, coronary flow reserve is a powerful marker of clinical risk, which helps refine clinical risk stratification and, potentially, direct therapy. In addition, PET enables noninvasive assessment of myocardial viability that helps identify myocardial viability and facilitates medical decision making in patients with severe left ventricular dysfunction due to coronary artery disease. During the last two decades, we have witnessed a significant improvement in the prevention and management of coronary artery disease (CAD) and its devastating consequences. Despite these efforts, however, cardiovascular disease (especially coronary artery disease and its sequelae) remains highly prevalent and it represents a healthcare burden in industrialized and developing countries. This has resulted in a continued expansion and refinement of our noninvasive imaging approaches to improve diagnosis and risk prediction. Positron-emission tomography (PET) is a powerful noninvasive imaging tool for phenotyping patients at risk or with known coronary artery disease that has been evolving over the past 30 years. One of the key advantages over other imaging modalities is its unique ability to quantify physiologic processes including myocardial blood flow (in mL/min/g), metabolism, and cardiac receptors and its high sensitivity for delineating and quantifying molecular targets in vivo using targeted imaging probes. The discussion that follows will review the principles of PET as well as its established and emerging clinical applications in cardiovascular disease.

14.1 Technical Considerations

PET is a nuclear medicine technique that uses positron-emitting radionuclides to obtain images of the heart and vasculature. Fortunately, atoms of high biologic significance (e.g., carbon, oxygen, and nitrogen) also have radionuclide species that decay by positron emission. Thus, the use of positron-emitting radionuclides allows obtaining unique quantitative information of important biologic processes in vivo (e.g., myocardial perfusion, glucose metabolism, fatty acid metabolism, cardiac innervation). The fundamental principle of positron tomography is that positron-emitting radionuclides (e.g., ^{11}carbon, ^{13}nitrogen, ^{15}oxygen, ^{18}fluorine) decay by emitting "positively" charged electrons (positrons). Once released from the nucleus, these positrons travel short distances in the tissue and annihilate with the encounter of nearby electrons. This annihilation releases energy in the form of two gamma rays or photons that are emitted in a characteristic opposite direction (i.e., 180° from each other). These opposite high-energy photons (511 keV) are captured externally by an array of detector elements (scintillators) in the PET gantry. The electronics of the PET system are arranged to facilitate detection of 511 keV photons arriving at opposite detectors within a narrow temporal window and rejection of scattered photons arriving outside the preset temporal window, thereby enhancing the spatial and contrast resolution of the PET images.

Several technical advantages account for the improved image quality and diagnostic ability of PET compared to SPECT including: (1) routine measured (depth independent) attenuation correction, which decreases false positives and, thus, increases specificity; (2) high spatial and contrast resolution (heart-to-background ratio) that allows improved detection of small perfusion defects, thereby decreasing false negatives and increasing sensitivity; and (3) high temporal resolution that allows fast dynamic imaging of tracer kinetics, which makes absolute quantification of myocardial perfusion (in mL/min/g of tissue) possible. In addition, the use of short-lived radiopharmaceuticals allows fast, sequential assessment of regional myocardial perfusion (e.g., rest and stress), thereby improving laboratory efficiency and patient throughput.

14.1.1 Multidimensional PET/CT Imaging

All modern PET systems are now combined with a computed tomography (CT) scanner into hybrid PET/CT camera. Each component of the integrated system provides unique information for the evaluation of patients with known or suspected CAD as described below.

14.1.1.1 CT Scans

Low-dose CT scans (scout image or topogram) are used for positioning patients in the scanner field of view. A low-dose non-gated CT scan covering the heart region (transmission scan) is then used for correction of the inhomogeneities of radiotracer distribution in the PET images caused by overlapping soft tissue (e.g., breast, diaphragm). This post-processing step is known as attenuation correction and is mandatory for cardiac PET imaging. In selected patients (e.g., those without known CAD), a prospectively gated CT scan, in which the x-ray tube is "turned on" only during the end-diastolic phase of the cardiac cycle – typically 75–80 % of the R-R interval – with a higher tube current (~250 mA) acquired during inspiratory breathhold. This gated CT scan is used to calculate a coronary artery calcium (CAC) score (Agatston score). Finally, it is also possible to obtain a coronary CT angiogram (CCTA) immediately following the assessment of myocardial perfusion and/or metabolism. For the latter application, a hybrid PET scanner equipped with a 64-detector CT scanner or higher is required. The resulting added radiation from the CT scans is approximately 0.3–0.5 mSv for the transmission scan, 1.5–2.0 mSv for the calcium score, and 3.0–7.0 for the CCTA.

14.1.1.2 Emission Scans

Due to the short physical half-life of PET radiopharmaceuticals for the assessment of myocardial perfusion, approximately the same dose is injected for both the rest and stress myocardial perfusion studies (Table 14.1). Injected doses are adjusted according to the size of the patient and type of PET data acquisition (i.e.,

Table 14.1 Examples of PET radiopharmaceuticals in clinical practice and translational research

Radiopharmaceutical	Targeted biologic process	Uptake mechanism	Physical half-life	FDA-approved
^{15}O-water	Myocardial perfusion	Freely diffusible	2 min	No
^{13}N-ammonia	Myocardial perfusion	Metabolic trapping	10 min	Yes
^{82}Rubidium	Myocardial perfusion	Na/K ATPase	76 s	Yes
^{18}F-FDG	Myocardial metabolism	Metabolic trapping, glucose metabolism	110 min	Yes
^{62}Cu-PTSM	Myocardial perfusion	Intracellular binding	10 min	No
^{11}C-acetate	Myocardial metabolism	Krebs cycle flux, oxidative metabolism	20 min	No
^{11}C-palmitate	Myocardial metabolism	Fatty acid metabolism	20 min	No
^{11}C-glucose	Myocardial metabolism	Glucose metabolism	20 min	No
^{18}F-FTHA	Myocardial metabolism	Fatty acid metabolism	110 min	No
^{11}C-HED	Sympathetic innervation	Sympathetic uptake-1 and storage	20 min	No
^{11}C-epinephrine	Sympathetic innervation	Sympathetic storage	20 min	No
^{18}F-dopamine	Sympathetic innervation	Sympathetic uptake and function	20 min	No
^{11}C-CGP12177	β-Adrenoceptor density	Receptor binding	20 min	No

FDG fluorodeoxyglucose, *PTSM* pyruvaldehyde bis(N4-methylthiosemicarbazone), *FTHA* fluorothiaheptadecanoic acid, *HED* hydroxyephedrine

2-D vs. 3-D mode). List mode imaging has become standard practice with modern PET technology, which allows a comprehensive multidimensional examination illustrated in Fig. 14.1 including the assessment of myocardial perfusion, left ventricular ejection fraction (LVEF) and volumes, and quantitative coronary blood flow and flow reserve in the same setting. In selected patients with severe left ventricular dysfunction, metabolic imaging with FDG is used to assess myocardial viability.

14.1.2 Radiopharmaceuticals

Table 14.1 lists the most common radiopharmaceuticals used with PET in translational research and clinical practice.

14.2 Imaging Markers of Coronary Artery Disease from Hybrid PET/CT

The integrated PET/CT approach provides access to a comprehensive list of quantitative imaging markers that have been used successfully in clinical research and are quickly being incorporated into clinical practice.

14.2.1 Atherosclerotic Burden

ECG-gated scanning for coronary artery calcium (CAC) offers a reproducible, easy-to-perform method to reliably determine whether coronary calcification is present or absent, without the need of intravenous contrast administration. The extent and severity of calcification, reflecting the burden of atherosclerosis in the coronary arteries, can be quantified by validated scoring techniques (e.g., Agatston score). A score of 0 indicates no coronary calcification and portends very low risk of adverse cardiovascular events, whereas a score ≥400 indicates severe calcification and higher clinical risk [1]. Coronary calcium scanning is often performed in patients without known CAD undergoing myocardial perfusion PET/CT

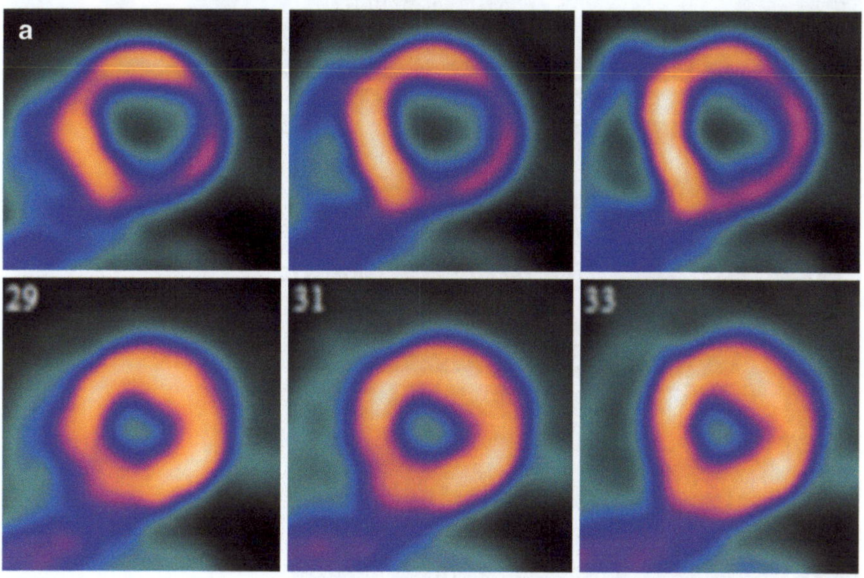

Fig. 14.1 Multidimensional PET protocol. *Panel A*: Stress and rest myocardial perfusion images delineating the extent of ischemia and scar. *Panel B*: ECG-gated images allow quantification of left ventricular volumes and ejection fraction at peak (or post) stress and at rest. *Panel C*: Multiframe or dynamic data allows tracer kinetic analysis and quantification of regional and global myocardial blood flow (in mL/min/g of tissue) and coronary flow reserve. *Panel D*: Metabolic imaging allows investigation of myocardial metabolism and tissue viability

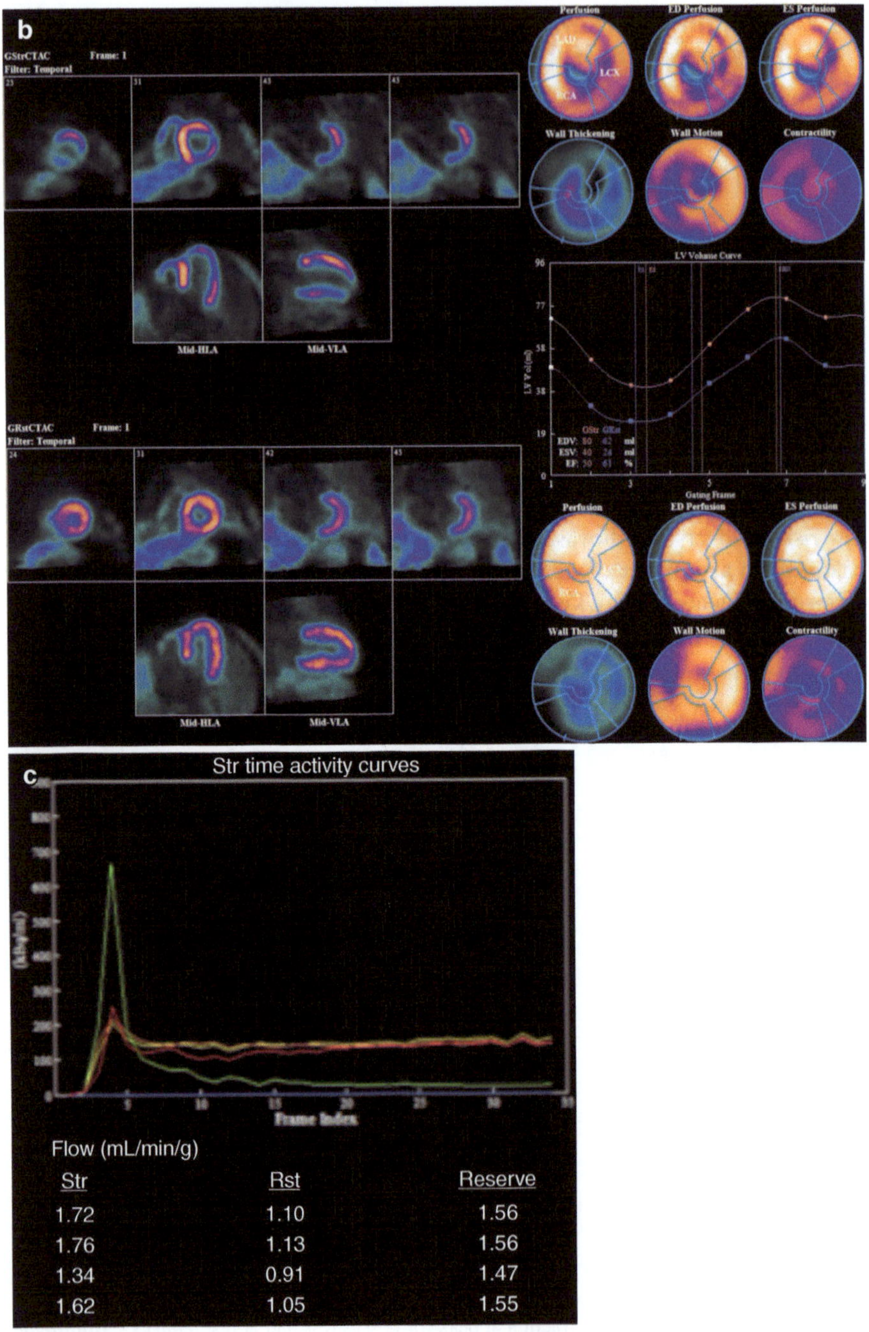

Fig. 14.1 (continued)

Fig. 14.1 (continued)

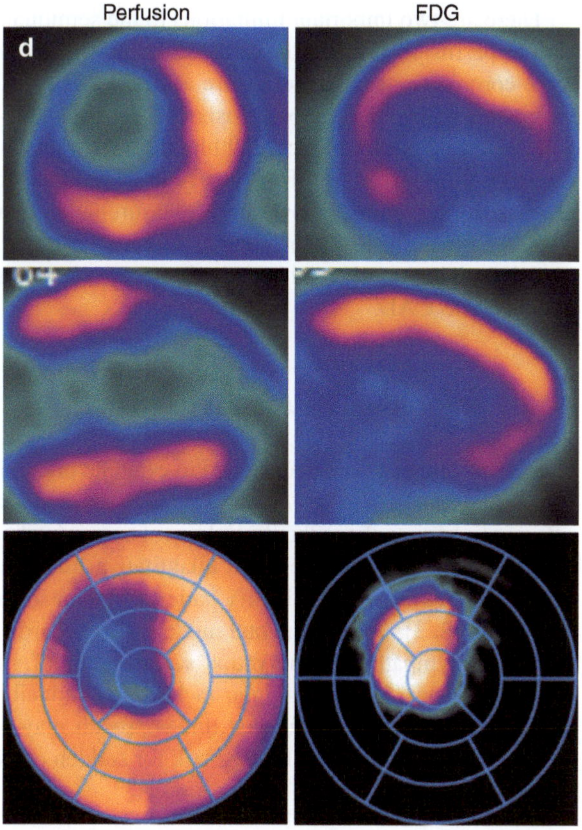

imaging. In selected patients, it is also possible to use ECG-gated CT imaging to obtain high-quality images of the coronary arteries after the administration of intravenous contrast, which allows visualization of both calcified and noncalcified plaques, as well as estimation of the severity of coronary artery narrowing resulting from those plaques.

14.2.2 Myocardial Perfusion and Metabolism

The myocardial perfusion imaging method is designed and targeted on the identification of flow-limiting stenoses. It is a robust approach to delineate flow-limiting CAD, quantify the magnitude of ischemic myocardium, and assess the extent of tissue viability. Semiquantitative assessments of ischemia and scar with radionuclide imaging are accurate and highly reproducible. In the integrated hybrid imaging approach, the assessment of ischemia provides instant feedback regarding the physiologic significance of upstream epicardial coronary stenosis, thereby guiding therapeutic management (i.e., selection of patients for revascularization).

There are two important limitations to the semiquantitative assessment of myocardial perfusion images: the underestimation of the extent of ischemia when all three coronary artery territories are affected and inability to characterize patients with nonobstructive atherosclerosis. At the moment, PET is the most validated technique to quantify myocardial blood flow (in mL/min/g of tissue) and estimate coronary flow reserve (CFR; as the ratio of peak myocardial blood flow over that at rest). As discussed below, these measurements of myocardial blood flow and CFR are powerful tools for clinical investigation and are emerging as clinically useful imaging markers that help improve diagnosis and risk stratification of patients with CAD.

14.2.3 Myocardial Neuronal Function

The use of imaging probes designed to evaluate pre- and postsynaptic targets of the cardiac autonomic nervous system allows quantification of autonomic function and offers insights into the pathophysiology of a variety of cardiovascular disorders. For example, recent data suggest that quantitative imaging of the cardiac sympathetic nervous system may help identify patients with heart failure at risk for sudden cardiac death [2, 3]. In experimental models of myocardial infarction, the presence of functional sympathetic denervation within areas of viable myocardium identifies sites at higher risk of ventricular tachycardia inducibility [4]. There is emerging clinical trial data suggesting that this approach may provide a useful method for identification of patients at highest risk for sudden cardiac death [2, 3].

14.2.4 Left Ventricular Function

Left ventricular ejection fraction is one the most powerful predictors of prognosis in cardiovascular medicine. ECG-gated myocardial perfusion imaging allows accurate and reproducible quantification of the left ventricular volumes and ejection fraction.

14.3 Use of PET/CT Imaging Markers in Translational Research and Clinical Practice with a Focus in Atherosclerosis

14.3.1 Preclinical Characterization of Atherosclerosis

14.3.1.1 Coronary Artery Calcification

Coronary artery calcification is part of the development of atherosclerosis. The process begins early and accelerates as the disease progresses. CAC occurs exclusively in atherosclerotic arteries and is absent in normal vessels. Although the extent of CAC correlates with the histologic plaque burden, its absence does not necessarily exclude atheromatous plaque especially in the young and in symptomatic populations. Because calcification is a surrogate measure of coronary atherosclerosis, clinical interest has focused on the usefulness of noninvasive detection of calcium as a coronary risk stratification tool. The Multiethnic Study of Atherosclerosis (MESA) involved 6,722 individuals with no known cardiovascular disease who were followed up for a median of nearly 4 years [1]. In comparison to participants without calcification (CAC score 0), those with a score >300 had a nearly sevenfold higher adjusted risk of a major coronary event. Importantly, the presence of coronary calcification provided predictive information beyond that derived from standard risk factors (i.e., Framingham risk score). Moreover, a recent study of 44,052 asymptomatic subjects followed for a median of 5 years demonstrated a stepwise increase in mortality risk with increasing CAC among individuals without traditional risk factors [5]. The observation that CAC improves risk prediction beyond that of conventional risk factor-based algorithms has been confirmed by multiple large observational studies, and guidelines now recommend the use of CAC for select low- to intermediate-risk individuals.

14.3.1.2 Coronary Vasomotor Dysfunction

Coronary vasomotor dysfunction is an early manifestation of atherosclerosis. As discussed above, PET allows direct measurements of coronary blood flow and flow reserve in response to vasodilator stress and cold pressor testing. There is an extensive literature documenting the presence of impaired coronary flow reserve in asymptomatic patients with coronary risk factors without obstructive CAD [6, 7]. These abnormalities have been associated with the deleterious effects of oxidative stress, hyperglycemia, low-level systemic inflammation, as well as the fluid dynamic effects of diffuse atherosclerosis and microvascular remodeling on coronary vasodilator function.

There is consistent evidence supporting quantitative CFR as a powerful marker of vascular health and, as such, a useful marker to improve diagnosis and risk stratification and to monitor response to treatment, particularly in the context of clinical trials. The accuracy of quantitative noninvasive PET measures of myocardial blood flow and flow reserve by PET has been extensively validated in experimental animals [8] and humans [9–12]. The reproducibility of this technique is also well established [11, 12]. PET is considered the gold standard for quantifying coronary blood flow and flow reserve. There is also growing evidence that quantitative CFR as a measure of coronary vascular dysfunction is a modifiable imaging biomarker, which has been tested in the context of clinical trials (Table 14.2) [13–21]. This suggests that CFR can also be used as a surrogate end point to assess efficacy of treatments aimed at reducing the burden of risk factors.

14.3.1.3 Interaction Between CAC and Coronary Vasomotor Dysfunction

Postmortem studies have shown that there are many noncalcified plaques for every calcified plaque [22]. Thus, it is unclear whether CAC itself increases the risk of adverse coronary outcomes or whether CAC deposition serves as a proxy for the

Table 14.2 Clinical trial experience using PET imaging end points

Author	Trial design	Setting	Cohort	Sample size	Intervention	Exposure	End point	Result	P value
Alexanderson [13]	Open label	Single center	Dyslipidemia w/o CAD	14	Ezetimibe/ simvastatin	8 weeks	CFR	13 %	NS
Ling [18]	RCT	Single center	Dyslipidemia w/CAD	72	Pravastatin, simvastatin, placebo	8 weeks	CFR	–	NS
Baller [14]	Open label	Single center	Dyslipidemia w/o CAD	23	Simvastatin	6 months	CFR	20 %	0.01
Guethlin [15]	Open label	Single center	Dyslipidemia w/ CAD	15	Fluvastatin	6 months	CFR	38 %	<0.05
Ilveskoski [16]	RCT	Single center	Dyslipidemia w/o CAD	44	Pravastatin	6 months	CFR	18 %	0.05
Lehtimaki [17]	RCT	Single center	Dyslipidemia w/o CAD	34	Pravastatin	6 months	CFR	18 %	0.002
Sdringola [21]	RCT	Multicenter	Dyslipidemia w/CAD	145	Atorvastatin	6 months	Semiquant TPD	–	NS
McMahon [19]	RCT	Single center	Type 2 DM w/o CAD	16	Pioglitazone	12 weeks	CFR	–	NS
Schelbert [20]	RCT	Multicenter	Dyslipidemia w/CAD	274	Atorvastatin + avasimibe vs. atorvastatin	12 months	CFR	–	NS
Adler (unpublished)	RCT	Single center	Type 2 DM w/o CAD	64	Spironolactone vs. HTCZ vs. placebo	6 months	CFR	15 %	0.006

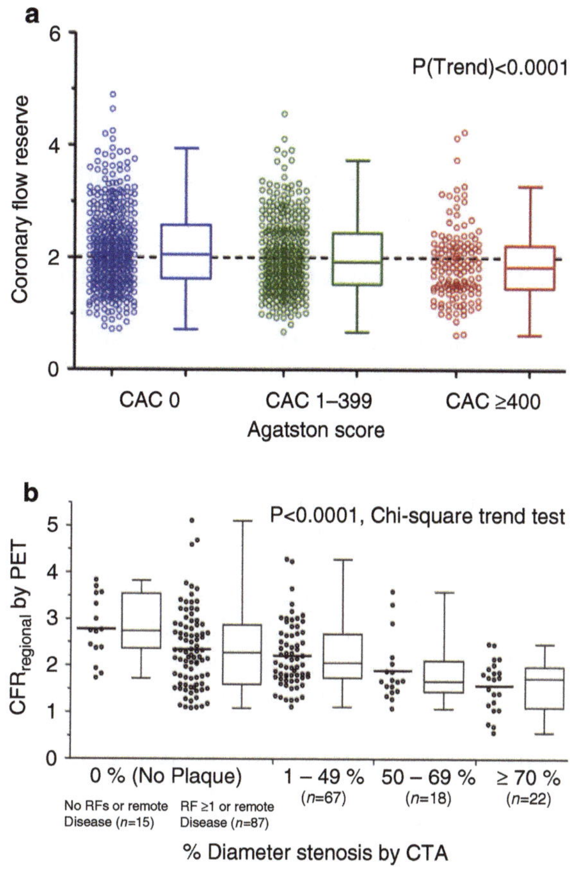

Fig. 14.2 Relationship between coronary flow reserve and atherosclerotic burden. *Panel A*: Coronary flow reserve across coronary artery calcium score categories (zero, 1–399, and ≥400). *Panel B:* Coronary flow reserve across categories of luminal angiographic stenosis by coronary CTA (Reproduced with permission from Refs. [23] and [24])

extent and magnitude of noncalcified atherosclerosis and its adverse functional consequence of coronary vasomotor function. Measures of coronary flow reserve (reflecting both endothelial and smooth muscle cell dysfunction) are weakly correlated with CAC and also with the total plaque burden as assessed by coronary CT angiography. Indeed, there is wide variability in abnormal coronary vasomotor function in each level of CAC score or luminal angiographic severity (Fig. 14.2) [23, 24]. The scatter of coronary flow reserve values within varying degrees of coronary plaque burden suggests that epicardial coronary plaque burden is not a complete reflection of overall disease activity within the coronary circulation. Indeed, circulating inflammatory biomarkers (including CRP, IL-6, fibrinogen, MMP-9, MCP-1, TNF-alpha, and others) were found to have only a weak association with the burden of coronary artery calcifications [25]. Moreover, a recent study demonstrates that for any level of coronary artery calcification, the presence of abnormal coronary flow reserve is consistently associated with a higher rate of adverse cardiac events [24]. Together, these findings may help explain the relatively low numbers of coronary events even among patients with high coronary artery calcium scores [1, 26] and support the notion that measures of CAC and coronary vasomotor function provide distinct and complementary information regarding the extent of anatomic atherosclerosis and its physiologic significance.

14.3.2 Evaluation of Symptomatic Patients with Suspected or Known CAD

14.3.2.1 Diagnosis of Obstructive Coronary Artery Disease

Two recent meta-analyses compared the diagnostic accuracy of PET and single-photon emission computed tomography (SPECT) myocardial perfusion imaging (MPI) for detecting obstructive CAD [27, 28]. The pooled mean sensitivity of PET was significantly higher than that of SPECT MPI (92.6 % and 90 % vs. 88.3 % and 85 %, respectively). However, no significant difference in specificity was observed between PET and SPECT (81.3 % and 88 % vs. 75.8 % and 85 %, respectively).

Despite its widespread use and acceptance, a recognized limitation of radionuclide myocardial perfusion imaging with PET (and SPECT) is that it often uncovers only coronary territories supplied by coronary arteries with the most severe stenosis, and, consequently, it is relatively insensitive to accurately delineate the extent of obstructive angiographic CAD especially in the setting of multivessel CAD [29, 30]. Two quantitative approaches with PET are used to help mitigate this limitation. One approach includes quantification of LVEF at rest and during peak stress. In normal subjects, LVEF increases during peak vasodilator stress [30]. In patients with obstructive CAD, however, the delta change in LVEF from baseline to peak stress (so-called LVEF reserve) is inversely related to the extent of obstructive angiographic CAD [30]. Indeed, patients with obstructive multivessel or left main disease show a frank drop in LVEF during peak stress even in the absence of apparent perfusion defects. In contrast, those without significant CAD or with single-vessel disease show a normal increase in LVEF. An adequate increase in LVEF during stress (≥6 % from baseline) has a high sensitivity and negative predictive value for excluding multivessel disease [30].

Another approach is to quantify myocardial blood flow (in mL/min/g) and CFR (calculated as the ratio of peak hyperemic myocardial blood flow over that at rest). A number of studies have demonstrated that among relatively young patients with modest coronary risk factor burden and predominantly single-vessel CAD, a relationship exists between myocardial blood flow or CFR and percent diameter stenosis on angiography [31–33]. These studies demonstrate that CFR is relatively preserved for lesions with less than 50 % stenosis. With increasing severity of stenosis beyond this level, however, there is progressive worsening of coronary flow reserve. These observations have served as the basis for the clinical use of quantitative myocardial blood flow to improve identification of obstructive CAD (Fig. 14.3) and especially to exclude the presence of angiographic multivessel CAD (Fig. 14.4) [34–36]. In the largest study to date [36], the presence of a relatively normal global CFR (>2.0) in patients with normal or abnormal myocardial perfusion scans was associated with a very low likelihood of high-risk angiographic CAD (NPV, 97 %).

Regadenoson-stress and rest ^{13}N ammonia PET

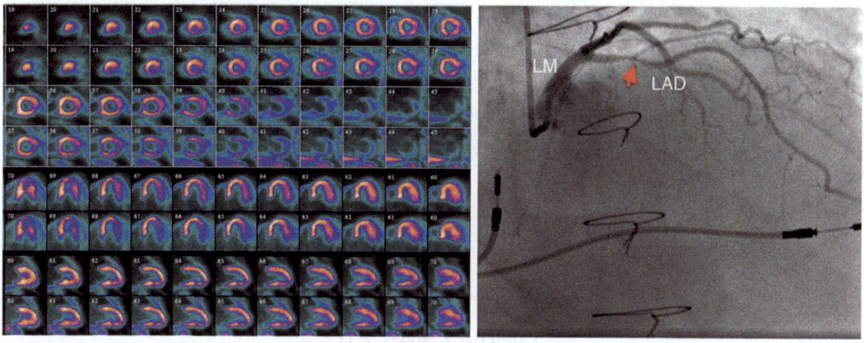

Myocardial blood flow and coronary flow reserve

Region	Stress	Rest	Reserve
LAD	1.67	1.09	1.53
LCX	2.80	0.92	3.04
RCA	2.54	0.96	2.64
TOT	2.06	1.00	2.05

Fig. 14.3 Example of a 58-year-old male patient status post cardiac transplantation 17 years prior to PET presenting with pre-syncope. The stress-rest myocardial perfusion images (*left upper panel*) demonstrated no evidence of flow-limiting stenosis. However, the quantitative coronary flow reserve (*left lower panel*) was abnormal in the left anterior descending (*red arrow in LAD*) coronary territory (1.53; normal value >2.0). Subsequent coronary angiography (*right upper panel*) demonstrated a significant stenosis in the proximal LAD coronary artery

14.3.2.2 Identification of Patients with Symptoms Due to Diffuse Atherosclerosis and Coronary Microvascular Dysfunction

There is increasing recognition that in many patients, the symptom of angina may not necessarily be caused by the presence of a focal coronary stenosis in the epicardial coronary arteries [37, 38]. Indeed, the presence of diffuse atherosclerosis without discrete narrowing of the coronary arteries as well as remodeling and dysfunction of the arteriolar circulation (invisible to coronary angiography) may result in abnormal myocardial perfusion and ischemia [39]. This syndrome of angina without obstructive CAD has been termed "syndrome X" or "microvascular angina" and has been linked to a higher incidence of adverse cardiovascular events [37, 40]. Quantification of myocardial blood flow and coronary flow reserve with PET integrates the hemodynamic effects of diffuse atherosclerosis and microvascular dysfunction on myocardial perfusion, thereby providing a practical, sensitive, and noninvasive method to diagnose whether angina symptoms are related to myocardial ischemia.

A recent study in a relatively large cohort of symptomatic patients without obstructive CAD demonstrated a high frequency (~50 %) of coronary vasomotor dysfunction (Fig. 14.5), reflecting preclinical coronary atherosclerosis, among women and men [40]. The severity of such vascular dysfunction is associated with

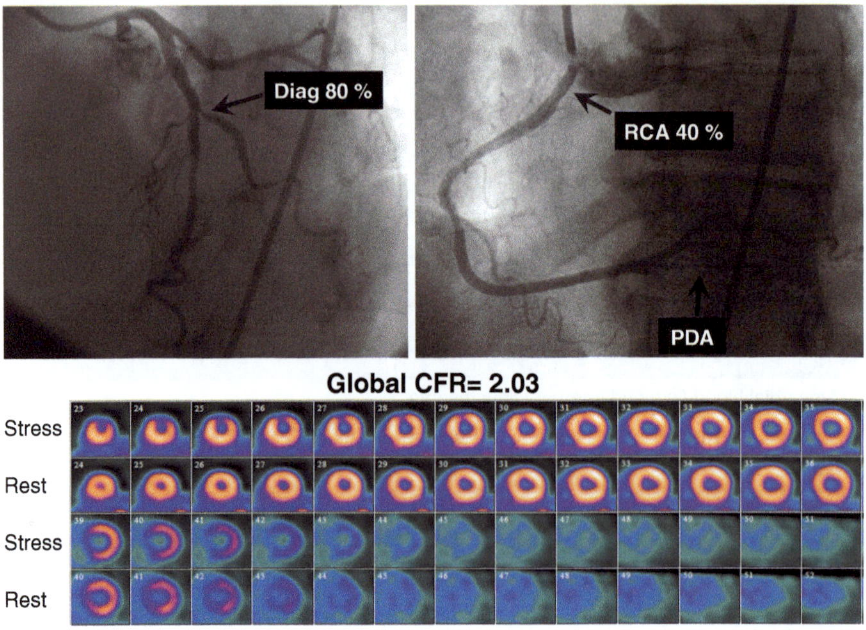

Fig. 14.4 A 66-year-old female patient with a history of high cholesterol and a family history of CAD referred for evaluation of atypical chest pain. The *top panel* presents selected coronary angiographic views of the left (**a**) and right (**b**) coronary arteries. There is severe disease in the first diagonal branch, moderate stenosis in the proximal RCA, and diffuse disease in the PDA. In the *lower panel* (**c**), the short axis stress-rest myocardial perfusion images demonstrate a small but severe perfusion defect involving the mid- and apical anterior wall, with complete reversibility. This patient's quantitative global CFR was 2.03 (Reproduced with permission from Ref. [36])

older age and the burden of coronary risk factors including hypertension, diabetes, and obesity. More importantly, the presence of coronary vasomotor dysfunction increases the risk of adverse events irrespective of gender. The mechanisms underlying the observed coronary vasomotor dysfunction are likely to be multifactorial and related to autonomic dysregulation, as well as the adverse effects of oxidative stress, adenosine, endothelin-1, angiotensin II, and low-level systemic inflammation, among other stimuli on endothelial and smooth muscle cell dysfunction.

14.3.2.3 Risk Stratification

The power of radionuclide myocardial perfusion imaging (including PET) for risk stratification is based on the fact that the major determinants of prognosis in patients with CAD are readily available from gated myocardial perfusion imaging. These include the amount of myocardial scar, the extent and severity of stress-induced ischemia, measurements of LV size (i.e., volumes), and ejection fraction. Optimal risk stratification is based on the concept that the risk associated with a normal study is sufficiently low that revascularization will not further improve patient outcomes. Hence, catheterization is an unlikely option after testing. Conversely, patients with abnormal stress imaging results are at greater risk of adverse events and, thus, are

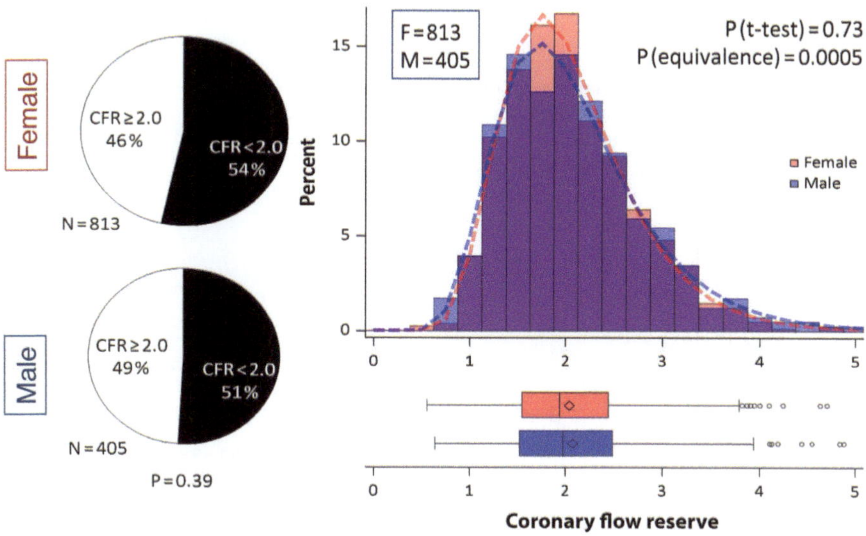

Fig. 14.5 Frequency and severity of microvascular dysfunction in women and men. *Left panel*: Pie charts demonstrating that more than 50 % of women and men showed abnormal coronary flow reserve (i.e., CFR<2.0). *Right panel*: Histogram (*top*) showing the distribution of coronary flow reserve for men (*blue*) and women (*red*). Areas of overlap are shown in *purple*. Fitted lognormal distribution for men (*dashed blue line*) and women (*dashed red line*) are also displayed. Similar data are also shown in box plots (*bottom*). No statistically significant difference was seen between genders using *t*-test with lognormal distribution ($P=0.73$). CFR was equivalent between the genders ($P=0.0005$ for <10 % difference) using two one-sided tests and lognormal distribution (Reproduced with permission from Ref. [40])

potential candidates for intervention, and the magnitude of their risk is related to the extent and severity of the imaging abnormalities.

There is emerging, consistent data that like SPECT MPI, stress myocardial perfusion PET also provides robust risk stratification. A recent review of the published literature suggests an elevated 5.1-fold (95 % CI 2.8–9.3) increase in risk of adverse cardiovascular events for patients with an abnormal as compared to normal stress myocardial perfusion PET scan [41]. These data have now been confirmed in a large multicenter registry that evaluated prognosis in 7,061 patients undergoing pharmacological stress ^{82}Rb PET myocardial perfusion imaging [42]. This registry demonstrated that for the prediction of cardiac death and all-cause death, an abnormal PET scan provided significant incremental prognostic value over pre-imaging data (Fig. 14.6). Patients with a severely abnormal stress PET MPI had almost a fivefold higher hazard of cardiac death compared with patients with a normal PET MPI. Importantly, the PET findings provided significant risk reclassification in 12 % of patients, confirming the clinical utility of PET perfusion imaging. A separate analysis from the same registry demonstrated a proportional relationship between CAD mortality and magnitude of perfusion deficit on stress Rb-82 PET for both men and women [43], as well as obese and nonobese individuals [44]. The confirmation of similar prognostic value regardless of sex is important as PET may offer advantages

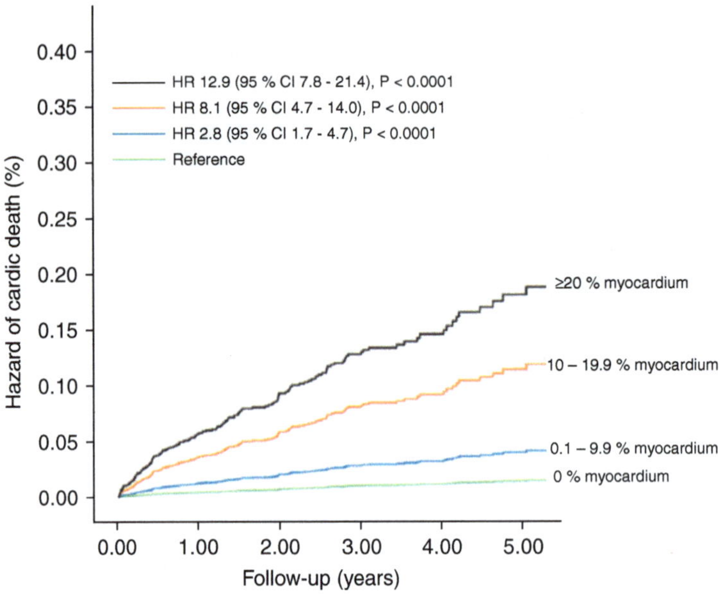

Fig. 14.6 Unadjusted risk of cardiac death by percent myocardium abnormal on vasodilator stress rubidium-82 PET. The risk of cardiac death (6,037 patients, 169 cardiac deaths) was lowest in patients with normal positron-emission tomography (*PET*) myocardial perfusion imaging (*MPI*) and increased gradually in patients with minimal, mild, moderate, and severe degrees of scan abnormality (Reproduced with permission from Ref. [42])

in the evaluation of women due to improved image quality and sensitivity for detection of obstructive CAD as well as improved safety profile with significantly lower radiation doses than other nuclear medicine techniques.

Incremental Value of Coronary Flow Reserve

In addition to the diagnostic utility of quantitative measures of myocardial blood flow discussed above, coronary flow reserve is also emerging as a powerful quantitative prognostic imaging marker of clinical cardiovascular risk. As discussed above, CFR provides a robust and reproducible clinical measure of the integrated hemodynamic effects of epicardial CAD, diffuse atherosclerosis, vessel remodeling, and microvascular dysfunction on myocardial tissue perfusion. Consequently, it is a more sensitive measure of myocardial ischemia and overall vascular health that provides unique information about clinical risk. The available data thus far suggests that CFR measurements by PET can distinguish patients at high risk for serious adverse events, including cardiac death [45–48]. Indeed, a severely reduced CFR (<1.5) was associated with a sixfold increased risk of cardiac death, even after adjusting for differences in clinical risk, the extent and severity of ischemia and scar, and LVEF, and led to a clinically meaningful risk reclassification of ~50 % of intermediate-risk patients [45]. Importantly, an abnormal CFR identified increased risk of cardiac death even among those normal scans by semiquantitative visual

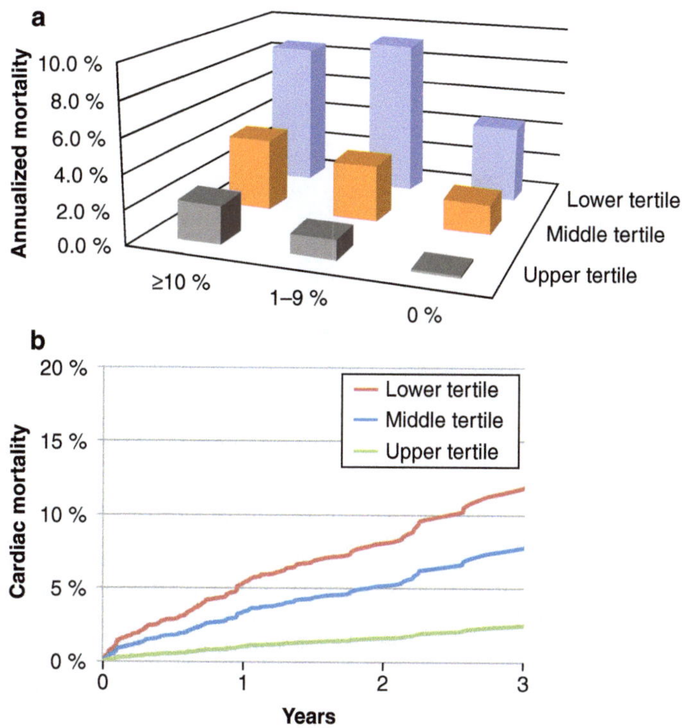

Fig. 14.7 *Panel A*: Unadjusted annualized cardiac mortality by percent myocardium ischemic and CFR tertiles showing that for each category of ischemia, CFR is able to separate populations at relatively higher and lower risks. *Panel B*: Incidence of cardiac mortality for tertiles of coronary flow reserve after adjustment for age, sex, BMI, hypertension, dyslipidemia, diabetes mellitus, family history of CAD, tobacco use, prior CAD, chest pain, dyspnea, early revascularization, rest LVEF, summed stress score, and LVEF reserve showing a significant association between CFR and cardiac mortality (Reproduced with permission from Ref. [45])

analysis (Fig. 14.7). These findings are also applicable to high-risk cohorts, including diabetes and chronic renal impairment [49, 50]. For example, a reduced global CFR is independently associated with higher rates of cardiac and all-cause mortality in a large cohort of patients with and without diabetes mellitus. Compared to diabetics with preserved CFR, those with reduced CFR experienced substantially higher cardiac mortality (Fig. 14.8) [49]. Importantly, diabetic patients without known CAD and with impaired CFR experienced a rate of cardiac death comparable to, and possibly higher than, that of nondiabetic patients with known CAD. These observations have implications for the classification of diabetes mellitus as a coronary disease risk equivalent [51]. Specifically, only among diabetics with impaired vascular function is prognosis comparable to nondiabetic patients with known CAD. Thus, differing levels of vascular health among previously studied cohorts may account for inconsistencies in relative mortality rates of diabetics without CAD and nondiabetics with CAD [52–54].

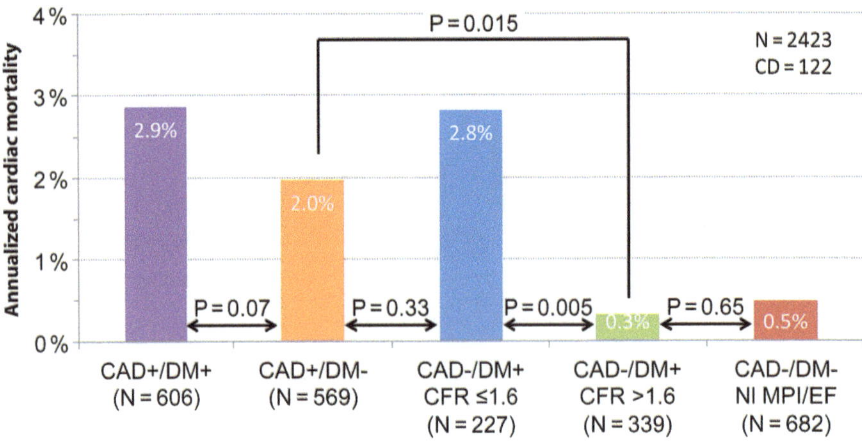

Fig. 14.8 Annualized cardiac mortality among patients with diabetes and/or CAD. Adjusted cardiac mortality among patients with coronary artery disease (CAD; i.e., history of coronary revascularization or myocardial infarction) without diabetes (*orange*), diabetic patients without CAD who have impaired CFR (*red*), diabetic patients without CAD who have preserved CFR (*blue*), and patients without diabetes or CAD with normal scans (no scar, ischemia or left ventricular dysfunction, *green*) presented as survival *curves* (*panel A*) and annualized cardiac mortality rates (*panel B*). Data for patients with CAD and diabetes are also presented for comparison (*purple*). The data demonstrates that in diabetics without overt CAD, a reduced CFR identifies a high-risk subgroup with comparable (and possibly higher) mortality than patients without diabetes with overt CAD. By contrast, a relatively preserved CFR in diabetics identifies low-risk patients with annual risk of cardiac death similar to those without diabetes or CAD (Reproduced with permission from Ref. [50])

Integrating CAC and CT Coronary Angiography and Myocardial Perfusion Imaging

As all modern PET scanners are combined with CT, we are beginning to understand the potential complementary roles between structure and function for diagnosis and management of CAD. There is growing evidence that coronary artery calcium scores are generally predictive of a higher likelihood of ischemia (reflecting obstructive CAD) on myocardial perfusion imaging [26, 55–57]. However, the relationship between the extent and severity of coronary calcification and measures of myocardial ischemia reflecting obstructive CAD is quite modest [23, 58]. Importantly, CAC scores <400, especially in symptomatic patients with intermediate likelihood of CAD, have limited sensitivity and negative predictive value to exclude CAD especially in young subjects and women [57, 59, 60].

The integration of CAC scores and ischemia information also offers a unique opportunity to refine the prognostic value of myocardial perfusion PET imaging. The CAC score, reflecting the anatomic extent of atherosclerosis [61], may offer an opportunity to improve the conventional models for risk assessment using nuclear imaging alone (especially in patients with normal perfusion), a finding that may serve as a more rational basis for personalizing the intensity and goals of medical therapy in a

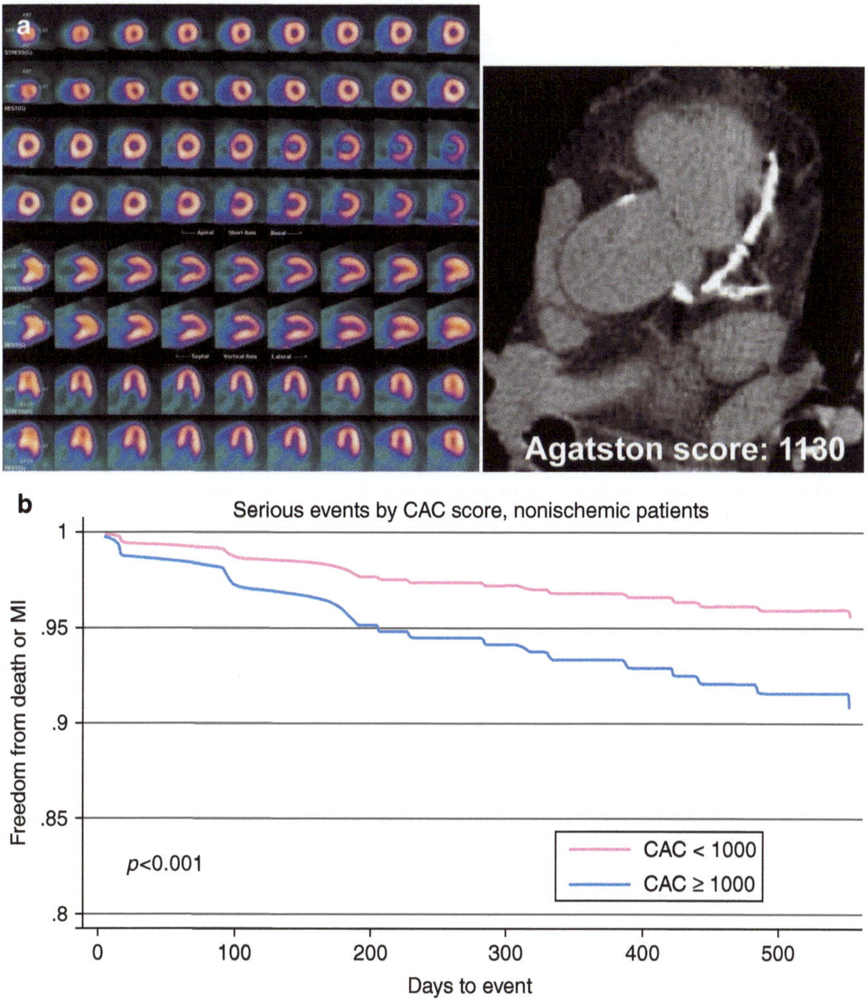

Fig. 14.9 *Panel A*: Example of a 68-year-old male with atypical angina. The stress-rest myocardial perfusion PET scan (*left*) is normal indicating no evidence of flow-limiting CAD. However, the gated non-contrast CT scan (*right*) demonstrates extensive coronary artery calcifications with a calculated Agatston score >1,000. *Panel B*: Adjusted survival in patients without ischemia by PET MPI is lower among patients with extensive coronary artery calcifications. This demonstrates the complementary value of myocardial perfusion imaging and calcium scoring for risk diagnosis and risk stratification (Adapted with permission from Ref. [57])

more cost-effective manner. For example, recent data suggest that quantification of CAC scores at the time of stress nuclear imaging using a dual-modality approach can enhance risk predictions in patients with suspected CAD [57]. Indeed, the presence of extensive coronary artery calcification identifies a higher risk cohort, which is independent of the magnitude of perfusion abnormality. This association is especially useful clinically in patients without evidence of ischemia on PET MPI (Fig. 14.9) [57].

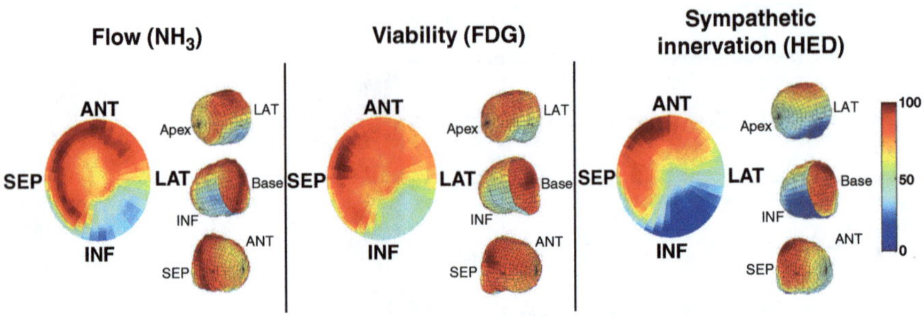

Fig. 14.10 Bull's-eye maps of myocardial perfusion (*left panel*), FDG viability (*middle panel*), and sympathetic innervation (*right panel*) in a patient that experienced sudden cardiac arrest (*SCA*). There is a large matched perfusion-metabolic defect involving the inferior and inferolateral walls, consistent with prior myocardial infarction. The HED images demonstrate a larger myocardial volume of sympathetic denervation (reduced HED uptake) compared to the scarred area. This mismatch between infarct size (reduced FDG) and the volume of sympathetic denervation (larger HED defect) has been identified as an imaging marker for ventricular arrhythmias. *ANT* anterior, *INF* inferior, *LAT* lateral, *SEP* septum (Courtesy of Dr. James A. Fallavollita, University of Buffalo, New York)

With the addition of intravenous contrast, CT coronary angiography further expands the role of hybrid PET/CT for diagnosis and management of CAD. There is evidence that hybrid imaging may offer superior diagnostic information with regard to identification of the culprit vessel [62–65]. Coronary CTA enhances the sensitivity for detecting multivessel CAD, while myocardial perfusion imaging improves the specificity and positive predictive value for delineation of flow-limiting coronary artery stenosis. The addition of coronary CTA is also quite helpful to help exclude severe coronary artery obstruction among patients with severely reduced coronary flow reserve [66].

Neuronal Imaging to Identify Patients at Risk for Sudden Cardiac Death

There is experimental and clinical evidence supporting the concept that sympathetic activation plays an important role as a potential trigger of ventricular arrhythmias after myocardial infarction. Indeed, myocardial infarction and ischemia can lead to sympathetic denervation in both the infarct and peri-infarct zones (Fig. 14.10). Viable but denervated myocardial regions show supersensitive shortening of effective refractory period in response to the infusion of norepinephrine and are more vulnerable to ventricular arrhythmias. This suggests that direct imaging of cardiac sympathetic innervation may have an important clinical role in risk stratification of patients after myocardial infarction.

The PAREPET (Prediction of ARrhythmic Events with Positron Emission Tomography) study was designed to test the hypothesis that the extent of inhomogeneity in myocardial sympathetic innervation and/or hibernating myocardium increased the risk of arrhythmic death independently of LV function in patients with ischemic cardiomyopathy (LVEF $\leq$35 %) [2]. The study included 204 patients who were eligible for primary prevention implantable cardiac defibrillators (ICDs). PET imaging was used to quantify myocardial sympathetic denervation (with ^{11}C-HED), perfusion, and metabolism. The primary end point was sudden cardiac arrest defined as arrhythmic death or ICD discharge for ventricular fibrillation or ventricular tachycardia >240 beats/min. Compared to patients in the lowest tertile of cardiac sympathetic denervation assessed by HED PET, those in the highest tertile showed a greater than sixfold increase in the risk of sudden cardiac arrest. In multivariable analysis, the extent of PET-defined sympathetic denervation, left ventricular end-diastolic volume index, and creatinine were significantly associated with the risk of sudden cardiac arrest.

14.3.2.4 Directing Therapy

Ischemia Burden to Guide Revascularization

The justification of stress imaging testing has hinged upon the ability of noninvasive estimates of myocardial ischemia to identify patients that may benefit from revascularization – that is, differentiating high-risk patients with extensive scar versus those with extensive ischemia. The advantages of this approach are clear – avoidance of unnecessary catheterizations that expose patients to risk and the potential for associated cost savings [67]. Evidence from large observational registries supports the notion of a significant association between the extent and severity of inducible myocardial ischemia by stress SPECT imaging and post-imaging treatment, such that in the setting of no or mild ischemia, patients undergoing medical therapy as their initial treatment had superior survival to those patients referred to revascularization. Conversely, in the setting of moderate to severe ischemia (>10 % of the total myocardium ischemic), patients undergoing revascularization had an increasing survival benefit over patients undergoing medical therapy. Patients with the highest clinical risk (e.g., diabetics) were found to have the greatest absolute benefit with revascularization over medical therapy in the setting of significant ischemia. There is preliminary evidence that a similar interaction between moderate–severe ischemia and revascularization may apply to patients undergoing stress PET imaging.

Myocardial Viability Imaging to Guide Revascularization in Patients with Ischemic Heart Failure

Metabolic imaging with PET has an established role in the evaluation of myocardial viability. Although several approaches have been documented [68–70], the use of ^{18}F-fluorodeoxyglucose (FDG) to assess regional myocardial glucose utilization (an index of tissue viability) is the most commonly used in clinical practice [71]. With this approach, specific abnormalities in myocardial metabolism reflecting viable and scarred myocardium have been described (Fig. 14.11). Contractile dysfunction is predicted to be reversible after revascularization in regions with increased FDG uptake or a *perfusion-FDG mismatch* and irreversible in those with reduced FDG uptake or a *perfusion-FDG match* pattern. Using these criteria, the average PPV for predicting improved segmental function after revascularization is 76 (range, 52–100 %), whereas the average NPV is 82 % (range, 67–100 %) [71].

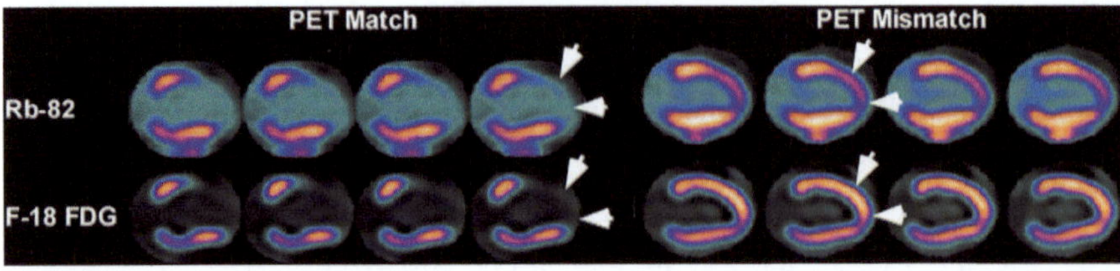

Fig. 14.11 PET patterns of myocardial viability. The *left panel* demonstrates concordant reductions in myocardial perfusion (rubidium-82) and glucose metabolism (FDG), reflecting myocardial infarction. The *right panel* demonstrates preserved glucose metabolism (FDG) in a territory with decreased myocardial perfusion (rubidium-82), reflecting complete tissue viability (Reproduced with permission from Ref. [90])

Several studies using different PET approaches have shown that the gain in global LVEF after revascularization is related to the magnitude of viable myocardium assessed preoperatively [72]. These data demonstrate that clinically meaningful changes in global LV function can be expected after revascularization only in patients with relatively large areas of hibernating and/or stunned myocardium (~20 % of the left ventricular mass). Similar to other noninvasive imaging modalities [73–75], the extent of nonviable or scarred myocardium by FDG PET correlates inversely with changes in LVEF after revascularization [76].

More importantly, there is consistent data from single-center, observational studies demonstrating that the presence of ischemic, viable myocardium among patients with severe LV dysfunction identifies patients at higher clinical risk and that prompt revascularization in selected patients is associated with improved LV function [77], symptoms [78], and survival [79, 80] as compared to medical therapy alone (Fig. 14.12). The randomized PARR-2 clinical trial demonstrated that image-guided decisions regarding revascularization could also help improve clinical outcomes following revascularization if treatment decisions adhere to imaging recommendations [81].

Nonetheless, the main criticism of those studies is that they were retrospective and medical therapy did not reflect current accepted management of heart failure nor was it standardized in any way. The results of the STICH trial [82], especially its ancillary viability [83] and ischemia [84] substudies, have challenged all prior data as they failed to demonstrate a significant interaction between ischemia or viability information, revascularization, and improved survival compared to optimal medical therapy. This casts significant uncertainty as to whether noninvasive characterization of ischemia, viability, and scar can actually provide useful information to guide management decisions. This issue is currently undergoing intense debate in the medical community [85, 86]. As we begin to incorporate the results of the STICH trial into our practice, it is important to consider the strengths and weaknesses of the STICH substudies.

The STICH viability and ischemia substudies are the largest reports to date relating myocardial viability and ischemia to clinical outcomes of patients with CAD and LV dysfunction associated with heart failure. They are also the firsts to assess these relationships prospectively among patients who were all eligible for

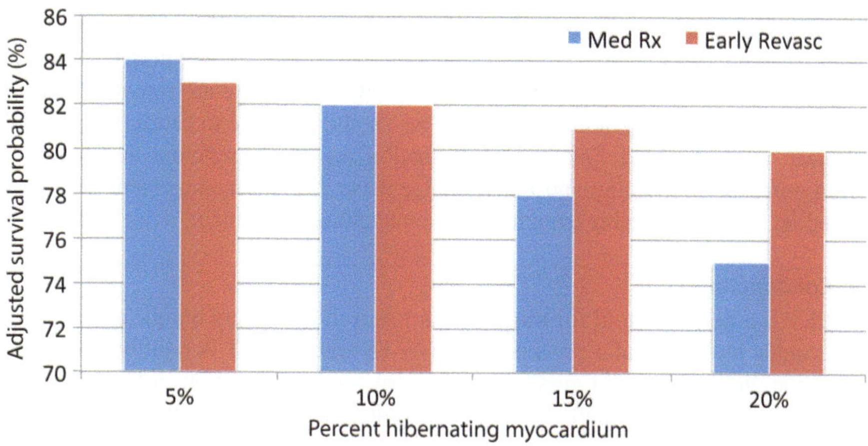

Fig. 14.12 Relationship between percent hibernating myocardium (as defined by a perfusion-FDG mismatch) and adjusted hazard ratio for patients treated with early revascularization (*red bars*) versus medical therapy (*blue bars*). Risk increases as a function of percent hibernating myocardium in medically treated patients. In patients referred to early revascularization, risk seems to be relatively unchanged across the range of values (Data for this graph obtained from Ref. [81])

CABG as well as optimal medical management alone. As mentioned above, medical therapy in the STICH trial was standardized and followed current published guidelines. However, these studies also have important limitations. First, viability data was only available in half and ischemia information in only a third of the STICH population, which is likely to introduce some selection bias. In fact, patients in the STICH viability study had higher prevalence of prior MI, lower frequency of limiting angina symptoms, lower LVEF, and more advanced LV remodeling as compared to those who did not receive viability imaging before randomization. Second, the definition of viability in STICH substudy was quite broad resulting in 81 % of the total study population being considered as having "viability" by study criteria. This number is quite higher from that seen in other studies such as the CHRISTMAS trial (59 %) [87], which used similar imaging modalities as the STICH trial and suggests that the definition may not have been sufficiently specific to identify patients with ischemia but viable from those with primarily nontransmural scar. Third, neither PET nor MRI was used to evaluate ischemia or viability. An important additional consideration to understand the generalizability of the STICH substudies is that patients in the main trial in general and those in the viability and ischemia studies in particular had end-stage LV remodeling. Indeed, the mean LV end-diastolic volume index (to body surface area) was greater than 120 mL/m2, and LV end-systolic volume index approached 100 mL/m2 [83]. This degree of advanced LV remodeling has generally been associated with poor outcomes regardless of the presence of ischemia or viability and treatment applied [88, 89]. In summary, the STICH trial and its imaging substudies suggest that among patients with *heart failure* and *end-stage LV remodeling*, identification of moderate ischemia or viability is not associated with a significant survival advantage from revascularization. While the benefits of optimal medical therapy in patients with ischemic cardiomyopathy are undeniable, we cannot and should not generalize the STICH findings to patients with heart failure, severe systolic dysfunction, but mild-to-moderate LV remodeling, as these patients were not studied in the STICH trial. As data from randomized clinical trials in such patients are limited, we should continue to carefully integrate clinical, anatomic, and functional information regarding ischemia and viability from noninvasive imaging and individualize these difficult management decisions based on the best available evidence and sound clinical judgment.

Conclusions

PET is a powerful tool for translational research that offers unique quantitative insights into molecular processes in vivo. Hybrid PET/CT is rapidly advancing our ability to image in great detail the structure and function in the heart and vasculature. By providing concurrent quantitative information about myocardial blood flow and metabolism with coronary and cardiac anatomy, PET/CT offers the opportunity for a comprehensive noninvasive evaluation of the consequences of atherosclerosis in the coronary arteries and the myocardium. This integrated platform for assessing anatomy and biology expands the potential for translating molecularly targeted imaging into humans. The goals of future investigation will be to refine these technologies, establish standard protocols for image acquisition and interpretation, address the issue of cost-effectiveness, and validate a range of clinical applications in large-scale clinical trials.

References

1. Detrano R, Guerci AD, Carr JJ, Bild DE, Burke G, Folsom AR, Liu K, Shea S, Szklo M, Bluemke DA, O'Leary DH, Tracy R, Watson K, Wong ND, Kronmal RA. Coronary calcium as a predictor of coronary events in four racial or ethnic groups. N Engl J Med. 2008;358: 1336–45.
2. Fallavollita JA, Heavey BM, Luisi Jr AJ, Michalek SM, Baldwa S, Mashtare Jr TL, Hutson AD, Dekemp RA, Haka MS, Sajjad M, Cimato TR, Curtis AB, Cain ME, Canty Jr JM. Regional myocardial sympathetic denervation predicts the risk of sudden cardiac arrest in ischemic cardiomyopathy. J Am Coll Cardiol. 2014;63:141–9.
3. Jacobson AF, Senior R, Cerqueira MD, Wong ND, Thomas GS, Lopez VA, Agostini D, Weiland F, Chandna H, Narula J, Investigators A-H. Myocardial iodine-123 meta-iodobenzylguanidine imaging and cardiac events in heart failure. Results of the prospective ADMIRE-HF (AdreView Myocardial Imaging for Risk Evaluation in Heart Failure) study. J Am Coll Cardiol. 2010;55:2212–21.
4. Sasano T, Abraham MR, Chang KC, Ashikaga H, Mills KJ, Holt DP, Hilton J, Nekolla SG, Dong J, Lardo AC, Halperin H, Dannals RF, Marban E, Bengel FM. Abnormal sympathetic innervation of viable myocardium and the substrate of ventricular tachycardia after myocardial infarction. J Am Coll Cardiol. 2008;51:2266–75.
5. Nasir K, Rubin J, Blaha MJ, Shaw LJ, Blankstein R, Rivera JJ, Khan AN, Berman D, Raggi P, Callister T, Rumberger JA, Min J, Jones SR, Blumenthal RS, Budoff MJ. Interplay of coronary artery calcification and traditional risk factors for the prediction of all-cause mortality in asymptomatic individuals. Circ Cardiovasc Imaging. 2012;5:467–73.
6. Campisi R, Di Carli MF. Assessment of coronary flow reserve and microcirculation: a clinical perspective. J Nucl Cardiol. 2004;11:3–11.

7. Camici PG, Crea F. Coronary microvascular dysfunction. N Engl J Med. 2007;356:830–40.
8. Kuhle WG, Porenta G, Huang SC, Buxton D, Gambhir SS, Hansen H, Phelps ME, Schelbert HR. Quantification of regional myocardial blood flow using 13N-ammonia and reoriented dynamic positron emission tomographic imaging. Circulation. 1992;86:1004–17.
9. Nitzsche EU, Choi Y, Czernin J, Hoh CK, Huang SC, Schelbert HR. Noninvasive quantification of myocardial blood flow in humans. A direct comparison of the [13N]ammonia and the [15O]water techniques. Circulation. 1996;93:2000–6.
10. Hutchins GD, Schwaiger M, Rosenspire KC, Krivokapich J, Schelbert H, Kuhl DE. Noninvasive quantification of regional blood flow in the human heart using N-13 ammonia and dynamic positron emission tomographic imaging. J Am Coll Cardiol. 1990;15:1032–42.
11. El Fakhri G, Kardan A, Sitek A, Dorbala S, Abi-Hatem N, Lahoud Y, Fischman A, Coughlan M, Yasuda T, Di Carli MF. Reproducibility and accuracy of quantitative myocardial blood flow assessment with (82)Rb PET: comparison with (13)N-ammonia PET. J Nucl Med. 2009;50:1062–71.
12. El Fakhri G, Sitek A, Guerin B, Kijewski MF, Di Carli MF, Moore SC. Quantitative dynamic cardiac 82Rb PET using generalized factor and compartment analyses. J Nucl Med. 2005;46:1264–71.
13. Alexanderson E, Garcia-Rojas L, Jimenez M, Jacome R, Calleja R, Martinez A, Ochoa JM, Meave A, Alexanderson G. Effect of ezetimibe-simvastatin over endothelial dysfunction in dyslipidemic patients: assessment by 13N-ammonia positron emission tomography. J Nucl Cardiol. 2010;17:1015–22.
14. Baller D, Notohamiprodjo G, Gleichmann U, Holzinger J, Weise R, Lehmann J. Improvement in coronary flow reserve determined by positron emission tomography after 6 months of cholesterol-lowering therapy in patients with early stages of coronary atherosclerosis. Circulation. 1999;99:2871–5.
15. Guethlin M, Kasel AM, Coppenrath K, Ziegler S, Delius W, Schwaiger M. Delayed response of myocardial flow reserve to lipid-lowering therapy with fluvastatin. Circulation. 1999;99:475–81.
16. Ilveskoski E, Lehtimaki T, Laaksonen R, Janatuinen T, Vesalainen R, Nuutila P, Laippala P, Karhunen PJ, Knuuti J. Improvement of myocardial blood flow by lipid-lowering therapy with pravastatin is modulated by apolipoprotein E genotype. Scand J Clin Lab Invest. 2007;67:723–34.
17. Lehtimaki T, Laaksonen R, Janatuinen T, Vesalainen R, Nuutila P, Mattila K, Ilveskoski E, Luomala M, Saikku P, Knuuti J, Hurme M. Interleukin-1B genotype modulates the improvement of coronary artery reactivity by lipid-lowering therapy with pravastatin: a placebo-controlled positron emission tomography study in young healthy men. Pharmacogenetics. 2003;13:633–9.
18. Ling MC, Ruddy TD, deKemp RA, Ukkonen H, Duchesne L, Higginson L, Williams KA, McPherson R, Beanlands R. Early effects of statin therapy on endothelial function and microvascular reactivity in patients with coronary artery disease. Am Heart J. 2005;149:1137.
19. McMahon GT, Plutzky J, Daher E, Bhattacharyya T, Grunberger G, DiCarli MF. Effect of a peroxisome proliferator-activated receptor-gamma agonist on myocardial blood flow in type 2 diabetes. Diabetes Care. 2005;28:1145–50.
20. Schelbert HR, Hassan A, Garner J, Di Carli M. Effects of ACAT inhibition by positron emission tomography measured myocardial blood flow: a double-blind, randomized, multicenter trial. J Am Coll Cardiol (Abstract). 2003;41:460A.
21. Sdringola S, Gould KL, Zamarka LG, McLain R, Garner J. A 6 month randomized, double blind, placebo controlled, multi-center trial of high dose atorvastatin on myocardial perfusion abnormalities by positron emission tomography in coronary artery disease. Am Heart J. 2008;155:245–53.
22. Rumberger JA, Sheedy 3rd PF, Breen JF, Schwartz RS. Coronary calcium, as determined by electron beam computed tomography, and coronary disease on arteriogram. Effect of patient's sex on diagnosis. Circulation. 1995;91:1363–7.

23. Naya M, Murthy VL, Blankstein R, Sitek A, Hainer J, Foster C, Gaber M, Fantony JM, Dorbala S, Di Carli MF. Quantitative relationship between the extent and morphology of coronary atherosclerotic plaque and downstream myocardial perfusion. J Am Coll Cardiol. 2011;58:1807–16.
24. Naya M, Murthy VL, Foster CR, Gaber M, Klein J, Hainer J, Dorbala S, Blankstein R, Di Carli MF. Prognostic interplay of coronary artery calcification and underlying vascular dysfunction in patients with suspected coronary artery disease. J Am Coll Cardiol. 2013;61: 2098–106.
25. Hamirani YS, Pandey S, Rivera JJ, Ndumele C, Budoff MJ, Blumenthal RS, Nasir K. Markers of inflammation and coronary artery calcification: a systematic review. Atherosclerosis. 2008;201:1–7.
26. Schepis T, Gaemperli O, Koepfli P, Namdar M, Valenta I, Scheffel H, Leschka S, Husmann L, Eberli FR, Luscher TF, Alkadhi H, Kaufmann PA. Added value of coronary artery calcium score as an adjunct to gated SPECT for the evaluation of coronary artery disease in an intermediate-risk population. J Nucl Med. 2007;48:1424–30.
27. Parker MW, Iskandar A, Limone B, Perugini A, Kim H, Jones C, Calamari B, Coleman CI, Heller GV. Diagnostic accuracy of cardiac positron emission tomography versus single photon emission computed tomography for coronary artery disease: a bivariate meta-analysis. Circ Cardiovasc Imaging. 2012;5:700–7.
28. Mc Ardle BA, Dowsley TF, DeKemp RA, Wells GA, Beanlands RS. Does rubidium-82 PET have superior accuracy to SPECT perfusion imaging for the diagnosis of obstructive coronary disease?: a systematic review and meta-analysis. J Am Coll Cardiol. 2012;60:1828–37.
29. Berman DS, Kang X, Slomka PJ, Gerlach J, de Yang L, Hayes SW, Friedman JD, Thomson LE, Germano G. Underestimation of extent of ischemia by gated SPECT myocardial perfusion imaging in patients with left main coronary artery disease. J Nucl Cardiol. 2007;14:521–8.
30. Dorbala S, Vangala D, Sampson U, Limaye A, Kwong R, Di Carli MF. Value of vasodilator left ventricular ejection fraction reserve in evaluating the magnitude of myocardium at risk and the extent of angiographic coronary artery disease: a 82Rb PET/CT study. J Nucl Med. 2007;48: 349–58.
31. Beanlands RS, Muzik O, Melon P, Sutor R, Sawada S, Muller D, Bondie D, Hutchins GD, Schwaiger M. Noninvasive quantification of regional myocardial flow reserve in patients with coronary atherosclerosis using nitrogen-13 ammonia positron emission tomography. Determination of extent of altered vascular reactivity. J Am Coll Cardiol. 1995;26:1465–75.
32. Di Carli M, Czernin J, Hoh CK, Gerbaudo VH, Brunken RC, Huang SC, Phelps ME, Schelbert HR. Relation among stenosis severity, myocardial blood flow, and flow reserve in patients with coronary artery disease. Circulation. 1995;91:1944–51.
33. Uren NG, Melin JA, De Bruyne B, Wijns W, Baudhuin T, Camici PG. Relation between myocardial blood flow and the severity of coronary-artery stenosis. N Engl J Med. 1994;330: 1782–8.
34. Fiechter M, Ghadri JR, Gebhard C, Fuchs TA, Pazhenkottil AP, Nkoulou RN, Herzog BA, Wyss CA, Gaemperli O, Kaufmann PA. Diagnostic value of 13N-ammonia myocardial perfusion PET: added value of myocardial flow reserve. J Nucl Med. 2012;53:1230–4.
35. Ziadi MC, Dekemp RA, Williams K, Guo A, Renaud JM, Chow BJ, Klein R, Ruddy TD, Aung M, Garrard L, Beanlands RS. Does quantification of myocardial flow reserve using rubidium-82 positron emission tomography facilitate detection of multivessel coronary artery disease? J Nucl Cardiol. 2012;19:670–80.
36. Naya M, Murthy VL, Taqueti VR, Foster CR, Klein J, Garber M, Dorbala S, Hainer J, Blankstein R, Resnic F, Di Carli MF. Preserved coronary flow reserve effectively excludes high-risk coronary artery disease on angiography. J Nucl Med. 2014;55:248–55.
37. Pepine CJ, Anderson RD, Sharaf BL, Reis SE, Smith KM, Handberg EM, Johnson BD, Sopko G, Bairey Merz CN. Coronary microvascular reactivity to adenosine predicts adverse outcome in women evaluated for suspected ischemia results from the National Heart, Lung and Blood Institute WISE (Women's Ischemia Syndrome Evaluation) study. J Am Coll Cardiol. 2010;55:2825–32.

38. Reis SE, Holubkov R, Conrad Smith AJ, Kelsey SF, Sharaf BL, Reichek N, Rogers WJ, Merz CN, Sopko G, Pepine CJ, Investigators W. Coronary microvascular dysfunction is highly prevalent in women with chest pain in the absence of coronary artery disease: results from the NHLBI WISE study. Am Heart J. 2001;141:735–41.
39. Gould KL, Nakagawa Y, Nakagawa K, Sdringola S, Hess MJ, Haynie M, Parker N, Mullani N, Kirkeeide R. Frequency and clinical implications of fluid dynamically significant diffuse coronary artery disease manifest as graded, longitudinal, base-to-apex myocardial perfusion abnormalities by noninvasive positron emission tomography. Circulation. 2000;101:1931–9.
40. Murthy VL, Naya M, Taqueti VR, Foster CR, Gaber M, Hainer J, Dorbala S, Blankstein R, Rimoldi O, Camici PG and Di Carli MF. Effects of gender on coronary microvascular dysfunction and cardiac outcomes. Circulation. 2014.
41. Shaw LJ, Hage FG, Berman DS, Hachamovitch R, Iskandrian A. Prognosis in the era of comparative effectiveness research: where is nuclear cardiology now and where should it be? J Nucl Cardiol. 2012;19:1026–43.
42. Dorbala S, Di Carli MF, Beanlands RS, Merhige ME, Williams BA, Veledar E, Chow BJ, Min JK, Pencina MJ, Berman DS, Shaw LJ. Prognostic value of stress myocardial perfusion positron emission tomography: results from a multicenter observational registry. J Am Coll Cardiol. 2013;61:176–84.
43. Kay J, Dorbala S, Goyal A, Fazel R, Di Carli MF, Einstein AJ, Beanlands RS, Merhige ME, Williams BA, Veledar E, Chow BJ, Min JK, Berman DS, Shah S, Bellam N, Butler J, Shaw LJ. Influence of sex on risk stratification with stress myocardial perfusion Rb-82 positron emission tomography: results from the PET (Positron Emission Tomography) Prognosis Multicenter Registry. J Am Coll Cardiol. 2013;62:1866–76.
44. Chow BJ, Dorbala S, Di Carli MF, Merhige ME, Williams BA, Veledar E, Min JK, Pencina MJ, Yam Y, Chen L, Anand SP, Ruddy TD, Berman DS, Shaw LJ, Beanlands RS. Prognostic value of PET myocardial perfusion imaging in obese patients. JACC Cardiovasc Imaging. 2014;7:278–87.
45. Murthy VL, Naya M, Foster CR, Hainer J, Gaber M, Di Carli G, Blankstein R, Dorbala S, Sitek A, Pencina MJ, Di Carli MF. Improved cardiac risk assessment with noninvasive measures of coronary flow reserve. Circulation. 2011;124:2215–24.
46. Ziadi MC, Dekemp RA, Williams KA, Guo A, Chow BJ, Renaud JM, Ruddy TD, Sarveswaran N, Tee RE, Beanlands RS. Impaired myocardial flow reserve on rubidium-82 positron emission tomography imaging predicts adverse outcomes in patients assessed for myocardial ischemia. J Am Coll Cardiol. 2011;58:740–8.
47. Fukushima K, Javadi MS, Higuchi T, Lautamaki R, Merrill J, Nekolla SG, Bengel FM. Prediction of short-term cardiovascular events using quantification of global myocardial flow reserve in patients referred for clinical 82Rb PET perfusion imaging. J Nucl Med. 2011;52:726–32.
48. Herzog BA, Husmann L, Valenta I, Gaemperli O, Siegrist PT, Tay FM, Burkhard N, Wyss CA, Kaufmann PA. Long-term prognostic value of 13N-ammonia myocardial perfusion positron emission tomography added value of coronary flow reserve. J Am Coll Cardiol. 2009;54:150–6.
49. Murthy VL, Naya M, Foster CR, Gaber M, Hainer J, Klein J, Dorbala S, Blankstein R, Di Carli MF. Association between coronary vascular dysfunction and cardiac mortality in patients with and without diabetes mellitus. Circulation. 2012;126:1858–68.
50. Murthy VL, Naya M, Foster CR, Hainer J, Gaber M, Dorbala S, Charytan DM, Blankstein R, Di Carli MF. Coronary vascular dysfunction and prognosis in patients with chronic kidney disease. JACC Cardiovasc Imaging. 2012;5:1025–34.
51. Executive summary of the third report of the National Cholesterol Education Program (NCEP) expert panel on detection, evaluation, and treatment of high blood cholesterol in adults (adult treatment panel III). J Am Med Assoc. 2001;285:2486–97.
52. Bulugahapitiya U, Siyambalapitiya S, Sithole J, Idris I. Is diabetes a coronary risk equivalent? Systematic review and meta-analysis. Diabet Med. 2009;26:142–8.

53. Schramm TK, Gislason GH, Kober L, Rasmussen S, Rasmussen JN, Abildstrom SZ, Hansen ML, Folke F, Buch P, Madsen M, Vaag A, Torp-Pedersen C. Diabetes patients requiring glucose-lowering therapy and nondiabetics with a prior myocardial infarction carry the same cardiovascular risk: a population study of 3.3 million people. Circulation. 2008;117:1945–54.
54. Wannamethee SG, Shaper AG, Whincup PH, Lennon L, Sattar N. Impact of diabetes on cardiovascular disease risk and all-cause mortality in older men: influence of age at onset, diabetes duration, and established and novel risk factors. Arch Intern Med. 2011;171:404–10.
55. He ZX, Hedrick TD, Pratt CM, Verani MS, Aquino V, Roberts R, Mahmarian JJ. Severity of coronary artery calcification by electron beam computed tomography predicts silent myocardial ischemia. Circulation. 2000;101:244–51.
56. Berman DS, Wong ND, Gransar H, Miranda-Peats R, Dahlbeck J, Arad Y, Hayes SW, Friedman JD, Kang X, Polk D, Hachamovitch R, Rozanski A. Relationship between stress-induced myocardial ischemia and atherosclerosis measured by coronary calcium tomography. J Am Coll Cardiol. 2004;44:923–30.
57. Schenker MP, Dorbala S, Hong EC, Rybicki FJ, Hachamovitch R, Kwong RY, Di Carli MF. Interrelation of coronary calcification, myocardial ischemia, and outcomes in patients with intermediate likelihood of coronary artery disease: a combined positron emission tomography/computed tomography study. Circulation. 2008;117:1693–700.
58. Curillova Z, Yaman BF, Dorbala S, Kwong RY, Sitek A, El Fakhri G, Anagnostopoulos C, Di Carli MF. Quantitative relationship between coronary calcium content and coronary flow reserve as assessed by integrated PET/CT imaging. Eur J Nucl Med Mol Imaging. 2009;36:1603–10.
59. Knez A, Becker A, Leber A, White C, Becker CR, Reiser MF, Steinbeck G, Boekstegers P. Relation of coronary calcium scores by electron beam tomography to obstructive disease in 2,115 symptomatic patients. Am J Cardiol. 2004;93:1150–2.
60. Vavere AL, Arbab-Zadeh A, Rochitte CE, Dewey M, Niinuma H, Gottlieb I, Clouse ME, Bush DE, Hoe JW, de Roos A, Cox C, Lima JA, Miller JM. Coronary artery stenoses: accuracy of 64-detector row CT angiography in segments with mild, moderate, or severe calcification–a subanalysis of the CORE-64 trial. Radiology. 2011;261:100–8.
61. Sangiorgi G, Rumberger JA, Severson A, Edwards WD, Gregoire J, Fitzpatrick LA, Schwartz RS. Arterial calcification and not lumen stenosis is highly correlated with atherosclerotic plaque burden in humans: a histologic study of 723 coronary artery segments using nondecalcifying methodology. J Am Coll Cardiol. 1998;31:126–33.
62. Gaemperli O, Schepis T, Koepfli P, Valenta I, Soyka J, Leschka S, Desbiolles L, Husmann L, Alkadhi H, Kaufmann PA. Accuracy of 64-slice CT angiography for the detection of functionally relevant coronary stenoses as assessed with myocardial perfusion SPECT. Eur J Nucl Med Mol Imaging. 2007;34:1162–71.
63. Namdar M, Hany TF, Koepfli P, Siegrist PT, Burger C, Wyss CA, Luscher TF, von Schulthess GK, Kaufmann PA. Integrated PET/CT for the assessment of coronary artery disease: a feasibility study. J Nucl Med. 2005;46:930–5.
64. Rispler S, Keidar Z, Ghersin E, Roguin A, Soil A, Dragu R, Litmanovich D, Frenkel A, Aronson D, Engel A, Beyar R, Israel O. Integrated single-photon emission computed tomography and computed tomography coronary angiography for the assessment of hemodynamically significant coronary artery lesions. J Am Coll Cardiol. 2007;49:1059–67.
65. Di Carli MF, Dorbala S, Curillova Z, Kwong RJ, Goldhaber SZ, Rybicki FJ, Hachamovitch R. Relationship between CT coronary angiography and stress perfusion imaging in patients with suspected ischemic heart disease assessed by integrated PET-CT imaging. J Nucl Cardiol. 2007;14:799–809.
66. Kajander S, Joutsiniemi E, Saraste M, Pietila M, Ukkonen H, Saraste A, Sipila HT, Teras M, Maki M, Airaksinen J, Hartiala J, Knuuti J. Cardiac positron emission tomography/computed tomography imaging accurately detects anatomically and functionally significant coronary artery disease. Circulation. 2010;122:603–13.
67. Shaw LJ, Hachamovitch R, Berman DS, Marwick TH, Lauer MS, Heller GV, Iskandrian AE, Kesler KL, Travin MI, Lewin HC, Hendel RC, Borges-Neto S, Miller DD. The economic

consequences of available diagnostic and prognostic strategies for the evaluation of stable angina patients: an observational assessment of the value of precatheterization ischemia. Economics of Noninvasive Diagnosis (END) Multicenter Study Group. J Am Coll Cardiol. 1999;33:661–9.
68. Gropler RJ, Geltman EM, Sampathkumaran K, Perez JE, Schechtman KB, Conversano A, Siegel BA. Comparison of carbon-11-acetate with fluorine-18-fluorodeoxyglucose for delineating viable myocardium by positron emission tomography. J Am Coll Cardiol. 1993;22:1587–97.
69. Rubin PJ, Lee DS, Davila-Roman VG, Geltman EM, Schechtman KB, Bergmann SR, Gropler RJ. Superiority of C-11 acetate compared with F-18 fluorodeoxyglucose in predicting myocardial functional recovery by positron emission tomography in patients with acute myocardial infarction. Am J Cardiol. 1996;78:1230–5.
70. Wolpers HG, Burchert W, van den Hoff J, Weinhardt R, Meyer GJ, Lichtlen PR. Assessment of myocardial viability by use of 11C-acetate and positron emission tomography. Threshold criteria of reversible dysfunction. Circulation. 1997;95:1417–24.
71. Di Carli MF. Advances in positron emission tomography. J Nucl Cardiol. 2004;11:719–32.
72. Di Carli MF. Predicting improved function after myocardial revascularization. Curr Opin Cardiol. 1998;13:415–24.
73. Ragosta M, Beller GA, Watson DD, Kaul S, Gimple LW. Quantitative planar rest-redistribution 201Tl imaging in detection of myocardial viability and prediction of improvement in left ventricular function after coronary bypass surgery in patients with severely depressed left ventricular function. Circulation. 1993;87:1630–41.
74. Perrone-Filardi P, Pace L, Prastaro M, et al. Dobutamine echocardiography predicts improvement of hypoperfused dysfunctional myocardium after revascularization in patients with coronary artery disease. Circulation. 1995;91:2556–65.
75. Kim RJ, Wu E, Rafael A, Chen EL, Parker MA, Simonetti O, Klocke FJ, Bonow RO, Judd RM. The use of contrast-enhanced magnetic resonance imaging to identify reversible myocardial dysfunction. N Engl J Med. 2000;343:1445–53.
76. Beanlands RS, Ruddy TD, deKemp RA, Iwanochko RM, Coates G, Freeman M, Nahmias C, Hendry P, Burns RJ, Lamy A, Mickleborough L, Kostuk W, Fallen E, Nichol G. Positron emission tomography and recovery following revascularization (PARR-1): the importance of scar and the development of a prediction rule for the degree of recovery of left ventricular function. J Am Coll Cardiol. 2002;40:1735–43.
77. Bax JJ, Poldermans D, Elhendy A, Boersma E, Rahimtoola SH. Sensitivity, specificity, and predictive accuracies of various noninvasive techniques for detecting hibernating myocardium. Curr Probl Cardiol. 2001;26:141–86.
78. Di Carli MF, Asgarzadie F, Schelbert HR, Brunken RC, Laks H, Phelps ME, Maddahi J. Quantitative relation between myocardial viability and improvement in heart failure symptoms after revascularization in patients with ischemic cardiomyopathy. Circulation. 1995;92: 3436–44.
79. Allman KC, Shaw LJ, Hachamovitch R, Udelson JE. Myocardial viability testing and impact of revascularization on prognosis in patients with coronary artery disease and left ventricular dysfunction: a meta-analysis. J Am Coll Cardiol. 2002;39:1151–8.
80. Ling LF, Marwick TH, Flores DR, Jaber WA, Brunken RC, Cerqueira MD, Hachamovitch R. Identification of therapeutic benefit from revascularization in patients with left ventricular systolic dysfunction: inducible ischemia versus hibernating myocardium. Circ Cardiovasc Imaging. 2013;6:363–72.
81. Beanlands RS, Nichol G, Huszti E, Humen D, Racine N, Freeman M, Gulenchyn KY, Garrard L, deKemp R, Guo A, Ruddy TD, Benard F, Lamy A, Iwanochko RM. F-18-fluorodeoxyglucose positron emission tomography imaging-assisted management of patients with severe left ventricular dysfunction and suspected coronary disease: a randomized, controlled trial (PARR-2). J Am Coll Cardiol. 2007;50:2002–12.
82. Velazquez EJ, Lee KL, Deja MA, Jain A, Sopko G, Marchenko A, Ali IS, Pohost G, Gradinac S, Abraham WT, Yii M, Prabhakaran D, Szwed H, Ferrazzi P, Petrie MC, O'Connor CM,

Panchavinnin P, She L, Bonow RO, Rankin GR, Jones RH, Rouleau JL. Coronary-artery bypass surgery in patients with left ventricular dysfunction. N Engl J Med. 2011;364: 1607–16.

83. Bonow RO, Maurer G, Lee KL, Holly TA, Binkley PF, Desvigne-Nickens P, Drozdz J, Farsky PS, Feldman AM, Doenst T, Michler RE, Berman DS, Nicolau JC, Pellikka PA, Wrobel K, Alotti N, Asch FM, Favaloro LE, She L, Velazquez EJ, Jones RH, Panza JA. Myocardial viability and survival in ischemic left ventricular dysfunction. N Engl J Med. 2011;364:1617–25.
84. Panza JA, Holly TA, Asch FM, She L, Pellikka PA, Velazquez EJ, Lee KL, Borges-Neto S, Farsky PS, Jones RH, Berman DS, Bonow RO. Inducible myocardial ischemia and outcomes in patients with coronary artery disease and left ventricular dysfunction. J Am Coll Cardiol. 2013;61:1860–70.
85. Velazquez EJ. Does imaging-guided selection of patients with ischemic heart failure for high risk revascularization improve identification of those with the highest clinical benefit?: myocardial imaging should not exclude patients with ischemic heart failure from coronary revascularization. Circ Cardiovasc Imaging. 2012;5:271–9. Discussion 279.
86. Mielniczuk LM, Beanlands RS. Does imaging-guided selection of patients with ischemic heart failure for high risk revascularization improve identification of those with the highest clinical benefit?: imaging-guided selection of patients with ischemic heart failure for high-risk revascularization improves identification of those with the highest clinical benefit. Circ Cardiovasc Imaging. 2012;5:262–70. Discussion 270.
87. Cleland JG, Pennell DJ, Ray SG, Coats AJ, Macfarlane PW, Murray GD, Mule JD, Vered Z, Lahiri A. Myocardial viability as a determinant of the ejection fraction response to carvedilol in patients with heart failure (CHRISTMAS trial): randomised controlled trial. Lancet. 2003;362:14–21.
88. Yamaguchi A, Ino T, Adachi H, et al. Left ventricular volume predicts postoperative course in patients with ischemic cardiomyopathy. Ann Thorac Surg. 1998;65:434–8.
89. Yamaguchi A, Ino T, Adachi H, Mizuhara A, Murata S, Kamio H. Left ventricular end-systolic volume index in patients with ischemic cardiomyopathy predicts postoperative ventricular function. Ann Thorac Surg. 1995;60:1059–62.
90. Di Carli MF, Hachamovitch R. New technology for noninvasive evaluation of coronary artery disease. Circulation. 2007;115(11):1464–80.

PET/CT Imaging of Inflammation and Calcification

15

Hamed Emami and Ahmed Tawakol

Contents

H. Emami, MD
Cardiac MR PET CT Program, Department of Imaging and Division of Cardiology, Massachusetts General Hospital and Harvard Medical School, 165 Cambridge Street, Suite 400, Boston, MA 02114-2750, USA

A. Tawakol, MD (✉)
Cardiac MR PET CT Program, Department of Imaging and Division of Cardiology, Massachusetts General Hospital and Harvard Medical School, 165 Cambridge Street, Suite 400, Boston, MA 02114-2750, USA

Division of Cardiology, Department of Medicine, Massachusetts General Hospital and Harvard Medical School, Boston, MA, USA
e-mail: atawakol@partners.org

E. Aikawa (ed.), *Cardiovascular Imaging: Arterial and Aortic Valve Inflammation and Calcification*, DOI 10.1007/978-3-319-09268-3_15

Abstract

The biological processes within atherosclerotic plaques are known to be critically important to the progression and rupture of plaques. Among them inflammation is thought to be a key participant in all stages of atherosclerosis, from plaque initiation to progression and atherothrombosis. Accordingly, imaging of inflammation may provide important insights into the atherosclerotic milieu.

^{18}F-fluorodeoxyglucose positron-emission tomography/computed tomography (FDG-PET/CT) imaging, originally developed as an imaging modality to evaluate oncologic processes, has evolved into a robust and reproducible modality for the quantification of arterial inflammation. Studies have shown that FDG uptake significantly correlates with arterial wall macrophage infiltration, high-risk morphological features of atherosclerotic plaques, expression of proinflammatory genes, and increased risk for future atherothrombotic events. Moreover, arterial FDG uptake is modifiable by anti-atherosclerotic treatments especially those with anti-inflammatory properties such as statins. Accordingly, FDG-PET/CT imaging is increasingly used as a surrogate imaging biomarker to monitor therapeutic efficacy of anti-atherosclerotic agents.

In this chapter, we review the basic cellular and molecular aspects of FDG-PET/CT imaging. Thereafter, we discuss the role of PET/CT imaging in noninvasive imaging of arterial inflammation, prediction of risk for progression of atherosclerosis, and risk assessment for subsequent atherothrombotic events. Furthermore, we discuss the utility of PET/CT imaging to evaluate the efficacy of new anti-atherosclerotic pharmacotherapies and review the results from recent imaging trials that employed PET/CT for this purpose. Lastly, we review the current state of the art and future directions for PET/CT imaging, with a review of coronary artery imaging, characterization of new targets, and recent improvements in camera and tracer technologies.

15.1 Introduction

A large body of evidence demonstrates that evaluation of coronary stenosis per se provides a relatively crude assessment of future risk of plaque rupture and cardiovascular events. This fact was emphasized, nearly 20 years ago, by a series of studies that evaluated the relationship between presence of coronary stenosis and subsequent atherothrombosis [1]. The study demonstrated that most culprit lesions do not cause significant luminal narrowing prior to cardiovascular events (Fig. 15.1). While plaques with greater degrees of luminal stenosis are more likely to progress to occlusion and/or give rise to infarction, most atherothrombotic events result from rupture of the plaques which are mildly to moderately obstructive, since the less obstructive plaques usually far outnumber severely obstructive plaques [1]. Accordingly, evaluation of coronary stenosis provides inadequate information in terms of risk assessment for subsequent cardiovascular events. The delineation of additional atherosclerotic features, such as vessel wall structure and biology, may provide important insights [2].

The paradigm of simultaneous assessment of structure and biology has been successfully performed for over a decade in the field of oncology. Two landmark papers

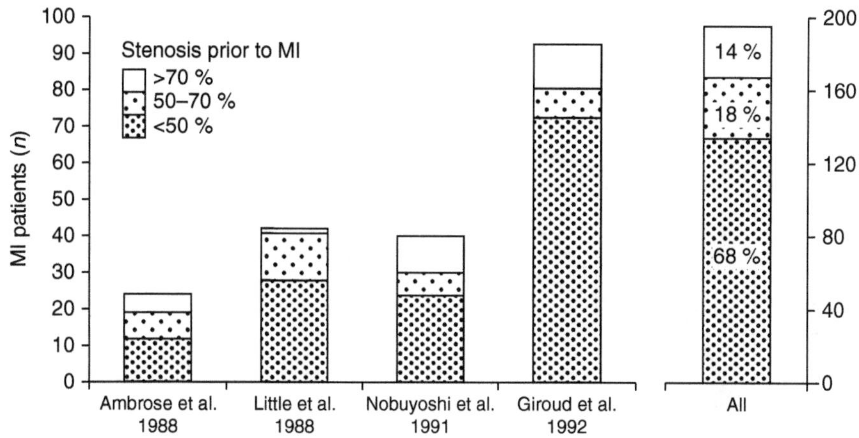

Fig. 15.1 Degree of coronary stenosis and subsequent cardiovascular events. In the coronary arteries, less obstructive plaques outnumber severely obstructive plaques. Vascular occlusions and cardiovascular events evolve most frequently from plaques that are only mildly to moderately obstructive months to years before infarction (Adapted with permission from a review article by Falk et al. [1])

in 2003 demonstrated that combined molecular and structural imaging, using PET and CT, is capable to localize and stage tumors more accurately compared to structural imaging alone [3, 4]. These observations led to the vast proliferation of PET/CT scans and have since fundamentally transformed the practice of oncology. In the study of cardiovascular disorders, the similar paradigm of simultaneous evaluation of structure and biology of atherosclerosis is relatively new and rapidly evolving.

Several features of atherosclerotic plaques that can be visualized noninvasively through imaging have been shown to be associated with a heightened risk of subsequent atherothrombosis [5]. These features include positive remodeling, high lipid content (low-attenuation plaque), thin fibrous cap, evidence of ulceration, intra-plaque hemorrhage, and microcalcification [5, 6]. The biological processes within plaques are also known to be critically important to the progression and rupture of plaques. Among them, inflammation is thought to be a key participant in all stages of atherosclerosis, from plaque initiation to plaque progression to atherothrombosis [7, 8]. Accordingly, imaging of inflammation may also provide important insights into the atherosclerotic milieu.

15.2 FDG-PET/CT Imaging of Oncologic Processes and Inflammation

The commonly employed PET/CT imaging agent, ^{18}F-fluorodeoxyglucose (FDG), is clinically used for identification of neoplasms, screening of tumor metastases, and assessment of response to antineoplastic therapies. Additionally, FDG-PET/CT imaging has been demonstrated to be clinically useful for imaging of various sources of inflammation, including evaluation of device infection, fever of unknown origin,

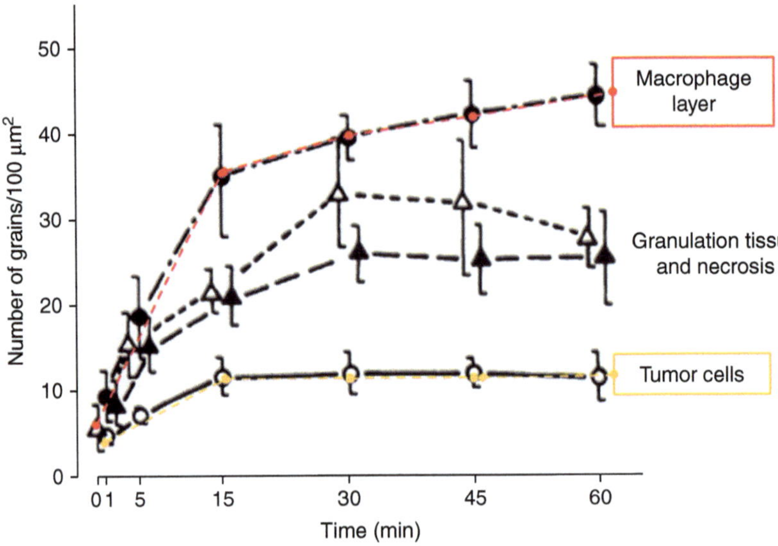

Fig. 15.2 High uptake of glucose analogs in tumor-associated macrophages. The uptake of tritium deoxyglucose (*[³H] DG*) is demonstrated over time in intra-tumoral cellular components of mammary carcinoma in mice. [³H] DG uptake is determined by microautoradiographic silver grain counting (Adapted with permission from Kubota et al. [9])

and sarcoidosis. Studies have shown that among the inflammatory cells, macrophages tend to have high uptake of FDG which is comparable to the amount of FDG uptake by tumor cell lines. Moreover, further investigations which were designed to reveal the source of intra-tumoral FDG uptake have demonstrated that the tumor-associated macrophages (TAMs) demonstrate even higher FDG uptake than the tumor cells [9] (Fig. 15.2). Accordingly, a substantial portion of the clinical utility of FDG-PET/CT scan for oncologic imaging relates to the uptake of FDG by macrophages.

The molecular mechanisms underlying FDG uptake by inflammatory cells have been well studied. FDG is a glucose analog that, similar to glucose, enters the cells through glucose transporters (GLUT), a group of membrane proteins that facilitate the transport of glucose over the plasma membrane. Within cells, FDG is phosphorylated by hexokinase to produce FDG-6-phosphate. Similarly, glucose is phosphorylated by the similar enzyme to become glucose-6-phosphate. Since the glucose-6-phosphatase enzyme is absent in most cells (except hepatocytes), the phosphorylated form of glucose/FDG cannot efflux from the cell. Glucose-6-phosphate, which is the natural substrate for the glycolysis pathway, becomes further phosphorylated and participates in glycolysis. However, FDG-6-phosphate is unable to participate further in glycolysis and thus accumulates within cells; hence, FDG accumulates in the cells and the quantity is in accordance with the rate of glycolysis (Fig. 15.3).

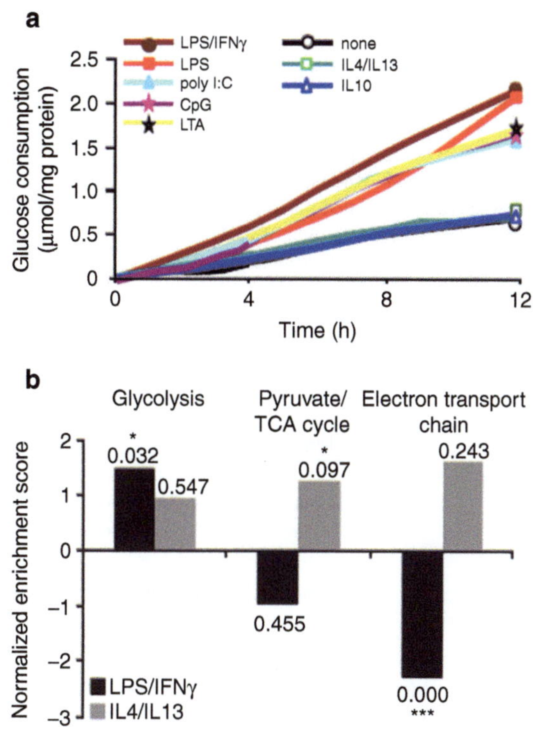

Fig. 15.3 Glycolytic flux in activated macrophages. (**a**) Metabolic flux (glucose uptake) is demonstrated in macrophages stimulated through the classic activation (induced by lipopolysaccharide and interferon-γ) and alternative activation pathways (induced by IL-4, IL-10, and IL-13). The time course of glucose consumption was determined by sampling the culture medium at periods of 2 h. (**b**) Gene set enrichment analysis. The normalized enriched scores are shown in the *bars*. Positive scores indicate upregulated genes, whereas negative normalized enriched scores correspond to downregulated genes (Modified with permission from Rodriguez-Prados et al. [10])

A broad body of research extending over three quarters of a century shows that myeloid cells including macrophages are highly dependent on glycolysis for energy metabolism [11, 12]. In resting macrophages, ATP is generated through the glycolytic and mitochondrial pathways in roughly equal proportions. Activated macrophages manifest a substantial upregulation of ATP production, the vast majority of which is produced through glycolysis. Further, the manner of macrophage stimulation has a significant impact on glycolytic flux [13]. While innate or classic activation (proinflammatory activation or M1 polarization) leads to increased glycolysis, alternative activation (anti-inflammatory activation or M2 polarization) does not [13]. Additionally, with M1 polarization, there is an upregulation of genes which encode glycolytic enzymes, which is accompanied by a downregulation of the genes that encode tricarboxylic acid cycle (TCA) and electron transport chain (ETC) proteins. The opposite occurs with M2 polarization (Fig. 15.4). In congruence with these findings, compared to resting macrophages, deoxyglucose uptake is increased in M1-polarized macrophages but is decreased in M2-polarized macrophages (Fig. 15.5) [14]. It should be noted that these findings are not without controversy. One study suggested that hypoxia, more than proinflammatory activation, drives macrophage glycolysis [16]. However, multiple groups have demonstrated that hypoxia itself is an important driver of both macrophage proinflammatory

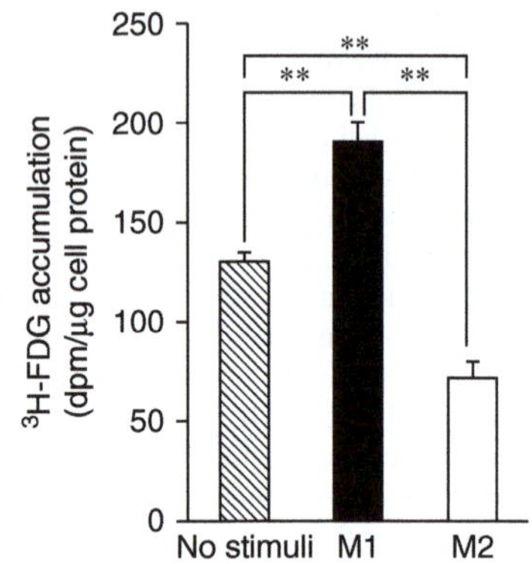

Fig. 15.4 Intracellular ^{3}H-FDG accumulations in human macrophages. Compared to un-stimulated macrophages, classically stimulated macrophages (M1 polarized) accumulate higher amounts of FDG, whereas in the alternatively stimulated macrophages (M2 polarized), the amount of FDG uptake is lower than un-stimulated macrophages (Modified with permission from Satomi et al. [14]. (Asterisks indicate statistical significance)

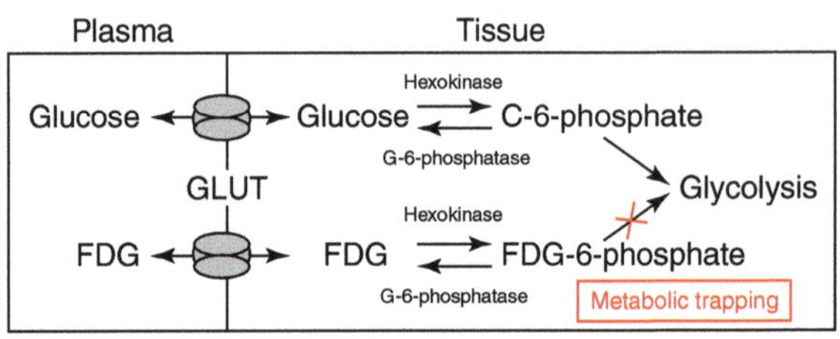

Fig. 15.5 Metabolic trapping of fluorodeoxyglucose. Fluorodeoxyglucose (*FDG*) enters the cells through glucose transporters (*GLUT*) and becomes phosphorylated by hexokinase to produce FDG-6-phosphate. Similarly, glucose is phosphorylated by the similar enzyme to become glucose-6-phosphate. Glucose-6-phosphate, which is the natural substrate for the glycolysis pathway, becomes further phosphorylated and participates in glycolysis. However, FDG-6-phosphate is unable to participate further in glycolysis and thus accumulates within cells; hence, FDG accumulates in the cells and the quantity is in accordance with the rate of glycolysis (Adapted with permission from Rudd et al. [15])

activation and glycolysis [17]. Moreover, it has been reported that across varying oxygen tensions, including hypoxic conditions, and through varying macrophage stimulatory conditions, a tight relationship exists between glycolytic flux and macrophage proinflammatory activation (measured as TNF alpha production) [18]. Accordingly, the glycolytic rate of macrophage-rich tissues (as assessed by FDG uptake) may provide an index of state of proinflammatory activation.

Given FDG accumulation in inflammatory cells, it follows that it may be useful for imaging inflammation. Indeed, in addition to its use as a tracer to characterize oncologic processes, FDG is clinically used for imaging of inflammation and infection. The clinical use of FDG-PET/CT for imaging of inflammation has substantially grown over the years, and recent guidelines provided by the Society of Nuclear Medicine and Molecular Imaging as well as the European Association of Nuclear Medicine suggest the clinical use of FDG imaging of inflammation and infection [19]. The current major inflammatory indications for FDG-PET/CT imaging include evaluation of fever of unknown origin, suspected spinal infections, vasculitides, osteomyelitis, sarcoidosis, device and prosthetic infections, and endocarditis [20].

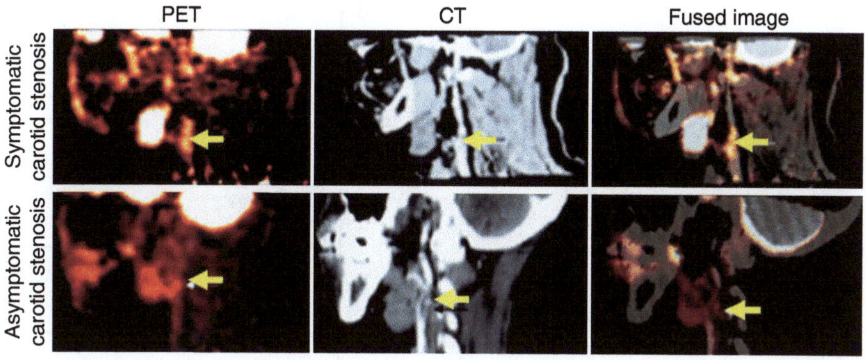

Fig. 15.6 FDG-PET/CT imaging of arterial inflammation. The *top row* (from left to right) shows PET, contrast-enhanced CT, and co-registered PET/CT images. These images are obtained from a 63-year-old man who had experienced two episodes of left-sided hemiparesis. The *bottom row* demonstrates a low level of FDG uptake in an individual with an asymptomatic carotid stenosis (Modified with permission from Rudd et al. [21])

15.3 FDG-PET/CT Imaging of Arterial inflammation

Imaging of atherosclerotic inflammation using FDG-PET was initially reported in humans in 2002 by Rudd et al. [21]. In their landmark study of individuals with recent strokes, they observed higher FDG uptake in the wall of the symptomatic carotid artery (compared to the contralateral carotid artery plaques; Fig. 15.6). In an analysis of an excised carotid plaque that was incubated with tritiated deoxyglucose, the authors furthermore observed that deoxyglucose localized to foamy macrophages within the lipid core, suggesting that the FDG signal may be reporting on macrophages. Thereafter, several groups reported in animal models that arterial FDG uptake correlates with inflammation which was confirmed by histology [22, 23]. Further, it was soon after shown in humans that PET imaging of FDG uptake within human carotid arteries provided an index of atherosclerotic plaque inflammation [24]. In that study, the authors measured the FDG uptake in carotid plaques of individuals who subsequently underwent carotid endarterectomy. They assessed the correlation between FDG uptake and the macrophage content, measured as CD68 staining by histopathology, on the same plaques that were excised during endarterectomy. In that study, the authors observed a significant correlation between FDG uptake and the macrophage content (Fig. 15.7). Several groups have replicated this observation, and some extended the concept by demonstrating that FDG uptake in the arterial wall also relates to the expression of proinflammatory genes [25, 26].

The accumulation of FDG within the arterial wall is inhomogeneous, as would be expected given the inhomogeneous distribution of atherosclerotic plaques and various stages of different atherosclerotic plaques. Figueroa et al. observed that arterial FDG uptake is especially prominent within the plaques that have morphological features suggestive of high-risk potential [27]. In their study, they recruited patients who were scheduled for carotid endarterectomy and performed arterial

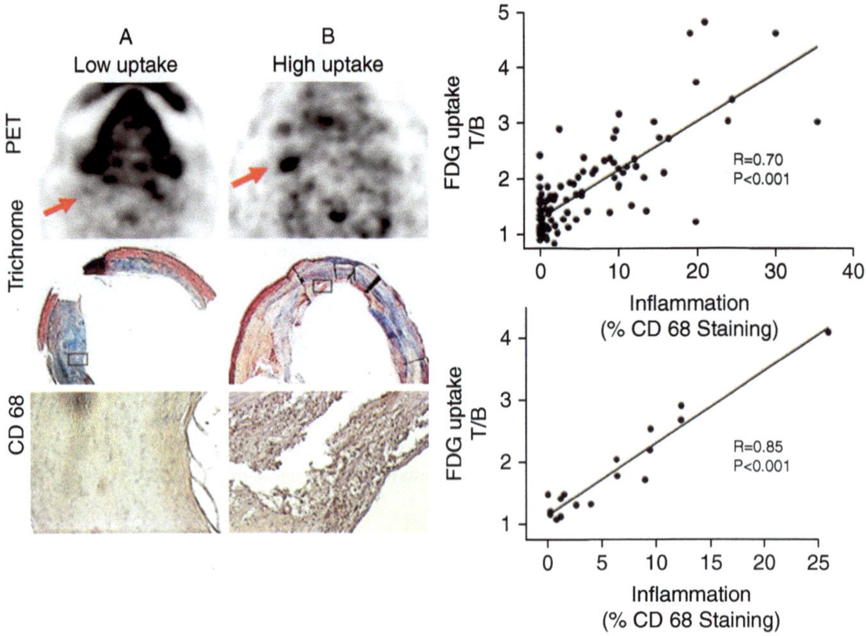

Fig. 15.7 FDG-PET imaging and macrophage content of atherosclerotic plaques. Axial positron-emission tomography (*PET*) images from two patients are demonstrated: Patient **A** manifested low FDG uptake in the region of the carotid plaque, whereas patient **B** had a high FDG uptake in that region. The region of the excised carotid plaque is noted with *arrows*. In patient A, the corresponding trichrome-stained histologic specimen demonstrates a collagen-rich plaque with low lipid content, and CD68 staining on the high-powered images demonstrates limited macrophage infiltration. In patient B, the corresponding trichrome-stained histologic specimen demonstrates a complex plaque with a necrotic core, and the CD68 staining demonstrates intense macrophage infiltration. The *boxes* in the trichrome-stained images indicate the regions corresponding to the high-powered CD68 stains. The *scatter plots* demonstrate that carotid plaque FDG uptake in carotid plaques significantly correlated with histologic measure of inflammation in the corresponding sections taken during carotid endarterectomy (Modified with permission from Tawakol et al. [24])

FDG-PET/CT and contrast-enhanced CT imaging prior to the procedure. They characterized plaque morphology using CT of the carotid arteries and defined high-risk morphological features as plaques with ulceration, low attenuation (which indicates lipid-rich locations), or positive remodeling. These features were selected based on a wealth of clinical data suggesting that those features are associated with an increased risk of subsequent plaque rupture and stroke. Additionally, following carotid endarterectomy, the carotid plaques were examined histopathologically. The authors demonstrated that the distribution of FDG uptake within the carotid arteries was heterogeneous; however, the amount of the FDG that localized to the arterial wall was associated with presence of atherosclerotic plaques. Moreover, they demonstrated that arterial inflammation as assessed by FDG uptake was higher in plaques with high-risk morphological features and depends on the number of high-risk features that each plaque contains (Fig. 15.8). Similarly, the macrophage

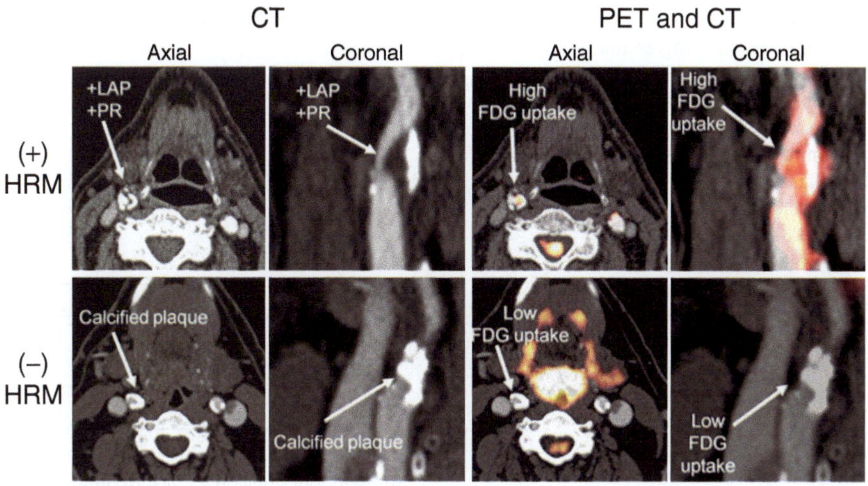

Fig. 15.8 Distribution of FDG uptake correlates with high-risk morphology of atherosclerotic plaques. Axial and coronal sections of computed tomography (*CT*) and positron-emission tomography/computed tomography (*PET/CT*) are demonstrated. *Top row* demonstrates that FDG uptake is higher in the regions of carotid artery with high-risk morphology (*HRM*) in the atherosclerotic plaques. Low-attenuation plaques (*LAP*) with positive remodeling (*PR*) are considered as HRM. The *bottom row* demonstrates that a predominantly calcified plaque without high-risk morphological feature (*HRM*) is associated with lower FDG uptake (Modified with permission from Figueroa et al. [27])

staining present within those plaques (as measured histopathologically after endarterectomy) also correlated with the number of high-risk morphological features. Accordingly, FDG uptake relates to both inflammation and the presence of high-risk morphological features, which are in turn interrelated.

15.4 Relationship Between Arterial Inflammation, Disease Progression, and Risk of Cardiovascular Events

Arterial inflammation has been shown to be predictive of subsequent plaque progression in human studies. Abdelbaky et al. observed that arterial wall locations with underlying inflammation (by FDG-PET/CT) subsequently manifested greater arterial calcification (quantified by CT imaging), compared to the locations with less inflammation [28] (Fig. 15.9). In that study, the authors observed that arterial FDG uptake was a strong predictor of subsequent arterial calcification (odds ratio [95 % CI]=2.59 [1.18–5.7]) after adjusting for other cardiovascular risk factors (e.g., age, hypertension, and dyslipidemia). Similarly, Fayad et al. demonstrated in a large prospective study that arterial segments with increased arterial inflammation (by PET/CT) experienced more volumetric expansion (measured by MRI) over the ensuing 18 months compared to segments with reduced inflammation [29]. These studies present insights about the local consequences of arterial inflammation and

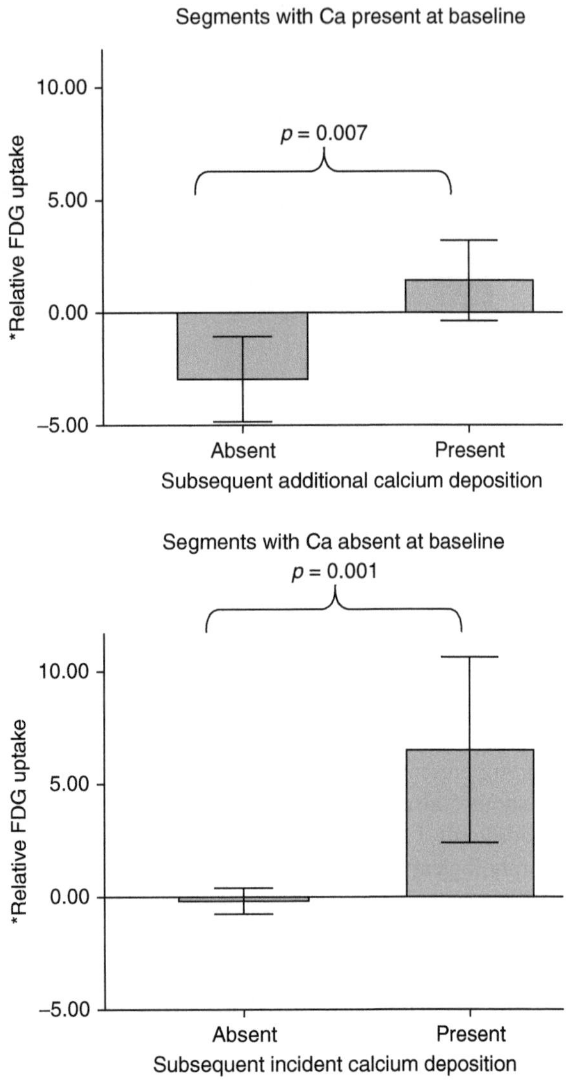

Fig. 15.9 Arterial inflammation and progression of atherosclerosis. This study evaluated the relationship between baseline arterial inflammation and subsequent calcification of the atherosclerotic plaques. The authors used a within-patient analysis where the segmental FDG uptake was expressed relative to the mean FDG uptake for the entire aorta within which that segment resides (as the percent difference between the individual segment SUV and the mean SUV of the whole aorta). They demonstrated that within each patient, the relative baseline SUV was higher in segments that manifested subsequent calcification. This held true in subset analyses of segments with calcium present at baseline ($P=0.007$) and segments without calcium at baseline ($P=0.001$) (Adapted with permission from Abdelbaky et al. [28])

thus provide a plausible explanation for observed increased risk of atherothrombotic events in individuals with heightened arterial inflammation.

Measures of arterial inflammation may provide an index of the risk of subsequent atherothrombotic events. In an early retrospective study of individuals who had undergone FDG-PET/CT imaging for clinical (mostly oncologic) indications, Rominger et al. initially demonstrated that arterial inflammation (FDG uptake) was predictive of event-free survival over a 40-month period [30]. However, that particular study did not identify the degree to which imaging of arterial inflammation may add to risk prediction over the standard risk prediction tools such as the Framingham

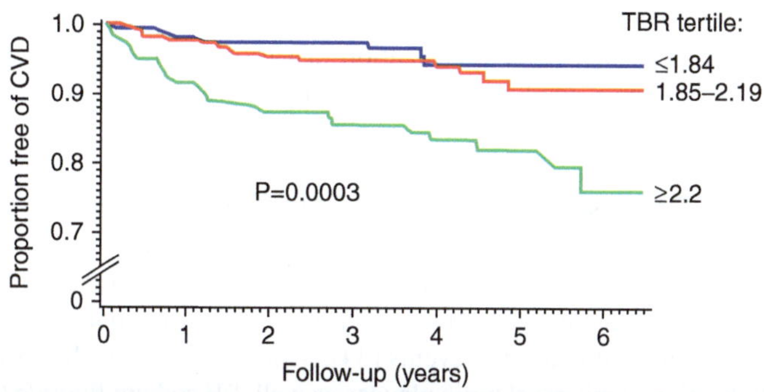

Risk categories	NRI [95% bootstrap CI]	Events correctly reclassified	Non-events correctly reclassified
<10 % risk 10–20 % risk >20 % risk	27.48 % [16.27,39.92]	12.66 %	14.82 %

Fig. 15.10 Quantification of arterial inflammation improves the risk assessment of cardiovascular events. Arterial FDG uptake (target-to-background ratio, *TBR*) is demonstrated to have a significant association with the risk of subsequent cardiovascular events. Moreover, authors showed that it improves the reclassification by 27 % when combined with the Framingham Risk Score (*FRS*) (Modified with permission from Figueroa et al. [32])

Risk Score (FRS). Indeed, studies have demonstrated an association between FRS and arterial inflammation (FDG uptake) [31]. Recently, one study evaluated the degree to which imaging measures of arterial inflammation (FDG-PET/CT imaging) may refine assessment of risk of cardiovascular beyond the FRS calculation [32]. In a study of 513 individuals who had undergone imaging for clinical indications but who were deemed to be free of active oncologic disease, FDG-PET/CT images were retrospectively analyzed. The authors of that study observed that arterial inflammation (measured as FDG uptake) independently predicted the risk of subsequent cardiovascular disease events. Moreover, they reported a net reclassification improvement of 27.5 % over FRS, with 12.7 % of events correctly reclassified and 14.8 % of nonevents correctly reclassified using noninvasive imaging (Fig. 15.10). Additionally, an association between vascular inflammation and the timing of cardiovascular events was observed, whereby individuals with events occurring within 6 months of imaging had the highest amount of FDG uptake in the index imaging. In contrast, the individuals with more remote events had lower initial arterial inflammatory signals, while those who never developed cardiovascular events had the lowest FDG uptake. In a separate small prospective study of 60 individuals with ischemic stroke, Marnane et al. sought to evaluate whether carotid FDG uptake after a stroke was associated with the risk of short-term (90 days) stroke recurrence. They found that in a Cox regression model including age and degree of stenosis (50–69 % or 70 %), mean plaque FDG uptake was the only independent predictor of stroke recurrence (adjusted hazard ratio, 6.1; 95 % CI,

1.3–28.8; $p=0.02$) [33]. While these studies suggest a promising role for PET/CT imaging in risk assessment and stratification in various patient populations, large prospective studies are needed to confirm these findings.

15.5 PET/CT Measures of Arterial Calcification

Large studies have demonstrated that measures of coronary artery calcification, such as the coronary calcium score (assessed by CT), provide potent prediction of subsequent incident cardiovascular events [34]. Molecular imaging has been used to identify calcification of atherosclerotic plaques as well. ^{18}F-sodium fluoride (^{18}F-NaF), which localizes formation of hydroxyapatite crystals in very early stages, has been suggested as a tracer for vascular imaging. Recently, Joshi et al. demonstrated that PET/CT imaging using ^{18}F-NaF might introduce a promising role for this noninvasive imaging modality to identify and localize high-risk coronary plaques [35] (Fig. 15.11). However, the relationship between ^{18}F-NaF uptake and the risk of cardiovascular events is yet undefined. Furthermore, it is still unknown whether arterial ^{18}F-NaF uptake provides an independent measure of risk when added to CT measures of calcium deposition such as the Agatston score. Dweck et al. have employed ^{18}F-NaF PET/CT imaging to identify active calcification and disease progression in aortic valve [36]. It is worth noting that these studies are performed in small patient populations and require larger studies to confirm their findings.

15.6 Utility of Noninvasive Imaging of Arterial Inflammation to Assess Effectiveness of Therapies

Arterial inflammation (FDG uptake using FDG-PET/CT imaging) is rapidly modifiable by interventions. Two preclinical studies evaluated the rate of change in arterial inflammation (using FDG-PET/CT) after pharmacotherapy. In one study, atherosclerotic inflammation decreased substantially within 2 days after administration of an anti-inflammatory drug [37]. Conversely, arterial FDG uptake increased within 3 days after administration of a proinflammatory cytokine [38]. Taken together, these preclinical findings show that arterial inflammation can be rapidly modified through anti-atherosclerotic pharmacotherapy.

Fig. 15.11 PET/CT imaging of coronary arteries. ^{18}F-sodium fluoride (*^{18}F-NaF*) is a tracer that localizes formation of hydroxyapatite crystals in very early stages. (**a**) Significant stenosis of proximal segment of left anterior descending coronary artery (*LAD*) by invasive angiography; (**b**) high uptake of ^{18}F-NaF in the same coronary segment; (**c**) culprit lesion (*red arrow*; LAD) in a patient with non-ST elevation myocardial infarction and bystander non-culprit lesion (*white arrow*; circumflex artery) that were both stented during the admission; (**d**) only the culprit lesion had increased ^{18}F-NaF uptake PET/CT. (**e**) *Box plot* demonstrates that ^{18}F-NaF uptake was significantly higher in culprit coronary lesions compared with non-culprit lesions (Modified with permission from Joshi et al. [35])

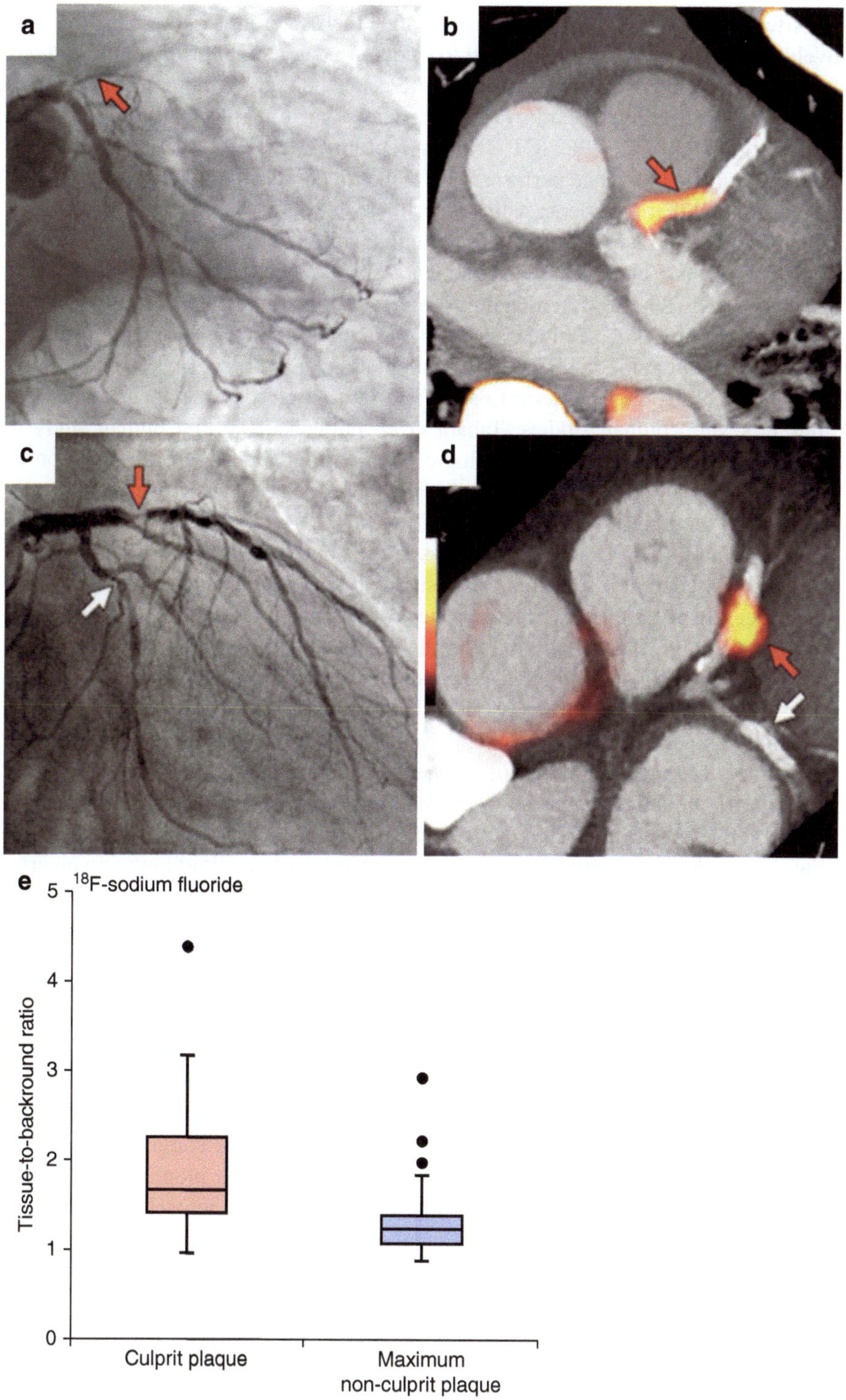
a
b
c
d
e
18F-sodium fluoride
Tissue-to-backround ratio
0
1
2
3
4
5
Culprit plaque
Maximum
non-culprit plaque

Arterial inflammation (FDG uptake) in the atherosclerotic plaques must be relatively stable and reproducible in order to be qualified as a monitoring tool for assessment of anti-atherosclerotic treatment effects. Rudd et al. demonstrated in 20 individuals with clinical cardiovascular disease that imaging measure of arterial inflammation by FDG-PET/CT scan is reproducible [39]. They prospectively enrolled study subjects and performed PET imaging at two timepoints 2 weeks apart and concluded that in patients with stable atherosclerosis who received stable treatment, the FDG signal was highly reproducible (Intraclass Correlation Coefficients of 0.79–0.92 and interobserver agreements of 0.92–0.97). Accordingly, the high sensitivity of FDG-PET/CT imaging for detection of treatment effects, along with its reproducibility under stable conditions in humans, provides rationale for use of FDG-PET/CT imaging to assess anti-inflammatory therapies.

FDG-PET/CT has been used to study anti-atherosclerotic therapeutic interventions in several human studies. Tahara et al. published the first human study to evaluate the impact of a pharmacologic intervention on arterial inflammation as measured by FDG-PET/CT imaging [40]. Using a single-center open-label study design, they compared simvastatin (5–20 mg) to diet management. By 3 months, arterial inflammation (FDG uptake) was significantly reduced in the simvastatin group compared to the group that was assigned to the diet management (Fig. 15.12). More recently, the anti-inflammatory effect of statins on arterial inflammation was studied in a multicenter double-blind trial [41]. In that study, 83 adults who were at risk or with established clinical atherosclerosis and were not taking high-dose statins were randomized to atorvastatin 10 mg versus 80 mg. Arterial FDG-PET/CT imaging was performed at baseline, 4 weeks, and 12 weeks after randomization. The authors reported that high-dose atorvastatin (80 mg daily) resulted in a significant relative reduction in arterial inflammation compared to atorvastatin 10 mg and that the reductions from baseline were seen as early as 4 weeks after randomization (Fig. 15.13). Most recently, the effect of non-pharmacologic lipid lowering on arterial inflammation was evaluated. In a study of individuals with familial hypercholesterolemia (FH), lipid lowering by lipoprotein apheresis resulted in a substantial reduction in arterial inflammation (FDG-PET/CT imaging) within 1 week of the intervention [42].

Additionally, FDG-PET/CT imaging has been used to study the effect on arterial inflammation of therapies that do not substantially impact serum LDL. Mizoguchi et al. studied the effect of pioglitazone (15–30 mg) versus glimepiride (0.5–4.0 mg) on arterial FDG uptake in glucose intolerant or diabetic patients who had carotid atherosclerosis [43]. They found that while both treatments comparably reduced fasting glucose concentrations and hemoglobin $A1_C$ values, pioglitazone but not glimepiride reduced arterial inflammation. Indeed, an anti-atherosclerotic effect of pioglitazone has been suggested by clinical endpoint studies as well, whereby several trials have suggested that the use of pioglitazone in diabetic patients is associated with a reduced incidence of atherothrombotic events [44, 45]. Hence, for statins as well as pioglitazone, findings of reduced arterial inflammation in FDG-PET/CT imaging trials are consistent with the findings of clinical endpoint trials.

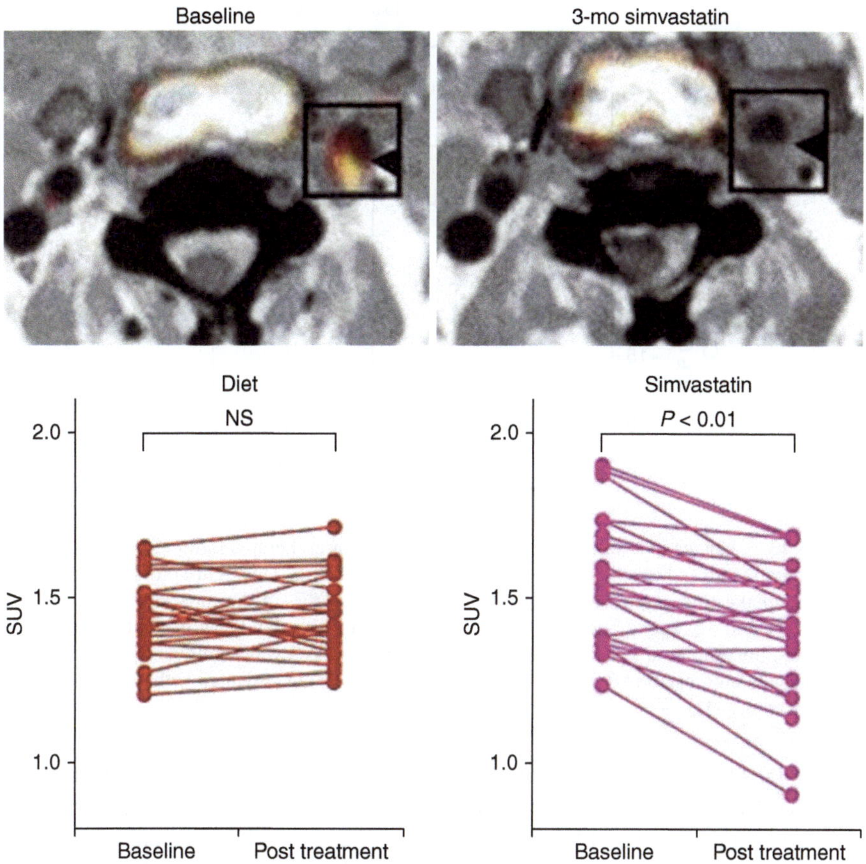

Fig. 15.12 Determination of simvastatin treatment effect by FDG-PET/CT imaging. Representative FDG-PET images at baseline and after 3 months of simvastatin therapy (posttreatment) are compared with dietary intervention. Baseline images demonstrate FDG uptake within a common carotid plaque (*square*). A substantial reduction in plaque. FDG uptake is seen after 3 months of simvastatin therapy (*top*). The *bottom panel* demonstrates per-subject data for baseline and posttreatment values in the diet and simvastatin groups. There was a significant reduction in vascular FDG uptake after simvastatin therapy but not after dietary modification. *NS* not significant (Modified with permission from Tahara et al. [40])

Recently, multicenter FDG-PET/CT studies have been performed to evaluate therapeutic efficacy of novel pharmacologic agents. The results of two large clinical endpoint studies have recently been published and provided an opportunity to compare the results of the imaging trials to those of the clinical endpoint trials. The first novel drug was dalcetrapib, a cholesteryl ester transfer protein (CETP) modulator. The dal-PLAQUE trial used multimodality imaging to evaluate the safety and efficacy of dalcetrapib on atherosclerotic disease [29]. In that phase 2b double-blind multicenter trial, 130 individuals with or at risk for coronary heart disease were

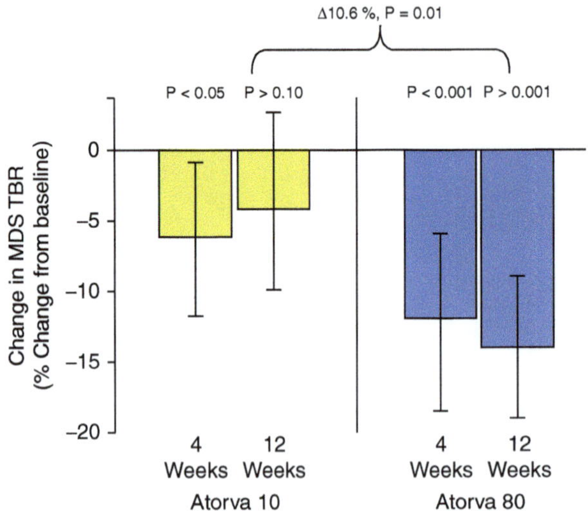

Fig. 15.13 Changes in arterial inflammation following statin therapy. In this multicenter study, statin therapy induced a rapid reduction in arterial inflammation. This figure provides the change in FDG uptake (measured as target-to-background ratio, *TBR*, in the most diseased segment, *MDS*) at 4 and 12 weeks after initiation of therapy with high- and low-dose atorvastatin. At 12 weeks, inflammation (TBR) in the MDS of the index vessel was significantly reduced from baseline with atorvastatin 80 mg, but not with atorvastatin 10 mg (Adapted with permission from Tawakol et al. [41])

randomized to placebo versus dalcetrapib. FDG-PET/CT imaging was performed at baseline and 6 months after randomization. In that study, there was no significant difference in the primary FDG-PET/CT imaging endpoint between dalcetrapib and placebo ($p=0.51$). The subsequently published dal-OUTCOMES trial evaluated the effect of dalcetrapib versus placebo by the composite outcome of death from coronary heart disease, nonfatal myocardial infarction, ischemic stroke, unstable angina, or cardiac arrest with resuscitation in nearly 16,000 individuals with the recent acute coronary syndromes [46]. The authors reported that while dalcetrapib was associated with a 40 % increase in HDL cholesterol, it did not reduce the risk of recurrent cardiovascular events.

The second novel therapeutic agent to be evaluated separately in an FDG-PET/CT imaging trial as well as in clinical endpoint trials was rilapladib, an inhibitor of lipoprotein-associated phospholipase A2 (Lp-PLA$_2$). In a multicenter trial, FDG-PET/CT imaging was used to evaluate the effect of rilapladib on arterial inflammation in over 80 individuals randomized to rilapladib (250 mg once daily) versus placebo for 3 months [28]. While rilapladib significantly reduced Lp-PLA$_2$ activity by up to 80 %, it did not reduce arterial inflammation (FDG uptake). The recent clinical endpoint trial evaluating the related Lp-PLA$_2$ antagonist, darapladib, similarly showed no significant reduction in clinical events. The STABILITY trial of nearly 16,000 individuals with stable atherosclerotic disease showed no beneficial effect of darapladib to reduce the primary composite endpoint of cardiovascular death, myocardial infarction, or stroke [47].

Thus for all four drug classes for which there are both FDG-PET/CT data and clinical endpoint data (atorvastatin, darapladib, dalcetrapib, and pioglitazone), the imaging trial findings have been consistent with the results from clinical endpoint studies. Accordingly, the use of FDG-PET/CT imaging may provide a pathway for predicting the potential efficacy of cardiovascular therapeutics using a relatively small number of patients and with observation periods of 1–3 months.

15.7 Imaging of Arterial Inflammation to Develop Physiologic Insights

Noninvasive imaging of arterial inflammation has proven to be useful for developing pathophysiologic insights while studying patient populations. FDG-PET/CT imaging has been used to study diseases that have been hypothesized to be associated with arterial inflammation. Kim et al. demonstrated that arterial inflammation is increased in individuals with type 2 diabetes mellitus or impaired glucose tolerance compared to healthy controls [31]. Others have reported increased arterial inflammation in patients with chronic obstructive pulmonary disease (COPD) and patients with mild stable asthma [48, 49]. Further, in individuals with mild asthma, the degree of arterial inflammation relates to the severity of asthma as assessed by pulmonary function testing such that there was an inverse correlation between arterial FDG uptake and forced expiratory volume in the first second (FEV1) and peak expiratory flow (PEF). These studies support the hypothesis that the increased risk of cardiovascular events in these disease states might be in part related to higher arterial inflammation.

It has been previously demonstrated that patients with rheumatoid arthritis (RA) have higher risk of myocardial infarction. A suggested mechanism is that joint inflammation potentiates systemic inflammation, which in turn accelerates arterial inflammation and the risk of atherothrombosis. One study recently evaluated whether adult patients with RA have increased arterial inflammation and whether synovial activity correlates with arterial inflammation [50]. In that study, 66 individuals underwent FDG-PET/CT imaging: 33 individuals with and 33 individuals without RA (matched by age and gender). The individuals with RA had substantially increased levels of arterial inflammation even after adjusting for well-established risk factors of atherosclerosis such as FRS. Moreover, the authors in that study showed that arterial inflammatory signal strongly correlated with the degree of synovial activation assessed with FDG-PET/CT imaging. Recently, Mäki-Petäjä et al. demonstrated that treatment with an antitumor necrosis-α therapy reduces arterial inflammation in individuals with RA within 8 weeks [51]. Taken together, these studies suggest that arterial inflammation in rheumatoid arthritis is closely linked to synovial disease activity and that anti-inflammatory therapies that have primarily targeted synovial disease are effective at reducing arterial inflammation as well. Several groups are now assessing whether more aggressive targeting of synovial disease activity in rheumatoid arthritis patients would result in a reduction in arterial inflammation.

FDG-PET/CT imaging has been used to gain important physiologic insights in studying atherosclerosis in association with human immunodeficiency virus (HIV) infection. It has long been established that HIV is associated with an increased risk of cardiovascular disease events, which is not fully accounted for by traditional risk factors [52, 53]. Several lines of evidence support the concept that chronic immune cell activation may promote arterial inflammation leading to an increased high-risk plaque phenotype in patients with HIV. Subramanian et al. used FDG-PET/CT imaging to assess arterial inflammation in individuals who are infected with HIV [54]. To do so, the authors prospectively recruited 81 individuals, 27 of whom were HIV infected without any known cardiovascular diseases. In their study, they employed FDG-PET/CT imaging to compare arterial inflammation within individuals with versus without HIV who were matched by FRS. They found that arterial inflammation was higher in HIV versus FRS-matched control subjects but was similar when compared to patients with established atherosclerosis. Moreover, they demonstrated that the arterial inflammatory signal correlated with levels of the monocyte activation marker CD163. In a separate study, the interrelationship between arterial inflammation and high-risk morphological features of coronary atherosclerotic plaques was assessed in HIV-infected individuals [55]. In that study, the authors recruited 41 subjects with HIV who were on stable antiretroviral therapy and had asymptomatic coronary atherosclerotic plaques on coronary CT angiography. Thereafter, the investigators tested the hypothesis that the degree of arterial inflammation (FDG uptake) is related to high-risk plaque morphology. They demonstrated that among HIV-infected individuals with higher degrees of aortic inflammation, there was an increased prevalence of coronary plaques manifesting high-risk morphological features compared to patients with lower degrees of arterial inflammation. Taken together, these data suggest that arterial inflammation is increased in HIV-infected individuals, is related to markers of monocyte activation, and is associated with the presence of high-risk coronary plaque subtypes. Several studies are currently ongoing to assess whether anti-inflammatory strategies would reduce arterial inflammation as well as the burden of high-risk coronary plaque features in individuals with HIV.

15.8 Extra-arterial FDG-PET/CT Inflammatory Imaging

FDG-PET/CT imaging is routinely used clinically for evaluation of extravascular inflammation. Notably, FDG-PET/CT imaging is used routinely for evaluation of sarcoidosis, a cardiac inflammatory disorder. Lee et al. demonstrated in a preclinical model that FDG uptake in myocardial tissue correlates with the density of proinflammatory monocytes [56]. While this observation provides rationale for evaluating cardiac inflammatory disorders such as sarcoidosis, it must be noted that the uptake of FDG by noninflammatory cells such as myocytes can be substantial. However, because myocytes preferentially use fatty acids rather than glucose as the energy source, myocardial uptake of FDG can be suppressed through dietary manipulation, allowing imaging of the inflamed tissues associated with sarcoidosis.

Indeed, FDG-PET/CT imaging to assess cardiac sarcoidosis has become a routine procedure. Blankstein et al. demonstrated that cardiac PET enhances prognostic assessments of patient with suspected cardiac sarcoidosis [57]. They showed that the presence of focal FDG uptake allows identification of patients who are at higher risk of death or potentially fatal arrhythmias (such as ventricular tachycardia). More recently, it has been shown in a longitudinal cohort that reduction in FDG uptake on serial FDG-PET/CT imaging is associated with improved left ventricular ejection fraction in patients of sarcoidosis [58]. The authors have suggested that serial PET scanning may be useful to guide monitoring and titration of immunosuppressive therapy in patients with sarcoidosis to improve or prevent heart failure. Taken together, an emerging literature suggests a potential clinical role for FDG-PET/CT imaging in the assessment of cardiac sarcoidosis.

FDG-PET/CT imaging has also been used to study the interrelationships between arterial inflammation and the inflammatory processes in other tissues. For example, there has been substantial interest in understanding the potential link between periodontal disease (a common inflammatory disorder of gingiva) and atherosclerosis, since several studies have shown that individuals with periodontal disease are at an increased risk for atherosclerosis. One clinical study showed (using FDG-PET/CT imaging) that periodontal FDG uptake correlates with the extent of carotid atherosclerotic inflammation (by carotid histopathological analysis) [59]. A more recent clinical trial demonstrated that periodontal FDG uptake correlates with alveolar bone loss seen on periodontal CT imaging which is a well-established imaging surrogate for severity of periodontal inflammation. Moreover, that study demonstrated that high-dose atorvastatin therapy results in a reduction in periodontal inflammation and that the improvements in periodontal inflammation closely correlate with improvements in arterial inflammation. Those findings highlight a potentially novel pleiotropic effect of statins and raise the possibility that a portion of the benefit of statins on atherosclerosis may in part be related to their effect on extra-arterial inflammation.

Along similar lines, visceral adiposity is also known to be associated with arterial inflammation as well as an increased risk of atherothrombosis. Studies have shown that the volume of visceral adipose tissue (VAT) is strongly correlated with metabolic risk factors [60]. Other studies evaluated the metabolic activity of VAT. Christen et al. demonstrated that FDG-PET/CT imaging can be used to characterize the biological activity of visceral fatty tissue [61]. They demonstrated that FDG uptake is higher in VAT compared to subcutaneous adipose tissue. Additionally, they showed that FDG uptake in VAT is increased after exposure to TNF-α. Figueroa et al. used FDG-PET/CT imaging to demonstrate that arterial inflammation correlates with the metabolic activity of VAT [62]. Further, they demonstrated that the metabolic activity of VAT (FDG uptake) predicts subsequent risk of cardiovascular disease events. Two groups have recently evaluated the impact of systemic pharmacotherapies on VAT activity. Elkhawad et al. showed that a p38 mitogen-activated protein kinase (p38MAPK) inhibitor reduces the metabolic activity (FDG uptake) in visceral but not subcutaneous adipose tissue (relative to placebo) [63]. Similarly, another study demonstrated that pioglitazone but not glimepiride reduces visceral adipose tissue activity [64]. These studies suggest that imaging of visceral adipose tissue may yield important physiologic insights and provide a pathway to identify potentially fruitful therapeutics.

15.9 FDG-PET/CT Imaging of the Coronary Arteries and Future Directions

Imaging of arterial inflammation has been most commonly performed in the large vascular beds (aorta and carotids arteries). The vast majority of the validation studies have been performed in the carotid circulation, while most of the human arterial FDG-PET/CT imaging trials have focused on the aorta and carotid arteries. Nevertheless, there is substantial interest to use this imaging modality for assessment of atherosclerotic plaque inflammation in the coronary arteries since the majority of myocardial infarctions and sudden cardiac deaths result from the rupture of coronary plaques. However, several factors provide substantial obstacles to performing coronary FDG-PET/CT imaging. Those challenges include (1) the significant motion of the coronary arteries, (2) the relatively small size of coronary plaques, and (3) the high uptake of FDG by adjacent myocardial cells. Despite these limitations, several groups have provided early observations of FDG-PET/CT imaging of coronary plaques.

One of the earliest reports of FDG-PET/CT imaging of coronary arteries was provided by Dunphy et al. In that study, patients with (vs. without) a history of coronary artery disease (CAD) had a fourfold increased likelihood of manifesting high left main coronary FDG uptake [65]. Similarly, Wykrzykowska et al. studied 32 patients with CAD who underwent FDG-PET/CT imaging after active dietary suppression of myocardial FDG uptake (via a low-carbohydrate high-fat meal the night before imaging and administration of a vegetable oil drink in the morning prior to imaging) [66]. In that study, myocardial suppression was adequate in 63 % of the patients, and they identified coronary FDG uptake in roughly half of the patients. In a subsequent study, Rogers et al. performed the first prospective study evaluating coronary FDG uptake after myocardial infarction [67]. In that study, 10 individuals with and 15 subjects without ACS underwent both FDG-PET/CT imaging and coronary angiography. The authors observed higher arterial inflammation (FDG uptake) in association with culprit lesions compared to stable plaques (Fig. 15.14). Furthermore, coronary FDG uptake correlated with C-reactive protein levels. While others have likewise reported higher coronary FDG uptake after acute myocardial infarction [68], not all groups evaluating FDG uptake in the coronary arteries observed increased FDG localization to culprit lesions. Joshi et al. recently evaluated FDG ability to localize to coronary plaques [35]. In that study, no active methods (such as an oil-rich drink or heparin) were used on the day of the study to suppress the myocardial FDG uptake. Unsurprisingly, the authors reported that patchy myocardial uptake affected the majority of vessel territories and thus limited their evaluation of coronary FDG uptake. That study serves as an important reminder that substantial challenges remain for more widespread application of coronary FDG imaging.

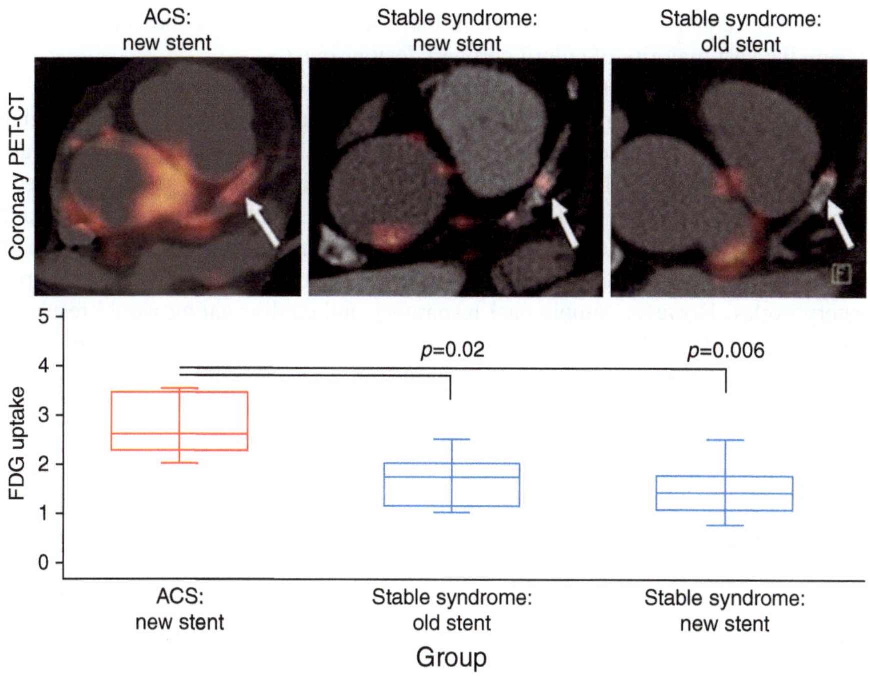

Fig. 15.14 FDG-PET/CT imaging of coronary arteries. *Upper panel* demonstrates three representative images from patients who presented with chest pain syndromes. The *left top panel* represents a patient with an acute coronary syndrome (*ACS*), and the *arrow* points to the stent placement site in the culprit lesion which has a substantial FDG uptake. The *middle top panel* represents a patient with a stable angina who had a stent placement at the culprit lesion. The FDG uptake associated with that lesion is relatively modest. The *right top panel* shows a remotely stented lesion for comparison. The *bottom panels* demonstrate quantitative values for FDG uptake and indicate that the post-ACS patients had higher FDG uptake in association with culprit lesions. The fact that FDG uptake in the stented stable angina group was not higher following the stent placement suggests that the increased FDG uptake in the post-ACS group is not the result of stenting procedure alone, but rather is due to the coronary syndrome (Adapted with permission from Rogers et al. [67])

The challenges notwithstanding, several groups have been investigating the effect of pharmacotherapies on coronary FDG uptake. Nitta et al. recently reported that pioglitazone decreases coronary artery inflammation measured with FDG-PET/CT imaging [69]. They studied 50 individuals with type 2 diabetes or impaired glucose tolerance that were randomized to pioglitazone versus glimepiride daily. The study subjects were imaged with FDG-PET/CT at baseline and 16 weeks after randomization. The authors analyzed the FDG uptake in the left main coronary artery. In that study, they demonstrated that FDG uptake in the coronary artery was substantially reduced in the pioglitazone group compared to the glimepiride group ($p=0.03$). Hence, initial studies suggest that pharmacotherapies with beneficial anti-atherosclerotic properties have the potential to modulate coronary FDG uptake, at least as assessed within the left main coronary artery. No study thus far has reported on changes in FDG uptake in more distal portions of the coronary tree where the vast majority of culprit coronary lesions exist.

More routine and extensive evaluation of coronary plaque inflammation will require several technological advances. Firstly, the challenges caused by substantial coronary motion will need to be overcome. To that end, several groups are investigating techniques to minimize the impact of coronary motion on the blurring of measured tracer activity. The PET images are obtained in List Mode, in which the data are acquired in multiple acquisition frames or bins. Thereafter, those bins are grouped according to external monitoring events based on electrocardiographic and/or respiratory cycles. However, simple dual respiratory and cardiac gating would result in loss of over 80 % of the acquired imaging data and would thus lead to an excessively low target-to-background ratio. Hence, alternative approaches are required to reduce the motion artifact without compromising image quality. One such approach that has been developed is the motion frozen technique [70]. This approach corrects for cardiac motion by tracking the left ventricle through all cardiac phases and then shifts the counts from most phases of the cardiac cycle into the end diastolic position by means of nonlinear image wrapping. Another approach to correct for motion uses the original projection data in a joint motion compensation and reconstruction process [71]. This process, termed Data-domain Cardiac Shape Tracking and Adjustment for Respiration (D-CSTAR), uses analysis of motion by evaluating the CT data to estimate the motion of PET activity and reconstructs the image without discarding any of the acquired PET data bins. Both general approaches have been shown to improve quantification methods, and both are being applied, in the research settings, for coronary PET/CT acquisitions. However, the intensive computing that is required to implement these techniques limits their utility at this time.

Another important advance that may allow for more routine coronary PET imaging is improvements in camera technology. In general, quantification of tracer activity, using PET, is possible due to the unique properties of positron-emitting tracers. A beta particle (positron) emitted from a tracer travels a short distance in tissue before encountering an electron and participating in an annihilation event. This annihilation event leads to the generation of two high-energy photons that are emitted at exactly 180° apart. In standard PET imaging, a detector system looks for photons that are separated by 180° when they are coincidentally (nearly simultaneously) detected by the detector system. Using the concept of coincidental detection, nearly simultaneously detected pairs of photons arriving 180° from one another are accepted as "true events," while non-coincidentally detected photons or those arriving at angles other than 180° apart are rejected (since they might have been subjected to scatter). This thus allows for the generation of a line of response between those two accepted photons to indicate the location of the line of origin of the annihilation event. As more pairs of photons are emitted from that tissue location, several intersecting lines will then pinpoint the origin of the annihilation events and the activity can be quantified. Time of flight (TOF) takes this concept further to additionally improve the quantification of PET signal. The TOF systems are able to not only identify photons that arrive at 180° apart but also to resolve the slight time differences between them. By doing so, the system need not to assume that the photons were admitted along a single line, but instead will calculate the difference in the time of flight between the two photons and derive a more precise location for where the photons were initially generated. Hence, TOF allows for even more precise quantification of PET activity. As TOF technology improves, quantification of PET signal will continue to improve as well.

Two additional advances that may expedite the development of coronary PET imaging are advances in PET/MR technologies and development of novel tracers. PET/MR is currently becoming widely available and provides new opportunities and challenges for evaluating the coronary tree. While MR is generally less well suited for coronary imaging compared to CT (due to its reduced temporal and spatial resolution), MR does provide certain advantages. One such advantage is that the MR acquisition may be derived simultaneously to the PET. Hence theoretically, attenuation correction (AC) algorithms that use MR data to correct the PET data may be superior to those derived from CT. The net impact on coronary PET imaging of MR-derived AC (relative to CT-based AC) is still under investigation.

Improvements in tracer technology may provide the most impactful advance in arterial PET/CT imaging. Several novel tracers targeting inflammation are currently under development. One such tracers (studied in clinical trials) targets the benzodiazepine receptors (which is upregulated in inflamed tissues) [72]. Another tracer which has been tested in preclinical models targets the adenosine receptor (which is also richly expressed in inflamed tissues) [73]. Moreover, novel tracers have been developed to differentially target M2-polarized (vs. M1-polarized) macrophages. One such tracer, F18 radiolabeled fluorodeoxymannose (FDM), targets the mannose receptor, which is highly expressed in M2-polarized macrophages [74]. It should be noted, however, that none of the tracers targeting inflammation are currently FDA approved, with the exception of FDG. Nonetheless, the eventual development and approval of tracers targeting inflammation may prove to be transformative for imaging atherosclerosis and in particular for imaging of coronary inflammation.

Conclusion

Measuring arterial inflammation is feasible using FDG-PET/CT imaging. The approach has been shown to correlate well with plaque inflammation in humans, is reproducible, and is rapidly modifiable by anti-inflammatory interventions. However, several obstacles limit application of PET imaging to the coronary arteries. Improvements in camera technologies, in reconstruction methods, and in novel tracers may provide a means to overcome these obstacles. Nonetheless, currently feasible assessment of large arterial inflammation (aorta and carotids) has been shown to enhance assessment of clinical risk, provide a better understanding of therapeutic efficacy of novel drugs, and may provide a window into inflammation within the coronary tree.

References

1. Falk E, Shah PK, Fuster V. Coronary plaque disruption. Circulation. 1995;92(3):657–71.
2. Sanz J, Fayad ZA. Imaging of atherosclerotic cardiovascular disease. Nature. 2008;451(7181): 953–7.

3. Lardinois D, Weder W, Hany TF, Kamel EM, Korom S, Seifert B, et al. Staging of non-small-cell lung cancer with integrated positron-emission tomography and computed tomography. N Engl J Med. 2003;348(25):2500–7.
4. Antoch G, Vogt FM, Freudenberg LS, Nazaradeh F, Goehde SC, Barkhausen J, et al. Whole-body dual-modality PET/CT and whole-body MRI for tumor staging in oncology. JAMA. 2003;290(24):3199–206.
5. Motoyama S, Sarai M, Harigaya H, Anno H, Inoue K, Hara T, et al. Computed tomographic angiography characteristics of atherosclerotic plaques subsequently resulting in acute coronary syndrome. J Am Coll Cardiol. 2009;54(1):49–57.
6. Kitagawa T, Yamamoto H, Horiguchi J, Ohhashi N, Tadehara F, Shokawa T, et al. Characterization of noncalcified coronary plaques and identification of culprit lesions in patients with acute coronary syndrome by 64-slice computed tomography. JACC Cardiovasc Imaging. 2009;2(2):153–60.
7. Libby P. Inflammation in atherosclerosis. Nature. 2002;420(6917):868–74.
8. Dutta P, Courties G, Wei Y, Leuschner F, Gorbatov R, Robbins CS, et al. Myocardial infarction accelerates atherosclerosis. Nature. 2012;487(7407):325–9.
9. Kubota R, Kubota K, Yamada S, Tada M, Ido T, Tamahashi N. Microautoradiographic study for the differentiation of intratumoral macrophages, granulation tissues and cancer cells by the dynamics of fluorine-18-fluorodeoxyglucose uptake. J Nucl Med. 1994;35(1):104–12.
10. Rodriguez-Prados JC, Traves PG, Cuenca J, Rico D, Aragones J, Martin-Sanz P, et al. Substrate fate in activated macrophages: a comparison between innate, classic, and alternative activation. J Immunol. 2010;185(1):605–14.
11. Fleischmann W, Kubowitz F. Über den Stoffwechsel der Leukocyten. Biochem Z. 1927;181:385.
12. Garedew A, Henderson SO, Moncada S. Activated macrophages utilize glycolytic ATP to maintain mitochondrial membrane potential and prevent apoptotic cell death. Cell Death Differ. 2010;17(10):1540–50.
13. Rodriguez-Prados JC, Traves PG, Cuenca J, Rico D, Aragones J, Martin-Sanz P, et al. Substrate fate in activated macrophages: a comparison between innate, classic, and alternative activation. J Immunol. 2010;185(1):605–14.
14. Satomi T, Ogawa M, Mori I, Ishino S, Kubo K, Magata Y, et al. Comparison of contrast agents for atherosclerosis imaging using cultured macrophages: FDG versus ultrasmall superparamagnetic iron oxide. J Nucl Med. 2013;54(6):999–1004.
15. Rudd JH, Narula J, Strauss HW, Virmani R, Machac J, Klimas M, et al. Imaging atherosclerotic plaque inflammation by fluorodeoxyglucose with positron emission tomography: ready for prime time? J Am Coll Cardiol. 2010;55(23):2527–35.
16. Folco EJ, Sheikine Y, Rocha VZ, Christen T, Shvartz E, Sukhova GK, et al. Hypoxia but not inflammation augments glucose uptake in human macrophages: implications for imaging atherosclerosis with 18fluorine-labeled 2-deoxy-D-glucose positron emission tomography. J Am Coll Cardiol. 2011;58(6):603–14.
17. Eltzschig HK, Carmeliet P. Hypoxia and inflammation. N Engl J Med. 2011;364(7):656–65.
18. Singh P, Tawakol A, Mojena M, Pimentel-Santillana M, Emami H, Vucic E, et al. Close interrelationship between macrophage pro-inflammatory activation and energy metabolism in an atherosclerotic environment. Meeting of American Heart Association, Dallas. 2013.
19. Jamar F, Buscombe J, Chiti A, Christian PE, Delbeke D, Donohoe KJ, et al. EANM/SNMMI guideline for 18F-FDG use in inflammation and infection. J Nucl Med. 2013;54(4):647–58.
20. Glaudemans AW, de Vries EF, Galli F, Dierckx RA, Slart RH, Signore A. The use of (18) F-FDG-PET/CT for diagnosis and treatment monitoring of inflammatory and infectious diseases. Clin Dev Immunol. 2013;2013:623036.
21. Rudd JH, Warburton EA, Fryer TD, Jones HA, Clark JC, Antoun N, et al. Imaging atherosclerotic plaque inflammation with [18F]-fluorodeoxyglucose positron emission tomography. Circulation. 2002;105(23):2708–11.
22. Tawakol A, Migrino RQ, Hoffmann U, Abbara S, Houser S, Gewirtz H, et al. Noninvasive in vivo measurement of vascular inflammation with F-18 fluorodeoxyglucose positron emission tomography. J Nucl Cardiol. 2005;12(3):294–301.

23. Hyafil F, Cornily JC, Rudd JH, Machac J, Feldman LJ, Fayad ZA. Quantification of inflammation within rabbit atherosclerotic plaques using the macrophage-specific CT contrast agent N1177: a comparison with 18F-FDG PET/CT and histology. J Nucl Med. 2009;50(6):959–65.
24. Tawakol A, Migrino RQ, Bashian GG, Bedri S, Vermylen D, Cury RC, et al. In vivo 18F-fluorodeoxyglucose positron emission tomography imaging provides a noninvasive measure of carotid plaque inflammation in patients. J Am Coll Cardiol. 2006;48(9):1818–24.
25. Pedersen SF, Graebe M, Fisker Hag AM, Hojgaard L, Sillesen H, Kjaer A. Gene expression and 18FDG uptake in atherosclerotic carotid plaques. Nucl Med Commun. 2010;31(5):423–9.
26. Graebe M, Pedersen SF, Borgwardt L, Hojgaard L, Sillesen H, Kjaer A. Molecular pathology in vulnerable carotid plaques: correlation with [18]-fluorodeoxyglucose positron emission tomography (FDG-PET). Eur J Vasc Endovasc Surg. 2009;37(6):714–21.
27. Figueroa AL, Subramanian SS, Cury RC, Truong QA, Gardecki JA, Tearney GJ, et al. Distribution of inflammation within carotid atherosclerotic plaques with high-risk morphological features: a comparison between positron emission tomography activity, plaque morphology, and histopathology. Circ Cardiovasc Imaging. 2012;5(1):69–77.
28. Abdelbaky A, Corsini E, Figueroa AL, Fontanez S, Subramanian S, Ferencik M, et al. Focal arterial inflammation precedes subsequent calcification in the same location: a longitudinal FDG-PET/CT study. Circ Cardiovasc Imaging. 2013;6(5):747–54.
29. Fayad ZA, Mani V, Woodward M, Kallend D, Abt M, Burgess T, et al. Safety and efficacy of dalcetrapib on atherosclerotic disease using novel non-invasive multimodality imaging (dal-PLAQUE): a randomised clinical trial. Lancet. 2011;378(9802):1547–59.
30. Rominger A, Saam T, Wolpers S, Cyran CC, Schmidt M, Foerster S, et al. 18F-FDG PET/CT identifies patients at risk for future vascular events in an otherwise asymptomatic cohort with neoplastic disease. J Nucl Med. 2009;50(10):1611–20.
31. Kim TN, Kim S, Yang SJ, Yoo HJ, Seo JA, Kim SG, et al. Vascular inflammation in patients with impaired glucose tolerance and type 2 diabetes: analysis with 18F-fluorodeoxyglucose positron emission tomography. Circ Cardiovasc Imaging. 2010;3(2):142–8.
32. Figueroa AL, Abdelbaky A, Truong QA, Corsini E, MacNabb MH, Lavender ZR, et al. Measurement of arterial activity on routine FDG PET/CT images improves prediction of risk of future CV events. JACC Cardiovasc Imaging. 2013;6(12):1250–9.
33. Marnane M, Merwick A, Sheehan OC, Hannon N, Foran P, Grant T, et al. Carotid plaque inflammation on 18F-fluorodeoxyglucose positron emission tomography predicts early stroke recurrence. Ann Neurol. 2012;71(5):709–18.
34. Detrano R, Guerci AD, Carr JJ, Bild DE, Burke G, Folsom AR, et al. Coronary calcium as a predictor of coronary events in four racial or ethnic groups. N Engl J Med. 2008;358(13):1336–45.
35. Joshi NV, Vesey AT, Williams MC, Shah AS, Calvert PA, Craighead FH, et al. 18F-fluoride positron emission tomography for identification of ruptured and high-risk coronary atherosclerotic plaques: a prospective clinical trial. Lancet. 2014;383(9918):705–13.
36. Dweck MR, Jenkins WS, Vesey AT, Pringle MA, Chin CW, Malley TS, et al. 18F-sodium fluoride uptake is a marker of active calcification and disease progression in patients with aortic stenosis. Circ Cardiovasc Imaging. 2014;7(2):371–8.
37. Lobatto ME, Fayad ZA, Silvera S, Vucic E, Calcagno C, Mani V, et al. Multimodal clinical imaging to longitudinally assess a nanomedical anti-inflammatory treatment in experimental atherosclerosis. Mol Pharm. 2010;7(6):2020–9.
38. Singh P, Tawakol A, Mojena M, Pimentel-Santillana M, Fayad Z, Rudd J, et al. GM-CSF enhances glycolytic activity in macrophages in vitro and improves detection of atherosclerotic inflammation in vivo. San Francisco: Meeting of American College of Cardiology; 2013.
39. Rudd JH, Myers KS, Bansilal S, Machac J, Pinto CA, Tong C, et al. Atherosclerosis inflammation imaging with 18F-FDG PET: carotid, iliac, and femoral uptake reproducibility, quantification methods, and recommendations. J Nucl Med. 2008;49(6):871–8.
40. Tahara N, Kai H, Ishibashi M, Nakaura H, Kaida H, Baba K, et al. Simvastatin attenuates plaque inflammation: evaluation by fluorodeoxyglucose positron emission tomography. J Am Coll Cardiol. 2006;48(9):1825–31.

41. Tawakol A, Fayad ZA, Mogg R, Alon A, Klimas MT, Dansky H, et al. Intensification of statin therapy results in a rapid reduction in atherosclerotic inflammation: results of a multicenter fluorodeoxyglucose-positron emission tomography/computed tomography feasibility study. J Am Coll Cardiol. 2013;62(10):909–17.
42. van Wijk D, Sjouke B, Figueroa A, Emami H, van der Valk F, MacNabb H, et al. Non-pharmacologic lipoprotein apheresis reduces arterial inflammation in patients with familial hypercholesterolemia: a pilot study. J Am Coll. Cardiol. 2014 (in press).
43. Mizoguchi M, Tahara N, Tahara A, Nitta Y, Kodama N, Oba T, et al. Pioglitazone attenuates atherosclerotic plaque inflammation in patients with impaired glucose tolerance or diabetes a prospective, randomized, comparator-controlled study using serial FDG PET/CT imaging study of carotid artery and ascending aorta. JACC Cardiovasc Imaging. 2011;4(10):1110–8.
44. Erdmann E, Dormandy JA, Charbonnel B, Massi-Benedetti M, Moules IK, Skene AM. The effect of pioglitazone on recurrent myocardial infarction in 2,445 patients with type 2 diabetes and previous myocardial infarction: results from the PROactive (PROactive 05) Study. J Am Coll Cardiol. 2007;49(17):1772–80.
45. Dormandy JA, Charbonnel B, Eckland DJ, Erdmann E, Massi-Benedetti M, Moules IK, et al. Secondary prevention of macrovascular events in patients with type 2 diabetes in the PROactive Study (PROspective pioglitAzone Clinical Trial In macroVascular Events): a randomised controlled trial. Lancet. 2005;366(9493):1279–89.
46. Schwartz GG, Olsson AG, Abt M, Ballantyne CM, Barter PJ, Brumm J, et al. Effects of dalcetrapib in patients with a recent acute coronary syndrome. N Engl J Med. 2012;367(22): 2089–99.
47. White HD, Held C, Stewart R, Tarka E, Brown R, Davies RY, et al. Darapladib for preventing ischemic events in stable coronary heart disease. N Engl J Med. 2014;370(18):1702–11.
48. Coulson JM, Rudd JH, Duckers JM, Rees JI, Shale DJ, Bolton CE, et al. Excessive aortic inflammation in chronic obstructive pulmonary disease: an 18F-FDG PET pilot study. J Nucl Med. 2010;51(9):1357–60.
49. Vijayakumar J, Subramanian S, Singh P, Corsini E, Fontanez S, Lawler M, et al. Arterial inflammation in bronchial asthma. J Nucl Cardiol. 2013;20(3):385–95.
50. Emami H, Vijayakumar J, Subramanian S, Vucic E, Singh P, MacNabb M, et al. Arterial inflammation in rheumatoid arthritis correlates with joint inflammation. Meeting of American Heart Association, Dallas. 2013.
51. Maki-Petaja KM, Elkhawad M, Cheriyan J, Joshi FR, Ostor AJ, Hall FC, et al. Anti-tumor necrosis factor-alpha therapy reduces aortic inflammation and stiffness in patients with rheumatoid arthritis. Circulation. 2012;126(21):2473–80.
52. Mehta N, Reilly M. Atherosclerotic cardiovascular disease risk in the HAART-treated HIV-1 population. HIV Clin Trials. 2005;6(1):5–24.
53. Rasmussen LD, Engsig FN, Christensen H, Gerstoft J, Kronborg G, Pedersen C, et al. Risk of cerebrovascular events in persons with and without HIV: a Danish nationwide population-based cohort study. AIDS (London, England). 2011;25(13):1637–46.
54. Subramanian S, Tawakol A, Burdo TH, Abbara S, Wei J, Vijayakumar J, et al. Arterial inflammation in patients with HIV. JAMA. 2012;308(4):379–86.
55. Tawakol A, Lo J, Zanni MV, Marmarelis E, Ihenachor EJ, MacNabb M, et al. Increased arterial inflammation relates to high-risk coronary plaque morphology in HIV-infected patients. J Acquir Immune Defic Syndr. 2014;66(2):164–71.
56. Lee WW, Marinelli B, van der Laan AM, Sena BF, Gorbatov R, Leuschner F, et al. PET/MRI of inflammation in myocardial infarction. J Am Coll Cardiol. 2012;59(2):153–63.
57. Blankstein R, Osborne M, Naya M, Waller A, Kim CK, Murthy VL, et al. Cardiac positron emission tomography enhances prognostic assessments of patients with suspected cardiac sarcoidosis. J Am Coll Cardiol. 2014;63(4):329–36.
58. Osborne MT, Hulten EA, Singh A, Waller AH, Bittencourt MS, Stewart GC, et al. Reduction in (18)F-fluorodeoxyglucose uptake on serial cardiac positron emission tomography is associated with improved left ventricular ejection fraction in patients with cardiac sarcoidosis. J Nucl Cardiol. 2014;21(1):166–74.

59. Fifer KM, Qadir S, Subramanian S, Vijayakumar J, Figueroa AL, Truong QA, et al. Positron emission tomography measurement of periodontal 18F-fluorodeoxyglucose uptake is associated with histologically determined carotid plaque inflammation. J Am Coll Cardiol. 2011;57(8):971–6.
60. Fox CS, Massaro JM, Hoffmann U, Pou KM, Maurovich-Horvat P, Liu CY, et al. Abdominal visceral and subcutaneous adipose tissue compartments: association with metabolic risk factors in the Framingham Heart Study. Circulation. 2007;116(1):39–48.
61. Christen T, Sheikine Y, Rocha VZ, Hurwitz S, Goldfine AB, Di Carli M, et al. Increased glucose uptake in visceral versus subcutaneous adipose tissue revealed by PET imaging. JACC Cardiovasc Imaging. 2010;3(8):843–51.
62. Figueroa AL, MacNabb M, Abdelbaky A, Corsini E, Lavender Z, Kaplan R, et al. Visceral adipose tissue activity independently predicts the risk of future cardiovascular events. Meeting of American Heart Association, Dallas. 2013.
63. Elkhawad M, Rudd JH, Sarov-Blat L, Cai G, Wells R, Davies LC, et al. Effects of p38 mitogen-activated protein kinase inhibition on vascular and systemic inflammation in patients with atherosclerosis. JACC Cardiovasc Imaging. 2012;5(9):911–22.
64. Kodama N, Tahara N, Tahara A, Honda A, Nitta Y, Mizoguchi M, et al. Effects of pioglitazone on visceral fat metabolic activity in impaired glucose tolerance or type 2 diabetes mellitus. J Clin Endocrinol Metab. 2013;98(11):4438–45.
65. Dunphy MP, Freiman A, Larson SM, Strauss HW. Association of vascular 18F-FDG uptake with vascular calcification. J Nucl Med. 2005;46(8):1278–84.
66. Wykrzykowska J, Lehman S, Williams G, Parker JA, Palmer MR, Varkey S, et al. Imaging of inflamed and vulnerable plaque in coronary arteries with 18F-FDG PET/CT in patients with suppression of myocardial uptake using a low-carbohydrate, high-fat preparation. J Nucl Med. 2009;50(4):563–8.
67. Rogers IS, Nasir K, Figueroa AL, Cury RC, Hoffmann U, Vermylen DA, et al. Feasibility of FDG imaging of the coronary arteries: comparison between acute coronary syndrome and stable angina. JACC Cardiovasc Imaging. 2010;3(4):388–97.
68. Cheng VY, Slomka PJ, Le Meunier L, Tamarappoo BK, Nakazato R, Dey D, et al. Coronary arterial 18F-FDG uptake by fusion of PET and coronary CT angiography at sites of percutaneous stenting for acute myocardial infarction and stable coronary artery disease. J Nucl Med. 2012;53(4):575–83.
69. Nitta Y, Tahara N, Tahara A, Honda A, Kodama N, Mizoguchi M, et al. Pioglitazone decreases coronary artery inflammation in impaired glucose tolerance and diabetes mellitus: evaluation by FDG-PET/CT imaging. JACC Cardiovasc Imaging. 2013;6(11):1172–82.
70. Suzuki Y, Slomka PJ, Wolak A, Ohba M, Suzuki S, De Yang L, et al. Motion-frozen myocardial perfusion SPECT improves detection of coronary artery disease in obese patients. J Nucl Med. 2008;49(7):1075–9.
71. Ambwani S. Joint cardiac and respiratory motion correction and super resolution reconstruction in coronary PET/CT. International symposium on biomedical imaging, Chicago. 2011.
72. Cuhlmann S, Gsell W, Van der Heiden K, Habib J, Tremoleda JL, Khalil M, et al. In vivo mapping of vascular inflammation using the translocator protein tracer 18F-FEDAA1106. Mol Imaging. 2014;13(0):1–10.
73. Elmaleh DR, Fischman AJ, Tawakol A, Zhu A, Shoup TM, Hoffmann U, et al. Detection of inflamed atherosclerotic lesions with diadenosine-5′,5′′′-P1, P4-tetraphosphate (Ap4A) and positron-emission tomography. Proc Natl Acad Sci U S A. 2006;103(43):15992–6.
74. Tahara N, Mukherjee J, de Haas HJ, Petrov AD, Tawakol A, Haider N, et al. 2-deoxy-2-[18F]fluoro-D-mannose positron emission tomography imaging in atherosclerosis. Nat Med. 2014;20(2):215–9.

Clinical Feasibility and Monitoring of the Effects of Anti-inflammatory Therapy in Atherosclerosis

16

Nobuhiro Tahara, Atsuko Tahara, and Sho-ichi Yamagishi

Contents

Abstract

Atherosclerosis and its thrombotic complications represent the major cause of morbidity and mortality of cardiovascular disease. The composition of atherosclerotic plaques rather than the degree of arterial stenosis has been linked to an increased risk of plaque rupture and subsequent acute clinical events associated with atherosclerotic cardiovascular disease. Vulnerable plaques have a large

N. Tahara, MD, PhD (✉) • A. Tahara, MD
Division of Cardiovascular Medicine, Department of Medicine,
Kurume University School of Medicine, Kurume, Japan
e-mail: ntahara@med.kurume-u.ac.jp

S.-i. Yamagishi, MD, PhD
Department of Pathophysiology and Therapeutics of Diabetic Vascular Complications,
Kurume University School of Medicine, Kurume, Japan

E. Aikawa (ed.), *Cardiovascular Imaging: Arterial and Aortic Valve Inflammation and Calcification*, DOI 10.1007/978-3-319-09268-3_16

lipid-rich necrotic core, a thin-fibrous cap, and numerous inflammatory and immune cells. Above all, macrophage activation plays a central role in vascular inflammation and plaque instability within the atherosclerosis. However, we have yet to clinically demonstrate vascular inflammation in atherosclerosis assessed by computed tomography angiography, magnetic resonance imaging, intravascular ultrasound, and optical coherence tomography. Molecular imaging is the tool best suited for identifying metabolically active macrophages. Positron-emission tomography (PET) imaging with ^{18}F-fluorodeoxyglucose (FDG) is capable of identifying and quantifying vascular inflammation characterized by macrophage activation within the atherosclerotic plaques. FDG-PET might be a feasible clinical tool for detecting vulnerable plaques and evaluating the efficacy of drugs in plaque instability. We would like to review the clinical utility of FDG-PET imaging in identifying patients at risk of plaque rupture and resultantly prone to cardiovascular disease.

16.1 Introduction

The composition of atherosclerotic plaques has been linked to an increased risk of plaque rupture and subsequent acute clinical events associated with atherosclerotic cardiovascular disease (CVD) [1]. Atherosclerotic CVD has been attributed to the subendothelial accumulation of lipids with oxidative, inflammatory, and immune reactions [2–6]. Evidence suggests that atherosclerosis is intrinsically an inflammatory disease [2–6]; therefore, local inflammation could be a surrogate marker to predict future cardiovascular events [7]. However, we have yet to clinically demonstrate that vascular inflammation in atherosclerosis plays a crucial role in cardiovascular events. X-ray contrast angiography is one of the gold standard imaging techniques that is used to evaluate atherosclerosis as well as the severity of luminal stenosis in arteries; however, it cannot provide information on the compositional characteristics of atherosclerotic plaques. Atherosclerotic plaques have been morphologically assessed using various noninvasive modalities including ultrasound, computed tomography (CT), and magnetic resonance imaging (MRI). Additional information has been obtained on plaque volume, plaque composition, or the thickness of the fibrous cap using invasive intravascular ultrasound (IVUS), IVUS-virtual histology, and optical coherence tomography (OCT) [8–11]. The imaging modalities used to evaluate therapeutic efficacy, such as measurements of carotid intima-media thickness (IMT) by ultrasound [12, 13], coronary plaque volume by IVUS [14, 15], and the thickness of the coronary fibrous cap by OCT [16], are also in clinical use.

Molecular imaging will provide further insights into atherosclerosis and lead to the development of novel clinical applications. Atherosclerotic plaque activity can be directly visualized using positron-emission tomography (PET). PET with ^{18}F-fluorodeoxyglucose (FDG), which measures inflammatory activity based on the metabolism of glucose, has been employed to noninvasively qualify and quantify plaque inflammation instead of plaque morphology [17–19]. FDG-PET can also detect changes in the metabolism of glucose in response to therapeutic interventions before the morphology of the plaque is altered [20] and has been used in multicenter clinical trials [21, 22]. In this chapter, we described the clinical feasibility and monitoring of the effects of anti-inflammatory therapy in atherosclerosis with a noninvasive imaging modality using FDG-PET.

16.2 Vulnerable Plaques

Atherosclerotic CVD is the leading cause of mortality and morbidity in the western world [23, 24]. In spite of major advances in the treatment of patients with CVD, a large number of apparently healthy subjects die suddenly due to cardiovascular events without prior symptoms [25, 26]. Previous studies reported that severe stenotic lesions detected by angiography were not necessarily the culprit lesions for atherosclerotic CVD [27, 28]. This discrepancy between the degree of stenosis and clinical outcomes was initially revealed by X-ray contrast angiography [27, 28] and illustrated by randomized controlled trials with 3-hydroxy-3-methylglutaryl-coenzyme A (HMG-CoA) reductase inhibitors (statins), which have been shown to markedly reduce acute cardiovascular events [29], but modestly improve stenosis [30–32].

The cellular structures within atherosclerotic plaques include smooth muscle cells, a collagen matrix, and endothelial cells that line the lumen and exist within the normal arterial wall. Other components include monocyte-derived macrophages, lymphocytes, mast cells, neutrophils, red blood cells, and platelets derived from the circulation. Atherosclerosis is initiated after blood monocytes and T lymphocytes are attracted to oxidized low-density lipoprotein (LDL) within the vessel wall. The expression of vascular cell adhesion molecule-1 (VCAM-1) and E- and P-selectins by the endothelium allows LDL to adhere to and enter the subendothelial space. Monocytes subsequently differentiate into mature macrophages, ingest excessively oxidized LDL, and become cholesterol-enriched foam cells. Smooth muscle cells promote proliferation, which enlarged the atherosclerotic lesion. Inflammatory cytokines such as interleukins, tumor necrosis factor-alpha (TNF-α), and monocyte chemotactic protein-1 (MCP-1) by foam cells and lymphocytes are released during chronic vascular inflammation. Interferon-gamma, which is secreted by T lymphocytes, inhibits the production of collagen by smooth muscle cells, while matrix metalloproteinases (MMPs), which are secreted by macrophages, directly degrade and thin the fibrous cap. Activated macrophages and inflammation induce necrosis in foam cells during the progression of atherosclerotic lesions. Some macrophage foam cells and smooth muscle cells can undergo apoptosis, which leads to the formation of a lipid-rich core. A larger lipid-rich core within a plaque and thinner fibrous cap are more prone to rupture. Coagulation factors also contribute through the development of atherothrombotic cardiovascular events.

A consensus has defined a number of criteria to diagnose vulnerable plaques in order to identify healthy subjects at risk of future cardiovascular events [26]. An atherosclerotic plaque, characterized by a lipid-rich necrotic core covered by a thin fibrous cap with macrophage-dense inflammation, is considered to be more prone to rupture [1, 25, 26]. Cardiovascular events are frequently initiated by a sudden rupture of a vulnerable plaque linked to an inflammatory process and result in either subsequent thrombotic occlusion at the site of rupture or distal embolization [33].

A complex cascade of CVD mechanisms is known to result in the transformation of a stable plaque into a vulnerable plaque that is prone to rupture. Vulnerable plaques also consist of inflammatory and immune cells that release cytokines and other effector molecules. Immune reactions have been shown to accelerate the progression of inflammatory activity in atherosclerotic lesions [34]. Previous studies demonstrated that activated macrophages played a key role in plaque rupture and the subsequent formation of thrombosis in atherosclerosis [1, 3, 25, 26, 35]. Atherosclerotic CVD has recently been recognized as an inflammatory process within the arterial wall.

16.3 Molecular Imaging

A vulnerable plaque often possesses a large lipid-rich necrotic core, a thin fibrous cap, and macrophage-dense inflammation [1, 25, 26]. Although the risk of rupture is higher for vulnerable plaques, there are currently no specific markers to identify them. High-risk plaques are often characterized by large necrotic core volumes, positive vascular remodeling, and the attenuation of fibrous caps using ultrasound, CT, MRI, IVUS, and OCT [10, 36, 37]. The remaining obligatory component of plaque vulnerability is inflammation, which cannot be visualized in a clinical setting.

Molecular imaging using single-photon emission computed tomography (SPECT) or positron-emission tomography (PET) has the potential to provide quantitative information regarding the specific biological aspects of developing atherosclerotic lesions. This requires the generation of highly specific plaque tracers. SPECT ligands designed to probe the various processes associated with atherosclerosis progression and rupture have been manufactured and applied for use in experimental and human studies [38]. These molecular approaches have employed radiolabeled autologous leukocytes [39], LDL [40, 41], and the Fc fragments of immunoglobulin [42] to target the scavenger receptor function of macrophages. More recent studies have employed the radiolabeled ligands of cytokine and adhesion molecules such as MCP-1 [43, 44], VCAM-1 [45], and MMPs to evaluate plaque instability [46]. Furthermore, radiolabeled arginine-glycine-aspartate peptides that target integrin $\alpha v\beta 3$ for angiogenesis [47, 48] and monoclonal antifibrin antibodies for thrombogenicity have also been applied to assess plaque vulnerability [49].

The molecular targeting approaches used to identify metabolically activated macrophages and plaque inflammation have recently been employed with varying degrees of success. FDG-PET imaging in particular has found an application in the detection of inflammatory lesions and has potential clinical utilities. FDG is a glucose analogue that is taken up by cells at the same rate as glucose and is phosphorylated by hexokinase, which prevents its return to the circulation. Once inside the cell, phosphorylated FDG is taken up by metabolic trapping through the glycolysis pathway [20]. Therefore, the uptake of FDG by cells is interpreted as a measure of metabolic activity. FDG-PET has recently confirmed the clinical feasibility of imaging in detecting vulnerable plaques [17–19]. The rationale behind the uptake of FDG for identifying vulnerable plaques is metabolic activity within the atherosclerotic plaque, which reflects the activity of macrophages [20]. Previous studies demonstrated that the uptake of FDG by macrophage-rich plaques was high [17, 18]. Another very recent ex vivo study demonstrated that hypoxia also augmented the uptake of FDG by human macrophages in atherosclerotic plaques [50]. Furthermore, FDG-PET can be used to visualize the early stage of foam cell formation due to changes in hexokinase activity within vulnerable plaques [51].

16.4 Vascular FDG-PET Imaging for Clinical Feasibility

FDG-PET was first used to examine atherosclerosis in patients with recent carotid-territory transient ischemic attack who were scheduled to undergo carotid endarterectomy [17]. The uptake of FDG by the symptomatic carotid artery was significantly higher than that in the contralateral asymptomatic artery, and autoradiography of excised plaques confirmed the accumulation of deoxyglucose and dense macrophages within the lesions [17]. In other studies, FDG activity in the carotid plaques was correlated with the intensity of macrophage staining from the corresponding histological section [18] and gene expression levels of markers for atherosclerotic plaque vulnerability [52]. FDG activity has not been correlated with plaque area, plaque thickness, or smooth muscle cell staining [18]. Hence, FDG activity can reveal the bioactivity of plaque inflammation associated with atherosclerosis.

16.5 FDG-Verified High-Risk Plaques

Atherosclerotic plaques that contain numerous inflammatory cells are at a higher risk of rupture [53]. FDG accumulates in macrophage-rich areas within atherosclerotic plaques [17, 18]; therefore, we have been able to noninvasively qualify and quantify plaque inflammation with FDG-PET. Evidence to show the relationship between vascular FDG activity with cardiovascular risk factors [54–58] and circulating inflammatory and thrombogenic biomarkers [59–65] is accumulating.

To the best of our knowledge, no clinically available imaging technique can completely evaluate plaque vulnerability within atherosclerotic lesions; hence, an increase in the activity of vascular FDG may emerge as the strongest predictor of a subsequent vascular event in oncologic patients [66–68] as well as in patients free of cancer [69]. Because the annual rate of cardiovascular events is relatively low in patients with subclinical atherosclerosis, future prospective trials with a large population need to be conducted in order to establish whether a decrease in vascular inflammation evaluated by FDG-PET in response to therapeutic interventions translates into a reduced risk of cardiovascular events.

The degree of plaque inflammation may be a promising biomarker for plaque vulnerability, the risk of plaque rupture, and subsequent cardiovascular events [25]. Thus, the presence of FDG-verified high-risk plaques may be a predictor of future cardiovascular events. Diagnostic modalities indicating plaque vulnerability may be of importance to expedite clinical applications. Because of its recent wide availability for clinical use, FDG-PET is a very attractive candidate for biological vascular imaging.

16.6 Efficacy of Drugs in the Treatment of Atherosclerosis

An assessment of vascular vessel wall changes defined by various imaging modalities may enhance understanding of the natural history and pathophysiological mechanisms of atherosclerosis. This would allow for a better risk stratification of atherosclerotic CVD, the identification of patients at risk and follow-up, and the selection of appropriate therapeutic strategies [70]. A number of invasive and non-invasive imaging modalities have been used clinically to detect the various features of atherosclerotic plaques. Conventional X-ray contrast angiographic images can detect the diameter of the lumen and stenosis, while other modalities can measure vessel wall thickness, plaque volume, and plaque characteristics. The inflammatory state and composition of atherosclerotic plaques, rather than the severity of stenosis, are currently recognized as the major contributing factors for acute cardiovascular events. Hence, the resolution of inflammation and reductions in necrotic core volumes has been associated with plaque stabilization and is the main target for the treatment of vulnerable plaques. The stabilization of atherosclerotic lesions, rather than percutaneous interventions or surgical procedures, provides a new therapeutic target. The development and validation of plaque-stabilizing therapies is one of the major challenges for most pharmaceutical industries but is hampered by the lack of surrogate markers to prove the efficacy of treatments for plaque instability.

16.6.1 HMG-CoA Reductase Inhibitors (Statins)

An elevated serum cholesterol level is a modifiable risk factor that significantly contributes to the risk of cardiovascular events [71]. Statins represent a powerful therapeutic option for lowering cholesterol and preventing major adverse cardiovascular events [72]. Medications that have been shown to be beneficial for plaque stabilization consist of statins. Statins act primarily to lower plasma LDL cholesterol (LDL-C) levels [73, 74]. Evidence to suggest that statins have beneficial effects on atherosclerotic disease progression in both animal models and humans is increasing [73, 74]. Previous randomized clinical trials demonstrated that statins reduced atherogenic lipoproteins, as well as cardiovascular morbidity and mortality in humans [72]. Statins may contribute to plaque stabilization via several different mechanisms (pleiotropic effects), including changes in plaque composition, the attenuation of inflammatory and immune responses, decreased thrombogenicity, and improvements in endothelial dysfunction. Previous studies reported that statins could alter the composition of plaques without necessarily impacting on their size or stenosis [29–32].

One of the underlying mechanisms involves an alteration in the composition of plaques by depleting plaque lipids, particularly the cholesterol ester. Lipid depletion and removal of the cholesterol ester from soft plaques with a concomitant increase in cholesterol monohydrate crystals may increase the mechanical strength of these plaques. Statins have also been shown to reduce inflammatory mediators and inflammatory cell activity, including the number of macrophage-rich foam cells [75]. C-reactive protein (CRP) has emerged as an important predictor and potential contributor to future cardiovascular events [76]. A previous study showed that statins reduced the levels of high-sensitivity CRP [2] and other inflammatory biomarkers [77]. In the Cholesterol and Recurrent Events (CARE) trial, a direct relationship was found between the degree of risk reduction and baseline values of CRP [78]. Pravastatin resulted in a higher relative risk reduction in coronary artery disease (CAD) in patients with elevated serum CRP than in those without elevated serum CRP [78]. Statins are also known to prevent the oxidation of LDL and consequently reduce the avidity with which macrophages ingest oxidized LDL, possibly through preserving the endogenous antioxidant superoxide dismutase [79]. Statins have also been shown to decrease the vascular expression of adhesion molecules, monocyte expression, and monocyte adhesion in hypercholesterolemic patients [80]. These anti-inflammatory properties of statins may be attributed to improvements in endothelial function. Statins have been shown to decrease the number of microvessels in the intima, which may represent a point entry for leukocytes and various other inflammatory cells. It has been thought that the microvessels are prone to leakage or hemorrhage. Subsequent thrombosis in situ may cause the release of substances such as thrombin [81]. Hence, a reduction in neovascularization by lipid-lowering statin therapy may also promote plaque stabilization. All of the actions of statins may contribute in varying degrees to the reduction in clinical events with lipid-lowering and pleiotropic effects. While it is presumed that some of these effects are independent of reductions in LDL-C levels, it currently remains unknown how much of the clinical data are truly independent of LDL-C reductions in humans. Some statins increase plasma high-density lipoprotein cholesterol (HDL-C) levels, which should conceivably present plaque-stabilizing effects in most data on plaque stabilization using statins.

16.6.2 Peroxisome Proliferator-Activated Receptor (PPAR) Agonists

Pioglitazone, one of the peroxisome proliferator-activated receptor-gamma agonists, is widely used in the treatment of type 2 diabetes. It improves insulin resistance and subsequently decreases plasma glucose as well as glycosylated hemoglobin A1c values in patients with diabetes [82]. Pioglitazone has been shown to exert other beneficial metabolic effects in diabetic patients; it not only decreases blood pressure levels but also improves lipid profiles [83, 84]. Furthermore, several clinical trials reported that pioglitazone may exhibit atheroprotective properties in humans [15, 85–88]. CHICAGO (Carotid Intima-Media Thickness in Atherosclerosis Using Pioglitazone) and PERISCOPE (Pioglitazone Effect on Regression of Intravascular Sonographic Coronary Obstruction Prospective Evaluation) trials revealed that pioglitazone was better than glimepiride, an insulin secretagogue, at preventing the progression of atherosclerosis in patients with diabetes [15, 88]. A large clinical trial designed to assess the effects of pioglitazone on ischemic cardiovascular outcomes (the PROactive, PROspective pioglitAzone Clinical Trial In macroVascular Events) did not find significant effects on primary composite outcomes (death/myocardial infarction/stroke/acute coronary syndrome/vascular intervention/amputation) [85]. When secondary composite outcomes were assessed, pioglitazone was found to markedly reduce the recurrence of stroke and acute coronary syndrome in high-risk diabetic patients shortly after starting the treatment, and these findings suggested the plaque-stabilizing effects of pioglitazone [86, 87].

PPAR-gamma activators inhibit the release of pro-inflammatory cytokines and matrix-degrading enzymes in monocytes and macrophages. PPAR-gamma activators modulate the expression of chemokines and endothelin in the endothelium, and PPAR-gamma ligands have been shown to reduce the secretion of interferon-gamma in T cells [89]. Clinical findings demonstrated that pioglitazone reduced the serum inflammatory markers of atherosclerosis [84, 90]. Pioglitazone has emerged as a promising target for attenuating vascular and atherosclerotic plaque inflammation.

16.7 Monitoring of the Effects of Anti-inflammatory Therapy on Atherosclerosis

Previous studies reported that FDG-PET was highly reproducible for the quantification of plaque instability in the carotid arteries and aorta with favorable inter- and intra-observer agreements [91, 92]. Hence, we could employ FDG-PET imaging to evaluate the efficacy of therapeutic interventions for vascular inflammation and atherosclerotic plaque vulnerability. The effects of therapeutic interventions have been clinically investigated in several studies by serial FDG-PET imaging [19, 22, 93–95] (Table 16.1).

The first randomized clinical study has been reported that vascular FDG uptake was attenuated by simvastatin or dietary modification for 3 months [19]. FDG activity in the carotid arteries and thoracic aorta was validated using merged FDG-PET and CT images (Fig. 16.1). The 3-month follow-up scan revealed the significant resolution of FDG activity within plaques in the simvastatin group, but not in the diet group (Fig. 16.2). Although simvastatin was found to reduce LDL-C levels by approximately 30 %, the extent of the reduction in FDG uptake within atherosclerotic plaques did not correlate with that of LDL-C levels (Fig. 16.3, upper right). These findings suggested that simvastatin could attenuate vascular inflammation in a LDL-C independent manner. The extent of the reduction in FDG activity in these plaques was positively correlated with that of the approximately 15 % increase in

Table 16.1 Effects of various metabolic modifiers on atherosclerosis

Interventions	Dose (mg)	Active comparator	Follow-up months	ΔLDL-C (%)	ΔHDL-C (%)	Target vessels	Reference number
Simvastatin	5–20	Diet management	3	−29.5	+14.9	Aorta, carotid arteries	[19]
Atorvastatin	20	Atorvastatin 5 mg	6	−38.5	+13.5	Aorta, femoral arteries	[94]
Atorvastatin	40	None	3	+11.1	0	Aorta, iliofemoral arteries	[95]
Atorvastatin	80	Atorvastatin 10 mg	12	−38.4	−0.4	Aorta, carotid arteries	[22]
Fluvastatin	20	None	3	−39.8	+36.0	Aorta, carotid arteries	[99]
Pitavastatin	4	None	3	+5.9	+46.4	Coronary artery	[110]
Pioglitazone	15–30	Glimepiride 0.5–4 mg	4	−1.8	+11.3	Aorta, carotid arteries	[100]
Pioglitazone	15–30	Glimepiride 0.5–4 mg	4	−1.8	+9.4	Coronary artery	[112]
Dalcetrapib	600	Placebo	12	+3.8	+33.9	Aorta, carotid arteries	[21]
Lifestyle modification	Dietary counseling, physical exercise	None	17	−6.5	+13.5	Aorta, carotid, subclavian, and iliac arteries	[93]

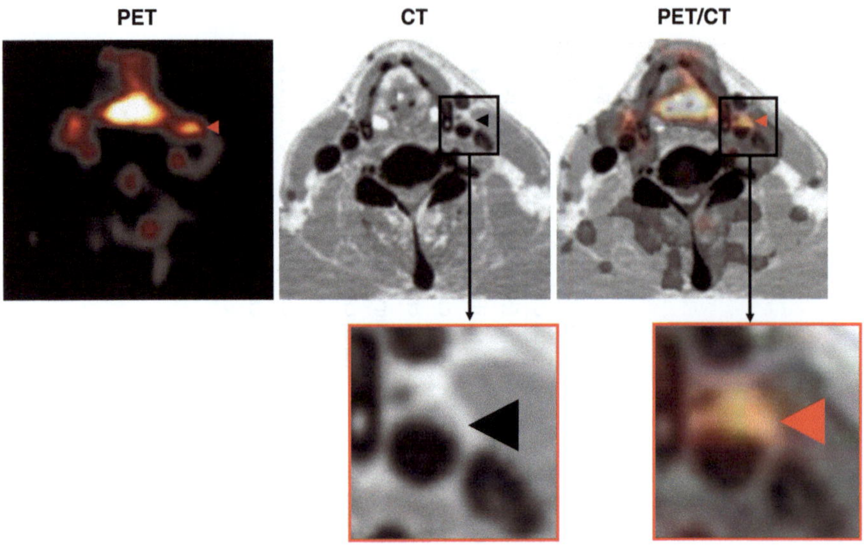

Fig. 16.1 Representative transaxial images of FDG-PET (*left*), enhanced CT (*middle*), and the co-registration of PET and CT (PET/CT) (*right*) showing FDG uptake in the right carotid plaque (*arrowheads*). *FDG* ^{18}F-fluorodeoxyglucose, *PET* positron-emission tomography, *CT* computerized tomography

HDL-C levels (Fig. 16.3, lower right) and led us to speculate about the anti-inflammatory properties of HDL-C and/or simvastatin [19]. Alternatively, lifestyle modifications have been shown to induce favorable effects on blood pressure and lipid profiles, thereby decreasing arterial FDG activity over 17 months in response to atherogenic risk reductions [93]. This study also demonstrated that the extent of reductions in arterial FDG activity correlated with the approximately 15 % increase in HDL-C levels [93]. Rosuvastatin was also found to decrease the volume of atheroma in association with the approximately 15 % increase in HDL-C levels in an IVUS study [96], which further suggested that the anti-inflammatory effects of statins may be partly mediated by elevations in HDL-C levels.

Statins have been shown to reduce the risk of cardiovascular morbidity and mortality in both primary and secondary prevention studies in proportion to reductions in LDL-C levels and the circulating markers of inflammation [97]. Furthermore, the intensification of statin therapy has also reduced the incidence of major cardiovascular events [98]. However, it remains unknown whether high-dose statin treatment could result in greater reductions in atherosclerotic inflammation than low-dose statins. Several very recent studies using PET/CT imaging demonstrated that atorvastatin produced significant dose-dependent reductions in vascular FDG activity [22, 94, 95]. In accordance with the findings of previous studies, changes in vascular FDG activity did not correlate with changes in LDL-C. Fluvastatin also attenuated the activity of FDG in the carotid arteries and thoracic aorta [99] (Fig. 16.4). Compared to atorvastatin, these favorable effects appear not to be class specific.

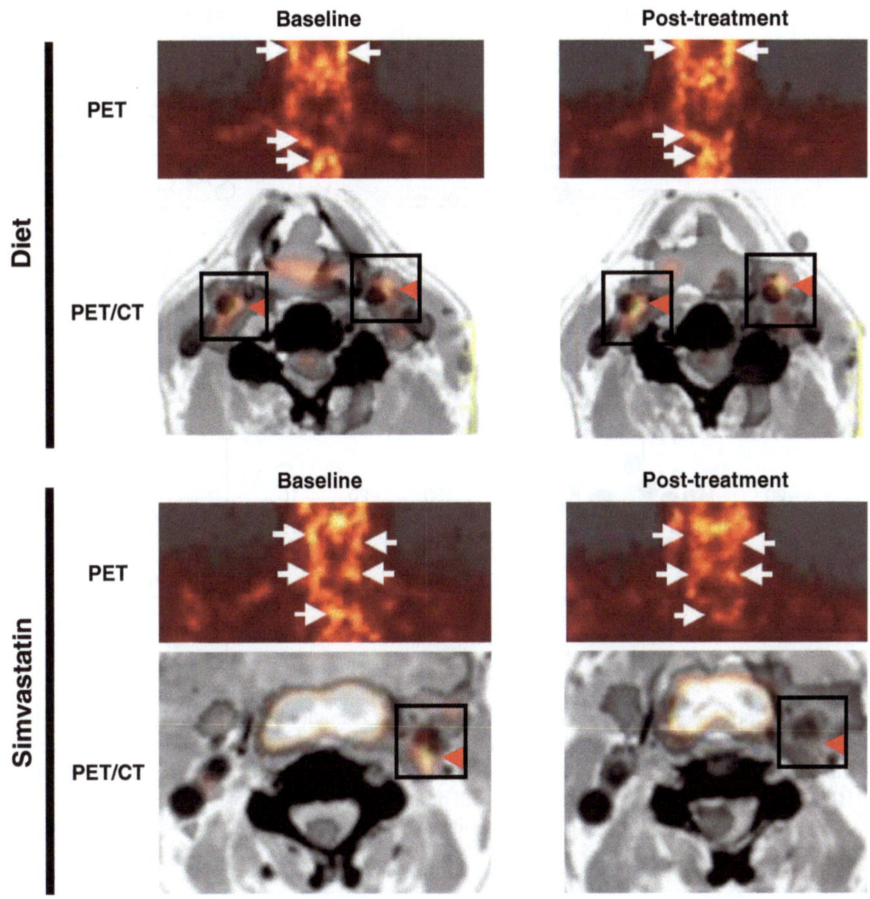

Fig. 16.2 FDG-PET images at baseline (*left*) and after 3 months of an intervention (*right*) with a dietary modification (*top*) or simvastatin therapy (*bottom*). The dietary modification alone had no effect on FDG uptake (*top*, *arrows*) in the carotid arteries and aortic arch. On the other hand, the uptake of FDG was markedly reduced by the simvastatin treatment (*bottom*, *arrows*). Serial co-registered PET and CT images allowed the identification of FDG localization in the carotid arteries (*red arrowheads*) (Reproduced, with permission, from Rudd and Tahara et al. [20]). *FDG* ^{18}F-fluorodeoxyglucose, *PET* positron-emission tomography, *CT* computerized tomography

These findings suggest that serial FDG-PET images can be used to monitor improvements in the inflammatory component of atherosclerotic lesions in response to therapeutic interventions.

PET is a promising modality for the future development of new therapeutic strategies including molecular targeted therapies and remains one of the most important tools for probing human disease processes. A previous study using FDG-PET imaging of the carotid arteries revealed that vascular inflammation was clearly associated with metabolic syndrome [54]; vascular FDG activity was independently associated with waist circumference, hypertension medication, carotid IMT, insulin resistance, CRP,

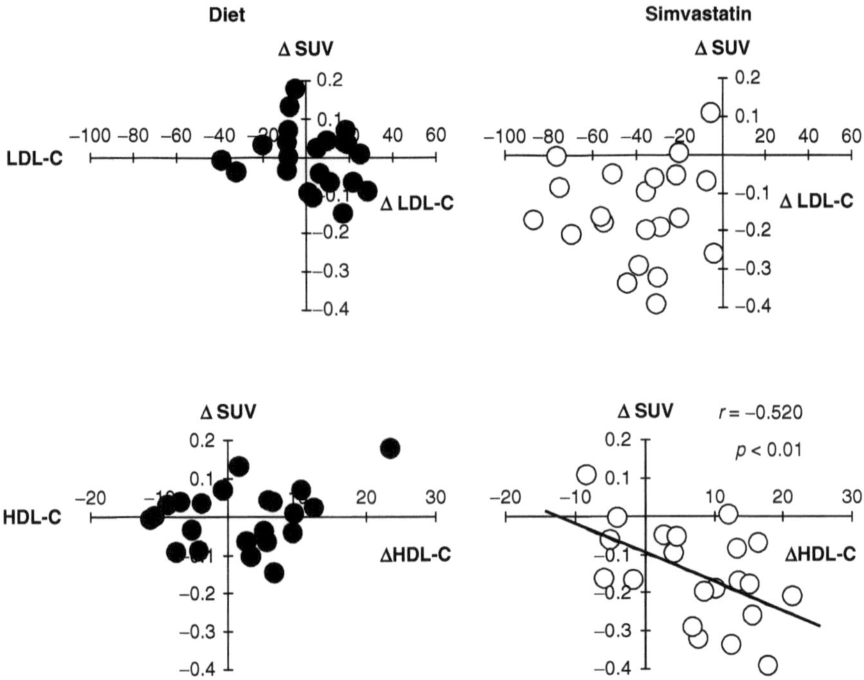

Fig. 16.3 Correlations between changes in plaque FDG activity and alterations in HDL cholesterol (Δ*HDL-C*) and LDL cholesterol (Δ*LDL-C*) after a 3-month treatment with dietary management alone (diet) or simvastatin. ΔSUV as FDG activity within plaques only correlated with ΔHDL-C in the statin group (Reproduced, with permission, from Tahara et al. [19]). *HDL-C* high-density lipoprotein cholesterol, *LDL-C* low-density lipoprotein cholesterol, *SUV* standardized uptake value

and HDL-C. Furthermore, age- and gender-adjusted vascular FDG activity increased in proportion to the number of conditions associated with metabolic syndrome [54].

Pioglitazone has been shown to exert other beneficial metabolic effects including not only improvements in insulin resistance, which has been implicated in metabolic syndrome, but also lipid profiles, such as increased HDL-C levels [83–88]. FDG-PET/contrasted CT has been used to evaluate the effects of pioglitazone on plaque inflammation [100]. A recent study reported that FDG activity in the carotid arteries and ascending aortas of the aortic arch in patients with impaired glucose tolerance or type 2 diabetes was significantly lower following a 4-month treatment with pioglitazone than with glimepiride in a glucose-lowering independent manner, whose changes were inversely associated with those in plasma HDL-C levels (Fig. 16.5) [100]. It is also well known that not only high levels of LDL-C but also low levels of HDL-C are significant predictors of atherosclerotic CVD [101]. These studies have provided a valuable insight into how patients with low levels of HDL-C become vulnerable to cardiovascular events at the vascular level [19, 93, 100].

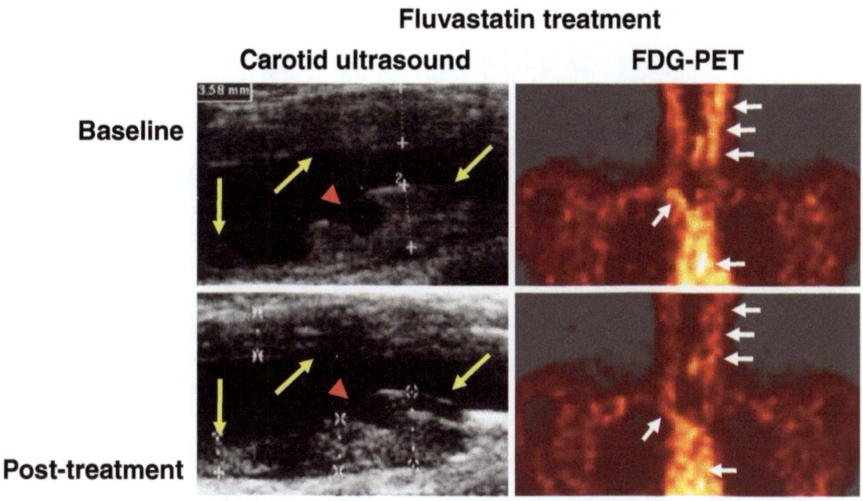

	LDL-C	HDL-C
Baseline	181.9 mg/dL	56.4 mg/dL
Post-treatment	109.5 mg/dL	76.7 mg/dL
%change	–40%	36%

Fig. 16.4 Carotid artery ultrasound imaging revealed carotid atherosclerosis in a patient with a recent history of acute cardiovascular events. The plaque had a homogeneous ultrasonic appearance with an irregular surface at baseline. A ruptured plaque showing discontinuity of the surface on the left carotid artery was detected (*arrowhead*). The patient received 20 mg fluvastatin, and a marked resolution of abnormal FDG uptake was observed after the treatment for 3 months (post treatment) with a concomitant reduction in LDL-C levels and elevation in HDL-C levels. *Yellow arrows* denote carotid plaques, and the *red arrowhead* denotes atherosclerotic plaque ulceration. *White arrows* indicate vascular FDG uptake (Reproduced and modified, with permission, from Tahara et al. [99]). *FDG* ^{18}F-fluorodeoxyglucose, *PET* positron-emission tomography, *CT* computerized tomography

16.8 New Drugs to Increase HDL-C Levels

Cholesteryl ester transfer protein (CETP) mediates the transfer of cholesteryl esters from HDL to other lipoproteins (e.g., LDL) and also the transfer of triglycerides to HDL. The inhibition of CETP has been shown to increase HDL-C levels and decrease LDL-C cholesterol levels [102]. Accordingly, the increase in HDL-C

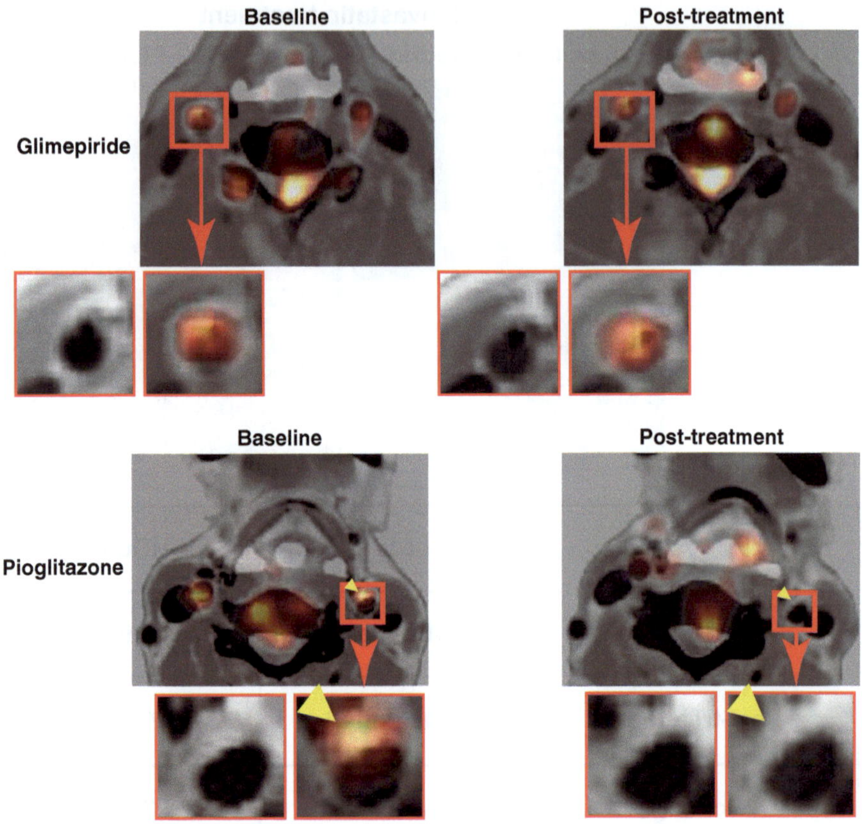

Fig. 16.5 Treatment effects of pioglitazone and glimepiride on FDG uptake in atherosclerotic plaques. Representative FDG-PET/CT with contrast media images (*left*) at baseline and (*right*) after a 4-month treatment with (*bottom*) pioglitazone or (*top*) glimepiride. A reduction was observed in the uptake of FDG by the atherosclerotic plaque with the pioglitazone treatment (*arrowheads*) (Reproduced, with permission, from Mizoguchi and Tahara et al. [100]). *FDG* ^{18}F-fluorodeoxyglucose, *PET* positron-emission tomography, *CT* computerized tomography

levels induced by the inhibition of CETP may represent an attractive approach for reducing vascular inflammation.

The first class CETP inhibitor, torcetrapib, did not cause atherosclerotic plaque regression, as established by both IVUS-derived percent atheroma volume [103] and carotid IMT [104], in spite of its potent effects including a more than 15 % relative decrease in LDL-C levels and a more than 50 % relative increase in HDL-C levels. However, the clinical development of torcetrapib was discontinued when the Investigation of Lipid Level Management to Understand its Impact in Atherosclerotic Events (ILLUMINATE) trial found that torcetrapib was associated with an increased risk of CVD events and all-cause death [105].

The second class CETP inhibitor, dalcetrapib, increased HDL-C levels by approximately 30 % without affecting LDL-C or triglyceride levels, and this was associated with a reduction in carotid arterial and aortic wall inflammation, as evaluated by FDG-PET/CT, over 6 months relative to that with the placebo (dal-PLAQUE) [21]. No significant differences were observed in blood pressure and the frequency of adverse events between dalcetrapib and the placebo. These findings indicated that dalcetrapib and/or HDL-C increases could have therapeutic effects on inflammatory activity in aortic wall vessels. However, a study on the effects of dalcetrapib on atherosclerotic disease in patients with coronary artery disease (dal-OUTCOMES) was terminated after an interim analysis of the trial revealed that dalcetrapib did not significantly reduce CVD events [106], which was similar to the findings of the ILLUMINATE trial [105].

The third class CETP inhibitor, anacetrapib, decreased LDL-C levels by 36 % and increased HDL-C levels by 38 % without increasing blood pressure [107]. Therefore, more potent CETP inhibitors may be able to improve the outcomes of patients with ACS. The REVEAL (randomized evaluation of the effects of anacetrapib through lipid modification, a large-scale, randomized placebo-controlled trial of the clinical effects of anacetrapib among people with established vascular disease) cardiovascular outcome study is currently ongoing to determine whether anacetrapib can reduce the incidence of major coronary events in statin-treated patients with a history of CVD [108].

HDL-C is believed to protect against atherosclerosis by promoting reverse cholesterol transport and anti-inflammatory effects. These multiple mechanisms of action make HDL-C a complex therapeutic target with potential for the treatment of patients with atherosclerosis. Not only an increase in the plasma levels of HDL-C but also improvements in HDL function are new therapeutic strategies currently being developed.

16.9 Measuring FDG Activity in the Coronary Artery

Measuring FDG activity in coronary arteries is limited by uptake into the myocardium; however, this can be reduced by a long fast and/or a low-carbohydrate and high-fat diet prior to an FDG scan. In a recent retrospective study, these preparations were found to adequately suppress the myocardial uptake of FDG in two thirds of patients [109]. FDG activity in the coronary arteries and aortic arch has been associated with the presence of angiographically proven coronary artery disease [109]. Cardiac or respiratory gating could greatly impact on spatial and temporal resolution for coronary artery FDG activity.

There is a recent report of a patient with Q-wave MI who had a right coronary artery aneurysm with a contrast-enhanced effect and focal FDG uptake in the aneurysm, as demonstrated by CT angiography and FDG-PET (Fig. 16.6, top) [110]. After a 3-month treatment of pitavastatin, an attenuation in the intense contrast effect and almost complete resolution of FDG uptake in the aneurysm were observed with a concomitant reduction in serum inflammatory markers and elevation in HDL-C levels (Fig. 16.6, bottom) [110]. These findings are encouraging and indicate that prospective and serial FDG-PET imaging, even for coronary artery inflammation, may become possible in the future.

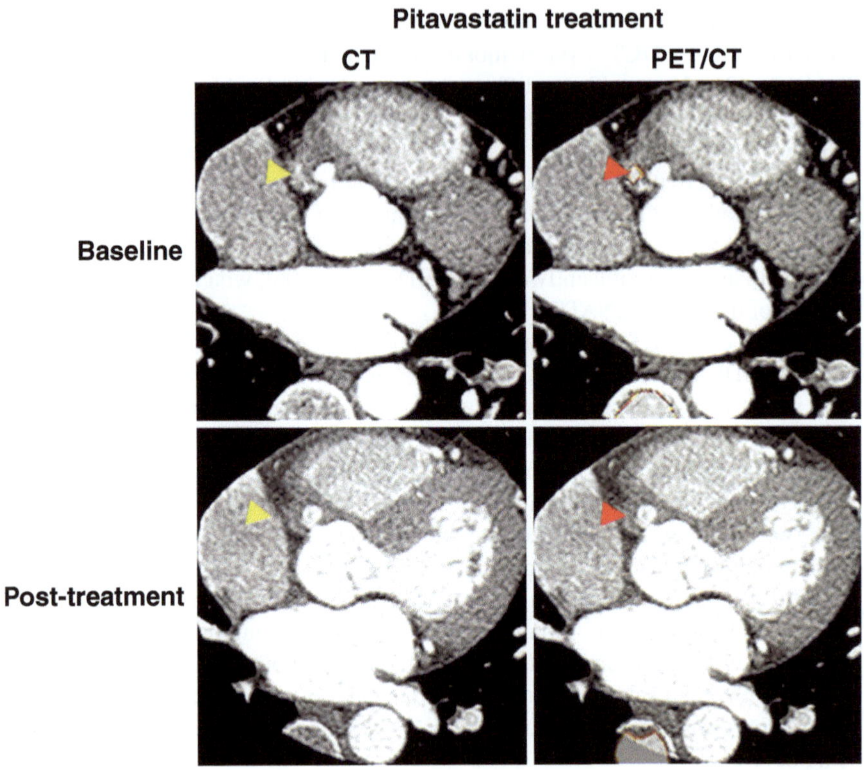

	LDL-C	HDL-C	CRP
Baseline	61.3 mg/dL	25.2 mg/dL	1.28 mg/dL
Post-treatment	64.9 mg/dL	36.9 mg/dL	0.61 mg/dL
%change	6 %	46 %	–52 %

Fig. 16.6 Multislice CT angiography revealed an RCA aneurysm and intense contrast effect in the aneurysm, which may have been indicative of inflammation (*left above*, *yellow arrowhead*). FDG-PET and co-registered CT scans revealed focal FDG uptake at the contrast-intense site in the RCA aneurysm (*left below*, *red arrowhead*). A 3-month treatment with 4 mg pitavastatin resolved the contrast intensity in the RCA aneurysm in follow-up CT angiography (*right above*, *yellow arrowhead*) and completely resolved abnormal FDG uptake in FDG-PET imaging (*right below*, *red arrowhead*) with a concomitant reduction in CRP levels and elevation in HDL-C levels (Reproduced and modified, with permission, from Tahara et al. [110]). *RCA* right coronary artery, *CRP* C-reactive protein, *PET* positron-emission tomography, *CT* computerized tomography, *LDL-C* low-density lipoprotein cholesterol

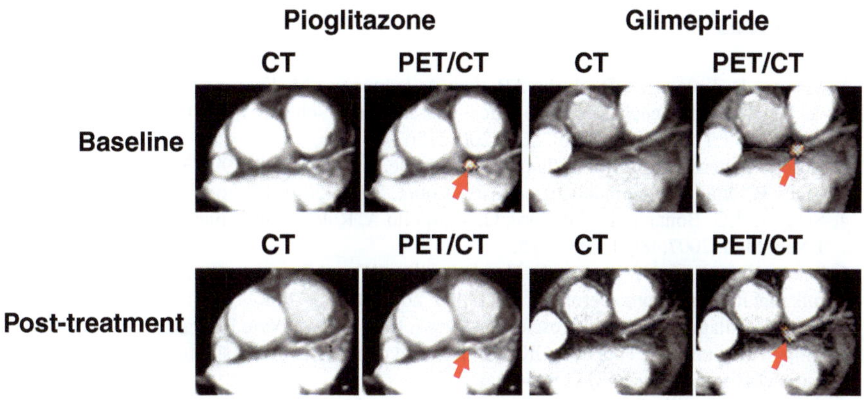

Fig. 16.7 Representative PET/CT fused images revealed the effects of pioglitazone and glimepiride on FDG uptake in the LM. A reduction was observed in FDG uptake in the LM with pioglitazone, but not with glimepiride (*arrows*) (Reproduced, with permission, from Nitta and Tahara et al. [112]). *LM* left main coronary artery, *PET* positron-emission tomography, *CT* computerized tomography

A recent prospective study demonstrated that FDG activity in the left main coronary artery was higher in patients with recent ACS than in those with stable disease [111]. Pioglitazone was very recently shown to attenuate FDG activity in the left main coronary artery in patients with impaired glucose tolerance or diabetes in a glucose-lowering independent manner, which suggests that pioglitazone may protect against cardiac events by suppressing coronary artery inflammation (Fig. 16.7) [112].

16.10 Concluding Remarks

The assessment of atherosclerotic plaques by imaging modalities is essential for the identification of atherosclerotic plaques in humans. Various invasive and noninvasive imaging modalities are currently available. Far from merely detecting stenosis, conventional imaging modalities can characterize plaque size and plaque composition, and most are employed as end points in therapeutic trials. The ultimate goal is to detect high-risk plaques that are vulnerable to rupture and thrombosis. The use of molecular imaging to provide functional and cellular information may enhance the risk stratification of atherosclerotic CVD beyond anatomical imaging. The area of molecular imaging has been rapidly advancing in recent years. The ability of noninvasive molecular imaging modalities such as FDG-PET to provide early insights into the efficacy of therapeutic interventions is more attractive than invasive morphological observations. Further studies will greatly facilitate the process of drug development and translate next-generation therapeutics into clinical medicine.

References

1. Virmani R, Kolodgie FD, Burke AP, Farb A, Schwartz SM. Lessons from sudden coronary death: a comprehensive morphological classification scheme for atherosclerotic lesions. Arterioscler Thromb Vasc Biol. 2000;20(5):1262–75.
2. Ross R. Atherosclerosis–an inflammatory disease. N Engl J Med. 1999;340(2):115–26.
3. Libby P. Inflammation in atherosclerosis. Nature. 2002;420(6917):868–74.
4. Spagnoli LG, Bonanno E, Sangiorgi G, Mauriello A. Role of inflammation in atherosclerosis. J Nucl Med. 2007;48(11):1800–15.
5. Tahara N, Imaizumi T, Virmani R, Narula J. Clinical feasibility of molecular imaging of plaque inflammation in atherosclerosis. J Nucl Med. 2009;50(3):331–4.
6. Libby P. Inflammation in atherosclerosis. Arterioscler Thromb Vasc Biol. 2012;32(9):2045–51.
7. Libby P, Ridker PM, Hansson GK. Progress and challenges in translating the biology of atherosclerosis. Nature. 2011;473(7347):317–25.
8. Rodriguez-Granillo GA, García-García HM, Mc Fadden EP, Valgimigli M, Aoki J, de Feyter P, Serruys PW. In vivo intravascular ultrasound-derived thin-cap fibroatheroma detection using ultrasound radiofrequency data analysis. J Am Coll Cardiol. 2005;46(11):2038–42.
9. Valgimigli M, Rodriguez-Granillo GA, Garcia-Garcia HM, Malagutti P, Regar E, de Jaegere P, de Feyter P, Serruys PW. Distance from the ostium as an independent determinant of coronary plaque composition in vivo: an intravascular ultrasound study based radiofrequency data analysis in humans. Eur Heart J. 2006;27(6):655–63.
10. Kubo T, Imanishi T, Takarada S, Kuroi A, Ueno S, Yamano T, Tanimoto T, Matsuo Y, Masho T, Kitabata H, Tsuda K, Tomobuchi Y, Akasaka T. Assessment of culprit lesion morphology in acute myocardial infarction: ability of optical coherence tomography compared with intravascular ultrasound and coronary angioscopy. J Am Coll Cardiol. 2007;50(10):933–9.
11. König A, Klauss V. Virtual histology. Heart. 2007;93(8):977–82.
12. Tahara N, Kai H, Nakaura H, Mizoguchi M, Ishibashi M, Kaida H, Baba K, Hayabuchi N, Imaizumi T. The prevalence of inflammation in carotid atherosclerosis: analysis with fluorodeoxyglucose-positron emission tomography. Eur Heart J. 2007;28(18):2243–8.
13. de Groot E, van Leuven SI, Duivenvoorden R, Meuwese MC, Akdim F, Bots ML, Kastelein JJ. Measurement of carotid intima-media thickness to assess progression and regression of atherosclerosis. Nat Clin Pract Cardiovasc Med. 2008;5(5):280–8.
14. Nissen SE, Tsunoda T, Tuzcu EM, Schoenhagen P, Cooper CJ, Yasin M, Eaton GM, Lauer MA, Sheldon WS, Grines CL, Halpern S, Crowe T, Blankenship JC, Kerensky R. Effect of recombinant ApoA-I Milano on coronary atherosclerosis in patients with acute coronary syndromes: a randomized controlled trial. JAMA. 2003;290(17):2292–300.
15. Nissen SE, Nicholls SJ, Wolski K, Nesto R, Kupfer S, Perez A, Jure H, De Larochellière R, Staniloae CS, Mavromatis K, Saw J, Hu B, Lincoff AM, Tuzcu EM, PERISCOPE Investigators. Comparison of pioglitazone vs glimepiride on progression of coronary atherosclerosis in patients with type 2 diabetes: the PERISCOPE randomized controlled trial. JAMA. 2008;299(13):1561–73.
16. Takarada S, Imanishi T, Kubo T, Tanimoto T, Kitabata H, Nakamura N, Tanaka A, Mizukoshi M, Akasaka T. Effect of statin therapy on coronary fibrous-cap thickness in patients with acute coronary syndrome: assessment by optical coherence tomography study. Atherosclerosis. 2009;202(2):491–7.
17. Rudd JH, Warburton EA, Fryer TD, Jones HA, Clark JC, Antoun N, Johnström P, Davenport AP, Kirkpatrick PJ, Arch BN, Pickard JD, Weissberg PL. Imaging atherosclerotic plaque inflammation with [18F]-fluorodeoxyglucose positron emission tomography. Circulation. 2002;105(23):2708–11.
18. Tawakol A, Migrino RQ, Bashian GG, Bedri S, Vermylen D, Cury RC, Yates D, LaMuraglia GM, Furie K, Houser S, Gewirtz H, Muller JE, Brady TJ, Fischman AJ. In vivo 18F-fluorodeoxyglucose positron emission tomography imaging provides a noninvasive measure of carotid plaque inflammation in patients. J Am Coll Cardiol. 2006;48(9):1818–24.

19. Tahara N, Kai H, Ishibashi M, Nakaura H, Kaida H, Baba K, Hayabuchi N, Imaizumi T. Simvastatin attenuates plaque inflammation: evaluation by fluorodeoxyglucose positron emission tomography. J Am Coll Cardiol. 2006;48(9):1825–31.
20. Rudd JH, Narula J, Strauss HW, Virmani R, Machac J, Klimas M, Tahara N, Fuster V, Warburton EA, Fayad ZA, Tawakol AA. Imaging atherosclerotic plaque inflammation by fluorodeoxyglucose with positron emission tomography: ready for prime time? J Am Coll Cardiol. 2010;55(23):2527–35.
21. Fayad ZA, Mani V, Woodward M, Kallend D, Abt M, Burgess T, Fuster V, Ballantyne CM, Stein EA, Tardif JC, Rudd JH, Farkouh ME, Tawakol A, dal-PLAQUE Investigators. Safety and efficacy of dalcetrapib on atherosclerotic disease using novel non-invasive multimodality imaging (dal-PLAQUE): a randomised clinical trial. Lancet. 2011;378(9802):1547–59.
22. Tawakol A, Fayad ZA, Mogg R, Alon A, Klimas MT, Dansky H, Subramanian SS, Abdelbaky A, Rudd JH, Farkouh ME, Nunes IO, Beals CR, Shankar SS. Intensification of statin therapy results in a rapid reduction in atherosclerotic inflammation: results of a multicenter fluorodeoxyglucose-positron emission tomography/computed tomography feasibility study. J Am Coll Cardiol. 2013;62(10):909–17.
23. Weintraub HS. Identifying the vulnerable patient with rupture-prone plaque. Am J Cardiol. 2008;101(12A):3F–10.
24. Go AS, Mozaffarian D, Roger VL, Benjamin EJ, Berry JD, Borden WB, Bravata DM, Dai S, Ford ES, Fox CS, Franco S, Fullerton HJ, Gillespie C, Hailpern SM, Heit JA, Howard VJ, Huffman MD, Kissela BM, Kittner SJ, Lackland DT, Lichtman JH, Lisabeth LD, Magid D, Marcus GM, Marelli A, Matchar DB, McGuire DK, Mohler ER, Moy CS, Mussolino ME, Nichol G, Paynter NP, Schreiner PJ, Sorlie PD, Stein J, Turan TN, Virani SS, Wong ND, Woo D, Turner MB, American Heart Association Statistics Committee and Stroke Statistics Subcommittee. Executive summary: heart disease and stroke statistics–2013 update: a report from the American Heart Association. Circulation. 2013;127(1):143–52.
25. Naghavi M, Libby P, Falk E, Casscells SW, Litovsky S, Rumberger J, Badimon JJ, Stefanadis C, Moreno P, Pasterkamp G, Fayad Z, Stone PH, Waxman S, Raggi P, Madjid M, Zarrabi A, Burke A, Yuan C, Fitzgerald PJ, Siscovick DS, de Korte CL, Aikawa M, Juhani Airaksinen KE, Assmann G, Becker CR, Chesebro JH, Farb A, Galis ZS, Jackson C, Jang IK, Koenig W, Lodder RA, March K, Demirovic J, Navab M, Priori SG, Rekhter MD, Bahr R, Grundy SM, Mehran R, Colombo A, Boerwinkle E, Ballantyne C, Insull Jr W, Schwartz RS, Vogel R, Serruys PW, Hansson GK, Faxon DP, Kaul S, Drexler H, Greenland P, Muller JE, Virmani R, Ridker PM, Zipes DP, Shah PK, Willerson JT. From vulnerable plaque to vulnerable patient: a call for new definitions and risk assessment strategies: part I. Circulation. 2003;108(14):1664–72.
26. Naghavi M, Libby P, Falk E, Casscells SW, Litovsky S, Rumberger J, Badimon JJ, Stefanadis C, Moreno P, Pasterkamp G, Fayad Z, Stone PH, Waxman S, Raggi P, Madjid M, Zarrabi A, Burke A, Yuan C, Fitzgerald PJ, Siscovick DS, de Korte CL, Aikawa M, Airaksinen KE, Assmann G, Becker CR, Chesebro JH, Farb A, Galis ZS, Jackson C, Jang IK, Koenig W, Lodder RA, March K, Demirovic J, Navab M, Priori SG, Rekhter MD, Bahr R, Grundy SM, Mehran R, Colombo A, Boerwinkle E, Ballantyne C, Insull Jr W, Schwartz RS, Vogel R, Serruys PW, Hansson GK, Faxon DP, Kaul S, Drexler H, Greenland P, Muller JE, Virmani R, Ridker PM, Zipes DP, Shah PK, Willerson JT. From vulnerable plaque to vulnerable patient: a call for new definitions and risk assessment strategies: part II. Circulation. 2003;108(15):1772–8.
27. Hackett D, Davies G, Maseri A. Pre-existing coronary stenoses in patients with first myocardial infarction are not necessarily severe. Eur Heart J. 1988;9(12):1317–23.
28. Nobuyoshi M, Tanaka M, Nosaka H, Kimura T, Yokoi H, Hamasaki N, Kim K, Shindo T, Kimura K. Progression of coronary atherosclerosis: is coronary spasm related to progression? J Am Coll Cardiol. 1991;18(4):904–10.
29. Velasco JA. After 4S, CARE and LIPID–is evidence-based medicine being practised? Atherosclerosis. 1999;147 Suppl 1:S39–44.
30. Topol EJ, Nissen SE. Our preoccupation with coronary luminology. The dissociation between clinical and angiographic findings in ischemic heart disease. Circulation. 1995;92(8):2333–42.

31. Corti R, Fayad ZA, Fuster V, Worthley SG, Helft G, Chesebro J, Mercuri M, Badimon JJ. Effects of lipid-lowering by simvastatin on human atherosclerotic lesions: a longitudinal study by high-resolution, noninvasive magnetic resonance imaging. Circulation. 2001;104(3):249–52.
32. Corti R, Fuster V, Fayad ZA, Worthley SG, Helft G, Smith D, Weinberger J, Wentzel J, Mizsei G, Mercuri M, Badimon JJ. Lipid lowering by simvastatin induces regression of human atherosclerotic lesions: two years' follow-up by high-resolution noninvasive magnetic resonance imaging. Circulation. 2002;106(23):2884–7.
33. Fayad ZA, Fuster V. Clinical imaging of the high-risk or vulnerable atherosclerotic plaque. Circ Res. 2001;89(4):305–16.
34. Hansson GK. Inflammation, atherosclerosis, and coronary artery disease. N Engl J Med. 2005;352(16):1685–95.
35. Kolodgie FD, Burke AP, Farb A, Gold HK, Yuan J, Narula J, Finn AV, Virmani R. The thin-cap fibroatheroma: a type of vulnerable plaque: the major precursor lesion to acute coronary syndromes. Curr Opin Cardiol. 2001;16(5):285–92.
36. Motoyama S, Kondo T, Anno H, Sugiura A, Ito Y, Mori K, Ishii J, Sato T, Inoue K, Sarai M, Hishida H, Narula J. Atherosclerotic plaque characterization by 0.5-mm-slice multislice computed tomographic imaging. Circ J. 2007;71(3):363–6.
37. Motoyama S, Kondo T, Sarai M, Sugiura A, Harigaya H, Sato T, Inoue K, Okumura M, Ishii J, Anno H, Virmani R, Ozaki Y, Hishida H, Narula J. Multislice computed tomographic characteristics of coronary lesions in acute coronary syndromes. J Am Coll Cardiol. 2007;50(4):319–26.
38. Langer HF, Haubner R, Pichler BJ, Gawaz M. Radionuclide imaging: a molecular key to the atherosclerotic plaque. J Am Coll Cardiol. 2008;52(1):1–12.
39. Virgolini I, Müller C, Fitscha P, Chiba P, Sinzinger H. Radiolabelling autologous monocytes with 111-indium-oxine for reinjection in patients with atherosclerosis. Prog Clin Biol Res. 1990;355:271–80.
40. Lees RS, Lees AM, Strauss HW. External imaging of human atherosclerosis. J Nucl Med. 1983;24(2):154–6.
41. Virgolini I, Rauscha F, Lupattelli G, Angelberger P, Ventura A, O'Grady J, Sinzinger H. Autologous low-density lipoprotein labelling allows characterization of human atherosclerotic lesions in vivo as to presence of foam cells and endothelial coverage. Eur J Nucl Med. 1991;18(12):948–51.
42. Fischman AJ, Rubin RH, Khaw BA, Kramer PB, Wilkinson R, Ahmad M, Needelman M, Locke E, Nossiff ND, Strauss HW. Radionuclide imaging of experimental atherosclerosis with nonspecific polyclonal immunoglobulin G. J Nucl Med. 1989;30(6):1095–100.
43. Ohtsuki K, Hayase M, Akashi K, Kopiwoda S, Strauss HW. Detection of monocyte chemoattractant protein-1 receptor expression in experimental atherosclerotic lesions: an autoradiographic study. Circulation. 2001;104(2):203–8.
44. Hartung D, Petrov A, Haider N, Fujimoto S, Blankenberg F, Fujimoto A, Virmani R, Kolodgie FD, Strauss HW, Narula J. Radiolabeled monocyte chemotactic protein 1 for the detection of inflammation in experimental atherosclerosis. J Nucl Med. 2007;48(11):1816–21.
45. Sadeghi MM, Schechner JS, Krassilnikova S, Gharaei AA, Zhang J, Kirkiles-Smith N, Sinusas AJ, Zaret BL, Bender JR. Vascular cell adhesion molecule-1-targeted detection of endothelial activation in human microvasculature. Transplant Proc. 2004;36(5):1585–91.
46. Fujimoto S, Hartung D, Ohshima S, Edwards DS, Zhou J, Yalamanchili P, Azure M, Fujimoto A, Isobe S, Matsumoto Y, Boersma H, Wong N, Yamazaki J, Narula N, Petrov A, Narula J. Molecular imaging of matrix metalloproteinase in atherosclerotic lesions: resolution with dietary modification and statin therapy. J Am Coll Cardiol. 2008;52(23):1847–57.
47. Haubner R. Alphavbeta3-integrin imaging: a new approach to characterise angiogenesis? Eur J Nucl Med Mol Imaging. 2006;33 Suppl 1:54–63.
48. Laitinen I, Saraste A, Weidl E, Poethko T, Weber AW, Nekolla SG, Leppänen P, Ylä-Herttuala S, Hölzlwimmer G, Walch A, Esposito I, Wester HJ, Knuuti J, Schwaiger M. Evaluation of alphavbeta3 integrin-targeted positron emission tomography tracer 18F-galacto-RGD for imaging of vascular inflammation in atherosclerotic mice. Circ Cardiovasc Imaging. 2009; 2(4):331–8.

49. Greco C, Di Loreto M, Ciavolella M, Banci M, Taurino M, Cerquetani E, Chiavarelli R, Naro F, Cusella-De Angelis G, Mele A, et al. Immunodetection of human atherosclerotic plaque with 125I-labeled monoclonal antifibrin antibodies. Atherosclerosis. 1993;100(2):133–9.
50. Folco EJ, Sheikine Y, Rocha VZ, Christen T, Shvartz E, Sukhova GK, Di Carli MF, Libby P. Hypoxia but not inflammation augments glucose uptake in human macrophages: Implications for imaging atherosclerosis with 18fluorine-labeled 2-deoxy-D-glucose positron emission tomography. J Am Coll Cardiol. 2011;58(6):603–14.
51. Ogawa M, Nakamura S, Saito Y, Kosugi M, Magata Y. What can be seen by 18F-FDG PET in atherosclerosis imaging? The effect of foam cell formation on 18F-FDG uptake to macrophages in vitro. J Nucl Med. 2012;53(1):55–8.
52. Pedersen SF, Graebe M, Fisker Hag AM, Højgaard L, Sillesen H, Kjaer A. Gene expression and 18FDG uptake in atherosclerotic carotid plaques. Nucl Med Commun. 2010;31(5):423–9.
53. Lombardo A, Biasucci LM, Lanza GA, Coli S, Silvestri P, Cianflone D, Liuzzo G, Burzotta F, Crea F, Maseri A. Inflammation as a possible link between coronary and carotid plaque instability. Circulation. 2004;109(25):3158–63.
54. Tahara N, Kai H, Yamagishi S, Mizoguchi M, Nakaura H, Ishibashi M, Kaida H, Baba K, Hayabuchi N, Imaizumi T. Vascular inflammation evaluated by [18F]-fluorodeoxyglucose positron emission tomography is associated with the metabolic syndrome. J Am Coll Cardiol. 2007;49(14):1533–9.
55. Saam T, Rominger A, Wolpers S, Nikolaou K, Rist C, Greif M, Cumming P, Becker A, Foerster S, Reiser MF, Bartenstein P, Hacker M. Association of inflammation of the left anterior descending coronary artery with cardiovascular risk factors, plaque burden and pericardial fat volume: a PET/CT study. Eur J Nucl Med Mol Imaging. 2010;37(6):1203–12.
56. Rudd JH, Myers KS, Bansilal S, Machac J, Woodward M, Fuster V, Farkouh ME, Fayad ZA. Relationships among regional arterial inflammation, calcification, risk factors, and biomarkers: a prospective fluorodeoxyglucose positron-emission tomography/computed tomography imaging study. Circ Cardiovasc Imaging. 2009;2(2):107–15.
57. Kim TN, Kim S, Yang SJ, Yoo HJ, Seo JA, Kim SG, Kim NH, Baik SH, Choi DS, Choi KM. Vascular inflammation in patients with impaired glucose tolerance and type 2 diabetes: analysis with 18F-fluorodeoxyglucose positron emission tomography. Circ Cardiovasc Imaging. 2010;3(2):142–8.
58. Bucerius J, Mani V, Moncrieff C, Rudd JH, Machac J, Fuster V, Farkouh ME, Fayad ZA. Impact of noninsulin-dependent type 2 diabetes on carotid wall 18F-fluorodeoxyglucose positron emission tomography uptake. J Am Coll Cardiol. 2012;59(23):2080–8.
59. Wu YW, Kao HL, Chen MF, Lee BC, Tseng WY, Jeng JS, Tzen KY, Yen RF, Huang PJ, Yang WS. Characterization of plaques using 18F-FDG PET/CT in patients with carotid atherosclerosis and correlation with matrix metalloproteinase-1. J Nucl Med. 2007;48(2):227–33.
60. Yoo HJ, Kim S, Park MS, Choi HY, Yang SJ, Seo JA, Kim SG, Kim NH, Baik SH, Choi DS, Choi KM. Serum adipocyte fatty acid-binding protein is associated independently with vascular inflammation: analysis with (18)F-fluorodeoxyglucose positron emission tomography. J Clin Endocrinol Metab. 2011;96(3):E488–92.
61. Choi HY, Kim S, Yang SJ, Yoo HJ, Seo JA, Kim SG, Kim NH, Baik SH, Choi DS, Choi KM. Association of adiponectin, resistin, and vascular inflammation: analysis with 18F-fluorodeoxyglucose positron emission tomography. Arterioscler Thromb Vasc Biol. 2011;31(4):944–9.
62. Yoo HJ, Kim S, Park MS, Yang SJ, Kim TN, Seo JA, Kim SG, Kim NH, Seo HS, Baik SH, Choi DS, Choi KM. Vascular inflammation stratified by C-reactive protein and low-density lipoprotein cholesterol levels: analysis with 18F-FDG PET. J Nucl Med. 2011;52(1):10–7.
63. Tahara N, Yamagishi S, Tahara A, Nitta Y, Kodama N, Mizoguchi M, Mohar D, Ishibashi M, Hayabuchi N, Imaizumi T. Serum level of pigment epithelium-derived factor is a marker of atherosclerosis in humans. Atherosclerosis. 2011;219(1):311–5.
64. Tahara N, Yamagishi S, Tahara A, Ishibashi M, Hayabuchi N, Takeuchi M, Imaizumi T. Adiponectin is inversely associated with ratio of serum levels of AGEs to sRAGE and vascular inflammation. Int J Cardiol. 2012;158(3):461–2.

65. Tahara N, Yamagishi S, Takeuchi M, Honda A, Tahara A, Nitta Y, Kodama N, Mizoguchi M, Kaida H, Ishibashi M, Hayabuchi N, Matsui T, Imaizumi T. Positive association between serum level of glyceraldehyde-derived advanced glycation end products and vascular inflammation evaluated by [(18)F]fluorodeoxyglucose positron emission tomography. Diabetes Care. 2012;35(12):2618–25.
66. Paulmier B, Duet M, Khayat R, Pierquet-Ghazzar N, Laissy JP, Maunoury C, Hugonnet F, Sauvaget E, Trinquart L, Faraggi M. Arterial wall uptake of fluorodeoxyglucose on PET imaging in stable cancer disease patients indicates higher risk for cardiovascular events. J Nucl Cardiol. 2008;15(2):209–17.
67. Rominger A, Saam T, Wolpers S, Cyran CC, Schmidt M, Foerster S, Nikolaou K, Reiser MF, Bartenstein P, Hacker M. 18F-FDG PET/CT identifies patients at risk for future vascular events in an otherwise asymptomatic cohort with neoplastic disease. J Nucl Med. 2009;50(10):1611–20.
68. Grandpierre S, Desandes E, Meneroux B, Djaballah W, Mandry D, Netter F, Wahl D, Fay R, Karcher G, Marie PY. Arterial foci of F-18 fluorodeoxyglucose are associated with an enhanced risk of subsequent ischemic stroke in cancer patients: a case-control pilot study. Clin Nucl Med. 2011;36(2):85–90.
69. Figueroa AL, Abdelbaky A, Truong QA, Corsini E, MacNabb MH, Lavender ZR, Lawler MA, Grinspoon SK, Brady TJ, Nasir K, Hoffmann U, Tawakol A. Measurement of arterial activity on routine FDG PET/CT images improves prediction of risk of future CV events. JACC Cardiovasc Imaging. 2013;6(12):1250–9.
70. Pasterkamp G, Falk E, Woutman H, Borst C. Techniques characterizing the coronary atherosclerotic plaque: influence on clinical decision making? J Am Coll Cardiol. 2000;36(1):13–21.
71. Grundy SM, Cleeman JI, Merz CN, Brewer Jr HB, Clark LT, Hunninghake DB, Pasternak RC, Smith Jr SC, Stone NJ, National Heart, Lung, and Blood Institute; American College of Cardiology Foundation; American Heart Association. Implications of recent clinical trials for the National Cholesterol Education Program Adult Treatment Panel III guidelines. Circulation. 2004;110(2):227–39.
72. Baigent C, Keech A, Kearney PM, Blackwell L, Buck G, Pollicino C, Kirby A, Sourjina T, Peto R, Collins R, Simes R, Cholesterol Treatment Trialists' (CTT) Collaborators. Efficacy and safety of cholesterol-lowering treatment: prospective meta-analysis of data from 90,056 participants in 14 randomised trials of statins. Lancet. 2005;366(9493):1267–78.
73. Crisby M, Nordin-Fredriksson G, Shah PK, Yano J, Zhu J, Nilsson J. Pravastatin treatment increases collagen content and decreases lipid content, inflammation, metalloproteinases, and cell death in human carotid plaques: implications for plaque stabilization. Circulation. 2001;103(7):926–33.
74. Sukhova GK, Williams JK, Libby P. Statins reduce inflammation in atheroma of nonhuman primates independent of effects on serum cholesterol. Arterioscler Thromb Vasc Biol. 2002;22(9):1452–8.
75. Aviram M, Dankner G, Cogan U, Hochgraf E, Brook JG. Lovastatin inhibits low-density lipoprotein oxidation and alters its fluidity and uptake by macrophages: in vitro and in vivo studies. Metabolism. 1992;41(3):229–35.
76. Ridker PM. Evaluating novel cardiovascular risk factors: can we better predict heart attacks? Ann Intern Med. 1999;130(11):933–7.
77. Cipollone F, Mezzetti A, Porreca E, Di Febbo C, Nutini M, Fazia M, Falco A, Cuccurullo F, Davì G. Association between enhanced soluble CD40L and prothrombotic state in hypercholesterolemia: effects of statin therapy. Circulation. 2002;106(4):399–402.
78. Sacks FM, Pfeffer MA, Moye LA, Rouleau JL, Rutherford JD, Cole TG, Brown L, Warnica JW, Arnold JM, Wun CC, Davis BR, Braunwald E. The effect of pravastatin on coronary events after myocardial infarction in patients with average cholesterol levels. Cholesterol and Recurrent Events Trial investigators. N Engl J Med. 1996;335:1001–9.
79. Chen L, Haught WH, Yang B, Saldeen TG, Parathasarathy S, Mehta JL. Preservation of endogenous antioxidant activity and inhibition of lipid peroxidation as common mechanisms of antiatherosclerotic effects of vitamin E, lovastatin and amlodipine. J Am Coll Cardiol. 1997;30(2):569–75.

80. Weber C, Erl W, Weber KS, Weber PC. HMG-CoA reductase inhibitors decrease CD11b expression and CD11b-dependent adhesion of monocytes to endothelium and reduce increased adhesiveness of monocytes isolated from patients with hypercholesterolemia. J Am Coll Cardiol. 1997;30(5):1212–7.
81. Moulton KS, Heller E, Konerding MA, Flynn E, Palinski W, Folkman J. Angiogenesis inhibitors endostatin or TNP-470 reduce intimal neovascularization and plaque growth in apolipoprotein E-deficient mice. Circulation. 1999;99(13):1726–32.
82. Aronoff S, Rosenblatt S, Braithwaite S, Egan JW, Mathisen AL, Schneider RL. Pioglitazone hydrochloride monotherapy improves glycemic control in the treatment of patients with type 2 diabetes: a 6-month randomized placebo-controlled dose-response study. The Pioglitazone 001 Study Group. Diabetes Care. 2000;23(11):1605–11.
83. Parulkar AA, Pendergrass ML, Granda-Ayala R, Lee TR, Fonseca VA. Nonhypoglycemic effects of thiazolidinediones. Ann Intern Med. 2001;134(1):61–71.
84. Pfützner A, Marx N, Lübben G, Langenfeld M, Walcher D, Konrad T, Forst T. Improvement of cardiovascular risk markers by pioglitazone is independent from glycemic control: results from the pioneer study. J Am Coll Cardiol. 2005;45(12):1925–31.
85. Dormandy JA, Charbonnel B, Eckland DJ, Erdmann E, Massi-Benedetti M, Moules IK, Skene AM, Tan MH, Lefèbvre PJ, Murray GD, Standl E, Wilcox RG, Wilhelmsen L, Betteridge J, Birkeland K, Golay A, Heine RJ, Korányi L, Laakso M, Mokán M, Norkus A, Pirags V, Podar T, Scheen A, Scherbaum W, Schernthaner G, Schmitz O, Skrha J, Smith U, Taton J, PROactive investigators. Secondary prevention of macrovascular events in patients with type 2 diabetes in the PROactive Study (PROspective pioglitAzone Clinical Trial In macroVascular Events): a randomised controlled trial. Lancet. 2005;366(9493):1279–89.
86. Wilcox R, Bousser MG, Betteridge DJ, Schernthaner G, Pirags V, Kupfer S, Dormandy J, PROactive Investigators. Effects of pioglitazone in patients with type 2 diabetes with or without previous stroke: results from PROactive (PROspective pioglitAzone Clinical Trial In macroVascular Events 04). Stroke. 2007;38(3):865–73.
87. Erdmann E, Dormandy JA, Charbonnel B, Massi-Benedetti M, Moules IK, Skene AM, PROactive Investigators. The effect of pioglitazone on recurrent myocardial infarction in 2,445 patients with type 2 diabetes and previous myocardial infarction: results from the PROactive (PROactive 05) Study. J Am Coll Cardiol. 2007;49(17):1772–80.
88. Mazzone T, Meyer PM, Feinstein SB, Davidson MH, Kondos GT, D'Agostino Sr RB, Perez A, Provost JC, Haffner SM. Effect of pioglitazone compared with glimepiride on carotid intima-media thickness in type 2 diabetes: a randomized trial. JAMA. 2006;296(21):2572–81.
89. Marx N, Kehrle B, Kohlhammer K, Grüb M, Koenig W, Hombach V, Libby P, Plutzky J. PPAR activators as antiinflammatory mediators in human T lymphocytes: implications for atherosclerosis and transplantation-associated arteriosclerosis. Circ Res. 2002;90(6):703–10.
90. Cominacini L, Garbin U, Fratta Pasini A, Campagnola M, Davoli A, Foot E, Sighieri G, Sironi AM, Lo Cascio V, Ferrannini E. Troglitazone reduces LDL oxidation and lowers plasma E-selectin concentration in NIDDM patients. Diabetes. 1998;47(1):130–3.
91. Rudd JH, Myers KS, Bansilal S, Machac J, Rafique A, Farkouh M, Fuster V, Fayad ZA. (18) Fluorodeoxyglucose positron emission tomography imaging of atherosclerotic plaque inflammation is highly reproducible: implications for atherosclerosis therapy trials. J Am Coll Cardiol. 2007;50(9):892–6.
92. Rudd JH, Myers KS, Bansilal S, Machac J, Pinto CA, Tong C, Rafique A, Hargeaves R, Farkouh M, Fuster V, Fayad ZA. Atherosclerosis inflammation imaging with 18F-FDG PET: carotid, iliac, and femoral uptake reproducibility, quantification methods, and recommendations. J Nucl Med. 2008;49(6):871–8.
93. Lee SJ, On YK, Lee EJ, Choi JY, Kim BT, Lee KH. Reversal of vascular 18F-FDG uptake with plasma high-density lipoprotein elevation by atherogenic risk reduction. J Nucl Med. 2008;49(8):1277–82.
94. Ishii H, Nishio M, Takahashi H, Aoyama T, Tanaka M, Toriyama T, Tamaki T, Yoshikawa D, Hayashi M, Amano T, Matsubara T, Murohara T. Comparison of atorvastatin 5 and 20 mg/d for reducing F-18 fluorodeoxyglucose uptake in atherosclerotic plaques on positron emission tomography/computed tomography: a randomized, investigator-blinded, open-label, 6-month

study in Japanese adults scheduled for percutaneous coronary intervention. Clin Ther. 2010; 32(14):2337–47.

95. Wu YW, Kao HL, Huang CL, Chen MF, Lin LY, Wang YC, Lin YH, Lin HJ, Tzen KY, Yen RF, Chi YC, Huang PJ, Yang WS. The effects of 3-month atorvastatin therapy on arterial inflammation, calcification, abdominal adipose tissue and circulating biomarkers. Eur J Nucl Med Mol Imaging. 2012;39(3):399–407.
96. Nissen SE, Nicholls SJ, Sipahi I, Libby P, Raichlen JS, Ballantyne CM, Davignon J, Erbel R, Fruchart JC, Tardif JC, Schoenhagen P, Crowe T, Cain V, Wolski K, Goormastic M, Tuzcu EM, ASTEROID Investigators. Effect of very high-intensity statin therapy on regression of coronary atherosclerosis: the ASTEROID trial. JAMA. 2006;295(13):1556–65.
97. Vaughan CJ, Gotto Jr AM, Basson CT. The evolving role of statins in the management of atherosclerosis. J Am Coll Cardiol. 2000;35(1):1–10.
98. van Herick A, Schuetz CA, Alperin P, Bullano MF, Balu S, Gandhi S. The impact of initial statin treatment decisions on cardiovascular outcomes in clinical care settings: estimates using the Archimedes Model. Clinicoecon Outcomes Res. 2012;4: 337–47.
99. Tahara N, Tahara A, Honda A, Nitta Y, Kodama N, Yamagishi SI, Imaizumi T. Molecular imaging of vascular inflammation. Curr Pharm Des. 2014;20(14):2439–47.
100. Mizoguchi M, Tahara N, Tahara A, Nitta Y, Kodama N, Oba T, Mawatari K, Yasukawa H, Kaida H, Ishibashi M, Hayabuchi N, Harada H, Ikeda H, Yamagishi S, Imaizumi T. Pioglitazone attenuates atherosclerotic plaque inflammation in patients with impaired glucose tolerance or diabetes a prospective, randomized, comparator-controlled study using serial FDG PET/CT imaging study of carotid artery and ascending aorta. JACC Cardiovasc Imaging. 2011;4(10):1110–8.
101. Natarajan P, Ray KK, Cannon CP. High-density lipoprotein and coronary heart disease: current and future therapies. J Am Coll Cardiol. 2010;55(13):1283–99.
102. Chapman MJ, Le Goff W, Guerin M, Kontush A. Cholesteryl ester transfer protein: at the heart of the action of lipid-modulating therapy with statins, fibrates, niacin, and cholesteryl ester transfer protein inhibitors. Eur Heart J. 2010;31(2):149–64.
103. Nissen SE, Tardif JC, Nicholls SJ, Revkin JH, Shear CL, Duggan WT, Ruzyllo W, Bachinsky WB, Lasala GP, Tuzcu EM, ILLUSTRATE Investigators. Effect of torcetrapib on the progression of coronary atherosclerosis. N Engl J Med. 2007;356(13):1304–16.
104. Vergeer M, Bots ML, van Leuven SI, Basart DC, Sijbrands EJ, Evans GW, Grobbee DE, Visseren FL, Stalenhoef AF, Stroes ES, Kastelein JJ. Cholesteryl ester transfer protein inhibitor torcetrapib and off-target toxicity: a pooled analysis of the rating atherosclerotic disease change by imaging with a new CETP inhibitor (RADIANCE) trials. Circulation. 2008; 118(24):2515–22.
105. Barter PJ, Caulfield M, Eriksson M, Grundy SM, Kastelein JJ, Komajda M, Lopez-Sendon J, Mosca L, Tardif JC, Waters DD, Shear CL, Revkin JH, Buhr KA, Fisher MR, Tall AR, Brewer B, ILLUMINATE Investigators. Effects of torcetrapib in patients at high risk for coronary events. N Engl J Med. 2007;357(21):2109–22.
106. Schwartz GG, Olsson AG, Abt M, Ballantyne CM, Barter PJ, Brumm J, Chaitman BR, Holme IM, Kallend D, Leiter LA, Leitersdorf E, McMurray JJ, Mundl H, Nicholls SJ, Shah PK, Tardif JC, Wright RS, dal-OUTCOMES Investigators. Effects of dalcetrapib in patients with a recent acute coronary syndrome. N Engl J Med. 2012;367(22):2089–99.
107. Bloomfield D, Carlson GL, Sapre A, Tribble D, McKenney JM, Littlejohn 3rd TW, Sisk CM, Mitchel Y, Pasternak RC. Efficacy and safety of the cholesteryl ester transfer protein inhibitor anacetrapib as monotherapy and coadministered with atorvastatin in dyslipidemic patients. Am Heart J. 2009;157(2):352–60.
108. Gutstein DE, Krishna R, Johns D, Surks HK, Dansky HM, Shah S, Mitchel YB, Arena J, Wagner JA. Anacetrapib, a novel CETP inhibitor: pursuing a new approach to cardiovascular risk reduction. Clin Pharmacol Ther. 2012;91(1):109–22.

109. Wykrzykowska J, Lehman S, Williams G, Parker JA, Palmer MR, Varkey S, Kolodny G, Laham R. Imaging of inflamed and vulnerable plaque in coronary arteries with 18F-FDG PET/CT in patients with suppression of myocardial uptake using a low-carbohydrate, high-fat preparation. J Nucl Med. 2009;50(4):563–8.
110. Tahara N, Tahara A, Narula J, Imaizumi T. Statin therapy resolves coronary artery inflammation. JACC Cardiovasc Imaging. 2013;6(10):1119–20.
111. Rogers IS, Nasir K, Figueroa AL, Cury RC, Hoffmann U, Vermylen DA, Brady TJ, Tawakol A. Feasibility of FDG imaging of the coronary arteries: comparison between acute coronary syndrome and stable angina. JACC Cardiovasc Imaging. 2010;3(4):388–97.
112. Nitta Y, Tahara N, Tahara A, Honda A, Kodama N, Mizoguchi M, Kaida H, Ishibashi M, Hayabuchi N, Ikeda H, Yamagishi S, Imaizumi T. Pioglitazone decreases coronary artery inflammation in impaired glucose tolerance and diabetes mellitus: evaluation by FDG-PET/CT imaging. JACC Cardiovasc Imaging. 2013;6(11):1172–82.

Index

E. Aikawa (ed.), *Cardiovascular Imaging: Arterial and Aortic Valve Inflammation and Calcification*, DOI 10.1007/978-3-319-09268-3

D

MIX
Papier aus verantwortungsvollen Quellen
Paper from responsible sources
FSC® C105338

If you have any concerns about our products,
you can contact us on
ProductSafety@springernature.com

In case Publisher is established outside the EU,
the EU authorized representative is:
Springer Nature Customer Service Center GmbH
Europaplatz 3, 69115 Heidelberg, Germany

Printed by Libri Plureos GmbH
in Hamburg, Germany